Neuroscience of Rule-Guided Behavior

Edited by
SILVIA A. BUNGE, Ph.D. and
JONATHAN D. WALLIS, Ph.D.

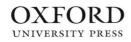

UNIVERSITY PRESS

2008

OXFORD
UNIVERSITY PRESS

Oxford University Press, Inc., publishes works that further
Oxford University's objective of excellence
in research, scholarship, and education.

Oxford   New York
Auckland   Cape Town   Dar es Salaam   Hong Kong   Karachi
Kuala Lumpur   Madrid   Melbourne   Mexico City   Nairobi
New Delhi   Shanghai   Taipei   Toronto

With offices in
Argentina   Austria   Brazil   Chile   Czech Republic   France   Greece
Guatemala   Hungary   Italy   Japan   Poland   Portugal   Singapore
South Korea   Switzerland   Thailand   Turkey   Ukraine   Vietnam

Published by Oxford University Press, Inc.
198 Madison Avenue, New York, New York 10016

www.oup.com

Oxford is a registered trademark of Oxford University Press

Library of Congress Cataloging-in-Publication Data
Neuroscience of rule-guided behavior / edited by
Silvia A. Bunge and Jonathan D. Wallis.
p. ; cm.
ISBN-13: 978-0-19-531427-4
1. Cognitive neuroscience.   2. Neuropsychology.   3. Rules (Philosophy)
I. Bunge, Silvia A.   II. Wallis, Jonathan D.
[DNLM: 1. Neurosciences—methods.   2. Behavior—physiology.
3. Brain—physiology.   4. Cognition—physiology.   5. Learning—physiology.
6. Social Conformity. WL 100 N495343 2007]
QP360.5.N4977 2007
612.8'233—dc22   2006102679

9 8 7 6 5 4 3 2 1

Printed in the United States of America
on acid-free paper

To Kevin and our family
S.A.B.

To Cathy, Maria, and Sam
J.D.W.

Preface

The idea for this book arose from a minisymposium on the neuroscience of rule-guided behavior that I chaired at the Society for Neuroscience conference in 2005. The speakers included Jonathan Wallis, as well as Marcel Brass, Eveline Crone, Eiji Hoshi, Amanda Parker, and Katsuyuki Sakai. The session presenters wrote a brief summary of the work presented at this minisymposium, which was published the week before the conference (Bunge et al., 2005).

Based on the success of this session, Joseph Burns from Springer suggested that I publish a book on this topic, and I promptly asked Jonathan Wallis to co-author it with me. After helpful discussions with Joe Burns as well as with Martin Griffiths from Cambridge University Press and Joan Bossert from Oxford University Press, we ultimately selected Oxford University Press as our publisher. However, we are grateful to all three publishers for their enthusiasm regarding this book topic.

The authors are to be commended on their interesting and scholarly contributions. I owe a great debt of gratitude to Christi Bamford, a graduate student in psychology at the University of California at Davis, for helping me to prepare the book manuscript and track our progress. Finally, we thank Joan Bossert for her instrumental support, as well as Mallory Jensen, Abby Gross, and Nancy Wolitzer from Oxford University Press for their expert assistance with this project.

Contents

Contributors *xi*
Introduction *xiii*

I. Rule Representation

1. Selection between Competing Responses Based on
   Conditional Rules *3*
   Michael Petrides

2. Single Neuron Activity Underlying Behavior-Guiding Rules *23*
   Jonathan D. Wallis

3. Neural Representations Used to Specify Action *45*
   Silvia A. Bunge and Michael J. Souza

4. Maintenance and Implementation of Task Rules *67*
   Katsuyuki Sakai

5. The Neurophysiology of Abstract Response Strategies *81*
   Aldo Genovesio and Steven P. Wise

6. Abstraction of Mental Representations: Theoretical
   Considerations and Neuroscientific Evidence *107*
   Kalina Christoff and Kamyar Keramatian

II. Rule Implementation

7. Ventrolateral and Medial Frontal Contributions to
   Decision-Making and Action Selection *129*
   Matthew F. S. Rushworth, Paula L. Croxson,
   Mark J. Buckley, and Mark E. Walton

8. Differential Involvement of the Prefrontal, Premotor,
   and Primary Motor Cortices in Rule-Based Motor Behavior *159*
   Eiji Hoshi

9. The Role of the Posterior Frontolateral Cortex in
   Task-Related Control *177*
   Marcel Brass, Jan Derrfuss, and D. Yves von Cramon

10. Time Course of Executive Processes: Data from
     the Event-Related Optical Signal   *197*
     Gabriele Gratton, Kathy A. Low, and Monica Fabiani

III.   Task-Switching

11. Task-Switching in Human and Nonhuman Primates:
     Understanding Rule Encoding and Control from Behavior
     to Single Neurons   *227*
     Gijsbert Stoet and Lawrence Snyder

12. Neural Mechanisms of Cognitive Control in Cued
     Task-Switching: Rules, Representations, and Preparation   *255*
     Hannes Ruge and Todd S. Braver

13. Dopaminergic and Serotonergic Modulation of Two
     Distinct Forms of Flexible Cognitive Control: Attentional
     Set-Shifting and Reversal Learning   *283*
     Angela C. Roberts

14. Dopaminergic Modulation of Flexible Cognitive Control:
     The Role of the Striatum   *313*
     Roshan Cools

IV.   Building Blocks of Rule Representation

15. Binding and Organization in the Medial Temporal Lobe   *337*
     Paul A. Lipton and Howard Eichenbaum

16. Ventrolateral Prefrontal Cortex and Controlling Memory
     to Inform Action   *365*
     David Badre

17. Exploring the Roles of the Frontal, Temporal, and
     Parietal Lobes in Visual Categorization   *391*
     David J. Freedman

18. Rules through Recursion: How Interactions between the
     Frontal Cortex and Basal Ganglia May Build Abstract,
     Complex Rules from Concrete, Simple Ones   *419*
     Earl K. Miller and Timothy J. Buschman

19. The Development of Rule Use in Childhood   *441*
     Philip David Zelazo

     Index   *457*

Contributors

DAVID BADRE, Ph.D.
Helen Wills Neuroscience Institute
University of California, Berkeley
Berkeley, California

MARCEL BRASS, Ph.D.
Max Planck Institute of Cognitive
    Neuroscience
Leipzig, Germany
Department of Experimental
    Psychology
Ghent University
Ghent, Belgium

TODD S. BRAVER, Ph.D.
Department of Psychology
Washington University
St. Louis, Missouri

MARK J. BUCKLEY, D.Phil.
Department of Experimental Psychology
University of Oxford
Oxford, United Kingdom

SILVIA A. BUNGE, Ph.D.
Department of Psychology and Helen
    Wills Neuroscience Institute
University of California, Berkeley
Berkeley, California &
Center for Mind and Brain
University of California at Davis
Davis, California

TIMOTHY J. BUSCHMAN, B.S.
The Picower Institute of Learning
    and Memory
Massachusetts Institute of Technology
Cambridge, Massachusetts

KALINA CHRISTOFF, Ph.D.
Department of Psychology
University of British Columbia
Vancouver, British Columbia, Canada

ROSHAN COOLS, Ph.D.
Department of Experimental Psychology
Behavioural and Clinical Neuroscience
    Institute
University of Cambridge
Cambridge, United Kingdom

PAULA L. CROXSON, M.Sc.
Department of Experimental
    Psychology
University of Oxford
Oxford, United Kingdom

JAN DERRFUSS, Ph.D.
Institute of Medicine
Research Center Juelich
Juelich, Germany

HOWARD EICHENBAUM, Ph.D.
Department of Psychology
Center for Memory and Brain
Boston University
Boston, Massachusetts

MONICA FABIANI, Ph.D.
Beckman Institute
University of Illinois
Urbana, Illinois

DAVID J. FREEDMAN, Ph.D.
Department of Neurobiology
Harvard Medical School
Boston, Massachusetts

ALDO GENOVESIO, Ph.D.
Section on Neurophysiology
National Institute of Mental Health
Bethesda, Maryland

GABRIELE GRATTON, M.D., Ph.D.
Beckman Institute
University of Illinois
Urbana, Illinois

EIJI HOSHI, M.D., Ph.D.
Brain Science Research Center
Tamagawa University Research Institute
Machida, Japan

KAMYAR KERAMATIAN, M.D.
Neuroscience Program
University of British Columbia
Vancouver, British Columbia, Canada

PAUL A. LIPTON, Ph.D.
Department of Psychology
Center for Memory and Brain
Boston University
Boston, Massachusetts

KATHY A. LOW, Ph.D.
Beckman Institute
University of Illinois
Urbana, Illinois

EARL K. MILLER, Ph.D.
Picower Institute for Learning
    and Memory
Massachusetts Institute of Technology
Cambridge, Massachusetts

MICHAEL PETRIDES, Ph.D.
Montreal Neurological Institute
McGill University
Montreal, Quebec
Canada

ANGELA C. ROBERTS, Ph.D.
Department of Anatomy
University of Cambridge
Cambridge, United Kingdom

HANNES RUGE, Ph.D.
Department of Psychology
Dresden Institute of Technology
Dresden, Germany

MATTHEW F. S. RUSHWORTH, D.Phil.
Department of Experimental
    Psychology
University of Oxford
Oxford, United Kingdom

KATSUYUKI SAKAI, M.D., Ph.D.
Department of Cognitive Neuroscience
Graduate School of Medicine
University of Tokyo
Tokyo, Japan

LAWRENCE H SNYDER, M.D., Ph.D.
Department of Anatomy and
    Neurobiology
Washington University School
    of Medicine
St. Louis, Missouri

MICHAEL J. SOUZA, M.A.
Center for Mind and Brain
University of California at Davis
Davis, California

GIJSBERT STOET, Ph.D.
Institute of Psychological Sciences
University of Leeds
Leeds, United Kingdom

D. YVES VON CRAMON, Ph.D.
Max Planck Institute for Human Cognitive
    and Brain Sciences
Leipzig, Germany

JONATHAN WALLIS, Ph.D.
Department of Psychology and Helen Wills
    Neuroscience Institute
University of California, Berkeley
Berkeley, California

MARK E. WALTON, D.Phil.
Department of Experimental Psychology
University of Oxford
Oxford, United Kingdom

STEVEN P. WISE, Ph.D.
Section on Neurophysiology
National Institute of Mental Health
Bethesda, Maryland

PHILIP DAVID ZELAZO, Ph.D.
Institute of Child Development
University of Minnesota
Minneapolis, Minnesota

Introduction

Silvia A. Bunge and Jonathan D. Wallis

Meaningful stimuli that we encounter in our daily lives trigger the retrieval of associations, that is, links that we have previously made between these stimuli and other stimuli, potential responses, heuristics for responding, or rewards. We often use these associations to select an appropriate course of action for a given situation in which we find ourselves. As such, much of our behavior is guided by *rules*, or "prescribed guide[s] for conduct or action" (Merriam-Webster, 1974).

We rely on a variety of rules, including both simple *stimulus-response (S-R) associations* (e.g., a red light means that you should stop) and rules with *response contingencies* (e.g., a carpool sign means that you can use the lane if two or more people are in the car, but not otherwise). Rules are explicit constructs, but we can learn them either explicitly, as in the case of arbitrary symbols, such as road signs that are associated with specific meanings, or implicitly, as in the case of unspoken rules for social interaction. Rules also govern some of our highest-level behaviors, involving very abstract concepts, such as "a defendant is innocent until proven guilty."

To understand how we use rules to determine our actions, it is critical to learn more about how we select responses based on associations in long-term memory. In the setting of a neuroscience laboratory, the most tractable way to investigate the interface between memory and action is to study the neural representation of explicit and simple rules for behavior.

This volume provides an overview of the current state of knowledge about the neural systems involved in various aspects of rule use: acquisition, long-term storage, retrieval, maintenance, and implementation. The book features a variety of experimental approaches. In particular, the contributors summarize findings from neuropsychological and anatomical studies, single-unit recordings, electroencephalography (EEG), functional magnetic resonance imaging (fMRI), neuropharmacology, transcranial magnetic stimulation, and behavioral studies in children. Additionally, in Chapter 10, Gratton, Low, and Fabiani provide an overview of their research involving near-infrared spectroscopy, focusing in particular on a novel analytic approach enabling them to detect event-related optical signals with high spatial and temporal resolution.

LATERAL PREFRONTAL CORTEX AND RULE REPRESENTATION

Research on the neural substrates of rule representation has focused primarily on lateral prefrontal cortex (LatPFC), a region that includes mid-dorsolateral PFC (referred to here as "DLPFC"; Brodmann areas [BA] 9, 46) and ventro-lateral PFC (VLPFC; BA 44, 45, 47). Many of the first studies of the function of LatPFC examined its role in working memory, a limited capacity system responsible for the temporary storage and manipulation of information. The first deficit to be associated specifically with damage to the frontal lobes was discovered using the spatial delayed response task. In this task, the monkey sees a reward hidden at one of two locations, and then, after a brief delay, is allowed to retrieve it. Monkeys with large PFC lesions act as if they forgot where the reward was hidden, even after short delays of just a few seconds (Jacobsen, 1936). Subsequent experiments showed that very restricted activity in LatPFC could produce the same deficit (Funahashi et al., 1993).

Neurophysiologists also discovered that a high proportion of neurons in LatPFC increased their firing rate when working memory was used to bridge a task delay (Fuster and Alexander, 1971; Kubota and Niki, 1971). Later studies showed that the firing properties of these neurons were selective for the specific memorized cue (Funahashi et al., 1989; Constantinidis et al., 2001). These firing patterns became synonymous with the notion of a "neuronal representation" of the cue, because the neuronal activity appeared to represent the cue, even when the cue was no longer present in the environment.

Despite this focus, working memory alone provided an unsatisfactory account of some of the deficits observed in humans and monkeys after PFC damage. Monkeys with LatPFC lesions were impaired at certain cognitive tasks, even when those tasks were specifically designed so that they did not have a working memory component (Rushworth et al., 1998). Many of the tasks sensitive to PFC damage in humans also did not have an obvious working memory component. For example, the Wisconsin Card Sorting Task (WCST), one of the first neuropsychological tests of PFC function in humans, requires patients to sort a deck of cards based on different abstract rules (e.g., "sort according to color" or "sort according to shape"). Patients had particular problems switching between these different rules (Milner, 1963). Deficits in rule implementation also occur when a subject must override a strongly pre-potent response tendency in favor of a recently learned rule. For example, patients with LatPFC damage are impaired on the Stroop task, where one must inhibit the tendency to name a word, and instead name the color of the ink in which the word is printed (Perret, 1974).

This disparity between the findings from neurophysiology and neuropsychology endured until the last decade or so of research. Neurophysiologists began to find that the delay selectivity in LatPFC neurons encoded more than just memorized cues. For example, they also encoded which task the monkey was currently performing (White and Wise, 1999; Asaad et al., 2000; Hoshi et al., 2000). Single neurons in LatPFC were also capable of encoding high-

level, abstract rules, such as "choose the picture that is the same as this one" (Wallis et al., 2001).

Thus, PFC neurons appeared to be capable of representing rules in addition to simple cues and responses. This finding helped to explain why patients have difficulty with tasks such as the WCST. This research is discussed further in Chapter 2, where Wallis compares the distribution of rule-encoding neurons in LatPFC with other frontal lobe regions, striatal regions, and posterior sensory areas of the brain. Consistent with these studies, fMRI studies examining active rule maintenance in humans consistently show that PFC is involved in maintaining rules online. However, the particular subregions that are implicated vary from study to study. As argued in Chapter 3 by Bunge and Souza, the type of rule that is being maintained is a critical factor in determining which PFC subregions are involved. Indeed, as argued by Christoff and Keramatian in Chapter 6, there may be a hierarchy of rule representations in LatPFC. The idea of a hierarchy of rules is further developed in Chapter 19 by Zelazo, with reference to the stages of rule learning in childhood.

Several recent studies have examined a related research topic, namely, the neural substrates of strategy use. Strategies are open-ended rules that govern choices at an abstract level, without defining the specific response to a given stimulus. Gaffan and colleagues (2002) trained monkeys to select specific stimuli, either persistently or only sporadically, to receive a reward, and showed that the use of these strategies relies on interactions between PFC and the temporal lobe. Neurophysiological studies in monkeys support these findings. As discussed in Chapter 5 by Genovesio and Wise, PFC neurons represent high-level behavioral strategies, such as a "repeat-stay" or "change-shift" strategy (Genovesio et al., 2005). Some of these neurons had strategy effects that were selective for a specific visual target, whereas others did not, suggesting that different levels of abstraction are coded in different sets of prefrontal neurons.

A further related cognitive construct is the notion of "task set." A task set is a neurocognitive state in which an upcoming task is prospectively configured. It consists of information about which stimulus attributes to attend to, the important conceptual criterion, goal states, and condition-action rules. It reflects not only which items a subject is preparing to process, but also how the subject plans to process the items and the rules of the to-be-performed task.

As described in Chapter 4 by Sakai, Sakai and Passingham collected fMRI data while subjects performed a task in which they received instructions in advance of the task stimuli (Sakai and Passingham, 2003, 2006). The authors performed functional connectivity analyses showing that anterior PFC (BA 10) activation closely correlates with that of different prefrontal regions, depending on which task the subject is preparing to perform. These data suggest that anterior PFC assists in preparing for an upcoming task by coordinating with brain regions that will be needed to carry out that task. Additional fMRI research indicates that this region represents high-level rules composed of several lower-level rules, consistent with the hypothesis that VLPFC and anterior

PFC are hierarchically organized, with the latter integrating across representations held in the former (Bunge et al., 2003; Crone et al., 2005).

Although LatPFC seems to be a critical area for the representation of rules, it is unlikely to be the long-term repository of memories for rules. Neuropsychological observations suggest that patients with LatPFC damage can sometimes tell the experimenter what the appropriate task rule is, even while being unable to implement it correctly (Shallice and Burgess, 1991). The developmental literature makes similar observations, suggesting that the growth of knowledge sometimes proceeds faster than the ability to control behavior (Zelazo et al., 1996). Patients with compromised LatPFC function are overly reliant on well-learned rules, to the extent that they have difficulty overriding these rules in favor of weaker, but more contextually appropriate rules (e.g., Cohen and Servan-Schreiber, 1992; Miller and Cohen, 2001; Braver and Barch, 2002). As discussed in Chapter 16 by Badre, the idea that LatPFC retrieves and implements rules for behavior from long-term stores in other brain regions is consistent with the long-term memory literature, which implicates VLPFC in strategic or controlled memory retrieval rather than in long-term mnemonic storage (Gershberg and Shimamura, 1995; Gabrieli et al., 1998; Wagner et al., 2001; Sylvester and Shimamura, 2002).

The question of where rule representations are stored in the brain has received little attention in the literature up to now. The lateral temporal lobes are a likely candidate for rule storage, given that they have been implicated in the long-term storage of both semantic and nonsemantic associations (Martin and Chao, 2001; Messinger et al., 2001; Bussey et al., 2002; Thompson-Schill, 2003). The parietal lobes are an equally likely candidate, given their involvement in representing actions associated with the environment (Goodale and Milner, 1992; Snyder et al., 2000). Other structures involved in motor planning, such as premotor cortex (Wallis and Miller, 2003), supplementary motor area (SMA), and pre-SMA (Picard and Strick, 1996, 2001), also merit consideration. A distributed network for rule representation would be consistent with the attribute specificity model of semantic knowledge, whereby different features (e.g., visual or functional) of a stimulus are stored in a distributed manner across brain regions involved in encoding these features (see Thompson-Schill, 2003, for a review). Further discussion of the issue of long-term storage of rules appears in Chapter 3 by Bunge and Souza.

TASK-SWITCHING

As mentioned earlier, patients with PFC damage seem to have particular difficulty in switching between different rules, a process that is generally believed to rely on LatPFC (for a review, see Bunge, 2004). In Chapter 12, Ruge and Braver discuss the neuronal mechanisms that might underlie this ability, and in particular, the role that simpler associations, such as S-R mappings and reward associations, may play in the reconfiguration that underlies a task switch.

Two chapters focus on the neuropharmacological underpinnings of task-switching. In Chapter 13, Roberts reviews the evidence from a series of neuropsychological and pharmacological studies in marmoset monkeys. These studies show that switching between different rules (specifically, different attentional sets) depends on the integrity of LatPFC, and in particular, its dopaminergic innervation. This contrasts with orbitofrontal cortex, where damage produces deficits in more reward-based switching and depends on serotonergic innervation. These studies are complemented by those of Cools (Chapter 14), who has performed a series of studies looking at the switching ability of patients with Parkinson's disease. These studies also highlight the importance of dopamine for flexible switching.

Studies in humans, using fMRI and EEG, additionally implicate parietal cortex and pre-supplementary motor cortex in task-switching (pre-SMA; medial BA 6) in task-switching (e.g., Sohn et al., 2000; Dreher and Berman, 2002; Rushworth et al., 2005). Both of these are areas with heavy connections to LatPFC. In addition, transcranial magnetic stimulation studies in humans have shown that transient stimulation of parietal cortex or pre-SMA/medial wall leads to a slowing in the ability to switch from one task to another (Rushworth et al., 2002, 2003).

In Chapter 11, Stoet and Snyder examine the neuronal properties in parietal cortex while monkeys performed a task-switching paradigm. The investigators have found that many neurons in parietal cortex, particularly in the lateral bank of intraparietal sulcus, tended to encode the overarching rules of the task. In addition, the latency of selectivity in these neurons correlated with the behavioral reaction times of the animals, indicating that they had a direct role in controlling the animal's performance on the task.

A recent fMRI study provides evidence that LatPFC is engaged when there is a need to access a less recently retrieved task rule, whereas pre-SMA/SMA and basal ganglia are primarily involved in overriding the tendency to perform the previously performed task (Crone et al., 2005, 2006). Further, in Chapter 9, Marcel Brass and colleagues discuss an EEG study in humans showing that activity in LatPFC precedes activity in parietal cortex during the updating of task rules (Brass et al., 2005b). These data support the hypothesis that LatPFC provides an abstract task representation that is then transmitted to, or further specified in, posterior cortices (see also Stoet and Snyder, 2004).

In addition to the VLPFC and DLPFC regions discussed earlier, Brass and colleagues have shown, using fMRI in humans, that a more posterior region in LatPFC is also involved in rule use. This region is located at the junction of inferior frontal sulcus and inferior precentral sulcus, and has therefore been termed the "inferior frontal junction." As summarized in Chapter 9, these investigators have conducted a series of studies suggesting that this region is involved in the environmentally guided updating of task rules (Brass et al., 2005a).

LEARNING RULES

Having explored how rules are represented and stored in the brain, and how we flexibly switch between different rules and task sets as our circumstances require, we will then turn our attention to looking at how rules are learned in the first place. One possibility is that high-level rules build on simpler S-R associations. For example, we learn the rules behind telephones by first acquiring a simple S-R association: "When the telephone rings, answer it." However, more sophisticated telephone usage requires us to take into account the context in which the ringing takes place (Miller and Cohen, 2001). For example, if the ringing telephone is in someone else's home, answering it may be inappropriate.

Research in a variety of species implicates the striatum and its dopaminergic inputs in learning S-R associations (reviewed in Packard and Knowlton, 2002). The frontal lobe and striatum are heavily interconnected, and recent studies have explored this interaction during the learning of S-R associations (Pasupathy and Miller, 2005). In Chapter 18, Miller and Buschman describe this research and focus on how the interactions between the striatum and frontal cortex may underlie the ability to use S-R associations to acquire higher-level rules.

In addition, LatPFC has been implicated in the acquisition of S-R associations. In Chapter 7, Rushworth and colleagues review the evidence that LatPFC, in particular, the VLPFC region, is particularly important for action selection based on external stimuli and according to learned arbitrary rules. In particular, VLPFC lesions in monkeys severely impair learning on *conditional visuomotor* tasks, which require subjects to use one of several arbitrary S-R mappings to respond to a visual stimulus (Murray et al., 2000; Passingham et al., 2000; Bussey et al., 2001). VLPFC receives its visual input from inferotemporal cortex (Pandya and Yeterian, 1998); therefore, disruption of the white matter tracts connecting VLPFC and ipsilateral temporal cortex also leads to impaired visuomotor learning (Parker and Gaffan, 1998; Bussey et al., 2002). In their chapter, Rushworth and colleagues contrast this type of learning with that which occurs in anterior cingulate cortex, where action control seems to be more reward-dependent.

Unlike in VLPFC, DLPFC damage causes little or no impairment in learning conditional tasks in either humans or nonhuman primates (see Murray et al., 2000). The exception to this is posterior DLPFC (BA 8), as discussed in Chapter 1. Petrides reviews patient and fMRI studies, and examines whether posterior DLPFC is particularly important for well-learned conditional rules, particularly those that indicate that a specific motor response should be performed. In contrast, he argues that VLPFC is more important for the initial learning of the conditional rule, indicative of its role in actively controlling the retrieval of information from memory critical to solving the task.

Rules might also build on learning taking place in posterior sensory systems. "Perceptual categorization" refers to our ability to group stimuli

meaningfully, based on sensory features. It seems to share many similarities with rule learning, which in some sense, involves grouping response contingencies into meaningful categories. In Chapter 17, Freedman explores the neuronal mechanisms taking place in LatPFC, parietal cortex, and temporal cortex that underlie perceptual categorization. The neuronal properties in these areas that are involved in categorization indeed look remarkably similar to those that underlie rule learning.

INTERACTIONS WITH OTHER BRAIN SYSTEMS

It appears that, to control behavior effectively, multiple brain systems must have access to rule representations. One such system is episodic memory instantiated by medial temporal lobe. There appear to be commonalities in the mechanisms underlying episodic memory and rule learning. In Chapter 15, Lipton and Eichenbaum discuss a model whereby the medial temporal system is responsible for abstracting information regarding the similarities and differences between discrete experiences that enables episodic memories to be formed. This is similar to the manner in which LatPFC abstracts the regularities between experiences to form overarching behavior-guiding rules and principles, and the interaction between these two systems may be a key component of the control of goal-directed behavior.

Once a rule representation has been activated, it must interact with the motor system if it is to control behavior. In Chapter 8, Hoshi examines the neuronal mechanisms that enable this to occur. In particular, he examines evidence that there is a hierarchical organization within the frontal lobe for controlling the motor system, by comparing neuronal responses in primary motor cortex, premotor cortex, and LatPFC. Neurons in LatPFC encoded the rules of the task, whereas neurons in premotor cortex and primary motor cortex were more involved in the planning and execution of the movement, respectively.

CONCLUSION

Research on humans and nonhuman primates has led to the identification of a set of brain regions that mediate flexible rule-guided behavior. An important next step will be to characterize the temporal dynamics of interactions between these regions, to gain further insight into the neural mechanisms of rule use. Accordingly, studies involving simultaneous electrophysiological recordings at several sites would prove useful, as would a brain imaging technique with high spatial and temporal resolution, such as combined fMRI/EEG. There is also a need for theoretical models of rule-guided behavior that can be tested empirically (O'Reilly et al., 2002).

An important challenge will be to determine whether the distinctions drawn between various types of rule representations are honored at the level of brain mechanisms. By studying how rules are retrieved from memory and

used to guide action in specific situations, we will make progress in understanding the interface among perception, memory, and motor control.

Finally, further research is needed to explore the role of language in rule representation. Such explorations may bear on research focusing on the development of rule use in early childhood, as discussed in Chapter 19 by Zelazo. Additionally, the role of language in rule use may help to explain behavioral and neuroanatomical differences in rule use between species (Stoet and Snyder, 2003).

The ability to learn and implement rules is critical for behaving meaningfully in the world. We rely on rules to plan our daily activities, carry out mental operations, and interact with others (Burgess et al., 2000; Goel et al., 2004). Investigations of rule use are relevant to several lines of cognitive research, including routine action selection (Botvinick and Plaut, 2004), cognitive control (e.g., Miller and Cohen, 2001; Bunge, 2004), decision-making (Ridderinkhof et al., 2004), and arguably, problem-solving (e.g., Zelazo and Muller, 2002; Fantino et al., 2003; Cherubini and Mazzocco, 2004). As such, the study of how rules are represented and used by the brain will enrich our understanding of behavior.

REFERENCES

Asaad WF, Rainer G, Miller EK (2000) Task-specific neural activity in the primate prefrontal cortex. Journal of Neurophysiology 84:451–459.

Botvinick M, Plaut DC (2004) Doing without schema hierarchies: a recurrent connectionist approach to normal and impaired routine sequential action. Psychological Review 111:395–429.

Brass M, Derrfuss J, Forstmann B, von Cramon DY (2005a) The role of the inferior frontal junction area in cognitive control. Trends in Cognitive Sciences 9:314–316.

Brass M, Ullsperger M, Knoesche TR, von Cramon DY, Phillips NA (2005b) Who comes first? The role of the prefrontal and parietal cortex in cognitive control. Journal of Cognitive Neuroscience 17:1367–1375.

Braver TS, Barch DM (2002) A theory of cognitive control, aging cognition, and neuromodulation. Neuroscience and Biobehavioral Reviews 26:809–817.

Bunge SA (2004) How we use rules to select actions: a review of evidence from cognitive neuroscience. Cognitive, Affective, and Behavioral Neuroscience 4:564–579.

Bunge SA, Kahn I, Wallis JD, Miller EK, Wagner AD (2003) Neural circuits subserving the retrieval and maintenance of abstract rules. Journal of Neurophysiology 90:3419–3428.

Bunge, S.A., Wallis, J.D., Parker, A., Brass, M., Crone, E.A., Hoshi, E., & Sakai, K. Neural circuitry underlying rule use in humans and non-human primates. Journal of Neuroscience 9;25:10347-50, 2005.

Burgess PW, Veitch E, de Lacy Costello A, Shallice T (2000) The cognitive and neuroanatomical correlates of multitasking. Neuropsychologia 38:848–863.

Bussey TJ, Wise SP, Murray EA (2001) The role of ventral and orbital prefrontal cortex in conditional visuomotor learning and strategy use in rhesus monkeys (*Macaca mulatta*). Behavioral Neuroscience 115:971–982.

Bussey TJ, Wise SP, Murray EA (2002) Interaction of ventral and orbital prefrontal cortex with inferotemporal cortex in conditional visuomotor learning. Behavioral Neuroscience 116:703–715.

Cherubini P, Mazzocco A (2004) From models to rules: mechanization of reasoning as a way to cope with cognitive overloading in combinatorial problems. Acta Psychologica (Amsterdam) 116:223–243.

Cohen J, Servan-Schreiber D (1992) Context, cortex, and dopamine: a connectionist approach to behavior and biology in schizophrenia. Psychological Review 99:45–77.

Constantinidis C, Franowicz MN, Goldman-Rakic PS (2001) The sensory nature of mnemonic representation in the primate prefrontal cortex. Nature Neuroscience 4:311–316.

Crone EA, Donohue SE, Honomichl R, Wendelken C, Bunge SA (2006) Brain regions mediating flexible rule use during development. Journal of Neuroscience 26:11239–11247.

Crone EA, Wendelken C, Donohue SE, Bunge SA (2005) Neural evidence for dissociable components of task-switching. Cerebral Cortex 16:475–486.

Dreher JC, Berman KF (2002) Fractionating the neural substrate of cognitive control processes. Proceedings of the National Academy of Sciences U S A 99:14595–14600.

Fantino E, Jaworski BA, Case DA, Stolarz-Fantino S (2003) Rules and problem solving: another look. American Journal of Psychology 116:613–632.

Funahashi S, Bruce CJ, Goldman-Rakic PS (1989) Mnemonic coding of visual space in the monkey's dorsolateral prefrontal cortex. Journal of Neurophysiology 61:331–349.

Funahashi S, Chafee MV, Goldman-Rakic P (1993) Prefrontal neuronal activity in rhesus monkeys performing a delayed anti-saccade task. Nature 365:753–756.

Fuster JM, Alexander GE (1971) Neuron activity related to short-term memory. Science 173:652–654.

Gabrieli JD, Poldrack RA, Desmond JE (1998) The role of left prefrontal cortex in language and memory. Proceedings of the National Academy of Sciences U S A 95:906–913.

Gaffan D, Easton A, Parker A (2002) Interaction of inferior temporal cortex with frontal cortex and basal forebrain: double dissociation in strategy implementation and associative learning. Journal of Neuroscience 22:7288–7296.

Genovesio A, Brasted PJ, Mitz AR, Wise SP (2005) Prefrontal cortex activity related to abstract response strategies. Neuron 47:307–320.

Gershberg FB, Shimamura AP (1995) Impaired use of organizational strategies in free recall following frontal lobe damage. Neuropsychologia 33:1305–1333.

Goel V, Shuren J, Sheesley L, Grafman J (2004) Asymmetrical involvement of frontal lobes in social reasoning. Brain 127:783–790.

Goodale MA, Milner AD (1992) Separate visual pathways for perception and action. Trends in Neuroscience 15:20–25.

Hoshi E, Shima K, Tanji J (2000) Neuronal activity in the primate prefrontal cortex in the process of motor selection based on two behavioral rules. Journal of Neurophysiology 83:2355–2373.

Jacobsen CF (1936) Studies of cerebral function in primates, I. The functions of the frontal association areas in monkeys. Comparative Psychological Monographs 13:1–60.

Kubota K, Niki H (1971) Prefrontal cortical unit activity and delayed alternation performance in monkeys. Journal of Neurophysiology 34:337–347.

Martin A, Chao LL (2001) Semantic memory and the brain: structure and processes. Current Opinion in Neurobiology 11:194–201.

Merriam-Webster Dictionary (1974) New York: Pocket Books.

Messinger A, Squire LR, Zola SM, Albright TD (2001) Neuronal representations of stimulus associations develop in the temporal lobe during learning. Proceedings of the National Academy of Sciences U S A 98:12239–12244.

Miller EK, Cohen JD (2001) An integrative theory of prefrontal cortex function. Annual Review of Neuroscience 24:167–202.

Milner B (1963) Effects of different brain lesions on card sorting. Archives of Neurology 9:90–100.

Murray EA, Bussey TJ, Wise SP (2000) Role of prefrontal cortex in a network for arbitrary visuomotor mapping. Experimental Brain Research 133:114–129.

O'Reilly RC, Noelle DC, Braver TS, Cohen JD (2002) Prefrontal cortex and dynamic categorization tasks: representational organization and neuromodulatory control. Cerebral Cortex 12:246–257.

Packard MG, Knowlton BJ (2002) Learning and memory functions of the basal ganglia. Annual Review of Neuroscience 25:563–593.

Pandya DN, Yeterian EH (1998) Comparison of prefrontal architecture and connections. In: The prefrontal cortex (Roberts AC, Robbins TW, Weiskrantz L, eds.), pp 51–66. Oxford: Oxford University Press.

Parker A, Gaffan D (1998) Memory after frontal/temporal disconnection in monkeys: conditional and non-conditional tasks, unilateral and bilateral frontal lesions. Neuropsychologia 36:259–271.

Passingham RE, Toni I, Rushworth MF (2000) Specialisation within the prefrontal cortex: the ventral prefrontal cortex and associative learning. Experimental Brain Research 133:103–113.

Pasupathy A, Miller EK (2005) Different time courses of learning-related activity in the prefrontal cortex and striatum. Nature 433:873–876.

Perret E (1974) The left frontal lobe of man and the suppression of habitual responses in verbal categorical behaviour. Neuropsychologia 12:323–330.

Petrides M (1997) Visuo-motor conditional associative learning after frontal and temporal lesions in the human brain. Neuropsychologia 35:989–997.

Picard N, Strick PL (1996) Motor areas of the medial wall: a review of their location and functional activation. Cerebral Cortex 6:342–353.

Picard N, Strick PL (2001) Imaging the premotor areas. Current Opinion in Neurobiology 11:663–672.

Ridderinkhof KR, van den Wildenberg WP, Segalowitz SJ, Carter CS (2004) Neurocognitive mechanisms of cognitive control: the role of prefrontal cortex in action selection, response inhibition, performance monitoring, and reward-based learning. Brain and Cognition 56:129–140.

Rushworth MF, Hadland KA, Paus T, Sipila PK (2002) Role of the human medial frontal cortex in task switching: a combined fMRI and TMS study. Journal of Neurophysiology 87:2577–2592.

Rushworth MF, Johansen-Berg H, Gobel SM, Devlin JT (2003) The left parietal and premotor cortices: motor attention and selection. Neuroimage 20 (Suppl 1):S89–S100.

Rushworth MF, Nixon PD, Wade DT, Renowden S, Passingham RE (1998) The left hemisphere and the selection of learned actions. Neuropsychologia 36:11–24.

Rushworth MF, Passingham RE, Nobre AC (2005) Components of attentional set-switching. Experimental Psychology 52:83–98.

Sakai K, Passingham RE (2003) Prefrontal interactions reflect future task operations. Nature Neuroscience 6:75–81.

Sakai K, Passingham R (2006) Prefrontal set activity predicts rule-specific neural processing during subsequent cognitive performance. Journal of Neuroscience 26: 1211-1218

Shallice T, Burgess PW (1991) Deficits in strategy application following frontal lobe damage in man. Brain 114 (Pt 2):727–741.

Snyder LH, Batista AP, Andersen RA (2000) Intention-related activity in the posterior parietal cortex: a review. Vision Research 40:1433–1441.

Sohn MH, Ursu S, Anderson JR, Stenger VA, Carter CS (2000) Inaugural article: the role of prefrontal cortex and posterior parietal cortex in task switching. Proceedings of the National Academy of Sciences U S A 97:13448–13453.

Stoet G, Snyder LH (2003) Executive control and task-switching in monkeys. Neuropsychologia 41:1357–1364.

Stoet G, Snyder LH (2004) Single neurons in posterior parietal cortex of monkeys encode cognitive set. Neuron 42:1003–1012.

Sylvester CY, Shimamura AP (2002) Evidence for intact semantic representations in patients with frontal lobe lesions. Neuropsychology 16:197–207.

Thompson-Schill SL (2003) Neuroimaging studies of semantic memory: inferring 'how' from 'where.' Neuropsychologia 41:280–292.

Wagner AD, Pare-Blagoev EJ, Clark J, Poldrack RA (2001) Recovering meaning: left prefrontal cortex guides controlled semantic retrieval. Neuron 31:329–338.

Wallis JD, Anderson KC, Miller EK (2001) Single neurons in prefrontal cortex encode abstract rules. Nature 411:953–956.

Wallis JD, Miller EK (2003) Neuronal activity in primate dorsolateral and orbital prefrontal cortex during performance of a reward preference task. European Journal of Neuroscience 18:2069–2081.

White IM, Wise SP (1999) Rule-dependent neuronal activity in the prefrontal cortex. Experimental Brain Research 126:315–335.

Zelazo PD, Frye D, Rapus T (1996) An age-related dissociation between knowing rules and using them. Cognitive Development 11:37–63.

Zelazo PD, Müller U (2002) Executive function in typical and atypical development. In: Handbook of childhood cognitive development (Goswami U, ed.), pp. 445–469. Oxford: Blackwell.

I

RULE REPRESENTATION

1

Selection between Competing Responses Based on Conditional Rules

Michael Petrides

It is now well established that the frontal cortex plays a major role in the executive control of behavior and cognition (e.g., Stuss and Benson, 1986; Robbins, 1996; Shallice and Burgess, 1996; Petrides, 2000, 2005a). The frontal cortex is not a homogeneous part of the cerebral cortex, but consists of several areas that exhibit marked differences in cytoarchitecture and connection patterns with other parts of the cerebral cortex, as well as with subcortical neural structures (e.g., Petrides and Pandya, 2002, 2004). Clearly, neuronal activity in the various frontal cortical areas underlies different types of control processing on which flexibility of cognition and behavior depends, and there is considerable evidence for such specialization of function (e.g., Petrides, 2005a). One important aspect of the control of behavior is the selection of an appropriate action that is guided by learned rules (Bunge, 2004). For several years, my colleagues and I have studied one type of rule-guided behavior, namely, the selection between competing responses on the basis of learned conditional rules (e.g., if stimulus A, select response X, but if stimulus B, select response Y). Such rule-guided responses are termed "conditional associative responses" because they are explicitly learned associations. I have examined the performance of patients with unilateral frontal cortical excisions during the learning of such rules and also that of macaque monkeys with lesions restricted to particular sectors of the lateral frontal cortex. Because the work on macaque monkeys has recently been reviewed (Petrides, 2005b), this chapter will focus on the work with patients.

CONDITIONAL ASSOCIATIVE RESPONSE LEARNING IN PATIENTS WITH FRONTAL CORTICAL EXCISIONS

A number of studies have demonstrated that patients with lateral frontal cortical excisions are severely impaired in the learning and performance of conditional associative responses (Petrides, 1985a, 1990, 1997). The experimental tasks used in these studies are similar to those previously developed for

comparable studies in the macaque monkey (e.g., Petrides, 1982, 1985b). Basically, in these tasks, there are several alternative responses (e.g., six motor actions) and an equal number of instructional cues (e.g., six different color stimuli), each one of which instructs the subject to perform a particular one of those responses. The subject must learn the arbitrary conditional relations between the instructional cues and the responses over a series of trials, so that when a given stimulus is presented, the correct response will be produced. The essential feature of these tasks is the selection, in each trial, of a specific response from among several other equally probable and competing responses on the basis of learned conditional relations between instructional cues and responses.

In the studies described here, the performance on conditional tasks of patients with unilateral excisions from the frontal cortex is compared with that of patients with unilateral excisions from the anterior part of the temporal lobe, as well as that of unoperated normal control subjects. The extent and precise locus of the frontal excisions varied from subject to subject, but in all cases, the motor cortex on the precentral gyrus was spared, and when the operation was carried out in the left hemisphere, Broca's speech area was also spared (Fig. 1–1). Such excisions of the frontal cortex do not cause any motor or somatosensory defects and do not impair performance on conventional intelligence tests and a large variety of perceptual, linguistic, and memory tasks that have proven to be sensitive indicators of posterior cortical or medial

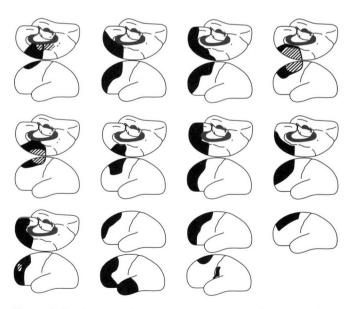

Figure 1–1 Diagrams showing examples of cortical excisions from the left frontal cortex.

temporal lobe damage (e.g., Milner, 1975; Petrides, 2000). However, despite the normal performance of these patients with frontal cortical excisions on standard intelligence, perception, memory, and language tests, many of them show poor adjustment to everyday life, partly because they cannot regulate their behavior by various explicit and implicit signals received from the environment. The deficits exhibited in learning to select among competing alternatives based on acquired conditional rules clearly contributes to the problems that these patients encounter in everyday life. The temporal lobe excisions studied always included the anterior part of the temporal neocortex and the amygdaloid nucleus, and in some cases, they extended posteriorly to include a large part of the hippocampus and parahippocampal cortex. Thus, a distinction is made between those left or right temporal lobe excisions resulting in little or no damage to the hippocampal system (LTh, RTh) and those in which the hippocampal system was removed to a considerable extent (LTH, RTH) [Fig. 1–2].

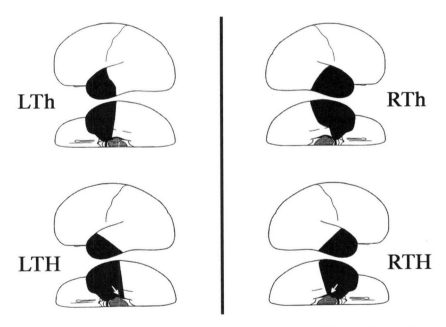

Figure 1–2 Diagrams showing examples of anterior temporal lobe excisions in four patients. LTh and RTh refer to patients with left (L) or right (R) temporal lobe excisions involving the anterior temporal neocortex, the amygdala and its surrounding cortex, but with little damage to the hippocampal system. LTH and RTH refer to patients with left (L) or right (R) temporal lobe excisions that involve the same areas that are affected in the patients designated as LTh and RTh, but with additional extensive damage to the parahippocampal cortex and the hippocampus. The *arrows* indicate the location of the additional damage in these cases.

Conditional Associative Response Learning: Motor Responses

One of the early experiments examined the question of whether patients with frontal cortical excisions would be impaired in learning to select between different motor responses on the basis of arbitrary conditional relations with instructional cues (Petrides, 1985a). In this experiment, the subjects first watched the experimenter demonstrate six different hand postures (Fig. 1–3). Subjects were then asked to demonstrate them from memory. All subjects could reproduce these six hand postures from memory after only a few demonstrations. Once this preliminary stage was completed, six stimuli of different colors were placed on the table in front of the experimenter and the subject was told that each one of those stimuli would be the cue for the performance

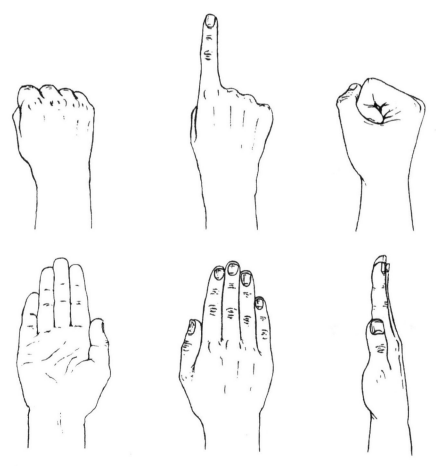

Figure 1–3 Schematic diagram illustrating the six hand postures that constituted the responses in the visual-motor conditional task.

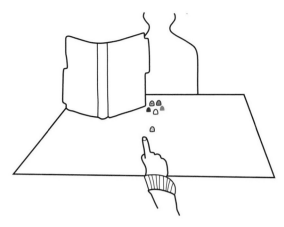

Figure 1–4 Schematic diagram of the experimental arrangement in the visual motor conditional task. The instructional cues were different colors, shown here as different shades (Reprinted from Petrides, *Neuropsychologia*, 23, 601–614. Copyright Elsevier, 1985).

of a specific hand posture. The subjects were told that they would have to learn which hand posture should be performed for each color cue on the basis of trial and error. Throughout testing, the stimuli remained on the table in full view of the subject. On each trial, one of the color stimuli (chosen pseudo-randomly) was placed in front of the others (Fig. 1–4). Subjects had to respond to the placement of one of the colors in front of the others by making the hand posture that they thought was indicated by that stimulus. If an incorrect posture was made, the subjects were told and had to try the other hand postures until the correct one was found. When the correct posture was produced, the trial was terminated by placing the stimulus back among the others. The relative position of the stimuli was changed by shuffling, and the next trial was administered by placing one of the color stimuli in front of the others. Thus, the subjects had to learn by trial and error the conditional relations between the instructional cues and the hand postures.

On this task, patients with either left or right frontal lobe excisions were severely impaired, many of them failing to learn the task within the limits of testing (Fig. 1–5). Patients with unilateral anterior temporal lobe excisions were not impaired, except for those who had sustained left temporal lobe excisions that involved extensive damage to the hippocampal region (Fig. 1–5). The involvement of the left hippocampal region in verbal memory is well known (e.g., Milner, 1975); therefore, the deficit of patients with left hippocampal damage in this task is probably due to its verbal memory component resulting from the tendency of many subjects to verbalize the associations between the color stimuli and the hand postures. It may also reflect the greater contribution of the left hemisphere to the control of certain types of motor

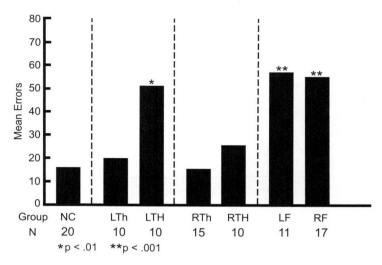

Figure 1–5 Mean error scores for the various groups of patients on the visual motor conditional task (trial-and-error testing procedure). NC, normal control; LTh, left temporal lobe group, limited hippocampal damage; LTH, left temporal lobe group, extensive hippocampal damage; RTh, right temporal lobe group, limited hippocampal damage; RTH, right temporal lobe group, extensive hippocampal damage; LF, left frontal lobe group; RF, right frontal lobe group (Reprinted from Petrides, *Neuropsychologia*, 23, 601–614. Copyright Elsevier, 1985).

action (Kimura and Archibald, 1974; DeRenzi et al., 1980) and, therefore, the greater involvement of the left hippocampal system in the learning of such motor acts.

A number of important points must be made. First, testing began only when subjects could reproduce the six hand postures from memory, a task that was extremely easy for all subjects. Second, on each trial, when an incorrect hand posture was produced in response to a particular instructional color stimulus, the subject was told by the experimenter that the selected response was incorrect and the subject had to perform the other hand postures until the correct one for that particular color stimulus was found. Only then was the next trial administered. Thus, *on every single trial*, the patients with frontal cortical lesions demonstrated that they knew and could perform from memory all six relevant hand postures, although they were severely impaired in selecting the correct response to the particular color stimulus presented. In other words, there was evidence on each trial that the problem of the patient was not in performing the hand postures or remembering what the relevant hand postures were, but rather in learning to select the particular responses required on the basis of the arbitrary conditional relations between color stimuli and hand postures. Thus, on every trial, there was clear evidence that there was no impairment in motor execution or generalized memory impairment after

these frontal lesions. Instead, the patients with frontal lesions were having trouble selecting between competing responses on the basis of learned arbitrary conditional relations (e.g., if A, select response X, but if B, select response Y).

In this experiment, learning of the conditional cues was by trial and error: On each trial, when the color instructional stimulus was presented, the subject had to perform the various hand postures with the experimenter providing feedback (correct or incorrect) after each hand posture until the correct one was performed. One question raised was whether this trial-and-error method of training was important for the impairment observed in patients with frontal excisions. Another study was therefore performed to determine whether the impairment in learning conditional associative tasks in patients with frontal excisions could be replicated using a modified testing procedure that did not involve trial and error (Petrides, 1997). In this new testing procedure, the associations between the color stimuli and the hand postures were demonstrated to the subjects by the experimenter. The experimenter placed one of the color stimuli in front of the others and performed with the right hand the posture that was associated with that particular color. The subject then performed the same hand posture with his or her right hand. The experimenter then replaced the color stimulus among the others, shuffled them to make their position irrelevant, selected one of the other colors according to a random order, placed it in front of the others, and performed the appropriate hand posture for that color. As before, the subject copied the hand posture made by the experimenter. This procedure was continued until all hand postures had been demonstrated. Immediately after this demonstration phase, a testing phase followed during which the experimenter placed one of the stimuli in front of the others and the subject had to perform the hand posture that was associated with it. If the subject made an error, the subject was told and the experimenter performed the correct posture. The subject also performed the same correct hand posture to strengthen his or her learning of the correct response. After a correct response or a correction of an erroneous response, the experimenter replaced the color stimulus among the others, shuffled them, and selected the next stimulus to be placed in front of the others, according to a random order. Again, the subject had to perform the hand posture associated with that stimulus, and if an error was made, the experimenter told the subject and demonstrated the correct response, which the subject copied. Testing proceeded in this manner until all of the color stimuli and the hand postures associated with them were performed. Once this testing phase was completed, there was another demonstration phase, followed by a testing phase (as described earlier), until the end of the testing session. Despite these changes in the testing procedure (i.e., demonstration of the stimulus-response associations by the experimenter), the results were the same as those in the study in which the trial-and-error method was used. As before, patients with left or right frontal cortical excisions were severely impaired in learning the arbitrary stimulus-response relations (Fig. 1–6). Patients with anterior

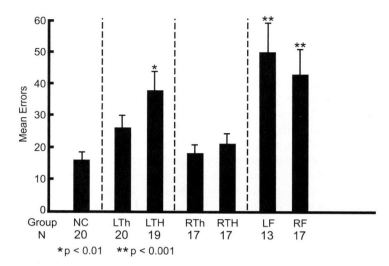

Figure 1–6 Mean error scores for the various groups of patients on the visual motor conditional task (demonstration testing procedure). NC, normal control; LTh, left temporal lobe group, limited hippocampal damage; LTH, left temporal lobe group, extensive hippocampal damage; RTh, right temporal lobe group, limited hippocampal damage; RTH, right temporal lobe group, extensive hippocampal damage; LF, left frontal lobe group; RF, right frontal lobe group (Reprinted from Petrides, *Neuropsychologia,* 35, 989–997. Copyright Elsevier, 1997).

temporal lobe excisions were not impaired, except for those with left anterior temporal lobe excisions that included extensive damage to the hippocampal system. Thus, regardless of whether testing used a trial-and-error method (Petrides, 1985a) or explicit demonstration of the stimulus-response relations (Petrides, 1997), patients with unilateral frontal cortical excisions were severely impaired in learning visual-motor conditional associative responses.

Conditional Associative Response Learning: Spatial Responses

Another series of experiments explored the question of whether the impairment in the learning of conditional associative relations between instructional cues and responses was restricted to the control of different movements (e.g., hand postures) or whether it was a more general impairment that involved other types of such arbitrary stimulus-response mappings. In one such study, the instructional cues were locations (i.e., six blue lamps that could only be distinguished by their location) and the responses were also spatial (i.e., six white cards arranged in a horizontal row in front of the subject) [Fig. 1–7]. The patients were required to learn arbitrary associations between the six

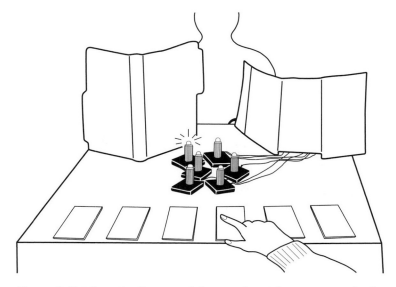

Figure 1–7 Schematic diagram of the experimental arrangement in the spatial conditional task (Reprinted from Petrides, *Neuropsychologia*, 23, 601–614. Copyright Elsevier, 1985).

spatial instructional cues and the six spatial responses (Petrides, 1985a). In this spatial conditional associative task, when one of the blue lamps was turned on, the subjects had to touch the card that they thought was indicated by the cue. If they touched the correct card, they were told that their response was correct and the lamp was turned off. If they touched an incorrect card, they were told that their response was wrong, the lamp remained lit, and they continued to touch other cards until they found the correct one. As can be seen in Figure 1–8, excisions from either the left or the right frontal cortex resulted in a severe impairment in learning this task. The severely impaired performance of the patients with frontal cortical excisions stood in marked contrast to that of patients with excisions from the left or right anterior temporal lobe. These patients learned this task at a normal rate, except for those patients with right temporal lobe excisions that included extensive damage to the hippocampal region. The impairment in performance on this spatial task after right hippocampal damage is consistent with other investigations that demonstrated the involvement of the right hippocampal system in spatial learning and memory (e.g., Milner, 1965; Smith and Milner, 1981). In yet another study, patients with excisions from the frontal cortex were impaired in learning conditional relations between color instructional cues and abstract designs (Petrides, 1990).

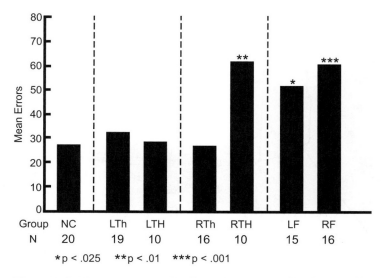

Figure 1–8 Mean error scores for the various groups of patients on the spatial conditional task. NC, normal control; LTh, left temporal lobe group, limited hippocampal damage; LTH, left temporal lobe group, extensive hippocampal damage; RTh, right temporal lobe group, limited hippocampal damage; RTH, right temporal lobe group, extensive hippocampal damage; LF, left frontal lobe group; RF, right frontal lobe group (Reprinted from Petrides, *Neuropsychologia*, 23, 601–614. Copyright Elsevier, 1985).

LEARNING AND PERFORMANCE OF CONDITIONAL ASSOCIATIVE RELATIONS DEPEND ON THE CAUDAL LATERAL FRONTAL CORTEX

The research with patients described earlier established the importance of the lateral frontal cortex in conditional associative learning and also provided strong clues that the deficit depended more on damage to the posterior lateral frontal region than on damage to the rostral dorsolateral prefrontal cortex. Such dissociations, however, are difficult to establish unambiguously in patient work because the lesions often included both regions. We therefore initiated a series of studies on macaque monkeys in which we compared the effects of excisions restricted to the mid-section of the dorsolateral prefrontal cortex versus its more caudal part (Fig. 1–9). The rostral lesions involved the mid-dorsolateral prefrontal cortex and included the cortex in the sulcus principalis and above it (i.e., areas 9, 46, and 9/46). The caudal lateral frontal lesions involved the cortex within the dorsal part of the arcuate sulcus and the immediately surrounding region, namely, rostral dorsal area 6 and area 8A. We called the latter lesions the "periarcuate lesions" because they involved the cortex within and surrounding the arcuate sulcus.

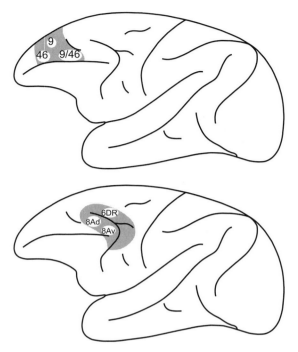

Figure 1–9 Schematic diagram of the mid-dorsolateral prefrontal lesions (areas 9, 46, and 9/46) and the posterior lateral frontal lesions (i.e., periarcuate lesions) [area 8 and rostral area 6].

Striking dissociations between the cognitive effects of lesions of the mid-dorsolateral prefrontal cortex versus those of the caudal lateral frontal cortex were established by the monkey work. Whereas lesions of the mid-dorsolateral prefrontal cortex caused a severe deficit in tasks that required monitoring (i.e., tracking) of information in working memory, caudal lateral frontal lesions did not affect performance on such tasks, but yielded a massive impairment in performance on conditional associative learning tasks comparable to those that we had administered to the patients. Thus, a double dissociation between the effects of mid-dorsolateral versus caudal lateral frontal lesions was established, providing the strongest possible evidence for specialized contribution along the rostral-caudal axis of the dorsolateral frontal cortex (see Petrides, 2005b for a recent review of this work).

An example from this work will be presented here. In one experiment, monkeys were tested on a visual-motor conditional task comparable to those used with patients (Petrides, 1982). The monkeys were required to learn to perform one of two actions (grip a stick or touch a button), depending on the visual stimulus that was shown on any given trial (Fig. 1–10). The monkeys

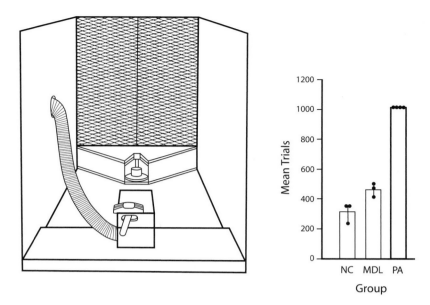

Figure 1–10 Left: Schematic diagram of the experimental arrangement in the visual motor conditional task used with monkeys. On each trial, the monkey must grip the stick or touch the button with the palm facing downward, depending on the object presented. The reward for a correct response is delivered through the tube that is connected to the box. When a correct response has been made and a reward has been delivered down the tube, the monkey pushes back the box to retrieve the reward. Right: Performance of monkeys on the visual motor conditional task. The animals with periarcuate lesions (PA) could not learn the task within the testing limit. The black dots on the histograms represent the performance of individual animals. NC, normal control; MDL, mid-dorsolateral prefrontal lesions; PA, periarcuate lesions. (Reprinted from Petrides, *Behavioural Brain Research*, 5, 407–413. Copyright Elsevier, 1982).

with posterior frontal lesions (i.e., periarcuate lesions) were severely impaired (Petrides, 1982). Further research showed that when the task requires the selection between distinct movements, area 6 is critical (Halsband and Passingham, 1982; Petrides, 1987). By contrast, when the animal has to select between visual stimuli on the basis of learned conditional relations with other visual stimuli, the critical region is area 8 (Petrides, 1987). These results are consistent with the anatomical connections of area 6 and area 8. Whereas area 6 is connected with motor cortical areas, area 8 is connected with cortical areas that control visual scanning in space (see Petrides and Pandya, 2002, 2004). Thus, area 6 is in a position to control the selection between different motor acts based on learned conditional relations with instructional cues, and area 8 is in a position to control attention to and thus the selection of different

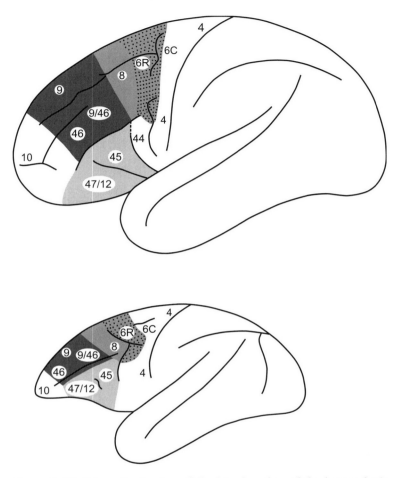

Figure 1–11 Schematic drawing of the lateral surface of the human brain (above) and that of the macaque monkey (below) to indicate the location of the mid-dorsolateral frontal region (areas 46, 9, and 9/46) and the mid-ventrolateral frontal region (areas 45 and 47/12). The term "mid-dorsolateral frontal cortex" is used to distinguish this region from the frontopolar cortex (area 10) and the posterior dorsolateral frontal cortex (area 8 and rostral area 6). In the human brain, the mid-dorsolateral frontal cortex occupies the mid-section of the middle and superior frontal gyri. The mid-ventrolateral frontal region occupies the pars triangularis (area 45) and pars orbitalis (area 47/12) of the inferior frontal gyrus.

objects scattered in the environment based on conditional relations (see also Petrides, 2005a).

The research with monkeys demonstrated that the caudal dorsolateral frontal cortex is a critical region for the learning and performance of conditional associative tasks that require selection between different responses based on

conditional rules. Control experiments showed that, like the patients with frontal lesions (discussed earlier), monkeys with caudal dorsolateral frontal lesions know and can perform the responses, although they are impaired in selecting between the alternative responses based on learned conditional relations. Furthermore, the monkeys (like the patients with frontal lesions) perform normally on many tasks of recognition and working memory, as well as on other tasks that require learning associations between stimuli. In other words, the deficit in performance on conditional associative tasks after caudal dorsolateral frontal lesions is not the result of a generalized impairment in learning, knowledge, or performance of the responses from which selections must be made.

WHAT IS THE ROLE OF THE MID-VENTROLATERAL PREFRONTAL CORTEX IN THE LEARNING AND PERFORMANCE OF CONDITIONAL ASSOCIATIVE RELATIONS?

What other structures within the lateral frontal cortex might be critical for the selection between alternative responses according to conditional rules? As discussed earlier, lesions of the mid-dorsolateral prefrontal cortex (areas 9, 46, and 9/46) had no effect or a negligible effect on the learning and performance of conditional associative responses (Petrides, 2005b). There is, however, some evidence that the mid-ventrolateral prefrontal cortex may play an important role (Fig. 1–11). Wang et al. (2000) found that bilateral injection of bicuculline (a gamma-aminobutyric acid–ergic antagonist) into the ventrolateral prefrontal cortex impaired the learning of novel visual-motor conditional associations, but did not affect the performance of preoperatively learned associations. Furthermore, infusions of bicuculline in the mid-dorsolateral prefrontal region did not affect the learning of novel visual-motor conditional associations or the performance of preoperatively learned associations, consistent with earlier work (Petrides, 1982, 2005b) that showed that the mid-dorsolateral prefrontal cortex is not a critical region for conditional associative learning. Bussey et al. (2001) examined the effect on conditional learning of massive lesions that involved not only the ventrolateral prefrontal cortex but also the orbitofrontal cortex as far as the medial orbital sulcus. These massive lesions caused impairment of rapid learning (i.e., within a session of 50 trials) of novel visual-motor conditional associations, although the monkeys could still learn the associations when trained gradually over several sessions. Because the lesions were not restricted to the mid-ventrolateral prefrontal cortex and the combined ventrolateral and orbital prefrontal lesions had disturbed several basic functions, this impairment in conditional learning is difficult to interpret. For instance, the monkeys with ventrolateral plus orbital frontal lesions had severe problems with the retention of preoperatively learned strategies and did not learn basic tasks, such as matching-to-sample. Thus, in these monkeys, the difficulty in learning conditional visual-motor tasks may have been secondary to other, more general cognitive

impairments. In conclusion, the available evidence suggests that the mid-ventrolateral prefrontal cortex may be important during the early stages of learning conditional responses, but not later, when the responses have been acquired. This pattern of deficits stands in sharp contrast to the specific effects of posterior lateral frontal lesions (i.e., periarcuate lesions). The monkeys with periarcuate lesions neither acquire novel conditional associations nor perform preoperatively learned ones, although they perform normally on matching-to-sample tasks, working memory tasks, and several other associative learning tasks (see Petrides, 1987, 2005b).

What might be the contribution of the mid-ventrolateral prefrontal cortex in conditional associative learning? The mid-ventrolateral prefrontal cortex is a critical region for the active controlled retrieval of information from memory in situations where relations between stimuli are ambiguous (Petrides, 2002, 2005a). It could be argued that, during the early stages of learning conditional associative relations, the task makes considerable demands on active controlled retrieval mechanisms because the relations between stimuli and responses are ambiguous. For instance, in the early stages of training, the traces of both responses X and Y in the context of both stimuli A and B will exist in the subject's memory because both X and Y were performed in the presence of A and B and the unambiguous links have not yet been established. Thus, in the early stages, the subject must retrieve actively from ambiguous memory relations by allocating attention to particular trials in memory, a control process emanating from the mid-ventrolateral prefrontal cortex. Rushworth et al. (1997) provided evidence from another domain, namely, the learning of a matching rule by monkeys, that the mid-ventrolateral prefrontal cortex may be important for the acquisition of rules, but not their subsequent performance (see also Chapter 7).

The critical importance of the caudal lateral frontal cortex (area 6), but not the ventrolateral prefrontal cortex, in the performance of well-learned conditional motor responses has also be shown in a recent functional neuroimaging study (Amiez et al., 2006). In this functional magnetic resonance imaging study, normal human subjects were scanned while they performed a conditional task requiring the selection among four different hand actions depending on previously learned arbitrary relations with visual color instructional stimuli. In relation to the control motor task, performance of the visual-motor conditional task resulted in significant, highly specific increases in activity within the superior branch of the precentral sulcus (i.e., dorsal premotor cortical region). The focus of the conditional task-related activity, which was anterior to the primary hand motor cortical representation and dorsal and posterior to the frontal eye field representation, was entirely consistent with the monkey lesion studies that identified dorsal premotor cortical area 6 as the critical region for visual-motor conditional responses.

A major finding of the functional magnetic resonance imaging study by Amiez et al. (2006) was the clear lack of any increase in activity in the mid-dorsolateral prefrontal cortex (areas 9, 46, and 9/46) or the ventrolateral

prefrontal cortex (areas 45 and 47/12) during the performance of these well-learned visual-motor conditional responses. These findings of a clear absence of activity in the mid-ventrolateral prefrontal cortex during the performance of well-learned conditional associative responses contrasts with earlier demonstrations of activity in this part of the prefrontal cortex during the learning of conditional relations to guide action (e.g., Toni et al., 2001; Bunge et al., 2003), again emphasizing the importance of the mid-ventrolateral prefrontal region in the learning, but not necessarily the performance, of such conditional responses.

INVOLVEMENT OF THE HIPPOCAMPAL SYSTEM IN CONDITIONAL ASSOCIATIVE LEARNING

The work with patients has clearly shown that the learning of conditional associative relations is subserved by a neural circuit that includes the lateral frontal cortex and the hippocampal region. The learning of conditional associations would be expected to involve the medial temporal lobe limbic region (i.e., hippocampal system) that is critical for the learning of explicit associations between stimuli (Milner, 1975; Eichenbaum, 1997; see also Chapter 15). Patients with anterior temporal lobe lesions that did not involve the hippocampal system learned conditional associations as well as normal control subjects, but patients who had extensive damage to the hippocampal system were impaired in acquiring these associations (Petrides, 1985a, 1997). Note that the hippocampal contribution was material-specific: Patients with right hippocampal damage were impaired in learning spatial conditional associative responses, whereas patients with left hippocampal damage were impaired in learning arbitrary stimulus-response mappings between color cues and hand postures. The importance of the hippocampal region in the learning of conditional associative relations has been confirmed in work with experimental animals. Findings from studies with both monkeys (Rupniak and Gaffan, 1987; Murray and Wise, 1996) and rats (Sziklas et al., 1996, 1998; Sziklas and Petrides, 2002) provide further evidence that the hippocampal system is necessary for the learning of conditional associations. In some studies with rats, lesions limited to the hippocampus gave rise to impairment in the performance of a visual-spatial conditional task only when a delay was interposed between the stimuli and the responses (Winocur, 1991; Marston et al., 1993). Single-cell recording studies in behaving monkeys have provided further support for the importance of the hippocampal system in the learning of conditional associations (Miyashita et al., 1989; Kita et al., 1995).

CONCLUDING COMMENT

The experiments with patients that were described earlier demonstrate that the lateral frontal cortex plays a major role in both the acquisition and the execution of conditional rules that enable the appropriate selection of a response

from several competing alternatives. Furthermore, studies with patients show that the learning of these conditional rules involves functional interaction between the frontal cortex and the hippocampal memory system. Experiments in macaque monkeys with lesions restricted to particular parts of the lateral frontal cortex have shown that the posterior lateral frontal cortical region (area 6 and area 8) is critical for both the acquisition and the operation of conditional rules for the appropriate selection of an action. Furthermore, it has been shown that, whereas rostral area 6 controls the selection between distinct motor acts on the basis of conditional rules, area 8 plays a major role in the selection between visual stimuli in the environment (see Petrides, 1987, and Petrides et al., 1993, for further discussion of this issue). There is also electrophysiological evidence for the involvement of these posterior frontal cortical areas in conditional response selection (e.g., Mitz et al., 1991; Chen and Wise, 1995; Wallis and Miller, 2003).

Recently, Brass et al. (2005) have examined, in the human brain, the role of the inferior frontal junction region in cognitive control. This region, which lies at the intersection of rostral area 6, area 8, and area 44, appears to be involved in contextually guided updating of task representations that may, in fact, be a more general application of conditional rules for the selection of action and for which the caudal lateral prefrontal cortex is critical (see also Chapter 9). Finally, both monkey lesion studies and functional neuroimaging studies in normal human subjects suggest that the mid-ventrolateral prefrontal cortex may be involved during the learning of conditional associative rules, but not necessarily during their execution. This involvement of the mid-ventrolateral prefrontal cortex in the learning of conditional associative relations may be a reflection of its role in active controlled memory retrieval.

ACKNOWLEDGMENTS Supported by the Canadian Institutes of Health Research (MOP-37753) and the Natural Sciences and Engineering Research Council of Canada (Grant 7466).

REFERENCES   •

Amiez C, Kostopoulos P, Champod A-S, Petrides M (2006) Local morphology predicts functional organization of the dorsal premotor region in the human brain. Journal of Neuroscience 26:2724–2731.

Brass M, Derrfuss J, Forstmann B, von Cramon DY (2005) The role of the inferior frontal junction area in cognitive control. Trends in Cognitive Science 9:314–316.

Bunge SA (2004) How we use rules to select actions: a review of evidence from cognitive neuroscience. Cognitive, Affective, and Behavioral Neuroscience 4:564–579.

Bunge SA, Kahn I, Wallis JD, Miller EK, Wagner AD (2003) Neural circuits subserving the retrieval and maintenance of abstract rules. Journal of Neurophysiology 90:3419–3428.

Bussey TJ, Wise SP, Murray EA (2001) The role of the ventral and orbital prefrontal cortex in conditional visuomotor learning and strategy use in rhesus monkeys (*Macaca mulatta*). Behavioral Neuroscience 115:971–982.

Chen LL, Wise SP (1995) Neuronal activity in the supplementary eye field during the acquisition of conditional oculomotor associations. Journal of Neurophysiology 73:1101–1121.

DeRenzi E, Motti R, Nichelli P (1980) Imitating gestures: a quantitative approach to ideomotor apraxia. Archives of Neurology 37:6–10.

Eichenbaum H (1997) Declarative memory: insights from cognitive neurobiology. Annual Review of Psychology 48:547–572.

Halsband U, Passingham R (1982) The role of premotor and parietal cortex in the direction of action. Brain Research 240:368–372.

Kimura D, Archibald Y (1974) Motor functions of the left hemisphere. Brain 97:337–350.

Kita T, Nishijo H, Eifuku S, Terasawa K, Ono T (1995) Place and contingency differential responses of monkey septal neurons during conditional place-object discrimination. Journal of Neuroscience 15:1683–1703.

Marston HM, Everitt BJ, Robbins TW (1993) Comparative effects of excitotoxic lesions of the hippocampus and septum/diagonal band on conditional visual discrimination and spatial earning. Neuropsychologia 31:1099–1118.

Milner B (1965) Visually guided maze learning in man: effects of bilateral hippocampal, bilateral frontal, and unilateral cerebral lesions. Neuropsychologia 3:317–338.

Milner B (1975) Psychological aspects of focal epilepsy and its neurosurgical management. In: Advances in neurology (Purpura DP, Penry JK, Walter RD, eds.) pp 299–321. New York: Raven Press.

Mitz AR, Godschalk M, Wise SP (1991) Learning-dependent neuronal activity in the premotor cortex of rhesus monkeys. Journal of Neuroscience 11:1855–1872.

Miyashita Y, Rolls ET, Cahusac PMB, Niki H, Feigenbaum JD (1989) Activity of hippocampal neurons in the monkey related to a conditional spatial response task. Journal of Neurophysiology 61:669–678.

Murray EA, Wise SP (1996) Role of the hippocampus plus subjacent cortex but not theamygdala in visuomotor conditional learning in rhesus monkeys. Behavioral Neuroscience 110:1261–1270.

Petrides M (1982) Motor conditional associative learning after selective prefrontal lesions in the monkey. Behavioural Brain Research 5:407–413.

Petrides M (1985a) Deficits on conditional associative-learning task after frontal- and temporal-lobe lesions in man. Neuropsychologia 23:601–614.

Petrides M (1985b) Deficits in non-spatial conditional associative learning after periarcuate lesions in the monkey. Behavioural Brain Research 16:95–101.

Petrides M (1987) Conditional learning and the primate frontal cortex. In: The frontal lobes revisited (Perecman E, ed.) pp 91–108. New York: IRBN Press.

Petrides M (1990) Nonspatial conditional learning impaired in patients with unilateral frontal but not unilateral temporal lobe excisions. Neuropsychologia 28:137–149.

Petrides M (1997) Visuo-motor conditional associative learning after frontal and temporal lesions in the human brain. Neuropsychologia 35:989–997.

Petrides M (2000) Frontal lobes and memory. In: Handbook of neuropsychology (Boller F, Grafman J, eds.), pp 67–84, 2nd edition, volume 2. Amsterdam: Elsevier.

Petrides M (2002) The mid-ventrolateral prefrontal cortex and active mnemonic retrieval. Neurobiology of Learning and Memory 78:528–538.

Petrides M (2005a) Lateral prefrontal cortex: architectonic and functional organization. Philosophical Transactions of the Royal Society B 360:781–795.

Petrides M (2005b) The rostral-caudal axis of cognitive control within the lateral frontal cortex. In: From monkey brain to human brain: a Fyssen Foundation symposium (Dehaene S, Duhamel J-R, Hauser MC, Rizzolatti G, eds.) pp 293–314. Cambridge, Massachusetts: MIT Press.

Petrides M, Alivisatos B, Evans AC, Meyer E (1993) Dissociation of human mid-dorsolateral from posterior dorsolateral frontal cortex in memory processing. Proceedings of the National Academy of Sciences U S A 90:873–877.

Petrides M, Pandya DN (2002) Association pathways of the prefrontal cortex and functional observations. In: Principles of frontal lobe function (Stuss DT, Knight RT, eds.) pp 31–50. New York: Oxford University Press.

Petrides M, Pandya DN (2004) The frontal cortex. In: The human nervous system (Paxinos G, Mai JK, eds.) pp 950–972, 2nd edition. San Diego: Elsevier Academic Press.

Robbins TW (1996) Dissociating executive functions of the prefrontal cortex. Philosophical Transactions of the Royal Society B 351:1463–1470.

Rupniak NMJ, Gaffan D (1987) Monkey hippocampus and learning about spatially-directed movements. Journal of Neuroscience 7:2331–2337.

Rushworth MFS, Nixon PD, Eacott MJ, Passingham RE (1997) Ventral prefrontal cortex is not essential for working memory. Journal of Neuroscience 17:4829–4838.

Shallice T, Burgess DF (1996) The domain of supervisory processes and temporal organization of behaviour. Philosophical Transactions of the Royal Society B 351:1405–1411.

Smith ML, Milner B (1981) The role of the right hippocampus in the recall of spatial location. Neuropsychologia 19:781–793.

Stuss DT, Benson DF (1986) The frontal lobes. New York: Raven Press.

Sziklas V, Lebel S, Petrides M (1998) Conditional associative learning and the hippocampal system. Hippocampus 8:131–137.

Sziklas V, Petrides M (2002) Effects of lesions to the hippocampus or the fornix on allocentric conditional associative learning in rats. Hippocampus 12:543–550.

Sziklas V, Petrides M, Leri F (1996) The effects of lesions to the mammillary region and the hippocampus on conditional learning by rats. European Journal of Neuroscience 8:106–115.

Toni I, Rushworth MFS, Passingham RE (2001) Neural correlates of visuomotor associations: spatial rules compared with arbitrary rules. Experimental Brain Research 141:359–369.

Wallis JD, Miller EK (2003) From rule to response: neuronal processes in the premotor and prefrontal cortex. Journal of Neurophysiology 90:1790–1806.

Wang M, Zhang H, Li B-M (2000) Deficit in conditional visuomotor learning by local infusion of bicuculline into the ventral prefrontal cortex in monkeys. European Journal of Neuroscience 12:3787–3796.

Winocur G (1991) Functional dissociation of the hippocampus and prefrontal cortex in learning and memory. Psychobiology 19:11–20.

2

Single Neuron Activity Underlying Behavior-Guiding Rules

Jonathan D. Wallis

Simple associations between environmental events and our behavioral responses can support much of our learning. For example, while learning to drive, we learn that we should brake when we encounter a red traffic light. Although such learning is clearly useful for our morning commute, it suffers from a number of disadvantages relative to more complex types of learning. First, it does not generalize very well, particularly if the relationship between the stimulus and the response is arbitrary, as in the case of traffic signals. Learning about red and green traffic lights, for example, tells you nothing about the red and green lights on your stereo. A second problem is that we need to learn stimulus-response associations through trial and error. Such learning necessarily involves errors, which can be costly. Errors may result in the lost opportunity for reward, or even physical harm. A third problem is that by dealing with the world in a literal fashion, we are potentially encoding it in an inefficient manner. There are so many potential combinations between stimuli and responses that we would be unable to remember all the possible combinations and their meanings.

A possible solution to these problems resides in our ability to abstract information across experiences. We learn to attend to the commonalities of a situation and ignore trivial differences. For example, after dining in a few restaurants, we learn to abstract the general rules that underlie ordering a meal, such as "wait to be seated," "order from the menu," and "pay the bill." Such rules are easy to generalize, and we can apply them to any restaurant that we subsequently visit. No two restaurants are physically identical, but because rules operate at a conceptual level, they are relevant to physically different situations. Furthermore, although we initially acquire the rules through trial-and-error learning (as we blunder our way through our first restaurant experience), once these rules have been established, we can use them to order a meal in a new restaurant. Finally, by abstracting the "gist" of a restaurant experience, we can substantially reduce the amount of information we need to store about restaurants.

Indeed, humans are so adept at storing information in an abstract form that we are often quite poor at remembering specific details. For example,

Bartlett found that subjects' recall of stories tended to be simpler than the original story (Bartlett, 1932). Similarly, if people recall their previous day at work, they tend to recall details, whereas if they recall a day at work from over a week ago, their recall consists of a "typical" day at work (Eldridge, 1994). Our memory system seems to be proficient at abstracting the generalities in the information it stores.

This chapter focuses on how the brain encodes abstract rules and compares and contrasts this with the encoding of stimulus-response associations. The discussion focuses particularly on prefrontal cortex (PFC), an area of the brain that has undergone a dramatic expansion in size and complexity across the course of mammalian evolution (Semendeferi et al., 2002). PFC reaches the pinnacle of its development in humans, where it accounts for approximately 30% of the cerebral cortex. Not surprisingly, this has led to the suggestion that PFC is responsible for those cognitive capacities that distinguish humans from animals, including the capacity to use abstract information. Therefore, PFC is a good place to begin looking for the neuronal mechanisms underpinning abstract rule use.

PREFRONTAL CORTEX AND COMPARATIVE PSYCHOLOGY

In anatomical terms, PFC is ideally suited to represent abstract, high-level rules. It receives input from all sensory modalities (Pandya and Yeterian, 1990; Barbas and Pandya, 1991), which is critical for organizing sensory information into supramodal concepts and rules. Furthermore, its neurons are responsive to a wide range of sensory modalities (Rolls and Baylis, 1994; Rao et al., 1997; Romo et al., 1999; Romanski and Goldman-Rakic, 2002). PFC also sends projections to a variety of secondary motor areas, including premotor cortex (PMC); these areas in turn project to more primary motor structures (Pandya and Yeterian, 1990; Barbas and Pandya, 1991). Thus, PFC appears to reside at the apex of the perception-action cycle, receiving highly processed sensory information and projecting to high-level motor areas (Fuster, 2002).

Yet, despite its size and location in the human brain, damage to PFC often appears to have surprisingly little effect. Sensorimotor abilities, language, memory, and intelligence are all intact, and in casual conversation, patients with PFC damage can appear remarkably normal. However, despite the superficial appearance of normality, the patients' everyday life is devastated. They have difficulty organizing and planning their behavior, are easily distracted, and tend to act in a disinhibited and impulsive manner. This pattern of deficits is called the "dysexecutive syndrome" because it reflects a breakdown in high-level, executive processes. One component of this syndrome is the inability to use high-level, abstract rules to control behavior. A classic test of PFC function is the Wisconsin Card Sorting Task. In this task, the patient has to sort a deck of cards according to different rules. The patient may need to sort them based on the number of shapes on each card, or according to the color or identity of the shapes. Patients with damage to PFC have difficulty performing this

task. In particular, they have difficulty switching between these different rules (Milner, 1963).

PREFRONTAL CORTEX AND RULE USE IN OTHER SPECIES

Exploring the neuronal processes that underlie these abilities is difficult in humans; for this, we need an animal model. Perhaps, though, we are pushing the limits of which animals are capable. Do they even have the capacity to use abstract information? It seems that at least some species do. One abstract rule that is relatively easy to demonstrate in animals is that of *sameness:* the matching-to-sample task tests this ability. A subject sees a sample stimulus, and then a short while later, it sees two test stimuli, one of which is the same as the sample. To get a reward, the subject must select the test stimulus that matches the sample stimulus. If an animal can successfully perform this task, it suggests that the animal can appreciate that the sample stimulus and the test stimulus are the same, and that this relationship controls the choice of the test stimulus.

However, there are potentially other explanations for this behavior. In particular, an animal might learn the task through specific configurations of the stimuli and responses. Consider the displays in Figure 2–1, which illustrate the various configurations between two pictures used in the task, and the correct response. Notice that the animal could learn this task by learning the correct motor response to a specific configuration of stimuli. For example, it could learn that the specific configuration of pictures in the upper left box instructs a motor response to the upper left. This type of learning shows nothing more than the acquisition of a stimulus-response association through trial and error. However, suppose that we were to use new stimuli on every trial. An animal relying on configural learning would not have the opportunity to learn by trial and error, and would have to guess. In contrast, an animal that understands the "same" rule would still be able to perform the task.

There is substantial evidence that some species understand the "same" rule and can solve the matching-to-sample task, even when every trial uses new stimuli. These species include chimpanzees (Nissen et al., 1948; Oden et al., 1988), rhesus monkeys (Mishkin et al., 1962), dolphins (Herman and Gordon, 1974) and sea lions (Kastak and Schusterman, 1994). The ability to use abstract rules is not limited to mammals. Corvids (the bird family that includes crows, rooks, jays, and jackdaws) and parrots all show the ability to perform the matching-to-sample task with novel stimuli (Wilson et al., 1985; Pepperberg, 1987). In contrast, although pigeons can learn the matching-to-sample task for small sets of stimuli, if novel stimuli are used on every trial, they perform at chance, suggesting that they are unable to abstract the rule (Wilson et al., 1985).

In terms of comparative psychology, other tasks that involve abstract rules yield similar results. One example is the formation of a "learning set." If primates learn a series of standard visual discriminations, where they see two pictures and must learn to select one of them to get a reward, their rate of

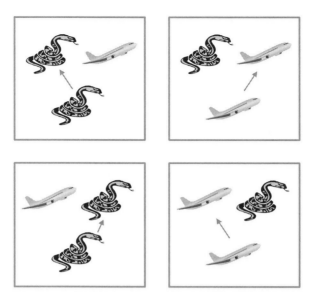

Figure 2–1 Possible configurations of stimuli and responses in a matching task. In each panel, the lower picture is the sample stimulus and the upper two pictures are the test stimuli. The *arrow* indicates the behavioral response. Although an animal could learn this task by abstracting the rule to choose the upper picture that matched the lower one, it could equally learn the task by memorizing the correct response to make to each of the four possible configurations of stimuli.

learning gets progressively better with each discrimination they solve (Harlow, 1949). Eventually, the monkey can learn the problem in a single trial: Performance on the first trial is necessarily at chance, but performance is virtually 100% correct on the second trial. The monkey has learned to extract the abstract rule "win-stay, lose-shift," which dramatically speeds performance (Restle, 1958). So, too, do corvids, but pigeons must solve each discrimination individually (Hunter and Kamil, 1971; Wilson et al., 1985). Interestingly, corvid brains differ from those of other birds, in that they have an enlarged mesopallium and nidopallium, areas that are analogous to PFC in mammals (Rehkamper and Zilles, 1991), prompting speculation that the capacity to use abstract information might have evolved at least twice in the animal kingdom (Emery and Clayton, 2004).

   In fact, the capacity to understand certain abstract concepts may be widespread. A recent study showed that even some insects can use "same" and "different" rules to guide their behavior (Giurfa, 2001). Investigators trained honeybees on a Y-maze. At the entrance to the maze was the sample stimulus, and at the entrance to the two forks in the Y-maze were two test stimuli. Bees

received a reward for choosing the arm with the matching test stimulus. Not only could the bees learn this task, but they also were able to apply the rule to novel stimuli. Furthermore, they were just as capable of learning to follow the "different" rule as they were the "same" rule. This study raises interesting questions. For example, why should the capacity to use an abstract rule be useful to bees, but not to pigeons? This capacity is not simply the ability to know that one flower is the "same" as another, a very simple (and useful) behavioral adaptation that can be solved through stimulus generalization and conditioning. Rather, it is using the relationship between two stimuli to govern behavior in an arbitrary fashion. Quite what use the bee finds for this ability is a mystery, but it does demonstrate that a remarkably simple nervous system, consisting of a brain of $1\,\mathrm{mm}^3$ and fewer than 1 million neurons (Witthöft, 1967) is capable of using abstract information. It remains an open question whether it can learn a variety of abstract information, as does the mammalian brain, or whether its abilities are more constrained.

These studies in neuropsychology and comparative psychology thus laid the groundwork for this exploration of the neuronal mechanisms that might underlie the use of abstract rules to guide behavior. They suggested a task that monkeys could perform to demonstrate their grasp of abstract rules and supported the notion that PFC would be an important brain region for the neuronal representation of such rules.

NEURONAL REPRESENTATION OF ABSTRACT RULES IN PREFRONTAL CORTEX

Behavioral Paradigm

Although the matching-to-sample task was useful for demonstrating behaviorally that monkeys could use abstract rules, this task presented several problems when it came to exploring the underlying neuronal mechanisms. First, the task made use of only one rule; to demonstrate neuronal selectivity, we need at least two rules. To see why this is the case, consider how we would define a neuron as encoding a face. We would want to show not only that the neuron responds to faces, but also that it does not respond to non-face stimuli. Otherwise, the neuron might be encoding any visual stimulus, rather than faces specifically. In an analogous fashion, to demonstrate that a neuron is encoding a specific rule, we need to show not only that it responds when the "same" rule is in effect, but also that it does not respond when other rules are in effect. The matching-to-sample task shows that monkeys can grasp the concept of "sameness." An obvious second rule to teach the monkey was that of "difference." Now, the monkey had to choose the test stimulus that did not match the sample stimulus.

We trained three monkeys to use both of these rules. A sample stimulus appeared on a computer screen, and we instructed the monkeys to follow either the "same" rule or the "different" rule. After a brief delay, one of two test

stimuli appeared. The monkey had to make a given response depending on which rule was in effect and whether the test stimulus matched or did not match the sample stimulus. This, of course, raises the following question: How do you instruct a monkey to follow a given rule? We did this by means of a cue that we presented simultaneously with the sample stimulus. If the monkey received a drop of juice, it knew that it should follow the "same" rule, and if it did not receive juice, it knew that it should follow the "different" rule. However, this method of cueing the currently relevant rule introduces a potential confounding factor. Any neuron that showed a difference in firing rate when the "same" or "different" rule was in effect might simply be encoding the presence or absence of juice. To account for this possibility, we had a second set of cues, drawn from a different modality. Thus, a neuron encoding the abstract rule should be one that shows a difference of activity, *irrespective* of the cue that we use to tell the monkey what to do. Figure 2–2 shows the full task; during the first delay period, the monkey must remember the sample picture as well as which rule is in effect, to perform the task correctly. Behavioral performance on this task was excellent (the monkeys typically performed approximately 90% of the trials correctly).

Each day, we used a set of four pictures that the monkey had not previously seen. We only used four pictures because we wanted to compare the number of neurons that encoded the sample picture and contrast it with the number of neurons that encoded the abstract rule. This meant that we needed multiple trials on which we used the same sample picture to estimate accurately the neuronal firing rate elicited by a given picture. Unfortunately, this repetition could conceivably allow the monkeys to learn the task through trial-and-error configural learning. For example, consider the trial sequence shown in the top row of Figure 2–2. The monkey might learn that the conjunction of the picture of a puppy and the cue that indicates the "same" rule (e.g., a drop of juice or a low tone) indicates that it should release the lever when it sees a picture of a puppy as a test stimulus. Further analysis of the monkeys' behavior showed that this is not how they learned the task (Wallis et al., 2001; Wallis and Miller, 2003a). First, they performed well above chance when applying the rules the first time they encountered a new picture (i.e., before trial-and-error learning could have occurred) [70% correct; 4 pictures × 55 recording sessions = 220 pictures; $p < 10^{-8}$; binomial test]. Second, in subsequent behavioral tests, the monkeys performed the task just as easily when new pictures were used on every trial (performing more than 90% of the trials correctly). Thus, the monkeys had to be solving the task by using the abstract rule.

Neurophysiological Results

Figure 2–3 shows the activity of a PFC neuron during performance of this task. This neuron shows a higher firing rate whenever the "same" rule is in effect. Furthermore, which of the four pictures the monkey is remembering does not affect the firing rate of the neuron, and neither does the cue that instructs the

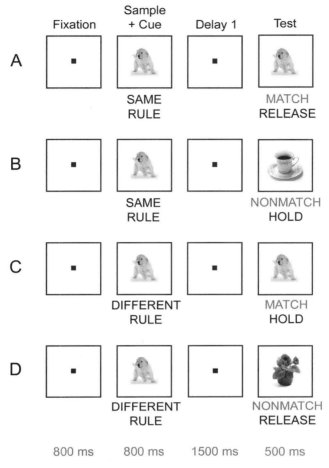

Fixation	Sample + Cue	Delay 1	Test

A

SAME
RULE

MATCH
RELEASE

B

SAME
RULE

NONMATCH
HOLD

C

DIFFERENT
RULE

MATCH
HOLD

D

DIFFERENT
RULE

NONMATCH
RELEASE

800 ms   800 ms   1500 ms   500 ms

Figure 2–2 Each row (A–D) indicates a sequence of possible events in the abstract rule task. A trial begins with the animal fixating on a central point on the screen. We then present a sample picture and a cue simultaneously. We use several cues drawn from different sensory modalities so that we can disambiguate neuronal activity to the physical properties of the cue from the abstract rule that the cue instructs. For our first monkey, we indicate the "same" rule using a drop of juice or a low tone and the "different" rule with no juice or a high tone. For the second monkey, juice or a blue border around the sample picture signifies "same," whereas no juice or a green border indicates "different." For the third monkey, juice or a blue border indicates "same," whereas no juice or a pink border indicates "different." After a short delay, a test picture appears and the animal must make one of two behavioral responses (hold or release a lever), depending on the sample picture and the rule that is currently in effect.

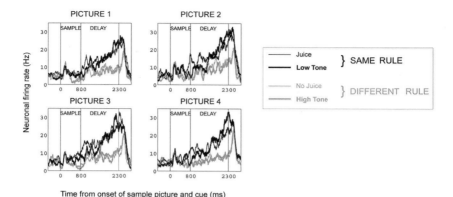

PICTURE 1   PICTURE 2

PICTURE 3   PICTURE 4

Time from onset of sample picture and cue (ms)

Figure 2–3 A prefrontal cortex neuron encoding an abstract rule. Neuronal activity is consistently higher when the "same" rule is in effect, as opposed to the "different" rule. We see the same pattern of neuronal activity irrespective of which picture the monkey is remembering or which cue instructs the rule.

rule. In addition, the monkey does not know whether the test stimulus will or will not match the sample stimulus; consequently, it does not know whether it will be holding or releasing the lever. As such, the activity of the neuron during the delay cannot reflect motor preparation processes. Finally, factors relating to behavioral performance cannot account for the firing rate, such as differences in attention, motivation, or reward expectancy. Behavioral performance was virtually identical in the "same" and "different" trials (0.1% difference in the percentage of correct trials and 7 ms difference in behavioral reaction time). The only remaining explanation is that single neurons in PFC are capable of encoding high-level abstract rules.

We used a three-way analysis of variance (ANOVA) to identify neurons whose average firing rate during the sample and delay epochs varied significantly with trial factors (evaluated at $p < 0.01$). The factors in the ANOVA were the modality of the cue, the rule that the cue signified ("same" or "different"), and which of the four pictures was presented as the sample. We defined rule-selective neurons as those that showed a significant difference in firing rate between the two different rules, regardless of either the cue that was used to instruct the monkey or the picture that was used as the sample stimulus. Likewise, picture-selective neurons were identified as those that showed a significant difference in firing rates between the four pictures, regardless of either the cue or the rule.

We recorded data simultaneously from three major PFC subregions: dorsolateral PFC, consisting of areas 9 and 46; ventrolateral PFC, consisting of area 47/12; and orbitofrontal cortex, consisting of areas 11 and 13. The pattern of neuronal selectivity was similar across the three areas: The most prevalent selectivity was encoding of the abstract rule, observed in approximately 40% of

Table 2–1 Percentage of Neurons Encoding the Various Factors Underlying
Performance of the Abstract Rule Task in Either the Sample
or the Delay Epochs

	DLPFC	VLPFC	OFC	PFC	PMC	STR	ITC
N	182	396	150	728	258	282	341
Cue	31%	20%	25%	24%	26%	18%	21%
Rule	42%	41%	38%	41%	48%	27%	12%
Picture	7%	18%	8%	13%	5%	4%	45%
Cue × Rule	31%	27%	23%	27%	50%	20%	9%
Rule × Picture	2%	1%	0%	1%	0%	1%	6%
Cue × Picture	2%	5%	3%	4%	3%	1%	1%

Percentages exceed 100% because neurons could show different types of selectivity in the two epochs.
DLPFC, dorsolateral prefrontal cortex; VLPFC, ventrolateral prefrontal cortex; OFC, orbitofrontal
cortex; PFC, prefrontal cortex; PMC, premotor cortex; STR, striatum; ITC, inferior temporal cortex.

PFC neurons (Table 2–1). There was an even split between neurons encoding
the "same" rule and those encoding the "different" rule. No topographic organization was evident, and we often recorded the activity of "same" and "different" neurons on the same electrode. The second most prevalent type of
neuronal activity was a Cue × Rule interaction (27%). This occurred when a
neuron was most active to a single cue. This may simply reflect the physical
properties of the cue, although, in principle, it could also carry some rule
information. For example, such a neuron might be encoding rule information,
but only from a single modality. In contrast with the extent of rule encoding, a
much smaller proportion encoded which picture appeared in the sample
epoch (13%).

These results suggest that encoding of abstract rules is an important function of PFC, indeed, more so than the encoding of sensory information.
Having determined this, we wanted to ascertain whether the representation of
abstract rules was a unique property of PFC. We thus recorded from some of
its major inputs and outputs, with the aim of determining whether rule information arises in PFC.

ENCODING OF ABSTRACT RULES IN REGIONS
CONNECTED TO PREFRONTAL CORTEX

In the next study, we recorded data from three additional areas that are heavily
interconnected with PFC (Muhammad et al., 2006), namely, inferior temporal
cortex (ITC), PMC, and the striatum (STR). We recorded data from ITC
because it is the major input to PFC for visual information (Barbas, 1988;
Barbas and Pandya, 1991). This was of interest because the rule task requires
the monkey to apply the "same" and "different" rules to complex visual

pictures and ITC plays a major role in the recognition of such stimuli (Desimone et al., 1984; Tanaka, 1996). Furthermore, interactions between PFC and ITC are necessary for the normal learning of stimulus-response associations (Bussey et al., 2002). We also recorded data from PMC and STR because these are two of the major outputs of PFC. Within PMC, we recorded data from the arm area because the monkeys needed to make an arm movement to indicate their response. Within STR, we recorded data from the head and body of the caudate nucleus, a region known to contain many neurons involved in the learning of stimulus-response associations (Pasupathy and Miller, 2005; see Chapter 18).

To compare selectivity across the four brain regions, we performed a receiver operating characteristic (ROC) analysis. This analysis measures the degree of overlap between two response distributions. It is particularly useful for comparing neuronal responses in different areas of the brain because it is independent of the neuron's firing rate, and so it is easier to compare neurons with different baseline firing rates and dynamic ranges. It is also nonparametric and does not require the distributions to be Gaussian.

For each selective neuron, we determined which of the two rules drove its activity the most. We then compared the distribution of neuronal activity when the neuron's preferred rule was in effect and when its unpreferred rule was in effect. We refer to these two distributions as P and U, respectively. We then generated an ROC curve by taking each observed firing rate of the neuron (i.e., the unique values from the combined distribution of P and U) and plotting the proportion of P that exceeded the value of that observation against the proportion of U that exceeded the value of that observation. The area under the ROC curve was then calculated. A value of 0.5 would indicate that the two distributions completely overlap (because the proportion of U and P exceeding that value is equal), and as such, would indicate that the neuron is not selective. A value of 1.0, on the other hand, would indicate that the two distributions are completely separate (i.e., every value of U is exceeded by the entirety of P, whereas none of the values of P is exceeded by any of the values of U), and so the neuron is very selective. An intuitive way to think about the ROC value is that it measures the probability that you could correctly identify which rule was in effect if you knew the neuron's firing rate.

We used the ROC measure to determine the time course of neuronal selectivity and to estimate each neuron's selectivity latency. We computed the ROC by averaging activity over a 200-ms window that we slid in 10-ms steps over the course of the trial. To measure latency, we used the point at which the sliding ROC curve equaled or exceeded 0.6 for three consecutive 10-ms bins. We chose this criterion because it yielded latency values that compared favorably with values that we determined by visually examining the spike density histograms. Other measures yielded similar results, such as values reaching three standard deviations above the baseline ROC values.

As shown in Figure 2–4, the strongest rule selectivity was observed in the frontal lobe (PFC and PMC), and there was only weak rule selectivity in STR

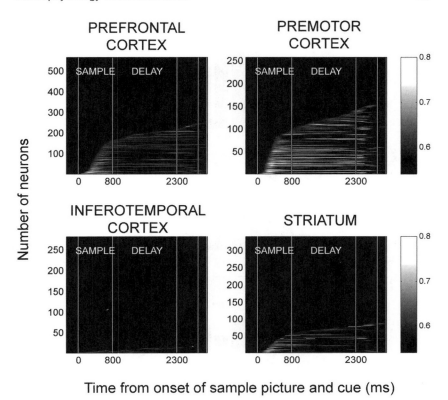

Time from onset of sample picture and cue (ms)

Figure 2–4 Time course of neuronal selectivity for the rule across the entire population of neurons from which we recorded. Each horizontal line consists of the data from
a single neuron, color-coded by its selectivity, as measured by a receiver operating
characteristic. We sorted the neurons according to their latency. The black area at the
top of each figure consists of the data from neurons that did not encode the rule. Rule
selectivity was strong in premotor cortex and prefrontal cortex, weak in striatum, and
virtually absent in inferotemporal cortex.

and ITC. Figure 2–4 illustrates the time course of rule selectivity across the
four neuronal populations from which we recorded. The x-axis refers to the
time from the onset of the sample epoch, and each horizontal line reflects data
from a single neuron. Color-coding reflects the strength of selectivity, as determined by the ROC analysis. We sorted the neurons along the y-axis so that
neurons with the fastest onset of neuronal selectivity are at the bottom of the
graph. The black area at the top of each graph indicates the neurons that did
not reach the criterion for determining their latency.

The analysis using a three-way ANOVA to define rule-selective neurons
confirmed the results displayed in Figure 2–4. There was a significantly greater
incidence of rule selectivity in the PMC (48% of all recorded neurons, or

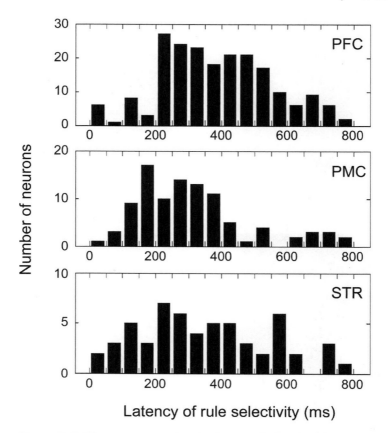

Figure 2–5 Histogram comparing the latency of rule selectivity across three of the areas from which we recorded. Rule selectivity appeared earlier in premotor cortex (PMC) [median = 280 ms] than in prefrontal cortex (PFC) [median = 370 ms], whereas striatum (STR) latencies (median = 350 ms) did not differ from those of PFC or PMC.

125/258) than in PFC (41%, or 297/728), a greater incidence in PFC than in STR (26%, or 89/341), and a greater incidence in STR than in ITC (12%, or 34/282; chi-square; all comparisons $p < 0.01$). In all areas, approximately half of the rule neurons showed higher firing rates to the "same" rule, whereas the other half showed higher firing rates to the "different" rule. There were also regional differences in terms of when rule selectivity first appeared. Figure 2–5 shows the distribution of latencies for neurons that reached the criterion for determining latency (ITC neurons are not included here because so few neurons showed a rule effect). On average, rule selectivity appeared significantly earlier in PMC (median = 280 ms) than in PFC (median = 370 ms; Wilcoxon's rank sum test; $p < 0.05$). STR latencies (median = 350 ms) were not significantly different from those of PFC or PMC.

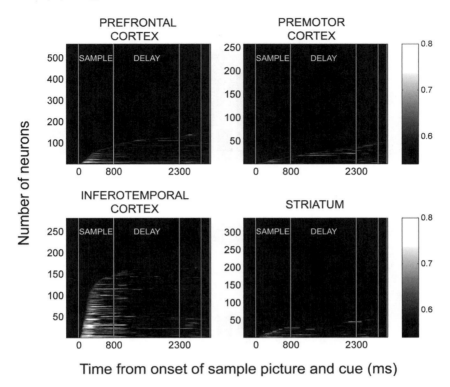

Figure 2–6 Time course of neuronal selectivity for the sample picture across the entire population of neurons from which we recorded. We constructed the figure in the same way as Figure 2–4. Picture selectivity was strong in inferotemporal cortex, weak in prefrontal cortex, and virtually absent in the striatum and premotor cortex.

When we compared the proportion of neurons with picture selectivity across regions, we saw a pattern that was quite different from that seen for rule selectivity. Picture selectivity was strongest in ITC (45% of all neurons, or 126/282), followed by PFC (13%, or 94/728), and finally, PMC (5%, or 12/258) and STR (4%, or 15/341). The incidence of picture selectivity in PMC and STR was not significantly different, but all other differences were (chi-square; $p < 0.01$). We saw a similar pattern of results with the sliding ROC analysis using the difference in activity between the most and least preferred pictures (Fig. 2–6). Once again, each line corresponds to one neuron, and we sorted the traces by their picture selectivity latency. Picture selectivity was strongest in ITC, followed by PFC, and it was weak in both PMC and STR. We used the sliding ROC analysis to determine latencies for picture selectivity after sample onset (Fig. 2–7). The mean latency for picture selectivity was significantly shorter in ITC (median = 160 ms) than in PFC (median = 220 ms; $p < 0.01$). Too few neurons reached the criterion in PMC and STR to allow for meaningful statistical comparisons.

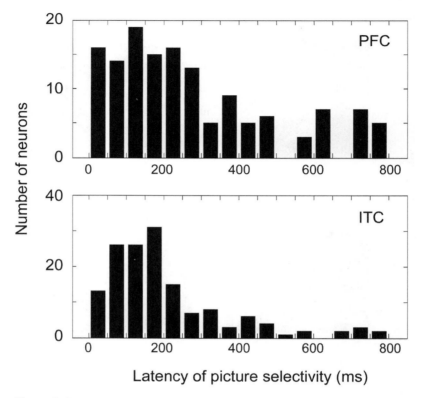

Figure 2–7 Histogram comparing the latency of picture selectivity in prefrontal cortex (PFC) and inferotemporal cortex (ITC). Picture selectivity appeared earlier in ITC (median = 160 ms) than in PFC (median = 220 ms).

In summary, PFC was the only area from which we recorded data that encoded all of the task-relevant information, namely, both the picture and the rule. In contrast, PMC and STR encoded the rule, but not the picture, whereas ITC encoded the picture, but not the rule. These results fit with the conceptualization of ITC, PFC, and PMC as cortical components of a perception-action arc (Fuster, 2002). Perceptual information was strongest and tended to appear earliest in ITC, a sensory cortical area long thought to play a central role in object recognition, and then in PFC, which receives direct projections from ITC. ITC does not project directly to PMC (Webster et al., 1994), and perceptual information was weakest in the PMC. By contrast, information about the rules was strongest and earliest in frontal cortex (PFC and PMC) and virtually absent in ITC.

One puzzling feature of our results is that PMC encodes rules more strongly and earlier than PFC, yet it is not a region that has previously been associated

with the use of abstract information. One possibility is that we observed stronger PMC rule effects because the rules were highly familiar to the animals; they had performed this task for more than a year. Evidence suggests that PFC is more critical for new learning than for familiar routines. PFC damage preferentially affects new learning; animals and humans can still engage in complex behaviors as long as they learned them before the damage occurred (Shallice and Evans, 1978; Shallice, 1982; Knight, 1984; Dias et al., 1997). PFC neurons also show more selectivity during new learning than during the performance of familiar cue-response associations (Asaad et al., 1998). Human imaging studies report greater blood flow to the dorsal PMC than to PFC when subjects are performing familiar versus novel tasks (Boettiger and D'Esposito, 2005) and greater PFC activation when subjects are retrieving newly learned rules versus highly familiar rules (Donohue, 2005). In addition, with increasing task familiarity, there is a relative shift in blood flow from areas associated with focal attention, such as PFC, to motor regions (Della-Maggiore and McIntosh, 2005). Therefore, it may be that STR is primarily involved in new learning, but with familiarity, rules become more strongly established in motor system structures.

A second possibility lies in the design of the task. The task we used ensured that the perceptual requirements were abstract: Monkeys had to make abstract judgments about the similarity of pictures. However, the motor requirements of the task were more concrete: The subjects always indicated their response with an arm movement. One could envision a version of the task in which the subject has to respond with an arm movement to one set of trials, as in the current task, and with an eye movement to other sets of trials. One might predict that in such a task, rule activity would only occur in PMC during the arm movement trials, and might occur in another frontal lobe structure, such as the frontal eye fields, during eye movement trials. In other words, we predict that rule activity in PFC would be effector-independent, which would not be the case for rule activity in PMC. PFC would be the only area to represent the rule in a genuinely abstract fashion, independent of *both* sensory input and the motor effector. These predictions should be tested in future research.

COMPARISON OF ABSTRACT RULES AND CONCRETE STIMULUS-RESPONSE ASSOCIATIONS

In the experiment described earlier, we found only weak rule selectivity in STR relative to the frontal cortex. Recently, very different results have emerged for the encoding of lower-level rules, such as the stimulus-response associations that underpin conditional rules. Pasupathy and Miller (2005) recorded data simultaneously from PFC and STR while monkeys learned stimulus-response associations (see Chapter 18). In their task, two stimuli (A and B) instruct one of two behavioral responses (saccade left or right). Both structures encoded the associations between the stimuli and the responses, but selectivity appeared earlier in learning in STR than in PFC. Despite this early neural correlate

of learning in STR, the monkey's behavior did not change until PFC encoded the associations. These results present us with a challenge: Why would the monkey continue to make errors, despite the fact that STR was encoding the correct stimulus-response associations? This finding suggests that not only is overt behavior under the control of PFC more so than under that of STR, but also that PFC will not necessarily use all of the information available to it to control behavior.

One possibility is that PFC is integrating information from many low-level learning systems, not just STR, and that some of these systems may not necessarily agree with STR as to the correct response. For example, consider the brain systems that acquire stimulus-reward associations or action-reward associations. It is impossible to learn stimulus-response associations using such stimulus-reward or action-reward associations because each action and each stimulus are rewarded equally often. However, this does not necessarily mean that these systems will be silent during the performance of a task dependent on stimulus-response associations. For example, perhaps after a reinforced leftward saccade, the action-reward system instructs PFC to make another leftward response, oblivious to the fact that on the next trial, the stimulus instructs a rightward response. PFC would need to learn that such information is not useful to solve the task, and ignore this system.

Lesion studies support the idea that these different low-level learning systems can compete with one another. For example, lesions of anterior cingulate cortex impair the learning of stimulus-*reward* associations (Gabriel et al., 1991; Bussey et al., 1997), but facilitate the learning of stimulus-*response* associations (Bussey et al., 1996). These findings suggest that in the healthy animal, anterior cingulate is responsible for learning stimulus-reward associations, and that removing the capacity to learn such associations can improve the ability to learn stimulus-response associations.

OTHER FORMS OF ABSTRACT ENCODING IN PREFRONTAL CORTEX

Recent studies have found that PFC neurons encode a variety of different kinds of abstract information relating to high-level cognition, including attentional sets (Mansouri et al., 2006), perceptual categories (Freedman et al., 2001; see Chapter 17), numbers (Nieder et al., 2002), and behavioral strategies (Genovesio et al., 2005; see Chapter 5). We have recently begun to explore whether abstract information might also have a role in lower-level behavioral control, to help guide simple decisions and choices. The neurophysiological studies discussed earlier used models derived from sensorimotor psychophysics and animal learning theory to make sense of the neuronal data. Over the last decade, however, there has been a growing realization that to understand the neuronal mechanisms underlying decision-making, it might help to widen the fields from which we construct our behavioral models (Glimcher, 2003; Glimcher and Rustichini, 2004; Schultz, 2004; Sanfey et al., 2006).

Evolutionary biologists and economists have constructed detailed models of the parameters that animals and humans use to make everyday decisions. These models emphasize the consideration of three basic parameters that must be considered in making a decision: the expected reward or payoff, the cost in terms of time and energy, and the probability of success (Stephens and Krebs, 1986; Loewenstein and Elster, 1992; Kahneman and Tversky, 2000). Determining the value of a choice involves calculating the difference between the payoff and the cost, and discounting this by the probability of success. One suggestion is that PFC integrates all of these parameters to derive an abstract measure of the value of a choice outcome (Montague and Berns, 2002).

To test this hypothesis about the representation of value, we examined whether PFC neurons encode an abstract representation of value by integrating the major decision variables of payoff, cost, and risk (Kennerley et al., 2005). We trained monkeys to choose between pictures while we simultaneously recorded data from multiple PFC regions. Each picture was associated with a specific outcome. Some pictures were associated with a fixed amount of juice, but only on a certain proportion of trials (risk manipulation). Other pictures were associated with varying amounts of juice (payoff manipulation). Finally, some pictures were associated with a fixed amount of juice, but the subject had to earn the juice by pressing a lever a certain number of times (cost manipulation). A large proportion of PFC neurons encoded the value of the choices under at least one of these manipulations (Table 2–2). Other neurons encoded the values under two of the manipulations, and still others encoded the value under all three manipulations, consistent with encoding an abstract representation of value. In other words, some PFC neurons encoded the value of the choice irrespective of how we manipulated its value. The majority of the selective neurons were located in medial PFC, where approximately half encoded the value of the choice outcome in some way.

The encoding of the value of a choice in an abstract manner has distinct computational advantages. When faced with two choices, A and B, we might imagine that it would be simpler to compare them directly rather than going through an additional step of assigning them an abstract value. The problem with this approach is that as the number of available choices increases, the number of direct comparisons increases exponentially. Thus, choosing among A, B, and C would require three comparisons (AB, AC, and BC), whereas choosing among A, B, C, and D requires six comparisons (AB, AC, AD, BC, BD, and CD). The solution quickly suffers from combinatorial explosion as the number of choices increases. In contrast, valuing each choice along a common reference scale provides a linear solution to the problem.

An abstract representation provides important additional behavioral advantages, such as flexibility and a capacity to deal with novelty. For example, suppose that an animal encounters a new type of food. If the animal relies on direct comparisons, then to determine whether it is worth choosing this new food over others, it must iteratively compare the new food with all previously encountered foods. By deriving an abstract value, on the other hand, the

Table 2–2 Percentage of Neurons Encoding Variables Underlying Choices in Different Prefrontal Cortex Subregions

N	Dorsolateral 108	Ventrolateral 52	Orbital 89	Medial 153
Risk	3%	2%	2%	20%
Payoff	2%	2%	6%	9%
Cost	1%	0%	0%	3%
Risk + Payoff	0%	0%	2%	13%
Risk + Cost	0%	0%	1%	4%
Payoff + Cost	0%	0%	0%	4%
All three	0%	0%	0%	15%

animal has only to perform a single calculation. By assigning the new food a value on the common reference scale, it knows the value of this foodstuff relative to all other foods. In addition, often it is not clear how to compare directly very different outcomes: How does a monkey decide between grooming a compatriot and eating a banana? Valuing the alternatives along a common reference scale helps with this decision. For example, although I have never needed to value my car in terms of bananas, I can readily do so because I can assign each item a dollar value.

CONCLUSIONS AND FUTURE RESEARCH

In conclusion, numerous studies now suggest that using abstract information to guide behavior is an important and potentially unique function of PFC. In turn, this capacity might underlie two of the hallmark functions of PFC, flexibility and the ability to deal with novelty. A key question that remains is how we learn such information in the first place. The mechanisms that underpin the learning of abstract information remain unclear. Traditionally, neurophysiologists record data from animals only once they have learned the task. There are good reasons for so doing. Collecting an adequate sample of neurons requires multiple recording sessions, and interpreting the data requires behavior to be stable across those sessions. Even in studies that have incorporated learning into the design, typically, monkeys are trained until there is a stable, asymptotic rate of learning (Wallis and Miller, 2003b; Pasupathy and Miller, 2005). However, this makes for a rather artificial model of behavior. In real life, behavior is rarely stable, but instead, constantly changes and adapts to the environment. Furthermore, the immense amount of training that the animals often require (usually lasting months, or even years) raises the possibility that the types of neuronal changes that we observe are not an accurate reflection of more natural learning, or are perhaps only reflective of the encoding of highly trained skills. Fortunately, recent advances in

neurophysiological studies, such as chronically implanted electrodes, and the increase in the number of neurons that can be recorded in a single session raise the possibility of recording during the learning of these tasks. These and other methodological advances will help us to understand how the brain achieves its impressive ability to abstract and generalize.

ACKNOWLEDGMENTS I would like to thank Earl Miller, in whose laboratory I completed the abstract rule experiments. Funds from NIH DA019028-01 and the Hellman Family Faculty Fund supported the abstract value experiments.

REFERENCES

Asaad WF, Rainer G, Miller EK (1998) Neural activity in the primate prefrontal cortex during associative learning. Neuron 21:1399-407.

Barbas H (1988) Anatomic organization of basoventral and mediodorsal visual recipient prefrontal regions in the rhesus monkey. Journal of Comparative Neurology 276:313–342.

Barbas H, Pandya D (1991) Patterns of connections of the prefrontal cortex in the rhesus monkey associated with cortical architecture. In: Frontal lobe function and dysfunction (Levin HS, Eisenberg HM, Benton AL, eds.), pp 35–58. New York: Oxford University Press.

Bartlett FC (1932) Remembering: a study in experimental and social psychology. Cambridge: Cambridge University Press.

Boettiger CA, D'Esposito M (2005) Frontal networks for learning and executing arbitrary stimulus-response associations. Journal of Neuroscience 25:2723–2732.

Bussey TJ, Muir JL, Everitt BJ, Robbins TW (1996) Dissociable effects of anterior and posterior cingulate cortex lesions on the acquisition of a conditional visual discrimination: facilitation of early learning vs. impairment of late learning. Behavioral Brain Research 82:45–56.

Bussey TJ, Muir JL, Everitt BJ, Robbins TW (1997) Triple dissociation of anterior cingulate, posterior cingulate, and medial frontal cortices on visual discrimination tasks using a touchscreen testing procedure for the rat. Behavioral Neuroscience 111:920–936.

Bussey TJ, Wise SP, Murray EA (2002) Interaction of ventral and orbital prefrontal cortex with inferotemporal cortex in conditional visuomotor learning. Behavioral Neuroscience 116:703–715.

Della-Maggiore V, McIntosh AR (2005) Time course of changes in brain activity and functional connectivity associated with long-term adaptation to a rotational transformation. Journal of Neurophysiology 93:2254–2262.

Desimone R, Albright TD, Gross CG, Bruce C (1984) Stimulus-selective properties of inferior temporal neurons in the macaque. Journal of Neuroscience 4:2051–2062.

Dias R, Robbins TW, Roberts AC (1997) Dissociable forms of inhibitory control within prefrontal cortex with an analog of the Wisconsin Card Sort Test: restriction to novel situations and independence from "on-line" processing. Journal of Neuroscience 17:9285–9297.

Donohue SE, Wendelken C, Crone EA, Bunge SA (2005) Retrieving rules for behavior from long-term memory. Neuroimage 26:1140–1149

Eldridge MA, Barnard PJ, Bekerian DA (1994) Autobiographical memory and daily schemas at work. Memory 2:51–74.

Emery NJ, Clayton NS (2004) The mentality of crows: convergent evolution of intelligence in corvids and apes. Science 306:1903–1907.

Freedman DJ, Riesenhuber M, Poggio T, Miller EK (2001) Categorical representation of visual stimuli in the primate prefrontal cortex. Science 291:312–316.

Fuster JM (2002) Cortex and mind. Oxford: Oxford University Press.

Gabriel M, Kubota Y, Sparenborg S, Straube K, Vogt BA (1991) Effects of cingulate cortical lesions on avoidance learning and training-induced unit activity in rabbits. Experimental Brain Research 86:585–600.

Genovesio A, Brasted PJ, Mitz AR, Wise SP (2005) Prefrontal cortex activity related to abstract response strategies. Neuron 47:307–320.

Giurfa M, Zhang S, Jenett A, Menzel R, Srinivasan MV (2001) The concepts of "sameness" and "difference" in an insect. Nature 410:930–933.

Glimcher PW (2003) Decisions, uncertainty, and the brain: the science of neuroeconomics. Cambridge: MIT Press.

Glimcher PW, Rustichini A (2004) Neuroeconomics: the consilience of brain and decision. Science 306:447–452.

Harlow HF (1949) The formation of learning sets. Psychological Review 56:51–65.

Herman LM, Gordon JA (1974) Auditory delayed matching in the bottlenose dolphin. Journal of the Experimental Analysis of Behavior 21:19–26.

Hunter MW, Kamil AC (1971) Object discrimination learning set and hypothesis behavior in the northern blue jay (Cyanocitta cristata). Psychonomic Science 22:271–273.

Kahneman D, Tversky A (2000) Choices, values and frames. New York: Cambridge University Press.

Kastak D, Schusterman RJ (1994) Transfer of visual identity matching-to-sample in two Californian sea lions (Zalophus californianus). Animal Learning and Behavior 22:427–453.

Kennerley SW, Lara AH, Wallis JD (2005) Prefrontal neurons encode an abstract representation of value. Society for Neuroscience Abstracts.

Knight RT (1984) Decreased response to novel stimuli after prefrontal lesions in man. Electroencephalography and Clinical Neurophysiology 59:9–20.

Loewenstein G, Elster J (1992) Choice over time. New York: Russell Sage Foundation.

Mansouri FA, Matsumoto K, Tanaka K (2006) Prefrontal cell activities related to monkeys' success and failure in adapting to rule changes in a Wisconsin Card Sorting Test analog. Journal of Neuroscience 26:2745–2756.

Milner B (1963) Effects of different brain lesions on card sorting. Archives of Neurology 9:100–110.

Mishkin M, Prockop ES, Rosvold HE (1962) One-trial object discrimination learning in monkeys with frontal lesions. Journal of Comparative and Physiological Psychology 55:178–181.

Montague PR, Berns GS (2002) Neural economics and the biological substrates of valuation. Neuron 36:265–284.

Muhammad R, Wallis JD, Miller EK (2006) A comparison of abstract rules in the prefrontal cortex, premotor cortex, inferior temporal cortex, and striatum. Journal of Cognitive Neuroscience 18:974–989.

Nieder A, Freedman DJ, Miller EK (2002) Representation of the quantity of visual items in the primate prefrontal cortex. Science 297:1708–1711.

Nissen HW, Blum JS, Blum RA (1948) Analysis of matching behavior in chimpanzees. Journal of Comparative and Physiological Psychology 41:62–74.

Oden DL, Thompson RK, Premack D (1988) Spontaneous transfer of matching by infant chimpanzees (Pan troglodytes). Journal of Experimental Psychology: Animal and Behavior Processes 14:140–145.

Pandya DN, Yeterian EH (1990) Prefrontal cortex in relation to other cortical areas in rhesus monkey: architecture and connections. Progress in Brain Research 85: 63–94.

Pasupathy A, Miller EK (2005) Different time courses of learning-related activity in the prefrontal cortex and striatum. Nature 433:873–876.

Pepperberg IM (1987) Interspecies communication: a tool for assessing conceptual abilities in the African Grey parrot (*Psittacus arithacus*). In: Cognition, language and consciousness: integrative levels (Greenberg G, Tobach E, eds.), pp 31–56. Hillsdale, NJ: Lawrence Erlbaum Associates Inc.

Rao SC, Rainer G, Miller EK (1997) Integration of what and where in the primate prefrontal cortex. Science 276:821–824.

Rehkamper G, Zilles K (1991) Parallel evolution in mammalian and avian brains: comparative cytoarchitectonic and cytochemical analysis. Cell and Tissue Research 263:3–28.

Restle F (1958) Toward a quantitative description of learning set data. Psychological Review 64:77–91.

Rolls ET, Baylis LL (1994) Gustatory, olfactory, and visual convergence within the primate orbitofrontal cortex. Journal of Neuroscience 14:5437–5452.

Romanski LM, Goldman-Rakic PS (2002) An auditory domain in primate prefrontal cortex. Nature Neuroscience 5:15–16.

Romo R, Brody CD, Hernandez A, Lemus L (1999) Neuronal correlates of parametric working memory in the prefrontal cortex. Nature 399:470–473.

Sanfey AG, Loewenstein G, McClure SM, Cohen JD (2006) Neuroeconomics: cross-currents in research on decision-making. Trends in Cognitive Sciences 10:108–116.

Schultz W (2004) Neural coding of basic reward terms of animal learning theory, game theory, microeconomics and behavioral ecology. Current Opinion in Neurobiology 14:139–147.

Semendeferi K, Lu A, Schenker N, Damasio H (2002) Humans and great apes share a large frontal cortex. Nature Neuroscience 5:272–276.

Shallice T (1982) Specific impairments of planning. Philosophical Transactions of the Royal Society London B Biological Sciences 298:199–209.

Shallice T, Evans ME (1978) The involvement of the frontal lobes in cognitive estimation. Cortex 14:294–303.

Stephens DW, Krebs JR (1986) Foraging theory. Princeton: Princeton University Press.

Tanaka K (1996) Inferotemporal cortex and object vision. Annual Review of Neuroscience 19:109–139.

Wallis JD, Anderson KC, Miller EK (2001) Single neurons in prefrontal cortex encode abstract rules. Nature 411:953–956.

Wallis JD, Miller EK (2003a) From rule to response: neuronal processes in the premotor and prefrontal cortex. Journal of Neurophysiology 90:1790–1806.

Wallis JD, Miller EK (2003b) Neuronal activity in primate dorsolateral and orbital prefrontal cortex during performance of a reward preference task. European Journal of Neuroscience 18:2069–2081.

Webster MJ, Bachevalier J, Ungerleider LG (1994) Connections of inferior temporal areas TEO and TE with parietal and frontal cortex in macaque monkeys. Cerebral Cortex 4:470–483.

Wilson B, Mackintosh NJ, Boakes RA (1985) Transfer of relational rules in matching and oddity learning by pigeons and corvids. Quarterly Journal of Experimental Psychology 37B:313–332.

Witthöft W (1967) Absolute anzahl und Verteilung der zellen im hirn der honigbiene. Zeitschrift fur Morphologie der Tiere 61:160–184.

3

Neural Representations Used to Specify Action

Silvia A. Bunge and Michael J. Souza

To understand how we use rules to guide our behavior, it is critical to learn more about how we select responses on the basis of associations retrieved from long-term memory and held online in working memory. Rules, or prescribed guide(s) for conduct or action (Merriam-Webster Dictionary, 1974), are a particularly interesting class of associations because they link memory and action. We previously reviewed the cognitive neuroscience of rule representations elsewhere (Bunge, 2004; Bunge et al., 2005). In this chapter, we focus mainly on recent functional brain imaging studies from our laboratory exploring the neural substrates of rule storage, retrieval, and maintenance. We present evidence that goal-relevant knowledge associated with visual cues is stored in the posterior middle temporal lobe. We further show that ventrolateral prefrontal cortex (VLPFC) is engaged in the effortful retrieval of rule meanings from long-term memory as well as in the selection between active rule meanings. Finally, we provide evidence that different brain structures are recruited, depending on the type of rule being represented, although VLPFC plays a general role in rule representation. Although this chapter focuses primarily on the roles of lateral prefrontal and temporal cortices in rule representation, findings in parietal and premotor cortices will also be discussed.

LONG-TERM STORAGE OF RULE KNOWLEDGE

Posterior Middle Temporal Gyrus Is Implicated in Rule Representation

In a previous functional magnetic resonance imaging (fMRI) study focusing on rule retrieval and maintenance, we observed activation of left posterior middle temporal gyrus (postMTG) [BA 21], as well as left VLPFC (BA 44/45/47), when subjects viewed instructional cues that were associated with specific rules (Bunge et al., 2003) [Fig. 3–1]. Although both postMTG and VLPFC were sensitive to rule complexity during the cue period, only VLPFC was sensitive to rule complexity during the delay.

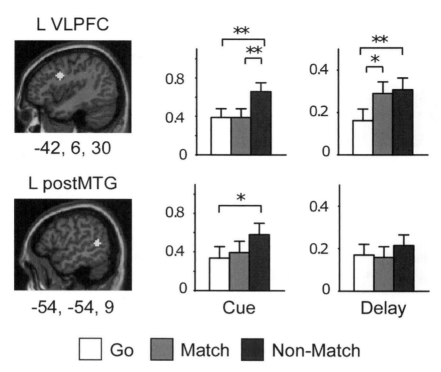

Figure 3–1 Brain activation related to the retrieval and maintenance of rules uncovered by functional magnetic resonance imaging (Bunge et al., 2003). Both left ventrolateral prefrontal cortex (L VLPFC) [BA 44/47] and left posterior middle temporal gyrus (L postMTG) [BA 21] were modulated by rule complexity during the Cue period, but only the left VLPFC continued this pattern into the Delay period. **$p < .01$; *$p < .05$. (Adapted from Bunge et al., 2003, *Journal of Neurophysiology*, 90:3419–3428, with permission from the American Physiological Society).

On the basis of evidence that semantic memories are stored in lateral temporal cortex and that VLPFC assists in memory retrieval (e.g., Gabrieli et al., 1998; Wagner et al., 2001), we proposed that left postMTG might store rule knowledge over the long term, and that VLPFC might be important for retrieving and using this knowledge (Bunge et al., 2003). However, it is clear that postMTG is not specifically involved in storing explicit rules for behavior; rather, the literature on tool use and action representation suggests that this region more generally represents action-related knowledge associated with stimuli in the environment (see Donohue et al., 2005).

In ongoing research, we aim to reconcile the disparate views of postMTG function emerging from the semantic memory literature (i.e., a general role in semantic memory) and the action representation literature (i.e., a more specific role in action-related semantic representation). A recent study from our

laboratory is consistent with the latter view, although a definitive answer awaits further experiments.

Intriguingly, our focus in left postMTG was close to a region that is believed to represent knowledge about actions associated with manipulable objects (Chao et al., 1999; Martin and Chao, 2001). A large body of research has shown that this region is active when subjects prepare to use a tool, mentally conceptualize the physical gestures associated with tool use, make judgments about the manipulability of objects, generate action verbs, or read verbs as opposed to nouns (for reviews, see Johnson-Frey, 2004; Lewis, 2006).

Although most of these studies involved visual stimuli (images or words), one group of researchers found that postMTG was engaged by meaningful relative to meaningless environmental sounds (Lewis et al., 2004), and for tools relative to animals (Lewis et al., 2005). Thus, the role of postMTG in storing mechanical or action-related knowledge about stimuli extends to the realm of auditory information; it is unclear whether it also extends to other modalities. Given that we likely acquire most of our action-related knowledge through vision and audition, one might expect that a region that specifically represents action-related knowledge would not be modulated by other modalities. However, the possibility that postMTG is engaged by other stimulus modalities remains an open issue, and we know of no functional brain imaging studies or studies of anatomical connectivity that speak to this issue.

In our rule study, unlike the action knowledge studies mentioned earlier, participants used recently learned arbitrary mappings between abstract cues (nonsense shapes or words) and task rules. This finding suggests that left postMTG plays a broader role in action knowledge than previously assumed. Rather than specifically representing actions that are non-arbitrarily associated with real-world objects, left postMTG also represents high-level rules that we learn to associate with otherwise meaningless symbols.

Explicitly Testing for Involvement of Left PostMTG in Rule Representation

We sought to further test the hypothesis that left postMTG represents rule knowledge in an fMRI study in which subjects viewed a series of road signs from around the world, and considered their meanings (Donohue et al., 2005). We had two reasons for selecting road signs as experimental stimuli: (1) they are associated with specific actions or with guidelines that can be used to select specific actions; and (2) they allow us to examine the retrieval of rule knowledge acquired long ago. As such, these stimuli enabled us to ask whether prefrontal cortex (PFC) [in particular, VLPFC] would be recruited during passive retrieval of action knowledge associated with well-learned symbols.

The road sign study involved "Old" signs that subjects had used while driving for at least 4 years, and "New" signs from other countries that they were unlikely to have been exposed to previously (Fig. 3–2A). Of these New signs, half were "Trained" (i.e., subjects were told their meaning before scanning, but

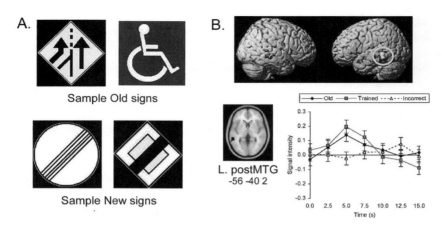

Figure 3–2 Retrieving well-known and recently learned behavioral rules from long-term memory (Donohue et al., 2005). *A.* Domestic, well-known ("Old") and foreign, generally unknown ("New," "Learned") signs were used in the study. *B.* Activation in left posterior middle temporal gyrus (L postMTG) [BA 21; *circled*] was identified in a group contrast comparing all correct trials relative to fixation. *Inset.* Activation in this region was specifically modulated by whether participants knew the meaning of the sign, *not* by when the participant learned the meaning of the sign. (Adapted from Donohue et al., 2005, *Neuroimage, 26,* 1140–1149, with permission from Elsevier).

had had no experience using them to guide their actions). The other half of the new signs were "Untrained"—in other words, subjects had viewed them before scanning, but were not given their meaning. We predicted that left postMTG would be active when subjects successfully accessed the meaning of Old and Trained signs, but not when subjects viewed signs whose meaning they did not know ("Incorrect" trials, of which the majority would be Untrained).

Just as predicted, left postMTG was more active when subjects passively viewed signs for which they knew the meaning than for signs that were familiar, but not meaningful to them (Fig. 3–2B). This contrast also identified several other regions, and all were located in the lateral temporal lobes. However, the largest and most significant focus was in the predicted region of left postMTG. Notably, unlike regions in lateral PFC, this region was insensitive to level of experience with the signs—it was engaged equally strongly for correctly performed Old and Trained signs (Fig. 3–2B, inset). Thus, it appears that left postMTG stores the meanings of arbitrary visual cues that specify rules for action, regardless of when these cues were originally learned or how much experience one has had with them. This pattern of activation suggests two points: (1) activation of the correct representation in temporal cortex contributes to remembering the sign's meaning; and (2) these temporal cortex representations can be activated either through effortful, top-down processes involving VLPFC or through

automatic, bottom-up means (controlled retrieval of rule-knowledge by VLPFC is discussed later).

PostMTG: Action Knowledge, Function Knowledge, or Both?

Although left postMTG has been implicated in tasks that promote retrieval of action knowledge, it has been noted that left postMTG is located near the posterior extent of the superior temporal sulcus, a region associated with representation of biological motion (Chao et al., 1999; Martin and Chao, 2001). Furthermore, this region is engaged when subjects think about how living entities move (Tyler et al., 2003). These observations raise the following question: Does left postMTG represent knowledge about specific *movements or actions* associated with a visual stimulus, or does it represent semantic memories associated with an object, such as—in the case of manipulable objects—knowledge about its *function?*

To address this question, we designed an fMRI study to investigate whether the left postMTG is sensitive to an object's function (functional knowledge) or how the object moves when one uses it (action knowledge) [Souza and Bunge, under review]. Participants viewed photographs of common household objects, such as a pair of scissors. The task was a 2 × 2 factorial design, manipulating whether or not one had to retrieve knowledge about a specific type of object, as well as the domain of cognitive processing required: verbal or visual-spatial (Fig. 3–3A).

Based on an instruction that they received on each trial, participants were asked to do one of the following: (1) imagine themselves using the object in a typical way (Imagery); (2) consider how they would describe the purpose of the object to another person (Function); (3) imagine themselves rotating the object 180 degrees along the surface (Rotate); or (4) identify and verbally rehearse the most prominent color of the object (Rehearse). The Function task required participants to retrieve information stored in long-term memory about the use of an object, whereas the Imagery task required participants to retrieve information about how to handle the object. The Rotate condition was devised as a control for the visual-spatial and movement-related demands of the Imagery task, and the Rehearse condition was devised as a control for the verbal demands of the Function task.

We posited that if left postMTG represents functions associated with objects, this region should be most active for the Function condition. In contrast, if this region represents action information, it should be most active for the Imagery condition. In fact, we found that left postMTG was engaged *specifically* when participants were asked to access function knowledge (Fig. 3–3B). These data indicate that postMTG represents semantic information about the function of an object, rather than how one interacts with it or how it typically moves when one uses it. In contrast to left postMTG, left inferior parietal lobule (IPL) [BA 40] (Fig. 3–3C) and dorsal premotor cortex (PMd) [BA 6]

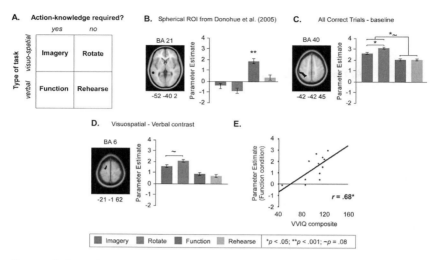

Figure 3–3 Brain regions associated with action representation with objects (Souza and Bunge, under review). *A.* The object study manipulated whether the action-knowledge was required and whether the task was primarily verbal or visual-spatial. *B.* A 6-mm spherical region-of-interest (ROI) was drawn, centered in the coordinates in left posterior middle temporal gyrus (postMTG; −56 −40 2) from Donohue et al. (2005). This ROI was *specifically* activated by the Function condition. *C.* Left inferior parietal (BA 40) activation was modulated by the task (visual-spatial > verbal) and in fact was greatest for Rotate. *D.* A similar pattern to that in left inferior parietal region was also found in left dorsal premotor cortex [BA 6]. *E.* Activation in left postMTG (BA 21) positively correlated with imagery ability as assessed by the Vividness of Visual Imagery Questionnaire (VVIQ) [Marks, 1973]. Note that VVIQ scores are reversed from the original scale such that higher scores reflect better visual imagery ability.

(Fig. 3–3*D*) were engaged more strongly in the Imagery than in the Function condition. Unlike PMd, ventral premotor cortex (PMv) [BA 6] was equally active across all four conditions. The roles of these regions in action representation are discussed further later.

Imagery and Semantic Retrieval: Two Routes to Retrieval of Object Knowledge

In this object knowledge study, we made an effort to direct participants to retrieve specific types of information associated with common household objects. Indeed, the fact that a number of brain regions were modulated by condition (and in opposite ways from other brain regions, in some cases) suggests that participants did tend to treat the conditions differently. In the real world, however, we most likely retrieve several types of information in parallel when we perceive a familiar object. Additionally, some individuals may tend to access one type of information more readily than another. In this study, we found that participants with better self-reported imagery ability—as measured by the

Vividness of Visual Imagery Questionnaire (VVIQ) [Marks, 1973]—engaged left postMTG more strongly when attempting to retrieve the function of an object (Fig. 3–3E), but not for the Motor Imagery, Rotate, or Rehearse conditions. Thus, participants may use visual imagery to assist in the retrieval of semantic knowledge about an object's function.

Action Representations in Premotor Cortex

Ventral Premotor Cortex

Similar to the postMTG, brain imaging studies of action knowledge have consistently reported activation in left PMv (BA 6/44) [for reviews, see Johnson-Frey, 2004; Kellenbach et al., 2003]. This region is active when subjects observe or copy movements, pretend to use tools, or generate verbs. As such, left PMv is believed to store movement representations, and to support the retrieval of motor information about tool use (Kellenbach et al., 2003).

In the road sign study described earlier (Donohue et al., 2005), the left PMv did not reflect rule knowledge, in that it was not more active for Correct than for Incorrect signs. However, PMv was significantly more active for Trained than for Old signs, and its response to Incorrect signs was intermediate to these (Fig. 3–4A). This finding was obtained regardless of the fact that subjects were not required to carry out any overt motor responses in the task. These results suggest that the PMv was engaged during attempts to retrieve action knowledge that does not come readily to mind. Additionally, as noted earlier with regard to the object knowledge study (Souza and Bunge, under review), PMv was engaged while participants considered pictures of artifacts—regardless of whether the type of information they were asked to retrieve about these artifacts was action-related (Fig. 3–4B). This result is consistent with the idea that PMv

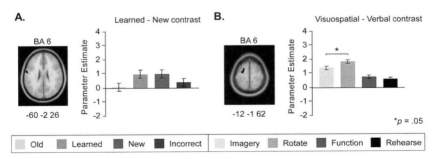

Figure 3–4 Involvement of premotor cortex in action knowledge. A. In the road sign study, a region of ventral premotor cortex (BA 6) showed maximal sensitivity to Learned (L) and New (N) signs, followed by Incorrect (I) and then Old (O) signs (Donohue et al., 2005). B. In the object study, we identified a cluster of dorsal premotor cortex activation (BA 6) that was significantly active for all conditions, but notably more so for the visual-spatial tasks (Souza and Bunge, under review).

is involved in the automatic retrieval of actions associated with manipulable objects (Kellenbach et al., 2003; Tranel et al., 2003; Johnson-Frey, 2004).

Dorsal Premotor Cortex

Left PMd (BA 6) is believed to support sensorimotor transformations (for reviews, see Picard and Strick, 2001; Chouinard and Paus, 2006). For example, it is active when participants are preparing to select between two movements relative to planning a single movement (Cavina-Pratesi et al., 2006). Lesion work shows that damage to PMd results in learning impairments for arbitrary sensorimotor associations in the monkey (Halsband and Passingham, 1982), as well as the human (Petrides, 1997). In the object knowledge study described earlier, we found that PMd activation was above baseline for all conditions, but was more active for the visuospatial tasks (Motor Imagery, Rotate > Function, Rehearse) [Fig. 3–4B], supporting the idea that this region aids in the planning of goal-directed movement.

Action Representations in Parietal Cortex

Another region that is often reported in the action knowledge literature is parietal cortex—in particular, the IPL and intraparietal sulcus (BA 40) [Johnson and Grafton, 2003; Johnson-Frey, 2004; Kellenbach et al., 2003]. Left IPL appears to be recruited only when subjects retrieve specific actions (Kellenbach et al., 2003), such as grasp-related movements associated with tools (Chao and Martin, 2000). This finding is consistent with the hypothesis that this region supports motor attention (Rushworth et al., 2001, 2003) and the literature on ideomotor apraxia indicating that patients with damage to this region have difficulty retrieving appropriate motor programs (Heilman et al., 1997).

In our initial rule study (Bunge et al., 2003), left IPL was sensitive to rule complexity during presentation of the instructional cue, as well as when subjects had to keep the rule in mind until they were prompted to select a response. In the object study, this region was most strongly modulated by the visual-spatial tasks, and in fact, was more active for Rotate than for Motor Imagery (Fig. 3–3C) [Souza and Bunge, under review], perhaps because participants could access familiar motor programs for the latter condition, but not for the former. Supporting a role in representing movements associated with objects, Motor Imagery–related activation in the left IPL was positively correlated with subsequent memory for having performed the imagery task on specific objects.

RETRIEVAL, SELECTION, AND MAINTENANCE OF RULE KNOWLEDGE

Studies Implicating VLPFC in Rule Learning and Rule Retrieval

Lesion studies in nonhuman primates demonstrate that VLPFC plays a critical role in rule learning and rule representation. VLPFC lesions in monkeys

severely impair learning on conditional visual-motor tasks that require that they use one of several arbitrary stimulus-response (S-R) mappings to respond to a visual stimulus (Murray et al., 2000; Passingham et al., 2000) [see Chapter 7]. These lesions impair both the ability to use associations learned preoperatively and the ability to learn new associations rapidly within a single session (Bussey et al., 2002). VLPFC lesions in monkeys also lead to a deficit in learning a match-to-sample rule, indicating that VLPFC is important for learning complex rules as well as simple associations (Bussey et al., 2002).

Consistent with the lesion studies in nonhuman primates, neuroimaging studies in humans have also implicated VLPFC in rule representation (Toni et al., 1998; Toni and Passingham, 1999; Toni et al., 2001; Brass et al., 2003; Bunge et al., 2003; Brass and von Cramon, 2004). More broadly, VLPFC is believed to be important for active, or *controlled*, memory retrieval under situations in which relevant associations do not spring readily to mind (i.e., when relations between representations are weak, unstable, or ambiguous) [Petrides, 2002; see also Miller and Cohen, 2001]. Animal studies indicate that VLPFC retrieves information from the temporal lobes (Eacott and Gaffan, 1992; Petrides, 1996; Hasegawa et al., 1999; Miyashita and Hayashi, 2000). Indeed, disruption of the white matter tracts connecting VLPFC and ipsilateral temporal cortex leads to impaired visual-motor learning (Bussey et al., 2002; Parker and Gaffan, 1998). This and other findings support the hypothesis that VLPFC is involved in the effortful retrieval of rule knowledge (as well as other associations) from temporal cortex.

Engagement of VLPFC during Effortful Rule Retrieval

We previously postulated that VLPFC has an inverted U relationship with associative memory strength (Bunge et al., 2004). According to this hypothesis, VLPFC is recruited when subjects engage retrieval processes that lead to the successful recollection of knowledge, more so when the recollection is effortful (Wagner et al., 2001). However, under situations in which initial recollection attempts are unsuccessful and subjects abandon the retrieval effort, one might observe diminished reliance on VLPFC processes (Dobbins et al., 2003). Thus, the inverted U model predicts greatest activation in VLPFC during effortful recollection, intermediate levels during less effortful recollection, and the least activation when subjects abandon early retrieval attempts.

We found some support for the inverted U model in the road sign study, in that right VLPFC and right dorsolateral PFC (DLPFC)—like PMv (see Fig. 3–4A)—were most strongly engaged by recently Trained signs than by either Old or New signs (Donohue et al., 2005). In contrast to left postMTG, PFC was not sensitive to rule knowledge: It exhibited no differences in activation between signs whose meaning a subject knew and signs whose meaning he or she didn't know. These results suggest that the associations between road signs and the rules that they indicate are stored in postMTG, and that right VLPFC is engaged as needed to assist with rule retrieval.

In contrast to right VLPFC, left VLPFC did not show an inverted U pattern in the road sign study. Rather, this region was strongly engaged for all signs, regardless of knowledge or experience. This finding surprised us, because our earlier work had implicated left VLPFC in rule retrieval and maintenance (Bunge et al., 2003). We considered it likely that the unconstrained viewing paradigm used in the road sign study led subjects to actively attempt to interpret each sign as it appeared on the screen, thereby leading to equal activation of left VLPFC across conditions. However, we sought to further examine the role of left VLPFC in rule representation in a subsequent study, by testing whether it might be involved in selecting between sign meanings instead of or in addition to retrieving them. The rationale for this next experiment was based on a debate in the long-term memory literature as to whether left VLPFC plays a role in memory retrieval (Wagner et al., 2001) or in selection between active memoranda (Thompson-Schill et al., 1997).

Left VLPFC: Controlled Rule Retrieval, Rule Selection, or Both?

In the road sign meaning-selection study, we sought to test whether left VLPFC would be sensitive to rule retrieval demands or to rule selection demands (Souza et al., 2005). We used a two-factorial task design: (1) whether subjects were to retrieve a newly learned meaning for a sign or a meaning that they had learned years ago (New/Old), and (2) whether a sign had one or two possible meanings.

On "Old" trials, subjects were cued for the original meaning for a domestic sign with only one meaning. On "New" trials, subjects were cued for the meaning of a foreign sign, which they were trained on before scanning. On "Relearned-Old" trials, subjects were cued for the original meaning for a domestic sign with *two* meanings (the other meaning having been taught before scanning). On "Relearned-New" trials, subjects were cued for the *new* meaning for a domestic sign with two meanings. On each trial, a red or green border instructed subjects to retrieve either an Old or a New meaning. For signs with two meanings, this border was *critical* in determining the appropriate meaning to be remembered.

First, we tested whether left VLPFC (BA 45) was sensitive to controlled retrieval demands (New > Old; Relearned-New > Relearned-Old). As predicted, this region—identified from all correct trials relative to baseline—was more active for New than for Old signs; this finding supports the idea that left as well as right VLPFC are involved in the active retrieval of sign meanings (Fig. 3–5). However, contrary to prediction, left VLPFC was equally active on Relearned-New and Relearned-Old trials. This surprising finding is discussed later.

Second, we tested whether left VLPFC showed competition effects when subjects were forced to select between two possible rule meanings (Relearned-New > other signs) [Thompson-Schill et al., 1997; Badre et al., 2005]. Indeed, left VLPFC (BA 45) was engaged more strongly by Relearned-New than by Old signs (Fig. 3–5), which is, on the surface, consistent with a selection account of

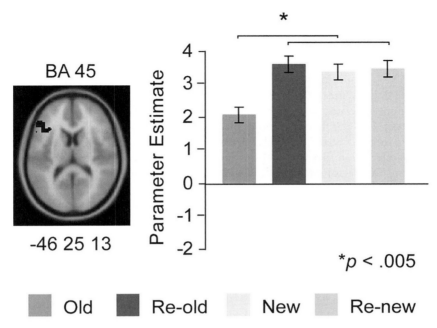

BA 45

-46 25 13

Old   Re-old   New   Re-new

Figure 3–5 Left ventrolateral prefrontal cortex (VLPFC): controlled retrieval or response selection (Souza and Bunge, under review)? A region in left VLPFC (BA 45), extracted from a group contrast comparing all correct meaning retrievals relative to baseline, revealed that activation in this region was not wholly consistent with a controlled retrieval (Wagner et al., 2001) or a response selection (Thompson-Schill et al., 1997) account. O, Old; Re-Old, Relearned-Old; N, New; Re-New, Relearned-New.

VLPFC function. However, greater activation was not observed for Relearned-New than for New trials, which would be predicted by a selection account.

In effect, left VLPFC was more active on Relearned-New, Relearned-Old, and New trials than on Old trials, but did not distinguish between the first three conditions. These data would be consistent with a controlled retrieval account if it were the case that subjects tended to retrieve both meanings for signs with two meanings. By this account, subjects would retrieve a New sign meaning for all signs except for the Old ones, and this effortful retrieval process would engage VLPFC.

On the whole, these data are more consistent with a controlled retrieval account than with a selection account for left VLPFC (BA 45) involvement in this task. However, it is certainly the case that left VLPFC also plays a role in selecting between competing mental representations (Jonides et al., 1998; Nelson et al., 2003). Further, Badre and colleagues (2005) [see Chapter 16] found that, within left VLPFC, mid-VLPFC (BA 45) is involved in resolving competition and anterior VLPFC (BA 47) is involved in controlled semantic retrieval.

To address the issue of possible functional dissociations within left VLPFC in our second traffic study, we conducted region of interest (ROI) analyses based on the precise regions identified by Badre and colleagues. Anterior VLPFC (BA 47), a 6-mm sphere centered on Montreal Neurological Institute (MNI) coordinates −45 27 −15, was not engaged on the task relative to baseline. Thus, the retrieval of sign meanings may not rely on anterior VLPFC, a region associated with controlled semantic retrieval (Wagner et al., 2001; Badre et al., 2005). However, an ROI analysis of Badre's mid-VLPFC region (a 6-mm sphere centered on MNI coordinates −45 27 −15 in BA 45) revealed the same interaction that we had previously observed with a larger ROI encompassing this region (Fig. 3–5). These and other findings suggest that mid-VLPFC may play a role in both the effortful retrieval of memory and the selection of relevant associations from among competing mnemonic representations.

VLPFC: Retrieval of Semantic Knowledge

In the object knowledge study discussed previously, subjects were asked to access semantic knowledge about an object (Function) or memory for the actions and movements associated with the use of the object (Imagery). The Rehearse and Rotate conditions were designed to control for verbal and visual-spatial task demands, respectively. Like postMTG, left VLPFC (BA 45) was activated by the following contrasts: Function > Rehearse and Function > Imagery (Fig. 3–6A). This finding is consistent with a large literature implicating left VLPFC in semantic memory (Vandenberghe et al., 1996; Gabrieli

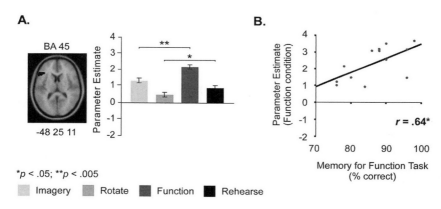

*p < .05; **p < .005

Imagery   Rotate   Function   Rehearse

Figure 3–6 Left ventrolateral prefrontal cortex (VLPFC) and the retrieval of action knowledge (Souza and Bunge, under review). A. A region of left VLPFC (BA 45), identified from a group contrast sensitive to action knowledge (Imagery, Function >Rotate, Rehearse), showed the greatest response to the Function condition. B. The level of activation in left VLPFC for the Function condition correlated with later accuracy for the Function items.

et al., 1998), and supports the hypothesis that VLPFC retrieves semantic information associated with objects from postMTG.

However, unlike postMTG, left VLPFC was more strongly engaged during imagery of object-specific actions (Imagery) than of actions that are not specifically associated with the objects (Rotate; see Fig. 3–6A). Thus, left VLPFC activation reflected retrieval of *both* functions and actions associated with objects. This region likely accesses multiple types of information from distinct brain regions, including object functions and rules from postMTG and information about how to interact with an object from parietal or premotor cortex. Collectively, these inputs provide contextual information that can inform the selection of goal-relevant and contextually appropriate actions.

VLPFC Activation Correlated with Subsequent Memory Performance

In the object knowledge study, subjects were given an incidental memory test after the scan session, in which they were asked to indicate which task they had performed on each of a series of objects (Imagery versus Function). Left VLPFC activation on the Function task was correlated with subsequent memory for thinking about the function of a specific object (Fig. 3–6B). In contrast, a correlation was not observed between VLPFC activation on the Imagery task and subsequent memory. Thus, although left VLPFC is active during performance of the Imagery task (albeit to a lesser extent than during the Function task), its engagement appears not to be necessary for later memory of this mental operation. Unlike VLPFC, postMTG, parietal, and premotor regions did not exhibit subsequent memory effects.

This finding is broadly consistent with earlier findings that greater engagement of left VLPFC during word encoding is associated with greater subsequent episodic memory for the presentation of those words (Wagner et al., 1998, 1999; Kirchhoff et al., 2000). These findings provide new insight into the role of VLPFC in rule learning: VLPFC can assist with rule learning by helping to retrieve not only specific associations with a stimulus (be it a real-world object or a symbol), but also memories for the *context* in which one had seen the stimulus previously, and how one had responded to the stimulus then.

Distinct Neural Representation for Different Types of Rules?

Neuroimaging studies in humans and electrophysiological recordings in nonhuman primates implicate both VLPFC and mid-DLPFC (BA 9, 46) in rule representation (for review, see Bunge, 2004). However, as noted earlier, neuropsychological studies in nonhuman primates implicate VLPFC, but not DLPFC, in rule representation. Damage to DLPFC causes little or no impairment on visual-motor conditional tasks in either humans or nonhuman primates (see Murray et al., 2000), with the exception of posterior DLPFC in humans (BA 8) [Petrides, 1997; Amiez et al., 2006; Monchi et al., 2006]. These apparent discrepancies raise two possibilities: (1) mid-DLPFC represents some types of

rules, but not others; and (2) DLPFC is engaged during rule representation without being *required* for adequate task performance.

In considering the types of rules that DLPFC may represent, two possibilities are suggested by the extant literature. First, DLPFC may be important for representing rules that require overriding a prepotent response tendency. Indeed, one study showed sustained mid-DLPFC (BA 9) activation while participants prepared to perform the Stroop task (MacDonald et al., 2000), and another showed that DLPFC (but not VLPFC) was more active when subjects were able to prepare to withhold a response on a go/no-go task than when they received no advance warning (Hester et al., 2004). Instead or additionally, DLPFC may not be engaged for low-level rules, such as stimulus-response associations, but may be recruited for more complex rules. Such a finding would be consistent with the hypothesis that DLPFC is recruited as needed to manage, monitor, or manipulate information kept active by VLPFC (D'Esposito et al., 1999; Rypma et al., 1999; Bor and Owen, 2006).

Our laboratory designed an experiment to test the hypothesis that VLPFC and DLPFC contribute differentially to rule representation (Donohue et al., under review). More generally, the aim of the second rule study was to investigate whether rules of different kinds are maintained differentially in the brain. To this end, participants performed two distinct tasks, at different levels of difficulty, during acquisition of event-related fMRI data. On each trial, an instructional cue appeared briefly on the screen, followed by a delay and a probe, during which a response occurred (Fig. 3–7A; see color insert). In the Stroop task, named after the classic test from which it was adapted, participants were cued to determine either the ink color or the color name associated with a word stimulus. The Ink condition was more challenging than the Word condition, because it involved overriding the automatic tendency to focus on the word's meaning. In the Memory task, participants were tested on their memory for pairs of color words learned before scanning. Participants had to retrieve four word pairs from long-term memory for each of two instructional cues (set A or set B; High memory load), and had to retrieve one word pair for each of two additional cues (set C or set D; Low memory load; Fig. 3–7B).

The more difficult condition in the Stroop task (Ink versus Word) involved suppression of response competition. However, in the Memory task, the more difficult condition (High load versus Low load) placed greater demands on long-term memory retrieval and working memory maintenance. Thus, we were able to test whether different regions in lateral PFC were modulated by response competition demands and memory demands during rule maintenance. We predicted that left VLPFC would be generally involved in rule representation, whereas DLPFC would specifically assist in the representation of inhibitory or complex rules.

As predicted, left VLPFC (BA 44/45) was engaged during the maintenance of all four types of rules, consistent with a general role in rule representation (Fig. 3–7C, *top*). This region was most strongly engaged by the High load. This finding extends the verbal working memory literature by showing

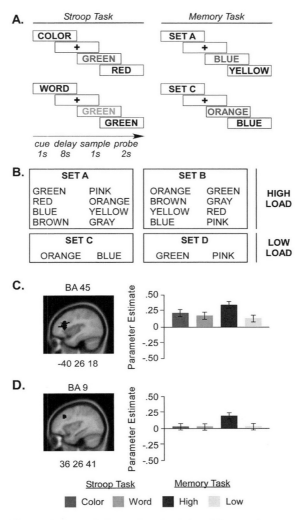

Figure 3–7 Retrieving and maintaining different rule types for future action (Donohue et al., under review). *A*. In the second rules study, participants memorized various set sizes of color pairings. *B*. On a given trial, a cue would indicate the type of rule to be followed. The delay was followed by a sample and a probe, and participants responded to the sample-probe pairing based on the instructional cue. *C*. During the Delay period, left ventrolateral prefrontal cortex (BA 45) was significantly activated for every condition. *D*. Right dorsolateral prefrontal cortex (BA 9), however, was specifically activated for the High-load condition.

load-dependent *rule* maintenance in VLPFC, in addition to load-dependent maintenance of other types of representations (see also Bunge et al., 2003). A homologous region in right VLPFC showed the same pattern, but was not as robustly engaged. In contrast to VLPFC, right DLPFC (BA 9; middle frontal gyrus [MFG]) was specifically engaged during the delay period for the maintenance of the High load rule (Fig. 3–7C, *bottom*). These findings are consistent with the prediction that DLPFC is not as generally involved in rule maintenance as VLPFC.

No region was preferentially engaged by the Ink condition during the delay period, suggesting that inhibitory rules are maintained online in a similar fashion to non-inhibitory rules. Conscious rule maintenance appears to rely on neural circuitry associated with verbal working memory, suggesting that rules do not enjoy special status relative to other types of information held online.

However, during the cue and probe periods, several control-related brain regions showed transient responses specifically for the Ink instruction, including right DLPFC (BA 9, MFG, inferior to the previous right DLPFC ROI) as well as right VLPFC, a region that has been implicated in response inhibition

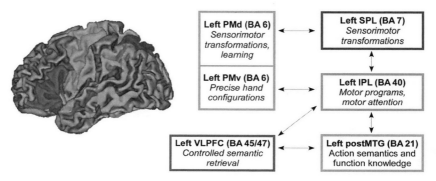

Figure 3–8 A theoretical framework for brain regions involved in action representation. Left ventrolateral prefrontal cortex (VLPFC) [BA 44/45/47] is involved in the controlled retrieval of semantics and rules (Wagner et al., 2001; Bunge et al., 2003). Left posterior middle temporal gyrus (postMTG) [BA 21] is involved in representing rules and action semantics (Bunge et al., 2003; Donohue et al., 2005; Souza and Bunge, under review). Ventral premotor cortex (PMv) [BA 6] is involved in precise hand grips required for object-related interactions (Kellenbach et al., 2003). Dorsal premotor cortex (PMd) [BA 6] is involved in sensorimotor learning and transformations (Petrides, 1997). Inferior parietal lobule (IPL) [BA 40] is involved in motor programs (Chao and Martin, 2000; Kellenbach et al., 2003) and motor attention (Rushworth et al., 2001, 2003). Superior parietal lobule (SPL) [BA 7] is involved in goal-directed sensorimotor transformations (Fogassi and Luppino, 2005). Left hemisphere fiducial rendering is from Caret 5.5 (Van Essen et al., 2001, 2002; http://brainmap.wustl.edu/caret). Regional demarkations are imprecise, and are meant for illustrative purposes only; the region encompassing the premotor cortex includes the primary motor cortex.

(Konishi et al., 1999; Garavan et al., 1999; Bunge et al., 2002; Aron et al., 2003). Thus, as predicted, two different types of rules were represented differentially in the brain—at least during rule retrieval and implementation, if not during maintenance.

Bunge and Zelazo previously hypothesized further neural dissociations in PFC with respect to rule representation (Bunge and Zelazo, 2006) [see Chapter 19]. According to this framework, orbitofrontal cortex represents values associated with specific stimuli or choices (see Chapter 2), whereas lateral PFC represents specific sets of response contingencies. Inspired by Kalina Christoff's model of prefrontal organization (Christoff and Gabrieli, 2002), we posited a hierarchy of rules represented in lateral PFC. Our framework posits that all manner of rules are represented in VLPFC and that rules of increasing structural complexity additionally rely on DLPFC or anterior PFC (BA 10). These proposed dissociations within PFC have yet to be tested explicitly. We have used this framework as a theoretical account of developmental improvements in rule use over childhood; the development of rule use is discussed further in Chapter 19.

CONCLUSION

We have focused here on several components of the neural mechanisms involved in rule representation (Fig. 3–8; see color insert). Extant data suggest that: (1) postMTG stores semantic knowledge associated with cues in the environment; (2) various regions in parietal and premotor cortices represent actions at different levels of abstraction; and (3) VLPFC is involved in controlled rule retrieval and conscious rule maintenance. Additionally, PFC subregions, including DLPFC and anterior PFC (not shown in Fig. 3–8), are involved in rule representation as needed, depending on the kind of rule. Indeed, rules can be actively maintained in verbal working memory, with the degree of engagement of lateral PFC depending on the amount of information to be held in mind. Future research on the neural mechanisms underlying rule retrieval, maintenance, and implementation will necessarily rely on brain imaging measures with higher temporal resolution than the blood-oxygen-level dependent (BOLD) signal measured with fMRI.

ACKNOWLEDGMENTS We thank Sarah Donohue for assistance with portions of the manuscript, and David Badre for helpful comments on an earlier version of the chapter. The studies presented here were funded by the National Science Foundation (NSF 00448844).

REFERENCES

Amiez C, Kostopoulos P, Champod AS, Petrides M (2006) Local morphology predicts functional organization of the dorsal premotor region in the human brain. Journal of Neuroscience 26:2724–2731.
Aron AR, Fletcher PC, Bullmore ET, Sahakian BJ, Robbins TW (2003) Stop-signal inhibition disrupted by damage to right inferior frontal gyrus in humans. Nature Neuroscience 6:115–116.

Badre D, Poldrack RA, Pare-Blagoev EJ, Insler RZ, Wagner AD (2005) Dissociable controlled retrieval and generalized selection mechanisms in ventrolateral prefrontal cortex. Neuron 47:907–918.

Bor D, Owen AM (2006) A common prefrontal-parietal network for mnemonic and mathematical recoding strategies within working memory. Cerebral Cortex 17:778–786.

Brass M, Ruge H, Meiran N, Rubin O, Koch I, Zysset S, Prinz W, von Cramon DY (2003) When the same response has different meanings: recoding the response meaning in the lateral prefrontal cortex. Neuroimage 20:1026–1031.

Brass M, von Cramon DY (2004) Decomposing components of task preparation with functional magnetic resonance imaging. Journal of Cognitive Neuroscience 16:609–620.

Bunge SA (2004) How we use rules to select actions: a review of evidence from cognitive neuroscience. Cognitive, Affective, and Behavioral Neuroscience 4:564–579.

Bunge SA, Burrows B, Wagner AD (2004) Prefrontal and hippocampal contributions to visual associative recognition: interactions between cognitive control and episodic retrieval. Brain and Cognition 56:141–152.

Bunge SA, Dudukovic NM, Thomason ME, Vaidya CJ, Gabrieli JD (2002) Immature frontal lobe contributions to cognitive control in children: evidence from fMRI. Neuron 33:301–311.

Bunge SA, Kahn I, Wallis JD, Miller EK, Wagner AD (2003) Neural circuits subserving the retrieval and maintenance of abstract rules. Journal of Neurophysiology 90:3419–3428.

Bunge SA, Wallis JD, Parker A, Brass M, Crone EA, Hoshi E, Sakai K (2005) Neural circuitry underlying rule use in humans and nonhuman primates. Journal of Neuroscience 25:10347–10350.

Bunge SA, Zelazo PD (2006) A brain-based account of the development of rule use in childhood. Current Directions in Psychological Science 15:118–121.

Bussey TJ, Wise SP, Murray EA (2002) Interaction of ventral and orbital prefrontal cortex with inferotemporal cortex in conditional visuomotor learning. Behavioral Neuroscience 116:703–715.

Cavina-Pratesi C, Valyear KF, Culham JC, Köhler S, Obhi SS, Marzi CA, Goodale M (2006) Dissociating arbitrary stimulus-response mapping form movement planning during preparatory period: evidence from event-related functional magnetic resonance imaging. Journal of Neuroscience 26:2704–2713.

Chao LL, Haxby JV, Martin A (1999) Attribute-based neural substrates in temporal cortex for perceiving and knowing about objects. Nature Neuroscience 2:913–919.

Chao LL, Martin A (2000) Representation of manipulable man-made objects in the dorsal stream. Neuroimage 12:478–484.

Christoff K, Gabrieli JDE (2002) The frontopolar cortex and human cognition: evidence for a rostrocaudal hierarchical organization within the human prefrontal cortex. Psychobiology 28:168–186.

Chouinard PA, Paud T (2006) The primary motor and premotor areas of the human cerebral cortex. The Neuroscientist 12:143–152.

D'Esposito M, Postle BR, Ballard D, Lease J (1999) Maintenance versus manipulation of information held in working memory: an event-related fMRI study. Brain and Cognition 41:66–86.

Dobbins IG, Rice HJ, Wagner AD, Schacter DL (2003) Memory orientation and success: separable neurocognitive components underlying episodic recognition. Neuropsychologia 41:318–333.

Donohue SE, Wendelken C, Bunge SA (under review) Keeping task-related information in mind: Neural correlates of inhibitory and non-inhibitory rule representations.

Donohue SE, Wendelken C, Crone EA, Bunge SA (2005) Retrieving rules for behavior from long-term memory. Neuroimage 26:1140–1149.

Eacott MJ, Gaffan D (1992) Inferotemporal-frontal disconnection: the uncinate fascicle and visual associative learning in monkeys. European Journal of Neuroscience 4: 1320–1332.

Fogassi L, Luppino G (2005) Motor functions of the parietal lobe. Current Opinion in Neurobiology 15:626–631.

Gabrieli JD, Poldrack RA, Desmond JE (1998) The role of left prefrontal cortex in language and memory. Proceedings of the National Academy of Sciences U S A 95: 906–913.

Garavan H, Ross TJ, Stein EA (1999) Right hemispheric dominance of inhibitory control: an event-related functional MRI study. Proceedings of the National Academy of Sciences U S A 96:8301–8306.

Halsband U, Passingham R (1982) The role of premotor and parietal cortex in the direction of action. Brain Research 240:368–372.

Hasegawa I, Hayashi T, Miyashita Y (1999) Memory retrieval under the control of the prefrontal cortex. Annals of Medicine 31:380–387.

Heilman KM, Maher LM, Greenwald ML, Rothi LJ (1997) Conceptual apraxia from lateralized lesions. Neurology 49:457–464.

Hester RL, Murphy K, Foxe JJ, Foxe DM, Javitt DC, Garavan H (2004) Predicting success: patterns of cortical activation and deactivation prior to response inhibition. Journal of Cognitive Neuroscience 16:776–785.

Johnson SH, Grafton ST (2003) From 'acting on' to 'acting with': the functional anatomy of object-oriented action schemata. Progress in Brain Research 142:127–139.

Johnson-Frey SH (2004) The neural bases of complex tool use in humans. Trends in Cognitive Science 8:71–78.

Jonides J, Smith EE, Marshuetz C, Koeppe RA (1998) Inhibition in verbal working memory revealed by brain activation. Proceedings of the National Academy of Sciences U S A 95:8410–8413.

Kellenbach ML, Brett M, Patterson K (2003) Actions speak louder than functions: the importance of manipulability and action in tool representation. Journal of Cognitive Neuroscience 15:30–46.

Kirchhoff BA, Wagner AD, Maril A, Stern CE (2000) Prefrontal-temporal circuitry for episodic encoding and subsequent memory. Journal of Neuroscience 20:6173–6180.

Konishi S, Nakajima K, Uchida I, Kikyo H, Kameyama M, Miyashita Y (1999) Common inhibitory mechanism in human inferior prefrontal cortex revealed by event-related functional MRI. Brain 122:981–991.

Lewis JW (2006) Cortical networks related to human use of tools. The Neuroscientist 12:211–231.

Lewis JW, Brefczynski JA, Phinney RE, Janik JJ, DeYoe EA (2005) Distinct cortical pathways for processing tool versus animal sounds. Journal of Neuroscience 25: 5148–5158.

Lewis JW, Wightman FL, Brefczynski JA, Phinney RE, Binder JR, DeYoe EA (2004) Human brain regions involved in recognizing environmental sounds. Cerebral Cortex 14:1008–1021.

MacDonald AW, Cohen JD, Stenger VA, Carter CS (2000) Dissociating the role of the dorsolateral prefrontal and anterior cingulate cortex in cognitive control. Science 288:1835–1838.

Marks DF (1973) Visual imagery differences in the recall of pictures. British Journal of Psychology 64:17–24.

Martin A, Chao LL (2001) Semantic memory and the brain: structure and processes. Current Opinion in Neurobiology 11:194–201.

Merriam-Webster Dictionary (1974) Pocket Books, New York.

Miller EK, Cohen JD (2001) An integrative theory of prefrontal cortex function. Annual Review of Neuroscience 24:167–202.

Miyashita Y, Hayashi T (2000) Neural representation of visual objects: encoding and top-down activation. Current Opinion in Neurobiology 10:187–194.

Monchi O, Petrides M, Strafella AP, Worsley KJ, Doyon J (2006) Functional role of the basal ganglia in the planning and execution of actions. Annals of Neurology 59:257–264.

Murray EA, Bussey TJ, Wise SP (2000) Role of prefrontal cortex in a network for arbitrary visuomotor mapping. Experimental Brain Research 133:114–129.

Nelson JK, Reuter-Lorenz PA, Sylvester CY, Jonides J, Smith EE (2003) Dissociable neural mechanisms underlying response-based and familiarity-based conflict in working memory. Proceedings of the National Academy of Sciences U S A 100:11171–11175.

Parker A, Gaffan D (1998) Memory after frontal/temporal disconnection in monkeys: conditional and non-conditional tasks, unilateral and bilateral frontal lesions. Neuropsychologia 36:259–271.

Passingham RE, Toni I, Rushworth MF (2000) Specialisation within the prefrontal cortex: the ventral prefrontal cortex and associative learning. Experimental Brain Research 133:103–113.

Petrides M (1996) Specialized systems for the processing of mnemonic information within the primate frontal cortex. Philosophical Transactions of the Royal Society of London Series B: Biological Sciences 351:1455–1461; discussion 1461–1452.

Petrides M (1997) Visuo-motor conditional associative learning after frontal and temporal lesions in the human brain. Neuropsychologia 35:989–997.

Petrides M (2002) The mid-ventrolateral prefrontal cortex and active mnemonic retrieval. Neurobiology of Learning and Memory 78:528–538.

Picard N, Strick PL (2001) Imaging the premotor areas. Current Opinion in Neurobiology 11:663–672.

Rushworth MF, Ellison A, Walsh V (2001) Complementary localization and lateralization of orienting and motor attention. Nature Neuroscience 4:656–661.

Rushworth MF, Johansen-Berg H, Gobel SM, Devlin JT (2003) The left parietal and premotor cortices: motor attention and selection. Neuroimage 20:S89–S100.

Rypma B, Prabhakaran V, Desmond JE, Glover GH, Gabrieli JD (1999) Load-dependent roles of frontal brain regions in the maintenance of working memory. Neuroimage 9:216–226.

Souza MJ, Donohue SE, Bunge SA (2005) What's your sign? Using functional MRI to uncover the storage and retrieval of rules. Presented at the annual meeting of the Cognitive Neuroscience Society in New York, NY, April 10–12.

Souza, MJ, Bunge, SA (under review) Representing actions and functions associated with objects.

Thompson-Schill SL, D'Esposito M, Aguirre GK, Farah MJ (1997) Role of the left inferior prefrontal cortex in retrieval of semantic knowledge: a reevaluation. Proceedings of the National Academy of Sciences U S A 94:14792–14797.

Toni I, Krams M, Turner R, Passingham RE (1998) The time course of changes during motor sequence learning: a whole-brain fMRI study. Neuroimage 8:50–61.

Toni I, Passingham RE (1999) Prefrontal-basal ganglia pathways are involved in the learning of arbitrary visuomotor associations: a PET study. Experimental Brain Research 127:19–32.

Toni I, Ramnani N, Josephs O, Ashburner J, Passingham RE (2001) Learning arbitrary visuomotor associations: temporal dynamic of brain activity. Neuroimage 14:1048–1057.

Tranel D, Kemmerer D, Adolphs R, Damasio H, Damasio AR (2003) Neural correlates of conceptual knowledge for actions. Cognitive Neuropsychology 20:409–432.

Tyler LK, Stamatakis EA, Dick E, Bright P, Fletcher P, Moss H (2003) Objects and their actions: evidence for a neurally distributed semantic system. Neuroimage 18:542–557.

Vandenberghe R, Price C, Wise R, Josephs O, Frackowiak RSJ (1996) Functional anatomy of a common semantic system for words and pictures. Nature 383:254–256.

Van Essen DC (2002) Windows on the brain: the emerging role of atlases and databases in neuroscience. Current Opinion in Neurobiology 12:574–579.

Van Essen DC, Dickson J, Harwell J, Hanlon D, Anderson CH, Drury HA (2001) An integrated software system for surface-based analyses of cerebral cortex. Journal of American Medical Informatics Association 41:1359–1378.

Wagner AD, Koutstaal W, Schacter DL (1999) When encoding yields remembering: insights from event-related neuroimaging. Philosophical Transactions of the Royal Society of London Series B: Biological Sciences 354:1307–1324.

Wagner AD, Pare-Blagoev EJ, Clark J, Poldrack RA (2001) Recovering meaning: left prefrontal cortex guides controlled semantic retrieval. Neuron 31:329–338.

Wagner AD, Schacter DL, Rotte M, Koutstaal W, Maril A, Dale AM, Rosen BR, Buckner RL (1998) Left prefrontal and temporal activation during human encoding is associated with whether experiences are remembered or forgotten. Science 281:1188–1191.

4

Maintenance and Implementation of Task Rules

Katsuyuki Sakai

We can respond to a stimulus more quickly when we have advance knowledge about the features of the stimulus or the types of movement we are to make. For example, the rate at which we press a button in response to a visual stimulus on a screen increases when we know in advance the location of stimulus to be presented. Such facilitation of behavior depends on the ability to represent the advance information in the form of an attention set. An attention set is mediated by the sustained activity in the frontoparietal network before task performance (Kanwisher and Wojciulik, 2000; Corbetta and Shulman, 2002). The network sends top-down signals to areas involved in actual task performance and facilitates the neural processing in those areas. In other words, the set activity guides subsequent task processing.

Similar mechanisms may take place in rule-guided behaviors. In some situations, we cannot anticipate specific stimuli or specific kinds of actions, but we can prepare our response to a stimulus based on the rule of the task. For example, if you are asked to raise your left hand when a red stimulus appears and to raise your right hand when a green stimulus appears, the rule is the specific association between the stimulus and the response. Alternately, the rule can be more abstract. For example, if you are asked to press the left button when two pictures are the same and to press the right button when the two pictures are different, the rule is not associated with any particular feature of the sensory stimuli.

In either case, one must represent the task rules before the task is actually performed. A "task set" refers to a sustained cognitive state where the task rules are maintained for subsequent use (Rogers and Monsell, 1995). In this chapter, I will discuss how task set activity guides behavior.

SINGLE-UNIT EVIDENCE OF TASK RULE REPRESENTATION

In electrophysiological studies of nonhuman primates, neurons can be considered to be involved in task set representation if they exhibit sustained activation before task performance that varies as a function of task rules. To identify such rule-specific neuronal activity, experimenters give monkeys task

instructions that specify the rule to be followed on a given trial, and then present the task items to be processed, based on this rule.

As described in Chapters 2 and 8, there are neurons in the prefrontal cortex that show rule-selective activity before task performance. For example, a neuron shows an increase in activity when monkeys are preparing to perform a Match task, but not a non-Match task, independent of the sensory features of the task items and the types of motor responses (Wallis et al., 2001). These and other studies have also shown that neurons coding different rules coexist within the same region (White and Wise 1999; Asaad et al., 2000; Hoshi et al., 2000; Wallis et al., 2001). This poses a problem when one wants to use brain imaging in human subjects to measure brain activation associated with the representation of different rules. It is possible, however, that neurons coding different rules project to different brain regions and influence the activity of the target neurons in these regions. If so, rule-specific activity in a single brain area might be associated with a rule-specific pattern of inter-regional interaction,

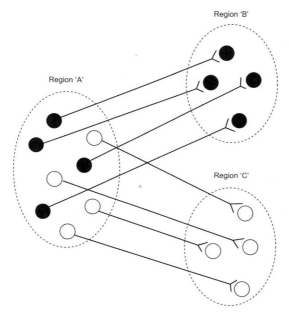

Figure 4–1 Schematic model of inter-regional interactions. Neurons representing different information are intermingled within region A, but each of the neuronal populations projects to different regions, B and C. When regions B and C are sufficiently separated in space, the information coded in region A can be identified as distinct patterns of inter-regional interaction with region B or C.

which we can identify using functional brain imaging techniques with human participants (Fig. 4–1).

RULE-SPECIFIC INTER-REGIONAL INTERACTION IDENTIFIED USING IMAGING

My colleagues and I used the logic outlined earlier to design a brain imaging study that focuses on task set representation in humans. In Sakai and Passingham (2003), healthy participants were asked to perform one of four tasks according to task instructions. The tasks involved remembering a sequence of locations of red squares in forward or backward order or remembering a sequence of letters in forward or backward order. The same stimulus set was used for all four tasks, and only the instructions given before each trial differed.

Using functional magnetic resonance imaging, we found sustained activity in the anterior prefrontal cortex (APF) [BA 10] for all four tasks during the delay period between the instruction and the presentation of the task items, which we call the "instruction delay." The peak of the activity was located in the lateral frontal convexity, just anterior to the frontomarginal sulcus. By contrast, other regions in the prefrontal cortex exhibited task-specific activation during the instruction delay. The posterior part of the superior frontal sulcus (SFS) [BA 8]—previously implicated in spatial working memory (Courtney et al., 1998)—exhibited sustained activation for both spatial tasks. Similarly, the left posterior inferior frontal gyrus (pIFG) [BA 44]—previously implicated in verbal working memory (Smith et al., 1998)—exhibited sustained activation for both verbal tasks. These activations did not differ between forward and backward remembering tasks (Fig. 4–2A and B).

By contrast, the patterns of prefrontal interaction changed not only according to whether the participants were to remember spatial or verbal items, but also according to whether they were to remember the items in forward or backward order. The correlation of the activity between the APF and SFS was significantly higher in the spatial backward condition than in other conditions. On the other hand, the correlation between the APF and pIFG was significantly higher in the verbal backward condition than in the others. Notably, such an increase in correlation values was observed when the task instruction was given, before the actual performance of the task (Fig. 4–2C).

Thus, the APF changed its partner of interaction according to the rule of the task to be performed. This study demonstrates the validity of functional connectivity analysis in identifying and discriminating between the rules that are represented by intermixed neuronal populations. Other studies have also shown that the prefrontal cortex interacts with different posterior regions according to the task being performed. The interaction pattern changes depending on whether the participants are paying attention to the color of the stimulus or the finger used to press a button (Rowe et al., 2005); whether the participants are imagining houses, chairs, or faces (Mechelli et al., 2004); or whether

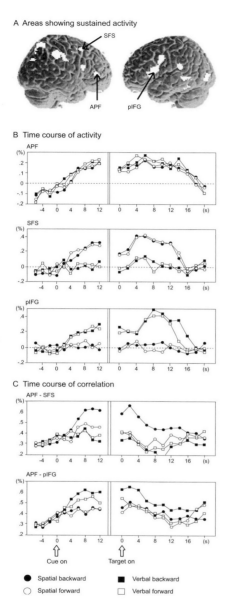

A Areas showing sustained activity

B Time course of activity

C Time course of correlation

Cue on   Target on

● Spatial backward   ■ Verbal backward
○ Spatial forward   □ Verbal forward

Figure 4–2 Neural correlates for task set for spatial and verbal working memory tasks. *A.* Areas that showed significant activity during the instruction delay (i.e., the period between task instruction and task items). *B.* Time course of activation in the active areas. *C.* Time course of correlation in the active areas. The *left panels* correspond to the pre-task period, and time "0" indicates the presentation of task instruction. The *right panels* correspond to the task execution period, and time "0" indicates the presentation of the first task item. SFS, superior frontal sulcus (BA 8); APF, anterior prefrontal cortex (BA 10); pIFG, posterior part of the inferior frontal gyrus (BA 45) [Adapted from Sakai and Passingham, *Nature Neuroscience,* 6, 75–81. Copyright Macmillan Publishers, 2003].

participants are making judgments based on spelling or rhyming of visually presented words (Bitan et al., 2005). Our finding (Sakai and Passingham, 2003) suggests that the inter-regional interaction pattern changes not only according to the task that is *currently being performed,* but also during a preparatory period, according to the task that is *about to be performed.*

FUNCTIONAL SIGNIFICANCE OF RULE REPRESENTATION

Such rule-specific patterns of prefrontal interaction during the instruction delay can be thought of as reflecting task sets. However, the issue of the functional significance of prefrontal activity and interaction remains. This issue
is important, given that neurons representing task rules are found in widely
distributed prefrontal areas as well as in premotor and parietal areas (Wallis
et al., 2001; Wallis and Miller, 2003; Stoet and Snyder, 2004; see Chapter 11).
Here we asked a specific question: Does the set activity in the APF have something to do with the subsequent task performance?

In this regard, Paul Burgess has shown that patients with lesions in the APF
are impaired in rule-based behaviors (Burgess et al., 2000). It remains open,
however, whether set activity in this region has functional significance. Burgess
et al. (2000) also showed that these patients are impaired in the implementation of rules rather than the maintenance of rules. This highlights another issue of the mechanisms of rule implementation, which I will discuss
later in this chapter.

Behaviorally, the functional significance of the set activity can be shown as
the presence of a preparation effect: When participants are tested on trials with
a very short instruction delay, their performance slows down. This effect might
be due to the fact that participants have insufficient time to establish the
task operations before the actual task performance (Rogers and Monsell, 1995;
Monsell, 2003; for other accounts, see Meiran et al., 2000; Wylie and Allport,
2000). Thus, the comparison between a task that shows a preparation effect
and a task without the effect would show that the neural correlates of task set
maintenance have functional significance.

In a new study, we sought to replicate and extend our earlier findings showing that the APF interacts with different brain regions, depending
on the task that participants are preparing to perform (Sakai and Passingham, 2006). The task was phonological, semantic, or visual case judgment
for a visually presented word. The task instructions were given before each
word, with an instruction delay of 0.3, 2, 4, 6, or 8 sec. We found that there
was a significant interaction between the length of instruction delay and task
conditions on the reaction time (RT) of the subsequent task performance
(Fig. 4–3). In the phonological and semantic conditions, there was an increase
in RT in trials with a delay length of 0.3 sec. The RT of the visual task, on
the other hand, was not affected by the length of the delay. In other words,
there was a preparation effect in the phonological and semantic tasks, but not
in the visual task.

The phonological condition involved covert reading of a word, and this
required transformation of the visual code (visually presented word) into a phonological code. The semantic condition involved thinking about the meaning of
a word, which required transformation of the visual code into a conceptual code.
By contrast, in the visual judgment condition, participants simply discriminated
among the visual features. Thus, the preparation effect observed in phonological

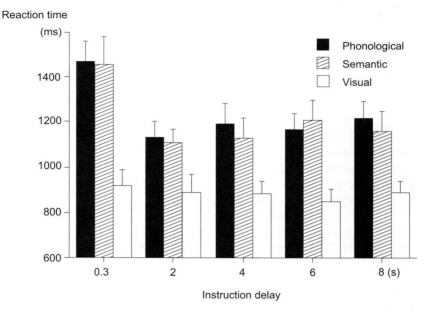

Figure 4–3 Behavioral preparation effect. Reaction times are plotted separately for the trials with different lengths of instruction delay. Note that there is an increase in reaction time in phonological and semantic tasks on trials with a delay length of 0.3 s; however, the effect is not observed in visual case judgment task (Adapted from Sakai and Passingham, *Journal of Neuroscience*, 26, 1211–1218. Copyright Society for Neuroscience, 2006).

and semantic tasks may be due to the preparatory process for the transformation between the codes.

Correspondingly, we found sustained activity during the delay in the APF that was significantly higher in the phonological and semantic conditions than in the visual condition (Fig. 4–4A). As in the previous study, the APF also interacted with posterior frontal regions in a rule-specific manner (Sakai and Passingham, 2003). During the instruction delay, the correlation between activation in the APF and the ventral part of the premotor cortex (PM) [BA 6] was significantly higher in the phonological condition than in the other conditions (Fig. 4–4B). By contrast, the correlation between activation in the APF and the anterior part of the inferior frontal gyrus (aIFG) [BA 47] during the delay was significantly higher in the semantic condition than in the other conditions. The PM and aIFG did not show significant sustained activity during the instruction delay, but showed phasic activity when a target word was presented.

The preparation effect observed in trials with a very short instruction delay may be due to a premature level at which these rule-specific patterns of interaction were established; in these trials, the rule-specific pattern of inter-

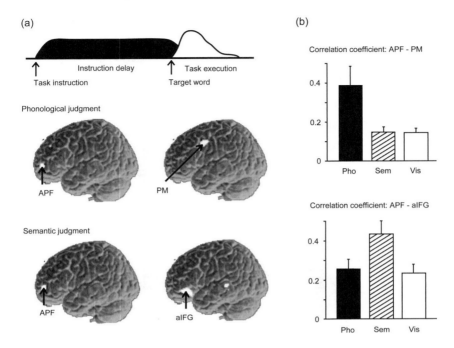

Figure 4–4 Neural correlates for task set for phonological and semantic tasks. *A.* Areas that showed significant activity during the instruction delay (*left*) and during task execution (*right*). *B.* Correlation coefficients between the active areas. The *error bar* indicates standard error across the 14 participants. APF, anterior prefrontal cortex (BA 10); PM, premotor cortex (BA 6); aIFG, anterior part of the inferior frontal gyrus (BA 47); Pho, phonological; Sem, semantic; Vis, visual.

regional interactions may be carried over into the task execution phase after presentation of a target word, thus causing an increase in RT.

SET ACTIVITY PREDICTS SUBSEQUENT BEHAVIORAL PERFORMANCE AND TASK ACTIVITY

In Sakai and Passingham (2006), we also found that the amount of set activity in the APF affected subsequent task performance. The set activity in the APF was inversely correlated with the RT of phonological and semantic performance (Fig. 4–5*A*). The activity was not correlated with the RT in the visual condition, suggesting the behavioral significance of the set activity in the APF in specific types of tasks.

The correlation between the set activity in the APF and RT suggests a causal link between rule representation and the performance based on that rule. Although neuronal activity representing task rules can be found all over the

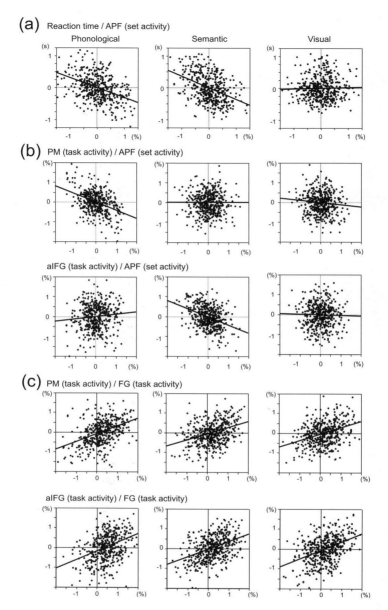

Figure 4–5 Correlations with anterior prefrontal cortex (APF) activation. *A.* Correlations between APF task set activity and reaction time. *B.* Correlation between APF task set activity and task activity in posterior areas, shown separately for the phonological, semantic, and visual case judgment tasks. *C.* Correlation between the task activity premotor cortex (PM) in the fusiform gyrus (FG) and the task activity in the PM and anterior part of the inferior frontal gyrus (aIFG). All plotted values were mean-adjusted across the three task conditions. (Adapted from Sakai and Passingham, *Journal of Neuroscience*, 26, 1211–1218. Copyright Society for Neuroscience, 2006).

prefrontal cortex (Wallis et al., 2001), these results suggest that, at least in the human brain, the APF may have a specialized role in the preparation of tasks that require item manipulation.

It is noteworthy that participants could still perform the task correctly, even with a short instruction delay or with a low level of set activity in the APF. This may suggest that the interactions between the APF and posterior frontal areas mediate implementation rather than maintenance of the task rule. This corresponds to the finding of impaired performance in task rule implementation, but not in task rule maintenance in patients with APF lesions (Burgess et al., 2000). This is also supported by the significant correlation between the set activity in the APF and the task activity in areas involved in actual task performance (Sakai and Passingham, 2006). The set activity in the APF was inversely correlated with activity in the PM during the task execution phase (task activity) [Fig. 4–5B]. The effect was observed in the phonological task, but not in other tasks. By contrast, the set activity in the APF was inversely correlated with task activity in the aIFG, and the effect was observed in the semantic task, but not in other tasks. Thus, the magnitude of the set activity in the APF had a negative influence on the magnitude of the task activity in areas that are involved in execution of the task specified by the instruction.

There was also a significant correlation between the task activity in the fusiform gyrus (FG) and task activity in the PM and aIFG (Fig. 4–5C). Unlike the effect of the set activity in the APF, the effect of the FG was positive and was nonspecific to the task. The activity in the FG was positively correlated with activity in the PM and aIFG in all three tasks.

In sum, online task processing evident in the task-specific posterior frontal areas, PM and aIFG, can be predicted by the set activity in the APF and task activity in the FG. Whereas the activity in the FG, which reflects visual processing of the words, influences the task processing in a nonspecific manner, the activity in the APF, which reflects endogenous signals related to a task rule, influences the task processing in a task-specific manner (Fig. 4–6). Such rule-specific inter-regional interactions may provide the mechanism by which task set activity guides rule-based behavior.

THE ROLE OF THE APF IN REPRESENTING HIGHER-ORDER TASK RULES

The APF is involved in specific instances of task set maintenance and implementation. The two studies described earlier suggest that the APF is involved in tasks where participants need to manipulate the task items (Sakai and Passingham 2003, 2006). The activity in the APF observed when participants were to perform a spatial or verbal working memory task may reflect preparation for transformation of the visual stimuli into covert eye movements or vocalization. The activity observed when participants were to perform a phonological or semantic task may reflect a preparatory process for transforming the visual stimuli into covert vocalization or their meaning.

Phonological judgment

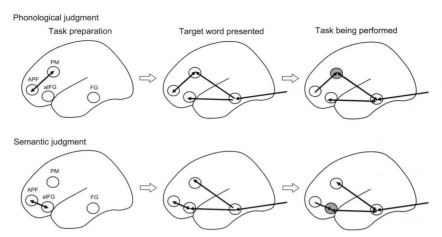

Figure 4–6 Schematic drawing of the neural mechanisms of task preparation (*left*), target word processing (*middle*), and task processing (*right*). Task set activity in the anterior prefrontal cortex (APF) establishes the pattern of inter-regional interaction specific to the task to be performed. The incoming information from a visually presented target word influences the activity in the fusiform gyrus (FG), and then in the premotor cortex (PM) and anterior part of the inferior frontal gyrus (aIFG) in the same manner across the tasks. Due to the pre-established task set pattern, the processing of the word occurs in areas associated with the task specified by the instruction.

Other studies also implicate the APF in the representation of higher-order task rules. For example, Bunge et al. (2003) have shown that the activity in the APF is significantly higher during the delay when participants prepare to perform a non-Match task than when they perform a Match or simple sensorimotor association task. In this study, the participants reported that they conceptualized a non-Match task as the reverse of a Match task, and the activity in the APF was believed to reflect elaboration of a default rule. In other studies, the APF was shown to be especially active when participants switched between two tasks based on different rules than when they performed a single task (Braver et al., 2003), and when participants need to activate delayed intentions to perform a secondary task during performance of another task (Koechlin et al., 1999; Burgess et al., 2003; Badre and Wagner, 2004).

The APF is also involved in guidance of memory control mechanisms (Lepage et al., 2000; Otten et al., 2006). Otten et al. (2006) used an electroencephalogram while participants performed an incidental encoding of words, and they found that the activity in the APF before the word presentation differed, depending on whether the word was subsequently remembered. Importantly, the participants were not required to remember the words, but simply to make judgments on the meaning of each word. The differential activity in the APF was observed when participants performed semantic judgments for visually presented words, but not when they performed orthographic judgments for

visually presented words or when they performed semantic judgments for auditorily presented words. Consistent with the studies described earlier, this finding suggests involvement of the APF in specific task sets. However, in this study, the set activity in the APF did not affect the RT for impending semantic judgment, but rather affected the subsequent recollection of the studied word 10 minutes later.

In addition to the APF, other areas are involved in task set maintenance and implementation. For example, Dosenbach et al. (2006) have shown that the anterior cingulate and anterior insular cortices show sustained activity during the instruction delay in all kinds of tasks. Although there is a possibility that the areas are involved in nonspecific arousal or attention to prepare for the subsequent task control, such a "core task set system" may interact with areas such as the APF to support the maintenance of specific types of task sets. The ventrolateral prefrontal cortex and inferior frontal junction area are also involved in task set maintenance, implementation, or both, as discussed in Chapters 3 and 9.

INTERACTION BETWEEN TONIC TOP-DOWN SIGNALS AND PHASIC BOTTOM-UP SIGNALS

We have shown that the influence from the APF over the posterior areas is rule-selective (Sakai and Passingham, 2006). This is potentially mediated by the positive influence of the APF over the posterior areas during the instruction delay. During this period, the APF might have primed the areas involved in task execution through positive and task-specific interactions, thereby reducing the online task-processing load before the task. It is possible, however, that influence from the APF is indirect and that other areas are also involved. In any case, the results show that the set activity in the APF is a good candidate for the source of the rule-specific causal influence on task-specific neural processing, although the direction of the influence remains an issue for future research.

The interaction between the tonic and phasic components of task processing has also been examined in Braver et al. (2003). Using a task-switching paradigm, they found that tonic activity in the APF is inversely correlated with phasic activity in the same region after the presentation of target items. This may suggest a carry-over of task set establishment processes into the task execution phase when tonic activity in the APF is low.

The mechanisms of the interaction between set activity and task processing have been examined in detail using visual attention tasks (Kanwisher and Wojciulik, 2000; Corbetta and Shulman, 2002). Attention is subserved by two separate, but inter-related components: a tonic increase of baseline activity before the stimulus and a gain control during stimulus presentation. The extrastriate visual areas involved in actual processing of the stimuli show an increase in baseline activity after the cue presentation, and this continues before the presentation of task stimuli. These areas show an additional increase of activity at the time of stimulus presentation. By contrast, the frontal and

parietal areas become active when a cue is presented, but they do not show an additional increase in activity during the task performance, suggesting that the main role of this activity is to maintain the attention set rather than to process sensory stimuli per se.

Similarly, in Sakai and Passingham (2003, 2006), the APF did not show an additional increase in activity at the start of task performance, even though the posterior frontal areas involved in task execution did show an increase in activity when the task was actually performed. Although maintenance of attention set is mediated by interactions with lower-order sensory areas, maintenance of task set seems to be mediated by interactions between higher-order prefrontal areas, probably because task set represents abstract rules rather than specific sensory features.

For tasks involving either attention set or task set, neural processing during the task execution can be thought of as an interaction between top-down signals from the frontoparietal network and bottom-up signals from task items. For example, Moore et al. (2003) have applied microstimulation to the frontal eye field (FEF) while monkeys performed a visual attention task. The activity in V4 neurons was enhanced when the visual target was presented within the receptive field of the neurons (bottom-up factor) and more so when the FEF neurons corresponding to that receptive field were stimulated (top-down factor). The study by Sakai and Passingham (2006) also shows that the task activity in the PM and aIFG is influenced by both the task activity in the FG (bottom-up factor) and the set activity in the APF (top-down factor). Generally speaking, a tonic endogenous drive from higher-order brain areas sets up a pattern of effective connectivity in a form that is suitable for goal-directed behavior, and an exogenous drive triggers the circuit to generate appropriate behavior.

SUMMARY

The maintenance of rules is not so difficult for humans. When we are asked to perform a semantic task, we can simply maintain the rule by verbally rehearsing the task instruction: "Press the right button when the word has abstract meaning; press the left button when the word has concrete meaning . . . right, abstract; left, concrete; right, abstract; left, concrete. . . ." Although such verbal coding is an efficient way of maintaining information, it may not be useful in speeding up the subsequent task performance. Instead, we must engage the computational mechanisms that are necessary for task execution and prepare for the rule-based processing of task items.

I have argued that sustained activity during the instruction delay reflects rule representations in an action-oriented form. The rules are represented through interactions with areas involved in actual performance of the task based on that rule. Our group and others have postulated that what is maintained during the delay of a working memory task is not the sensory information given in the past, but rather the information generated for prospective

use (Tanji and Hoshi, 2001; Passingham and Sakai, 2004). The same is true for the maintenance of task set.

The predictive nature of the set activity in the APF for task performance and task activity further suggests that this rule maintenance process operates as the process of implementing the rule for subsequent cognitive performance. The areas involved in task execution are primed in a task-specific manner before the task performance through rule-selective, inter-regional interactions during the active maintenance period. This is the way the prefrontal cortex prospectively configures and facilitates rule-based behavior.

ACKNOWLEDGMENTS The research was supported by grants from the Wellcome Trust and the Human Frontier Science Program. The author is grateful to Richard E. Passingham for an excellent collaboration.

REFERENCES

Asaad WF, Rainer G, Miller EK (2000) Task-specific neural activity in the primate prefrontal cortex. Journal of Neurophysiology 84:451–459.

Badre D, Wagner AD (2004) Selection, integration, and conflict monitoring: assessing the nature and generality of prefrontal cognitive control mechanisms. Neuron 41: 473–487.

Bitan T, Booth JR, Choy J, Burman DD, Gitelman DR, Mesulam MM (2005) Shifts of effective connectivity within a language network during rhyming and spelling. Journal of Neuroscience 25:5397–5403.

Braver TS, Reynolds JR, Donaldson DI (2003) Neural mechanisms of transient and sustained cognitive control during task switching. Neuron 39:713–726.

Bunge SA, Kahn I, Wallis JD, Miller EK, Wagner AD (2003) Neural circuits subserving the retrieval and maintenance of abstract rules. Journal of Neurophysiology 90: 3419–3428.

Burgess PW, Scott SK, Frith CD (2003) The role of the rostral frontal cortex (area 10) in prospective memory: a lateral versus medial dissociation. Neuropsychologia 41: 906–918.

Burgess PW, Veitch E, de Lacy Costello A, Shallice T (2000) The cognitive and neuroanatomical correlates of multitasking. Neuropsychologia 38:848–863.

Corbetta M, Shulman GL (2002) Control of goal-directed and stimulus-driven attention in the brain. Nature Review Neuroscience 3:201–215.

Courtney SM, Petit L, Maisog JM, Ungerleider LG, Haxby JV (1998) An area specialized for spatial working memory in human frontal cortex. Science 279:1347–1351.

Dosenbach NU, Visscher KM, Palmer ED, Miezin FM, Wenger KK, Kang HC, Burgund ED, Grimes AL, Schlaggar BL, Petersen SE (2006) A core system for the implementation of task sets. Neuron 50:799–812.

Hoshi E, Shima K, Tanji J (2000) Neuronal activity in the primate prefrontal cortex in the process of motor selection based on two behavioral rules. Journal of Neurophysiology 83:2355–2373.

Kanwisher N, Wojciulik E (2000) Visual attention: insights from brain imaging. Nature Review Neuroscience 1:91–100.

Koechlin E, Basso G, Pietrini P, Panzer S, Grafman J (1999) The role of the anterior prefrontal cortex in human cognition. Nature 399:148–151.

Lepage M, Ghaffar O, Nyberg L, Tulving E (2000) Prefrontal cortex and episodic memory retrieval mode. Proceedings of the National Academy of Sciences U S A 97: 506–511.

Mechelli A, Price CJ, Friston KJ, Ishai A (2004) Where bottom-up meets top-down: neuronal interactions during perception and imagery. Cerebral Cortex 14:1256–1265.

Meiran N, Chorev Z, Sapir A (2000) Component processes in task switching. Cognitive Psychology 41:211–253.

Monsell S (2003) Task switching. Trends in Cognitive Science 7:134–140.

Moore T, Armstrong KM (2003) Selective gating of visual signals by microstimulation of frontal cortex. Nature 421:370–373.

Otten LJ, Quayle AH, Akram S, Ditewig TA, Rugg MD (2006) Brain activity before an event predicts later recollection. Nature Neuroscience 9:489–491.

Passingham D, Sakai K (2004) The prefrontal cortex and working memory: physiology and brain imaging. Current Opinion in Neurobiology 14:163–168.

Rogers RD, Monsell S (1995) Costs of a predictable switch between simple cognitive tasks. Journal of Experimental Psychology General 124:207–231.

Rowe JB, Stephan KE, Friston K, Frackowiak RS, Passingham RE (2005) The prefrontal cortex shows context-specific changes in effective connectivity to motor or visual cortex during the selection of action or colour. Cerebral Cortex 15:85–95.

Sakai K, Passingham RE (2003) Prefrontal interactions reflect future task operations. Nature Neuroscience 6:75–81.

Sakai K, Passingham RE (2006) Prefrontal set activity predicts rule-specific neural processing during subsequent cognitive performance. Journal of Neuroscience 26: 1211–1218.

Smith EE, Jonides J, Marshuetz C, Koeppe RA (1998) Components of verbal working memory: evidence from neuroimaging. Proceedings of the National Academy of Sciences U S A 95:876–882.

Stoet G, Snyder LH (2004) Single neurons in posterior parietal cortex of monkeys encode cognitive set. Neuron 42:1003–1012.

Tanji J, Hoshi E (2001) Behavioral planning in the prefrontal cortex. Current Opinion in Neurobiology 11:164–170.

Wallis JD, Anderson KC, Miller EK (2001) Single neurons in prefrontal cortex encode abstract rules. Nature 411:953–956.

Wallis JD, Miller EK (2003) From rule to response: neuronal processes in the premotor and prefrontal cortex. Journal of Neurophysiology 90:1790–1806.

White IM, Wise SP (1999) Rule-dependent neuronal activity in the prefrontal cortex. Experimental Brain Research 126:315–335.

Wylie G, Allport A (2000) Task switching and the measurement of "switch costs." Psychological Research 63:212–233.

5

The Neurophysiology of Abstract Response Strategies

Aldo Genovesio and Steven P. Wise

The advent of a genuinely *cognitive* neurophysiology has been a long time coming. There have, of course, been many neurophysiological studies of perception, attention, memory, and the like, but rather little about the mechanisms of problem-solving or response-guiding rules and strategies, the pillars of intelligent, adaptive cognition. After all, "cognition" is just a word from Latin that means "knowledge," and knowledge takes many forms. Some forms, such as perception, attention, and memory, have received extensive consideration from neurophysiologists. Others, especially those involving advanced cognition, have gotten much less. So why has the neurophysiology of advanced cognition developed so slowly in relation to that of more primitive forms?

Among the impediments to progress in cognitive neurophysiology, the lingering influence of behaviorism remains surprisingly strong. According to Mario Bunge (2003), behaviorism is "the psychological school that studies only overt behavior," a research program synonymous with "S-R (stimulus-response) psychology." According to this doctrine, three factors—previously experienced stimuli, responses to those stimuli, and the outcomes of those actions—determine an animal's behavior. Some forms of behaviorism hold that advanced cognitive processes exist, but cannot be studied scientifically; others deny the reality of advanced cognition. Obviously, neither stance is particularly conducive to cognitive neurophysiology. Although behaviorism is "all but dead" as a philosophical matter (Bunge, 2003), there remains the suspicion among many neuroscientists that something must be wrong with any interpretation of neural activity beyond the bounds of stimuli, overt responses, or reinforcement outcomes.

This chapter reviews some neurophysiological results that involve a cognitive function considerably more advanced than those encompassed by S-R psychology: abstract response strategies (Genovesio et al., 2005). To that end, we begin with a seemingly simple question: What is a strategy?

WHAT IS A STRATEGY?

The term "strategy" derives from the Greek *strategos* (στρατηγός), which means "general," the military leader responsible for establishing objectives. In contrast to tactics, which involve the specific ways to achieve those objectives, the *strategos* selected them, and the ancient Greeks had separate leaders for strategy and tactics. In military science, therefore, strategy and tactics compose a dialectic. Unfortunately, cognitive scientists lack such a useful dialectic, and the concept of a strategy remains somewhat vague. In two of its senses, a strategy is either one among many solutions to some problem or—especially during learning—a partial solution.

To exemplify a strategy, imagine that you must respond to one of 12 illuminated numbers, arranged 1–12, as usual for an analog clock. But which one? In your task, that number brightens briefly at the beginning of each trial—the "3" at 3 o'clock, for example. However, you cannot respond at that time; instead, you must wait until that cue occurs again. In the meantime, any of the remaining 11 numbers might brighten from time to time, perhaps several times each, but you must withhold a response until the 3 brightens a second time. You might use one of three *strategies* to solve this problem: (1) You could use a verbal strategy by rehearsing the cued location as "3 o'clock . . . 3 o'clock . . . 3 o'clock . . .," and respond when the 3 brightens again. (2) You could encode the location nonverbally, simply remembering what the clock looked like when the 3 first brightened. Using that strategy, you could respond whenever the 3 brightens again to match your remembered image. (3) You could simply attend to the location of the 3—ignore all other places, remember and rehearse nothing, including the fact that the number 3 is at that location—and respond as soon as something brightens there. Any of these three strategies—which we can call "verbal," "mnemonic," and "attentional," respectively—will achieve your goal, and yet your overt behavior will be identical in each case.

Our laboratory's interest in strategies originated from a neurophysiological study of frontal cortex activity in monkeys (di Pellegrino and Wise, 1993a, b). We trained a monkey to perform a task much like the one just described. Psychologists would call that a "spatial matching-to-sample" task and would regard it as a test of spatial memory. Such names and interpretations, unfortunately, often obscure more than they illuminate. In our study, we found that cells in the prefrontal cortex signaled a location. But was it a remembered location or an attended one? The doctrine that spatial matching-to-sample tasks test spatial memory implied the former, but such an interpretation would depend on which strategy the monkey used. If the monkey used the attentional strategy described earlier, then an interpretation of neural activity in terms of memory would be unfounded. Accordingly, we began exploring ways in which strategies could be brought under experimental control. One path led to experiments that distinguished the neural activity underlying spatial attention, spatial memory, or both, and it turned out that only a minority of neurons in the prefrontal cortex encoded spatial memory. Most signaled an attended

location instead (Lebedev et al., 2004). The other path, the results of which form the basis of this chapter, led to a study of the neurophysiological correlates of abstract response strategies (Genovesio et al., 2005). Our experiment focused on two strategies, which we have named "Repeat-stay" and "Change-shift."

THE REPEAT-STAY AND CHANGE-SHIFT STRATEGIES

We first recognized the Repeat-stay and Change-shift strategies during a study of conditional motor learning (Murray and Wise, 1996). In this task, monkeys must solve problems of the following type: Symbolic cue A instructs response 1, and symbolic cue B instructs response 2 (Passingham, 1993). We can write A→1 and B→2 to describe these two conditional motor problems, sometimes called "mappings." Murray and Wise (1996) used a three-choice task: A→1, B→2, and C→3.

In the experiment that produced Figure 5–1 (see color insert), a computer selected one of three cues from the set (A, B, C) and presented it on a video screen. All three stimuli were novel at the beginning of a block of 50 trials. Each cue consisted of two characters, each of which was a letter, a number or some keyboard symbol: a small (3 cm) character of one color superimposed on a large (5 cm) character, usually of some other color. The monkeys grasped a joystick that could move in only three directions: left, right, or toward the monkey ("down"). Before a block of trials, the computer randomly paired each of the stimuli with one of those joystick movements. Thus, the set of three stimuli (A, B, C) mapped onto the set of three responses (left, right, down), according to the response rules A→left, B→right, and C→down. Accordingly, if cue A appeared on the first trial, the monkeys had a 67% chance of making an incorrect response (right or down) and a 33% of choosing the correct response (left). After a correct response, the monkeys received a reward, which motivated their performance. After an incorrect response, the monkeys got a second chance to respond to the same stimulus. This procedure usually led to a correct response in one or two additional attempts. The next trial began with the presentation of a cue selected randomly from the same set (A, B, C). Accordingly, in approximately one-third of the trials, the cue was the same as it had been in the previous trial, and in two-thirds, it differed. We called the former "repeat trials" and the latter "change trials."

The monkeys performed better in repeat trials than in change trials, especially early in the process of learning the cue-response mappings, and this difference led us to discern the strategies that they used in responding to novel stimuli. Figure 5–1A shows the grand mean learning curves for repeat trials (red) and change trials (blue), as four monkeys learned the three-choice conditional motor problems described earlier: A→left, B→right, and C→down. Each monkey learned the correct responses to 40 sets of novel cues, and Figure 5–1B shows that each of these four monkeys showed a similar performance difference between repeat and change trials. At the beginning of each block of 50 trials, the monkeys always performed better on repeat trials than

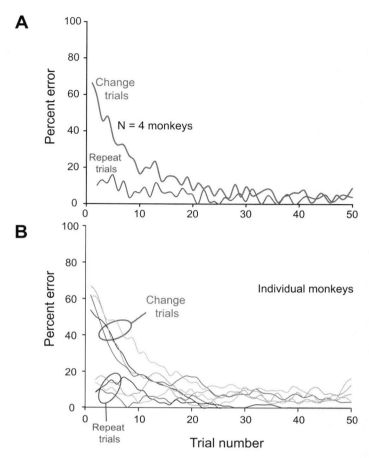

Figure 5–1 Conditional motor task. *A.* Performance rate for repeat
(red) and change (blue) trials during the learning of the task. The *curves*
show the grand means for four monkeys, each for data sets including 40
three-choice conditional motor problems. *B.* Individual scores for the
same four monkeys, with each monkey color-matched for the repeat and
change trials, bounded by the *ovals* in the early stages of learning.

on change trials. We could attribute the monkeys' superior performance on
repeat trials to an abstract response strategy, one that they could apply to novel
cues—before learning (Murray and Wise, 1996). On repeat trials, the monkeys
had learned to *stay* with the same response that they had made on the previous
trial, hence, the name: "Repeat-stay." Put another way, before the monkeys had
learned the mapping A → left, for example, they knew something important
about how to respond to novel cues. If their most recent exploratory response
had yielded a reward, then they remembered the cue (A) and their response
(left) over the intertrial interval. If the same cue reappeared in the next trial,

they simply repeated the response that they had just made. The monkeys also performed at better than the chance level of 67% incorrect in change trials. In those trials, the monkeys also remembered the cue (A) and their response (left) over the intertrial interval. When a different cue (B or C) appeared in the next trial, they had learned to *shift* from their previous response (left) to one of the two remaining possibilities (right or down), so we called that strategy "Change-shift."

In a three-choice task, perfect application of the Repeat-stay strategy would yield 0% incorrect (i.e., 100% correct) on repeat trials, and consistent use of the Change-shift strategy would lead to 50% incorrect in change trials, resulting in a score of 33% incorrect overall. Thus, by employing these two strategies perfectly, the monkeys could cut their error rate in half—from the 67% incorrect expected by chance, to only 33%—before learning which cue mapped to which response. They did not employ the strategies perfectly, but they came pretty close. In time, however, the monkeys did learn the cue–response mappings, as shown by the exponential decrease in errors in change trials, and the difference in performance between repeat and change trials disappeared after approximately 30 trials (Fig. 5–1).

The concept of applying the Repeat-stay and Change-shift strategies before the learning of mappings is not a simple one to grasp, at first. In fact, it took us quite a while to realize what the monkeys were doing. Perhaps an example from developmental linguistics will help to clarify this idea. According to Burling (2005), children sometimes produce a word before learning its meaning. Apparently, they learn the pronunciation of a word, and even the context in which they have heard it spoken by others, before they learn what the word means. When children do this, they must use an imitation strategy to generate the word, rather than a generative strategy that depends on selecting an appropriate word based on context and meaning. Later, they learn what the word means and use it, perhaps in the same sentence as previously, but summoned up with a different strategy. Similarly, when the monkeys use the Repeat-stay and Change-shift strategies, they make precisely the same response that they will later make to the identical stimulus, after they have learned the S-R mappings.

We have observed different combinations of the Repeat-stay and Change-shift strategies in individual monkeys (not illustrated). One monkey showed poor learning of the response instructed by each cue, and instead used the Repeat-stay and Change-shift strategies, alone, to exceed chance levels of performance. In fact, it was this monkey that led us to recognize the Repeat-stay and Change-shift strategies in the first place. Another monkey used Repeat-stay, but not Change-shift. Many other monkeys have solved conditional motor problems without adopting either of these two strategies.

To learn these strategies, the monkeys must have recognized the basic structure of the conditional motor task as we presented it to them, in particular, the fact that each of the three cues mapped uniquely to one correct response. The monkeys learned the Repeat-stay and Change-shift strategies

over a lengthy period of solving hundreds of conditional motor problems of this type, typically 40 sets of cues per week for several weeks.

Performance of the Repeat-stay and Change-shift strategies required several cognitive operations. (1) As noted earlier, the monkeys needed to remember the cue that had appeared on the previous trial. (2) They had to compare this remembered cue to the stimulus on the current trial and evaluate whether it had changed or repeated. In this respect, the Repeat-stay and Change-shift strategies required the same information-processing as a matching-to-sample or nonmatching-to-sample task (see Chapter 2). (3) The monkeys also needed to remember their response from the previous trial, or alternatively, they needed to remember the cue-response mapping. (4) The monkeys needed to use their decision about whether the cue repeated or changed to either stay with their previous response, in accord with the Repeat-stay strategy, or reject it, in accord with the Change-shift strategy. Of these four cognitive processes, two depend on short-term memory: the retention of the previous cue and the response to that cue. The monkeys needed to maintain these memories at least until they made the repeat-change decision and selected the next response.

Murray and Wise (1996) found that ablations of the hippocampus and subjacent cortex had no effect on the monkeys' capacity to employ the Repeat-stay and Change-shift strategies, notwithstanding the fact that these same monkeys had a severe deficit in learning new cue-response mappings. In contrast to this negative result, we later found that bilateral ablations of the orbital and ventral prefrontal cortex completely prevented monkeys from employing the Repeat-stay and Change-shift strategies (Bussey et al., 2001). Although we do not know whether the orbital or the ventral part of those lesions contributed most to the strategy deficit, some evidence involving reversible inactivations points to the ventral part (area 12) [Wang et al., 2000].

NEUROPHYSIOLOGY OF THE REPEAT-STAY AND CHANGE-SHIFT STRATEGIES

In our neurophysiological study (Genovesio et al., 2005), we operantly conditioned two monkeys to use the strategies that other monkeys, mentioned earlier, adopted spontaneously while engaged in conditional motor learning. Figure 5–2A illustrates the *strategy task* that we used. After a period of central fixation (converging dashed lines), a symbolic visual cue appeared on each trial, represented by the B in Figure 5–2A (second panel from the left). At the beginning of a block of approximately 100 trials, the monkeys had never seen that cue or either of the other two cues in the set (A, B, C). When the cue disappeared after an unpredictable period of 1.0 s, 1.5 s, or 2.0 s, the monkeys chose among three potential responses and expressed that choice by making a saccadic eye movement to fixate either the top, the left, or the right target. Figure 5–2A illustrates a response to the right target.

Figure 5–2B contrasts repeat trials and change trials. Before the end of each trial, we gave the monkeys an unlimited number of attempts to choose the

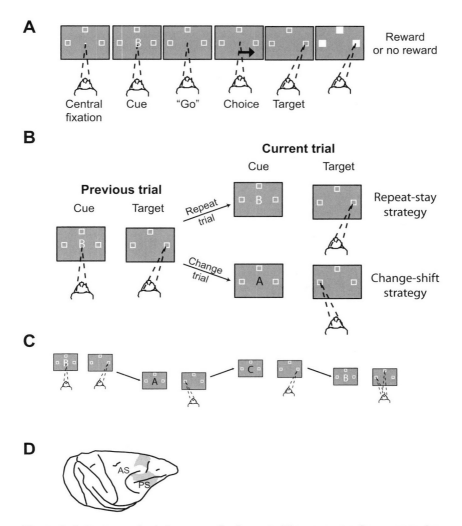

Figure 5–2 Strategy task. *A.* Sequence of task events. The *gray rectangles* represent the video screen; the *white squares* show the three potential response targets. The *white dot* at the center of the screen represents the fixation point, and the converging *dashed lines* indicate the gaze angle. After an initial fixation period, the cue appeared for 1–2 s, and its disappearance served as the trigger ("go") stimulus, after which the monkeys made a saccade (*solid arrow*) and maintained fixation at the chosen target. The target squares then filled with white, and reinforcement was delivered, when appropriate. *B.* Two trial types: repeat trials and change trials. *Top right.* The Repeat-stay strategy requires that the monkey choose the same target as on the previous trial. *Bottom right.* The Change-shift strategy requires the choice of a target other than the one chosen on the previous trial. *C.* Extension of the trial in *B* (*bottom right*) through two additional change trials. The response to the second *B* (*right*) cannot be to the right target, as it was for the first *B* (*second from left*). Either the left or the top target would be correct by the Change-shift strategy. *D.* The *gray shading* indicates the regions in the prefrontal cortex from which single neurons were sampled. AS, arcuate sulcus; PS, principal suclus.

response deemed correct. Thus, at the start of every *current trial,* the *previous trial* had always ended with a reward. Because the computer selected a stimulus pseudorandomly from the set (A, B, C), the cue from the previous trial (cue B in Fig. 5–2*B, left*), could either repeat, which occurred in one-third of the trials, or change, which happened in the remaining two-thirds of the trials. For a repeat trial, the monkeys produced a reward by choosing the same response as in the previous trial. In Figure 5–2*B*, this response was a saccade to the right target; for a change trial, the monkeys could have produced a reward only by choosing a different response, to either the top or the left target.

Unlike the conditional motor learning experiments described earlier (Fig. 5–1), in the strategy task, the monkeys could not learn a consistent relationship between a given cue and a particular response. Figure 5–2*C* illustrates the reason. Imagine that a trial with the C cue followed the one illustrated in the lower right of Figure 5–2*B*, which produced a reward. The monkey could not have chosen the left response after the C cue because, according to the Change-shift strategy, it had to reject its previous response, which was to the left. Now assume that the monkey chose the right response and that this, too, produced a reward. If the B cue followed next (Fig. 5–2*C, right*), a response to the right would have been precluded because the cue had changed and therefore the response had to shift to either the top or the left target. Thus, the first B cue in Figure 5–2*C* (left) led to a rightward response, but the second one could not. In this way, over the block of approximately 100 trials, each cue led to the choice of all three responses to a roughly equal extent.

Overall, both monkeys performed the strategy task correctly in more than 95% of the trials. As they did so, we monitored the discharge rates of single neurons in two parts of the prefrontal cortex, the dorsal prefrontal cortex (areas 6, 8, and 9) and dorsolateral prefrontal cortex (area 46) [Fig. 5–2*D*]. We found that the activity of many neurons reflected the strategy used on any given trial, both with and without response selectivity, and Figures 5–3 and 5–4 show one of each.

Figure 5–3 shows a prefrontal cortex neuron with activity that reflects the strategy used by the monkey on a particular trial, with a preference for the Change-shift strategy (Fig. 5–3*A* versus *B*). Note that there was no difference in activity for the three responses—top, left, or right—in either strategy. Because of this lack of response selectivity, we could not distinguish two correlates of this cell's activity: the fact that the stimulus changed from the previous trial or the fact that the monkey employed the Change-shift strategy. Note, as indicated in Figure 5–3*C*, that the difference between activity rates on change trials (*solid line*) and repeat trials (*dashed line*) developed in the period after the cue appeared. In the period just after the cue's onset, which occurred at time 0 in the plot (*solid vertical line*), there was a general increase in activity in both the repeat and change trials. Then, approximately 110 ms after cue onset (*dashed vertical line*), the average activity curves for this cell diverged, with activity on change trials reaching a slightly higher peak, but more impressively, demonstrating persistently higher activity during the period that the cue remained

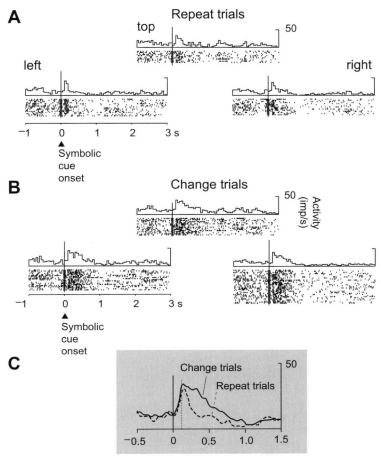

Figure 5–3 A cell exhibiting a strategy effect, but no target selectivity. *A.* The
cell's activity for the repeat trials appears in the top three displays, with each
raster line showing the time of an action potential (*tick mark*) in relation to a
temporal alignment point, the onset of the symbolic cue. Above each raster, a
histogram shows the average activity. Each trio of displays is arranged in the
pattern of the targets: left, top, and right. *B.* The cell's activity for the change trials
in the format of *A*. *C.* Activity for all three goals combined, separated for repeat
trials (*dashed line*) and change trials (*solid line*). The activity scale to the right of
each histogram gives mean discharge rates in impulses per second (imp/s).

visible (never less than 1.0 s). Note that the difference in activity between the
change and repeat trials decreased during the cue period, essentially disap-
pearing by 1.0 s after cue onset. Thus, this signal persisted for the time that
the monkeys needed to make a decision about what had occurred—change or
repeat—and which response to choose (or eliminate) on that basis. Like the

neuron shown in Figure 5–3, approximately 54% of the strategy-selective neurons in our prefrontal cortex sample lacked response selectivity. That is, they signaled whether the cue changed or repeated, or alternatively, whether the monkeys used the Change-shift or Repeat-stay strategy, but not what response the monkeys chose on that basis.

Figure 5–4 shows a more specific prefrontal cortex neuron. Like the neuron shown in Figure 5–3, this cell had higher activity on change trials (Fig. 5–4B) than on repeat trials (Fig. 5–4A). However, unlike the cell depicted in Figure 5–3, the one in Figure 5–4 could not simply have indicated that the cue had changed from the previous trial or that the Change-shift strategy was used: It showed virtually no activity modulation on change trials that led to rightward responses (Fig. 5–4B, right). Instead, the cell discharged when the monkey employed the Change-shift strategy for the other two responses. This finding shows that the cell had selectivity for the strategy as well as for the response

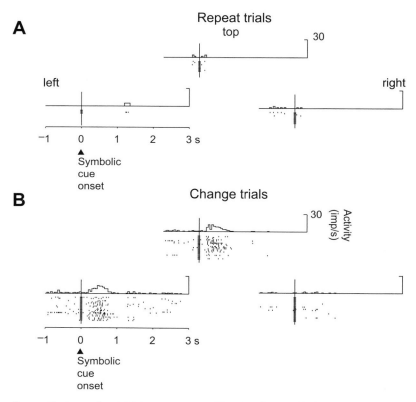

Figure 5–4 A cell exhibiting a strategy effect that is specific for one of the three potential goals. A. Activity for repeat trials in the format of Figure 5–3A. B. Activity for change trials in the format of Figure 5–3B. Note that the cell has a strong strategy effect (A versus B), but only for targets at the top and to the left.

selected on the basis of that strategy. It could not have signaled the response per se, because as shown in Figure 5–4A, the cell showed virtually no modulation when the monkey selected the left or top response on the basis of the Repeat-stay strategy. Approximately 46% of the strategy-selective neurons in our sample showed response selectivity of this sort.

The neuron illustrated in Figure 5–5 showed a different kind of strategy-related selectivity than the one shown in Figure 5–4. This cell's activity was specific for the cue that led to the Change-shift strategy. The boxed letters in Figure 5–5 (A, B, C) show the cues that appeared on both the previous trial and the current trial (as in Fig. 5–2B). This cell showed selectivity for the Change-shift strategy, like those illustrated in Figures 5–3 and 5–4. For

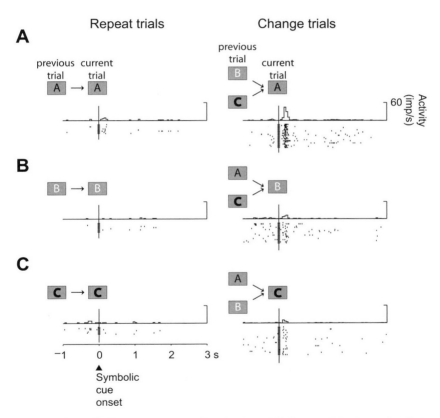

Figure 5–5 A cell showing a strategy effect that is specific for one of the three stimuli. *A.* Trials in which the stimulus on the current trial was designated "A." The format of each raster and histogram is as in Figures 5–3 and 5–4. *B.* Trials in which the stimulus on the current trial was designated "B." *C.* Trials in which the stimulus on the current trial was designated "C." *Left column.* Repeat trials. *Right column.* Change trials. Note that the cell has a strong strategy effect (left versus right column), but mostly for stimulus A.

example, when stimulus A appeared in the current trial (Fig. 5–5*A*), the cell discharged much more intensely on change trials (right) than on repeat trials (left). But unlike the neuron shown in Figure 5–4, which showed selectivity for the response during change trials, the neuron in Figure 5–5 showed selectivity for the cue (Fig. 5–5, *right, A versus B and C*). The cell did not simply respond to cue A, because had that been the case, it would not have shown any strategy selectivity. Nor did it simply reflect the fact that the stimulus had changed from the previous trial. Instead, this cell signaled the appearance of cue A only when it had not occurred on the previous trial, which meant that the monkey needed to employ the Change-shift strategy. The fact that this cell did not reflect the response selected on the current trial is not shown directly by Figure 5–5, but can be inferred from the trial-to-trial consistency in its activity for change trials with cue A. The cell discharged in a comparable way for all three responses. Approximately 20% of the strategy-selective neurons that were not selective for the response instead showed cue selectivity in the 400 ms after cue presentation.

Although all three of the cells illustrated in this chapter had a preference for the Change-shift strategy, this property was not characteristic of the population as a whole. Cells with a preference for the Repeat-stay and Change-shift strategies occurred in roughly equal numbers.

Figure 5–6 (see color insert) shows the average population activity for the neurons with strategy selectivity. In each of the four plots, the blue population averages show activity on change trials; the red averages show activity for the same cells on repeat trials. The cells were selected for each average on the basis of their having a statistically significant preference for either the change trials (Fig. 5–6*A*) or the repeat trials (Fig. 5–6*B*) in two monkeys. Before the onset of the cue, which occurred during a period of steady fixation on the video monitor (see Fig. 5–2*A*), neuronal activity was higher for the Change-shift–preferring cells than for the Repeat-stay–preferring cells. This fact is illustrated by the green dashed line marked *R* in Figure 5–6*A*, which corresponds to the activity level during the fixation period in Figure 5–6*B* for each monkey. Perhaps this difference reflected the fact that change trials occurred at twice the frequency of repeat trials; therefore, the overall population of prefrontal cortex neurons had a bias toward the Change-shift strategy. The cells preferring the Change-shift strategy (Fig. 5–6*A*) had a larger phasic activity increase on change trials (*green arrow*) than on repeat trials. In addition, on repeat trials, the level of activity quickly dropped below that during the fixation period, as shown by the red dashed line marked *F*, showing a net inhibition over the duration of the cue. The difference between the preferred and nonpreferred strategies persisted for at least as long as the shortest cue duration (1.0 s).

Figure 5–7 shows another way in which the population activity changed during the course of a trial. Cells encoding the cue decreased in proportion as the trial progressed, and those encoding the response increased concomitantly. Neurons encoding the strategy did not show any simple trend, but remained prevalent throughout the trial.

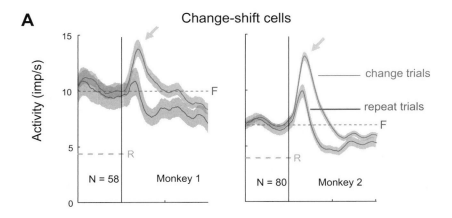

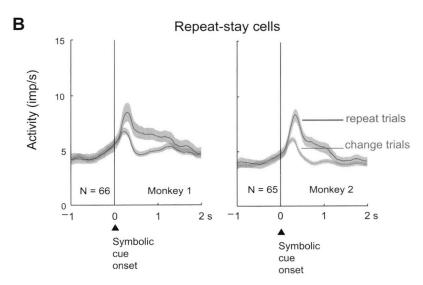

Figure 5–6 Population averages for neurons with selectivity for either the Change-shift strategy (*A*) or the Repeat-stay strategy (*B*), for two monkeys (left versus right column). The red curves show mean discharge rates for repeat trials; the blue curves show comparable data for change trials. The shading surrounding each curve shows activity rates±1 standard error of the mean. F, mean activity level for repeat trials during the fixation period; R, mean activity level during the fixation period for Repeat-stay cells.

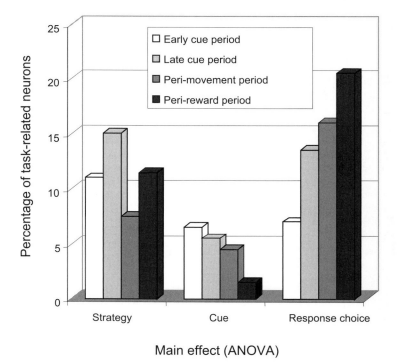

Main effect (ANOVA)

Figure 5–7 The proportion of cells with activity that reflects the main effects of strategy (*left*), cue (*middle*), and target (*right*), based on analysis of variance (ANOVA). Each set of four bars shows the proportion of the sample with the indicated main effect during four different periods of each trial (see Fig. 5–2A). The cue period was divided into an early part (up to 400 ms after cue onset) and a late part (from 400 ms until 1000 ms, the briefest of the three cue durations). The perimovement period extended from the "go" cue until the end of the saccade, and the perireward period began 420 ms before the reward delivery signal and lasted until 220 ms after the reward.

As noted earlier, implementation of the Repeat-stay and Change-shift strategies required the following:

1. Memory of the cue presented in the previous trial
2. Memory of the response chosen in the previous trial
3. Use of the cue memory to evaluate repeats and changes of the cue
4. Use of the response memory to reject or repeat the previous response

The activity of prefrontal cortex cells reflected three of these four cognitive processes. We found no evidence for cells storing information about the cue,

function 1, above, although such properties have been reported previously for neurons in prefrontal cortex (Rao et al., 1997; Rainer et al., 1998). Perhaps our recordings were too medial to observe such properties (see Fig. 5–2D). We did, however, find many cells related to the temporary storage of the previous response, function 2 (Genovesio et al., 2006). Some prefrontal neurons were selective for either the Repeat-stay or the Change-shift strategy, but showed no selectivity for the particular response chosen (Fig. 5–3). These characteristics coincide with function 3, above: the evaluation of stimulus repetition or change or selection of the correct strategy. Other cells were specific for the cue that either repeated or changed (Fig. 5–5). These cells could also have contributed to function 3. In yet other prefrontal cortex cells, the strategy-related activity was specific for a particular response (Fig. 5–4). These cells could contribute to function 4, which corresponds to the implementation of the abstract response strategy. So, of the four cognitive functions listed above, the prefrontal cortex neurons we sampled could support three, with memory of the previous cue depending on another region, perhaps the ventral prefrontal or sensory cortex.

STRATEGY VERSUS RULE ENCODING

We quantified the strength of the strategy effect by computing the receiver operating characteristic (ROC) for each prefrontal cortex neuron, using the mean firing rates across the period in which the cue appeared. Figure 5–8 shows the results of this analysis in comparison with rule-related activity from the same general regions of the prefrontal cortex (Wallis and Miller, 2003). ROC values measure the ability of an ideal, outside observer to decode which of the two strategies, in our experiment, or which of two rules, in the experiments from Wallis and Miller, occurred on any given trial. ROC values serve as a measure of strategy or rule selectivity, with 0.5 corresponding to no selectivity and higher values indicating progressively greater selectivity.

Comparing such measures between laboratories and experiments has several difficulties, but in both studies, the sample of neurons was collected on a "come-what-may" basis. We did our analysis in a way that matched theirs as closely as possible, although the number of trials collected for each rule or strategy differed. In our data, fewer trials were collected for each strategy, which biased our ROC analysis to produce lower values because of the increased influence of neural noise. Notwithstanding this disadvantage, Figure 5–8 shows that prefrontal cortex neurons reflected the Repeat-stay and Change-shift strategies more strongly than the matching and nonmatching rules studied by Wallis and Miller. Only 5% of their sample showed ROC values in excess of 0.7 for their rules, whereas approximately 20% of our neuronal sample did so for our strategies. The relative right shift of the *dashed lines* in Figure 5–8 indicates that the overall neuronal samples had the same tendency, which was highly statistically significant.

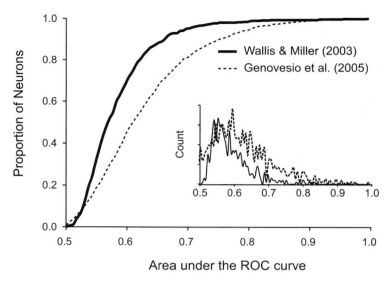

Figure 5–8 A comparison of rule encoding versus strategy encoding for prefrontal cortex cells. Data from the strategy task of Genovesio et al. (2005) [*dashed line*] and the rule task of Wallis and Miller (2003) [*solid line*]. *Inset.* A frequency distribution of the area under the receiver operating characteristic (ROC) curve for both neuronal samples (histograms of 100 bins, smoothed by spline interpolation). *Main plot.* Cumulative histogram of the same data. A high ROC value indicates that an ideal external observer could accurately estimate the rule or strategy that the monkey used, based on a single trial of neuronal activity, by comparing it with the overall distributions of activity levels for the two rules or the two strategies.

COMPARISON WITH OTHER STUDIES OF STRATEGIES AND RULES

Cortical Stimulation in Humans

The involvement of the prefrontal cortex in the use of different rules and strategies has also been supported by neuroimaging studies, as summarized by Bunge (2004), and in studies of event-related potentials (Folstein and Van Petten, 2004). We will not review these findings, which are covered in other chapters (see Chapters 3, 4, 9, 10, 12, and 16).

Beyond the neuroimaging data, however, one recent study showed that repetitive transcranial magnetic stimulation of the dorsolateral prefrontal cortex altered the decision-making strategy of participants engaged in a task that, by design, involved some choices that the participants perceived as unfair (van't Wout, 2005). This finding implicates the dorsolateral prefrontal cortex of humans, which is probably homologous to one of the regions that we studied in monkeys (Fig. 5–2D), in abstract response strategies.

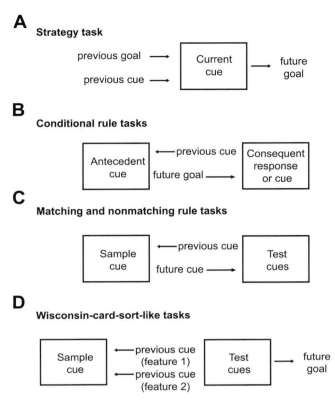

Figure 5–9 Comparison of rule and strategy tasks commonly used in neurophysiological studies of monkeys. *A.* The current strategy task (Genovesio et al., 2005). *B.* Tasks involving conditional motor learning or paired-associated learning. *C.* Matching-to-sample tasks and nonmatching-to-sample tasks, such as those used by Wallis and Miller (2003). *D.* Tasks derived from the Wisconsin Card Sorting task, such as that reported by Hoshi et al. (2000).

Neurophysiology in Monkeys

As reflected in other chapters in this volume (see Chapters 2, 11, 17, and 18), previous studies have also reported prefrontal cortex activity related to rules and strategies. Our findings on strategy-related neuronal activity in the prefrontal cortex agree, in general terms, with other studies of monkeys that indicate a role in either strategies or rules, at varying levels of abstraction (Collins et al., 1998; White and Wise, 1999; Wise and Murray, 1999; Asaad et al., 2000; Hoshi et al., 2000; Wallis and Miller, 2003; Barraclough et al., 2004). Figure 5–9 shows some of the tasks used in these previous studies (Fig. 5–9 *B* through *D*), in contrast with ours (Fig. 5–9*A*).

A representation of rules was found for location-matching and shape-matching rules (Hoshi et al., 2000), which resembled the Wisconsin Card Sorting Task (Fig. 5–9D). One previous study compared neuronal activity for spatial or object (Fig. 5–9C), and arbitrary, associative (Fig. 5–9B) rules and found many cells with activity that reflected each rule, even though the stimuli and responses did not differ (Asaad et al., 2000). Other studies have also compared arbitrary response rules (Fig. 5–9B) with spatial ones and have obtained similar results (White and Wise, 1999; Fuster et al., 2000). Barraclough et al. (2004) studied monkeys performing a task similar to the matching-pennies game, against a computer opponent. Their monkeys used both the Win-stay and Lose-shift strategies when the computer exploited only the biases in the monkeys' sequence of choices, but not when the computer exploited the biases in both the monkeys' choices and their reward history. Barraclough et al. (2004) found that signals related to the monkeys' past choices and their outcomes were combined in prefrontal cortex neurons, suggesting a role of the prefrontal cortex in optimizing decision-making strategies.

Neuropsychology in Monkeys

Gaffan et al. (2002) used a strategy task to demonstrate a deficit in strategy implementation after interruption of the connections between the frontal cortex and inferior temporal cortex. Their task differed from our strategy task in many ways, but perhaps the most important difference was that, in their task, the monkeys had to learn to classify visual, object-like stimuli into one of two categories, called "sporadic" and "persistent." Sporadic cues required the monkey to choose that cue only once to produce a reward, provided that they had just produced a reward by selecting a persistent cue. Persistent cues required four consecutive choices of that stimulus class to produce a reward. Thus, their task precluded the application of these strategies to novel stimuli; the monkeys first had to learn to classify the cues. In our strategy task, the monkeys responded by applying the Repeat-stay and Change-shift strategies to completely novel stimuli and could not associate any cue with a strategy or with differing amounts of effort needed to produce a reward.

Collins et al. (1998) used a spatial task to reveal a perseveration deficit after lateral frontal cortex lesions in marmosets. Their task was a spatial version of the self-ordered task, and it required these monkeys to choose each location, among a set of spatial targets, only once each to maximize the reward rate. The strategies that the monkeys adopted to perform this task consisted of choosing the targets in either a clockwise or a counterclockwise pattern, from one target to its nearest neighbor. Collins et al. (1998) found that, after ventral prefrontal cortex lesions (also known as the "lateral prefrontal cortex" in marmosets), these strategies broke down, which led to the perseveration that the investigators observed. This result supports the idea that the prefrontal cortex subserves the selection and implementation of response strategies. Like the

strategy task of Gaffan et al. (2002), described earlier, the task used by Collins et al. (1998) differed from ours in terms of cue novelty. Almost by definition, there were no novel places in their task. That is, the number of places was limited to a relatively small set. Although the pattern of locations that needed to be chosen on a given trial could occur in many combinations, and these combinations could be novel, the places per se quickly became familiar. This limitation is a feature of all spatial tasks: The number of places is limited by the size of the workspace and by the resolution required to distinguish one location from another. In contrast, in our task, each set of symbolic cues was novel in a way that spatial cues can never be, at least not in a task that requires many training and testing sessions. This difference is important because the ability to make decisions on the basis of completely novel inputs represents one of the key features of advanced cognition.

Together with the finding of Bussey et al. (2001), who showed that combined ventral and orbital prefrontal cortex lesions virtually abolished the Repeat-stay and Change-shift strategies, the fact that interfering with frontal cortex function caused strategy deficits in the two other tasks just mentioned, in both New World and Old World monkeys, suggests that a role in guiding decisions according to abstractions reflects a core function of the prefrontal cortex.

Having reviewed our neurophysiological results in comparison with other findings, we now turn to the final two questions: (1) How, if at all, do strategies differ from rules? (2) Are abstract response strategies the principal adaptive advantage conferred by the prefrontal cortex on primates?

DO STRATEGIES DIFFER FROM RULES?

Wise et al. (1996) proposed a distinction between higher-order and lower-order rules that might contribute to understanding some contrasts between strategies and rules. We pointed to evidence that the orbital prefrontal cortex mediates behavior-guiding rules based on objects and other object-like stimuli, especially those involving the linkage of objects with their biological value, sometimes called "affective valence" (Gaffan and Murray, 1990; Gaffan et al., 1993; Passingham, 1993). In contrast, monkeys with lesions restricted to the ventral prefrontal cortex fail on tests of object alternation; in nonmatching tasks with a single pair of objects (which differ very little from object alternation); and on delayed color-matching tasks with a single pair of colors (which differ very little from object non-alternation) [Passingham, 1975; Mishkin and Manning, 1978; Rushworth et al., 1997]. The tasks dependent on the orbital prefrontal cortex require decisions about the value of a given object, which monkeys can learn through response rules of the type "approach stimulus A" and "avoid stimulus B." The tasks dependent on the ventral prefrontal cortex require the use of rules based on abstract aspects of objects, rather than specific objects or their features. These tasks require choices based on objects, but

the object per se does not tell the monkey what to do. In one trial, a given object is to be chosen, but in the next trial, the same object is to be avoided.

This contrast with work in macaque monkeys is consistent with findings on marmosets, which discriminated compound stimuli consisting of colored shapes (one stimulus dimension) with white lines superimposed on them (a second dimension) [Dias et al., 1996a, b; Roberts and Wallis, 2000]. Marmosets with orbital prefrontal cortex lesions showed deficits on intradimensional shifts (choices based on object-like stimuli), whereas those with ventral prefrontal cortex lesions performed relatively poorly on extradimensional shifts (choices based on abstractions of stimuli). In the latter case, response rules, such as "approach object A" or "avoid object B," were inadequate. The monkeys must instead have learned a higher-order response rule that requires abstract information about objects, in words: "choose according to cue dimension."

Thus, Wise et al. (1996) put forward the idea that the orbital prefrontal cortex learns about specific objects (exemplars), whereas the ventral prefrontal cortex learns about abstractions concerning objects, and both use this knowledge in decision-making. For the former, termed "lower-order rules," objects can guide action. For the latter, termed "higher-order rules," a lower-order rule, such as "approach stimulus A," cannot do the job, and the monkeys must learn a higher-order rule that employs abstract information about objects. Thus, lower-order rules involve exemplars; higher-order rules involve abstractions.

As Pinker (1999) has pointed out, the dichotomy between memorized exemplars and abstractions is important, both scientifically and philosophically. Memorization plays a central role in associationist thought, including behaviorist traditions that emphasize simple S-R associations. In addition to associationist, behaviorist, and animal learning theory models of behavior, exemplar-based processing figures prominently in connectionist neural network theory, and broadly construed, in philosophical empiricism. Rules, strategies, and other behaviors based on abstractions figure prominently in cognitive neuroscience and computational models that manipulate symbols. Again, broadly construed, an emphasis on abstractions leads to philosophical rationalism. The interaction between empirical knowledge based on exemplars and rational knowledge based on analogies, inferences, categorizations, and other abstractions fuels advanced cognition in a way that neither could, alone.

In this context, the relationship between rules and strategies can be reconsidered. To a first approximation, the concepts of rules and strategies differ little. Both involve, as a dictionary definition holds, "a prescribed guide for conduct or action" (*Webster's New Collegiate Dictionary*, 1971). However, rules come in both higher-order and lower-order varieties, as distinguished earlier. As a practical matter, strategies do not: They depend on abstractions. Lower-order rules are based on memorized exemplars; higher-order rules and strategies are also "a prescribed guide for conduct or action," but are based on abstractions.

The incipient ability to base decisions on abstractions rather than exemplars must have been a powerful adaptive advantage to the animals that could do so, and the final section of this chapter addresses that issue.

ARE ABSTRACT RESPONSE STRATEGIES THE PRINCIPAL ADAPTIVE ADVANTAGE CONFERRED BY THE PREFRONTAL CORTEX ON PRIMATES?

Neurophysiological studies of the primate prefrontal cortex usually explore behavioral capabilities common to primates and other mammals. Yet, a body of evolutionary thought indicates that the largest part of the primate prefrontal cortex, the granular frontal cortex, is an evolutionary innovation of primates and, therefore, was not present in the ancestral condition (Preuss, 1995). If the selection and implementation of abstract response strategies depends on the prefrontal cortex, and the (granular) prefrontal cortex is a primate innovation, then could abstract response strategies be the principal adaptive advantage conferred by the prefrontal cortex on primates?

Neurophysiological studies have produced a list of roles for the prefrontal cortex, including categorization (Freedman et al., 2002, see also Chapter 17); predictive coding (Rainer et al., 1999); attentional control, especially of the top-down variety (Miller et al., 1996; Lebedev et al., 2004); the detection and generation of event sequences across time (Quintana and Fuster, 1999; Averbeck et al., 2002; Ninokura et al., 2003; Hoshi and Tanji, 2004), sometimes termed "cross-temporal contingencies" (Fuster, 1997); behavioral inhibition; and preparatory set (Fuster, 1997). Yet, each of these cognitive operations, not to mention those involving rules (Hoshi et al., 1998; White and Wise, 1999; Asaad et al., 2000; Wallis et al., 2001; Wallis and Miller, 2003), contributes to both the selection and the implementation of abstract response strategies. Decisions based on abstractions require a number of coordinated processes, including the top-down biasing of inputs to the prefrontal cortex; the categorization of contextual information, including sensory inputs, memories, and signals about internal states; the integration of contextual information with the actions and goals appropriate to that context; the choice among potential actions or goals, based on the predicted outcome of each possibility; and active maintenance of those choices or goals in memory, as a prospective code, without completely dispensing with the alternatives. The prefrontal cortex probably contributes to all of these functions, and all of them are necessary for the selection and implementation of abstract response strategies. Thus, it is not surprising that neurophysiological studies, each focused on one or a few of these functions, would find evidence for all of them.

Neuropsychological and neuroimaging research studies have produced several attempts to subsume prefrontal cortex function within a single construct. One holds that the principal function of the prefrontal cortex is working memory (i.e., maintaining information in short-term memory to manipulate it) [Goldman-Rakic, 1987]. Another proposes that the prefrontal cortex contributes to behavior whenever problems exceed a certain level of difficulty, requiring a departure from the automatic, or routine, functions of daily life (Duncan et al., 1996; Duncan and Owen, 2000; Gaffan, 2002). Yet another posits that the principal function of the prefrontal cortex is to attentively select

and monitor information in short-term memory, including plans and intentions (Owen et al., 1996; Rowe and Passingham, 2001; Petrides et al., 2002; Rowe et al., 2002; Lau et al., 2004).

Could these three ideas, too, be incorporated under the banner of "abstract response strategies"? They could, perhaps, if the emergence of the prefrontal cortex in the primate lineage is taken into account. (1) Many of the processes involved in strategies require working memory, which could foster the idea that working memory is the principal function of the prefrontal cortex. Working memory is not a primate innovation, but some forms of behavioral guidance by abstractions might be (Tomasello and Call, 1997), so the latter is probably more central to prefrontal function than the former. (2) Routine, or automatic, functions require few of the processes needed for abstract response strategies. Routine behaviors can run on autopilot control. Thus, the prefrontal cortex should become engaged whenever a difficult problem needs to be addressed and an abstract strategy needs to be employed. (3) Attentional selection (Rowe and Passingham, 2001; Rowe et al., 2002) and the monitoring of items in working memory (Owen et al., 1996; Petrides et al., 2002) cannot make a direct contribution to the inclusive fitness of monkeys. Instead, they must contribute indirectly, through their effects on adaptive actions, and this contribution likely takes the form of a contribution to the selection and monitoring of abstract response strategies.

It would be misguided, however, to substitute a different monolithic theory of prefrontal cortex function for those mentioned earlier. Even if a principal function of the prefrontal cortex is the selection and implementation of abstract response strategies, when experiments isolate the various cognitive processes that underlie this capacity, they will find evidence for each of them. As a whole, then, the current suggestion differs little from the proposal that the prefrontal cortex contributes to most, if not all, of the cognitive functions important to the life of primates (Gaffan, 2002). However, perhaps all of these functions have their largest biological importance when applied to the learning, implementation, and selection of abstract response strategies. In this way, the prefrontal cortex could contribute the key adaptive advantages in managing the cognitive challenges faced by primates.

ACKNOWLEDGMENTS We acknowledge the pivotal contribution that Dr. Peter Brasted made to our strategy experiment.

REFERENCES

Asaad WF, Rainer G, Miller EK (2000) Task-specific neural activity in the primate prefrontal cortex. Journal of Neurophysiology 84:451–459.

Averbeck BB, Chafee MV, Crowe DA, Georgopoulos AP (2002) Parallel processing of serial movements in prefrontal cortex. Proceedings of the National Academy of Sciences U S A 99:13172–13177.

Barraclough DJ, Conroy ML, Lee D (2004) Prefrontal cortex and decision making in a mixed-strategy game. Nature Neuroscience 7:404–410.

Bunge M (2003) Philosophical dictionary. New York: Prometheus.

Bunge SA (2004) How we use rules to select actions: a review of evidence from cognitive neuroscience. Cognitive, Affective and Behavioral Neuroscience 4:564–579.

Burling R (2005) The talking ape: how language evolved. Oxford, UK: Oxford University Press.

Bussey TJ, Wise SP, Murray EA (2001) The role of ventral and orbital prefrontal cortex in conditional visuomotor learning and strategy use in rhesus monkeys. Behavioral Neuroscience 115:971–982.

Collins P, Roberts AC, Dias R, Everitt BJ, Robbins TW (1998) Perseveration and strategy in a novel spatial self-ordered sequencing task for nonhuman primates: effects of excitotoxic lesions and dopamine depletions of the prefrontal cortex. Journal of Cognitive Neuroscience 10:332–354.

Dias R, Robbins TW, Roberts AC (1996a) Dissociation in prefrontal cortex of affective and attentional shifts. Nature 380:69–72.

Dias R, Robbins TW, Roberts AC (1996b) Primate analogue of the Wisconsin Card Sorting Test: effects of excitotoxic lesions of the prefrontal cortex in the marmoset. Behavioral Neuroscience 110:872–886.

di Pellegrino G, Wise SP (1993a) Effects of attention on visuomotor activity in the premotor and prefrontal cortex of a primate. Somatosensory and Motor Research 10:245–262.

di Pellegrino G, Wise SP (1993b) Visuospatial vs. visuomotor activity in the premotor and prefrontal cortex of a primate. Journal of Neuroscience 13:1227–1243.

Duncan J, Emslie H, Williams P, Johnson R, Freer C (1996) Intelligence and the frontal lobe: the organization of goal-directed behavior. Cognitive Psychology 30:257–303.

Duncan J, Owen AM (2000) Common regions of the human frontal lobe recruited by diverse cognitive demands. Trends in Neuroscience 23:475–483.

Folstein JR, Van Petten C (2004) Multidimensional rule, unidimensional rule, and similarity strategies in categorization: event-related brain potential correlates. Journal of Experimental Psychology: Learning, Memory and Cognition 30:1026–1044.

Freedman DJ, Riesenhuber M, Poggio T, Miller EK (2002) Visual categorization and the primate prefrontal cortex: neurophysiology and behavior. Journal of Neurophysiology 88:929–941.

Fuster JM (1997) The prefrontal cortex: anatomy, physiology and neuropsychology of the frontal lobe, 3rd edition. New York: Lippincott-Raven.

Fuster JM, Bodner M, Kroger JK (2000) Cross-modal and cross-temporal association in neurons of frontal cortex. Nature 405:347–351.

Gaffan D (2002) Against memory systems. Philosophical Transactions of the Royal Society of London B 357:1111–1121.

Gaffan D, Easton A, Parker A (2002) Interaction of inferior temporal cortex with frontal cortex and basal forebrain: double dissociation in strategy implementation and associative learning. Journal of Neuroscience 22:7288–7296.

Gaffan D, Murray EA (1990) Amygdalar interaction with the mediodorsal nucleus of the thalamus and the ventromedial prefrontal cortex in stimulus-reward associative learning in the monkey. Journal of Neuroscience 10:3479–3493.

Gaffan D, Murray EA, Fabre-Thorpe M (1993) Interaction of the amygdala with the frontal lobe in reward memory. European Journal of Neuroscience 5:968–975.

Genovesio A, Brasted PJ, Mitz AR, Wise SP (2005) Prefrontal cortex activity related to abstract response strategies. Neuron 47:307–320.

Genovesio A, Brasted PJ, Wise SP (2006) Representation of future and previous spatial goals by separate neural populations in prefrontal cortex. Journal of Neuroscience 26:7281–7292.

Goldman-Rakic PS (1987) Circuitry of primate prefrontal cortex and regulation of behavior by representational memory. In: Handbook of physiology: the nervous system, (Plum F, Mountcastle VB, eds.), pp 373–417, volume 5. Bethesda: American Physiological Society.

Hoshi E, Shima K, Tanji J (1998) Task-dependent selectivity of movement-related neuronal activity in the primate prefrontal cortex. Journal of Neurophysiology 80: 3392–3397.

Hoshi E, Shima K, Tanji J (2000) Neuronal activity in the primate prefrontal cortex in the process of motor selection based on two behavioral rules. Journal of Neurophysiology 83:2355–2373.

Hoshi E, Tanji J (2004) Area-selective neuronal activity in the dorsolateral prefrontal cortex for information retrieval and action planning. Journal of Neurophysiology 91:2707–2722.

Lau HC, Rogers RD, Ramnani N, Passingham RE (2004) Willed action and attention to the selection of action. Neuroimage 21:1407–1415.

Lebedev MA, Messinger A, Kralik JD, Wise SP (2004) Representation of attended versus remembered locations in prefrontal cortex. Public Library of Science: Biology 2:1919–1935.

Miller EK, Erickson CA, Desimone R (1996) Neural mechanisms of visual working memory in prefrontal cortex of the macaque. Journal of Neuroscience 16:5154–5167.

Mishkin M, Manning FJ (1978) Non-spatial memory after selective prefrontal lesions in monkeys. Brain Research 143:313–323.

Murray EA, Wise SP (1996) Role of the hippocampus plus subjacent cortex but not amygdala in visuomotor conditional learning in rhesus monkeys. Behavioral Neuroscience 110:1261–1270.

Ninokura Y, Mushiake H, Tanji J (2003) Representation of the temporal order of visual objects in the primate lateral prefrontal cortex. Journal of Neurophysiology 89: 2868–2873.

Owen AM, Evans AC, Petrides M (1996) Evidence for a two-stage model of spatial working memory processing within the lateral frontal cortex: a positron emission tomography study. Cerebral Cortex 6:31–38.

Passingham RE (1975) Delayed matching after selective prefrontal lesions in monkeys. Brain Research 92:89–102.

Passingham RE (1993) The frontal lobes and voluntary action. Oxford, UK: Oxford University Press.

Petrides M, Alivisatos B, Frey S (2002) Differential activation of the human orbital, midventrolateral, and mid-dorsolateral prefrontal cortex during the processing of visual stimuli. Proceedings of the National Academy of Sciences U S A 99:5649–5654.

Pinker S (1999) Word and rules. New York: Basic Books.

Preuss TM (1995) Do rats have a prefrontal cortex? The Rose-Woolsey-Akert program reconsidered. Journal of Cognitive Neuroscience 7:1–24.

Quintana J, Fuster JM (1999) From perception to action: temporal integrative functions of prefrontal and parietal neurons. Cerebral Cortex 9:213–221.

Rainer G, Asaad WF, Miller EK (1998) Memory fields of neurons in the primate prefrontal cortex. Proceedings of the National Academy of Sciences U S A 95:15008–15013.

Rainer G, Rao SC, Miller EK (1999) Prospective coding for objects in primate prefrontal cortex. Journal of Neuroscience 19:5493–5505.

Rao SC, Rainer G, Miller EK (1997) Integration of what and where in the primate prefrontal cortex. Science 276:821–824.

Roberts AC, Wallis JD (2000) Inhibitory control and affective processing in the prefrontal cortex: neuropsychological studies in the common marmoset. Cerebral Cortex 10:252–262.

Rowe J, Friston K, Frackowiak R, Passingham R (2002) Attention to action: specific modulation of corticocortical interactions in humans. Neuroimage 17:988–998.

Rowe JB, Passingham RE (2001) Working memory for location and time: activity in prefrontal area 46 relates to selection rather than maintenance in memory. Neuroimage 14:77–86.

Rushworth MFS, Nixon PD, Eacott MJ, Passingham RE (1997) Ventral prefrontal cortex is not essential for working memory. Journal of Neuroscience 17:4829–4838.

Tomasello M, Call J (1997) Primate cognition. New York: Oxford University Press.

van't Wout M (2005) Repetitive transcranial magnetic stimulation over the right dorsolateral prefrontal cortex affects strategic decision-making. Neuroreport 16:1849–1852.

Wallis JD, Anderson KC, Miller EK (2001) Single neurons in prefrontal cortex encode abstract rules. Nature 411:953–956.

Wallis JD, Miller EK (2003) From rule to response: neuronal processes in the premotor and prefrontal cortex. Journal of Neurophysiology 90:1790–1806.

Wang M, Zhang H, Li BM (2000) Deficit in conditional visuomotor learning by local infusion of bicuculline into the ventral prefrontal cortex in monkeys. European Journal of Neuroscience 12:3787–3796.

White IM, Wise SP (1999) Rule-dependent neuronal activity in the prefrontal cortex. Experimental Brain Research 126:315–335.

Wise SP, Murray EA (1999) Role of the hippocampal system in conditional motor learning: mapping antecedents to action. Hippocampus 9:101–117.

Wise SP, Murray EA, Gerfen CR (1996) The frontal cortex-basal ganglia system in primates. Critical Reviews in Neurobiology 10:317–356.

6

Abstraction of Mental Representations: Theoretical Considerations and Neuroscientific Evidence

Kalina Christoff and Kamyar Keramatian

The ability to conceive of highly abstract concepts is a fundamental feature of human cognition. Using abstract mental representations, we can organize perceptions garnered from disparate experiences, develop novel solutions to problems we encounter, and predict future outcomes based on past experiences. All of these faculties have been shown to rely on the integrity of the lateral prefrontal cortex (e.g., Milner, 1964; Luria, 1966; Shallice, 1982; Duncan et al., 1995). Understanding abstract thought and the nature of abstract mental representations, therefore, may provide a useful framework for understanding the functions and organization of lateral prefrontal cortex.

In this chapter, we focus on the evidence and implications for an organization of prefrontal cortex according to different levels of abstraction in representational content. In the first section, we offer a historical review of some of the central concepts found in philosophical theories of abstraction and discuss how they motivate contemporary investigation in the field of cognitive neuroscience.

In the second section, we describe two recent functional neuroimaging experiments that examine the role of abstract representations in terms of lateral prefrontal cortex organization. The results of these experiments suggest a topographical organization of lateral prefrontal regions according to the level of abstraction in representational content (Fig. 6–1). This topography appears to follow an arcuate[1] posterior-to-anterior direction, with concrete working memory representations corresponding to posterior prefrontal regions and representations at increasing levels of abstraction corresponding to progressively anterior regions.

HISTORICAL DEVELOPMENT IN THEORIES OF ABSTRACTION

Discussions of abstraction are ubiquitous in cognitive neuroscience literature, with terms such as "abstract cognitive abilities," "abstract thought," and

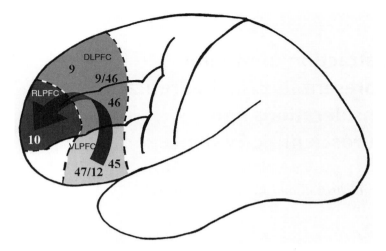

Figure 6–1 Proposed arcuate topography in the human lateral prefrontal cortex. The arrow depicts the direction of the proposed gradient of abstraction, with increasing levels of abstraction in working memory representation located toward the anterior prefrontal cortex. Numbers indicate Brodmann areas in lateral prefrontal cortex. DLPFC, dorsolateral prefrontal cortex; RLPFC, rostrolateral prefrontal cortex; VLPFC, ventrolateral prefrontal cortex.

"abstract rules" almost invariably employed when lateral prefrontal functions are discussed (e.g., Milner, 1963; Luria, 1966; Baker et al., 1996; Christoff and Gabrieli, 2000; O'Reilly et al., 2002; Bunge et al., 2003; Miller et al., 2003; Sakai and Passingham, 2003). Despite this widespread use, there is considerable ambiguity concerning the meaning of this term. Sometimes "abstractness" is equated with difficulty of comprehension or lack of intrinsic form; oftentimes, the term is simply left undefined. For our purposes, we hearken back to its roots in the Latin *abstrahere,* meaning "to drag away," and emphasize that abstract concepts are removed from specific instances.

The manner in which abstract concepts are "dragged away" from the specific has been the subject of much debate among thinkers. As George Berkeley wrote, "He who is not a perfect stranger to the writings and disputes of philosophers, must needs acknowledge that no small part of them are spent about abstract ideas" (Berkeley, 1734/1998). Here we review the development of some of the central philosophical concepts concerning abstraction.

Philosophical Theories of Abstraction

The idea for a distinction between abstract and concrete entities emerged as early as the time of Plato (c. 427–347 BCE), who contributed an early notion of

abstraction with his theory of forms (Plato, 360 BCE/2003). Plato believed that separate from the flawed, imperfect realm of sensation is a perfect realm of forms, such as "beauty," "goodness," "equality," "likeness," "sameness," and "difference," which give structure to our world. In Plato's view, "sensibles," or objects of sensation, draw their characteristics from forms. Many beautiful objects exist, but all draw their common characteristic from a single form, namely, beauty.

Plato's view that forms and sensibles occupy different realms has been opposed by those who believe that forms and sensibles must inform each other, and as such, cannot be so completely separated. Aristotle (384–322 BCE), Plato's student, was one thinker who believed that sensation and form are inseparable. In Aristotle's view, form is embedded in sensation, and separating form from the sensory world, therefore, is a dubious matter (Aristotle, 350 BCE/2002). This idea of dynamic and interactive abstract and concrete concepts is important to cognitive theories of abstraction today.

Plato and Aristotle saw abstractness in objective terms, viewing forms and sensibles as entities that existed in the absolute. Later philosophers, such as John Locke and George Berkeley, viewed abstraction as a mental concept, and accordingly framed the discussion of the abstract-concrete distinction within the mind. In his *Essay Concerning Human Understanding*, John Locke distinguishes between particular and general ideas. Particular ideas are constrained to specific contexts in space and time. General ideas are free from such restraints and thus can be applied to many different situations. In Locke's view, abstraction is the process in which "ideas taken from particular beings become general representatives of all of the same kind" by dint of the mind's removing particular circumstances from an idea (Locke, 1690/1979).

Locke's idea of abstraction faced criticism from later thinkers, such as George Berkeley (1685–1753). In the introduction to his *Treatise Concerning the Principles of Human Knowledge*, Berkeley attacks Locke's notion that one individual quality of an object can be isolated from other qualities (Berkeley, 1734/1998). For example, he argued, it is impossible to imagine the motion of an object without also imagining its shape, color, and direction.

As an alternative to Locke's account, Berkeley argues that abstraction occurs through a shift in attention. In this view, a particular object can represent a group of objects when we focus attention on one of its qualities. For example, the image of a particular triangle, regardless of whether it is equilateral, isosceles, scalene, right, obtuse, or acute, can be used to represent all possible triangles when attention is focused on its feature of having three connecting line segments.

Berkeley thus introduced the notion that attention plays an important role in the process of extracting abstract ideas. The idea that abstraction occurs through focusing attention on a particular feature—a process today referred to as "selective attention"—has inspired many subsequent empirical developments and is central to a number of present-day theories of abstraction.

Cognitive Theories of Abstraction

The study of abstract ideas has more recently become a subject of investigations in the empirical disciplines of cognitive science, psychology, linguistics, and cognitive neuroscience. Contemporary thinkers in these fields have extended philosophical theories of abstraction by incorporating ideas of attention, perception, and neural connectivity.

One cognitive theory, developed in a series of works by George Lakoff and Mark Johnson, argues for a dichotomy of abstract and concrete concepts based on metaphorical understanding (Lakoff and Johnson, 1980a, b, 1999). More concrete concepts, such as "up," "down," "front," "back," "substance," "container," "motion," and "food," are understood directly from bodily experience. More abstract concepts, such as "time," "emotions," "communication," "mind," and "ideas," are understood and structured in terms of more concrete and embodied concepts. For example, the abstract concept of "idea" can be understood metaphorically through the more concrete concepts of "commodity" ("How you package your ideas is important") or "food" ("This idea is hard to digest").

Notably, even the relatively concrete concepts described by Lakoff and Johnson are abstracted from more specific instances. For example, "food" is more abstract than the specific instances of "burrito" or "cheesecake." We can thus interpret Lakoff and Johnson's theory as part of a three-tier hierarchy of abstraction. Abstract concepts are understood by metaphorically mapping them onto relatively less abstract concepts, which in turn are learned by abstracting specific concrete instances encountered through sensation. Evidence for a similar three-level system of abstraction in representation is suggested by the neuroimaging findings presented later in this chapter.

In Lakoff and Johnson's theory, the way in which highly abstract concepts are specifically mapped onto less abstract ones is determined by which metaphorical features are emphasized and which are de-emphasized, a process the authors refer to as "highlighting" and "hiding" (Lakoff and Johnson, 1980b). When we think of an argument in terms of war ("She shot down my argument," "He attacked the weak points of my argument"), we highlight the combative aspects and hide the cooperative aspects of the situation. We have a different understanding of an argument if we think of it in terms of a process of achieving mutual understanding ("He responded to each point in my argument"), thus highlighting its cooperative aspects and hiding its combative aspects. Whereas Berkeley posited an idea of mapping concrete to abstract concepts with selective attention, Lakoff and Johnson emphasize the role of selective attention in mapping highly abstract, metaphorical concepts to relatively less abstract, nonmetaphorical concepts.

Other contemporary cognitive theories of abstraction do not rely on metaphor. For example, Lawrence Barsalou (1999) criticizes Lakoff and Johnson's theory on the grounds that metaphorical mappings alone cannot produce adequate conceptual understanding. Knowing that an idea is like a commodity

and like food, for example, is hardly sufficient for understanding the concept of "idea." Furthermore, Barsalou notes that Lakoff and Johnson ignore the possibility that much of what they denote "conceptual metaphor" may actually just function as polysemy. For instance, in the sentence "He attacked the weak points in my argument," the word "attack" may function in two distinct ways— as both a physical action intended to cause harm and an attempted logical criticism.

Instead, Barsalou advocates for a theory wherein connections between concrete and abstract concepts are direct and nonmetaphorical. In this theory, concepts take the form of simulators, which are semantic clusters that can generate infinite further examples of a concept. As we encounter examples of objects, we encode their perceptual features and store them in our memories. These features will form into clusters, which eventually become simulators, with a frame of previously encountered common features and a set of infinite possible simulations that the frame can generate. For instance, our perceptual experience with various chairs has helped us form a concept of "chair." We can now use this concept to simulate infinite further examples of chairs.

An abstract concept is understood in this system through three sequential processes. First, the concept is put into context by simulating an event sequence, or a system of projected actions associated with the concept. When we represent the abstract concept of "magic," for example, we may simulate the actions of wand-waving, disappearance, and spontaneous transformation. Next, selective attention will extract features of this event sequence that are relevant to an understanding of the concept and to the internal state of the conceptual thinker. Thus, a skeptic may emphasize more the agents of artifice in his event simulations of the concept, whereas a believer may emphasize the miraculous features. Finally, introspective perceptual systems are employed in the interpretation of these selective concept attributes. These systems include emotional states; cognitive operations, such as search and comparison; and idiosyncratic systems of perceptual construal.

Barsalou's theory provides a viable mechanism for concept dynamism and unconscious abstract representation. In addition, it builds on findings from neuroscience. Research showing the existence of neurons selective for certain object properties, such as color, orientation, and velocity, supports Barsalou's proposed mechanism of conceptual clustering (Hubel and Wiesel, 1968; Wandell, 1995; Simoncelli and Heeger, 1998). This framework thus provides a promising preliminary link between theories of abstract thought and findings in neuroscience.

NEUROSCIENTIFIC EVIDENCE FOR ABSTRACTION OF REPRESENTATIONS IN LATERAL PREFRONTAL CORTEX

In the previous section, we reviewed some of the major theories concerning abstract notions and how these notions are represented in the mind. In this section, we will discuss how these abstract concepts are represented in the

brain. As mentioned earlier, our focus in this part will be on lateral prefrontal cortex and its functional organization. In particular, we argue that lateral prefrontal cortex is organized according to working memory representations at different levels of abstraction, with the most anterior part corresponding to the highest level of abstraction. In the following paragraphs, we will present some experimental results providing support for this conceptualization of prefrontal function.

Several studies on nonhuman primates have shown that prefrontal cortex plays a key role in abstract rule-guided behaviors (Wallis et al., 2001; Nieder et al., 2002; Bunge et al., 2003; Miller et al., 2003; see also Chapters 2 and 18). Single neurons in the monkey prefrontal cortex encode abstract rules and not simply the physical properties of the stimuli (Wallis et al., 2001). It has also been suggested that different prefrontal subregions deal distinctively with abstract and concrete information (Dias et al., 1996, 1997; see also Chapter 13). Dias and colleagues reported such distinction by using the intradimensional-extradimensional dynamic categorization task in marmoset monkeys. Deficits in intradimensional reversals, which require feature-level representation, were associated with orbitofrontal lesions, whereas deficits in extradimensional shifts, which require dimension-level representation, corresponded to dorsolateral prefrontal cortex (DLPFC) lesions. Building on the results from this study, O'Reilly and colleagues designed a computational model using a combination of activation-based working memory and frontal representations organized according to two different levels of abstraction (O'Reilly et al., 2002). Together, these studies introduced a distinction between concrete and abstract working memory representations in the brains of nonhuman primates.

Humans, however, appear capable of higher forms of abstraction in mental representation than those exhibited by nonhuman primates. Examples of such higher-level abstraction in mental processing include integrating multiple relations simultaneously (Halford, 1984; Thompson et al., 1997) and solving analogies (Holyoak and Kroger, 1995; Gentner et al., 2001). Results from neuroimaging studies show that behaviors that require the use of abstract rules, such as reasoning and problem-solving, specifically activate the most anterior part of lateral prefrontal cortex, also known as rostrolateral prefrontal cortex (RLPFC), or lateral Brodmann area (BA) 10 (Baker et al., 1996; Christoff and Gabrieli, 2000; Christoff et al., 2001, 2003; Bunge et al., 2003; Bunge et al., 2005). This region is activated during the processing of highly abstract mental representations, such as internally generated information (Christoff and Gabrieli, 2000; Christoff et al., 2003), future task operations (Sakai and Passingham, 2003), abstract hierarchies of goals (Koechlin et al., 1999; Braver and Bongiolatti, 2002) and even meta-awareness during mind-wandering (Christoff et al., 2004; Smith et al., 2006). Comparative studies of BA 10 in human and nonhuman primates have revealed that this area occupies a proportionally larger volume of brain in humans than in other primates (Semendeferi et al., 2001), although the extent of this difference continues to be debated (Holloway, 2002).

When combined, the evidence from studies in humans and nonhuman primates suggests a possible organization of lateral prefrontal cortex based on the level of abstraction in working memory representation, a theory that we have recently proposed (Christoff, 2003). Here we describe two recent experiments designed to test this hypothesis directly.

Following Rules at Different Levels of Abstraction: The Role of Lateral Prefrontal Cortex

To examine the possibility that rule-guided behavior at different levels of abstraction activates different prefrontal subregions, we constructed a task that involved rule-guided behavior and rule reversal at three levels of abstraction (Christoff et al., manuscript under review-a). Thirteen healthy volunteers were recruited to undergo functional magnetic resonance imaging (fMRI) scanning while performing the task. The experiment comprised three sessions, each containing 140 trials grouped into three different conditions: concrete rule, first-order abstract rule, and second-order abstract rule (Fig. 6–2). In the concrete condition, the target was a single circle whose black side was oriented in one of four directions—right, left, up, or down—as determined by a cue at the beginning of each block. In the first-order abstract rule, the cue identified the target as a pair of circles whose orientation could be either "same" or "different." Finally, in the second-order abstract condition, the target consisted of two pairs of circles that could be either "related" (two pairs that were either "same"- "same" or "different"- "different") or "unrelated" ("same"- "different" or "different"- "same").

Each condition started with a cue that determined both the level of abstraction (condition) and the applicable rule at each level, followed by a series of visual stimuli. In all conditions, the stimuli were two pairs of circles separated by a vertical line. Each circle consisted of one white and one black semicircle. In each condition, after a number of successive trials, the rule reversed (Fig. 6–3). There were five reversals per session. In all conditions, participants pressed the left button to indicate that the target was present on the screen, or the right button to indicate that the target was not present. Their response was followed by immediate feedback on every trial.

Statistical parametric mapping analysis was performed to determine which areas of the brain are activated during reversals at each level of abstraction (i.e., concrete, first order of abstraction, and second order of abstraction). The effects of reversal were modeled using parametric modulation within an event-related model (Buchel et al., 1998). Each reversal was modeled as an event, and a parametric regressor was then constructed using "time prior to reversal" (i.e., the time elapsed after the last reversal). This allowed us to model the effects of stronger engagement of executive control at reversals occurring after larger number of trials spent following the same rule (i.e., looking for the same target).

The areas of prefrontal cortex that were activated during reversals at each level of abstraction are shown in Figure 6–4 (see color insert). In the concrete

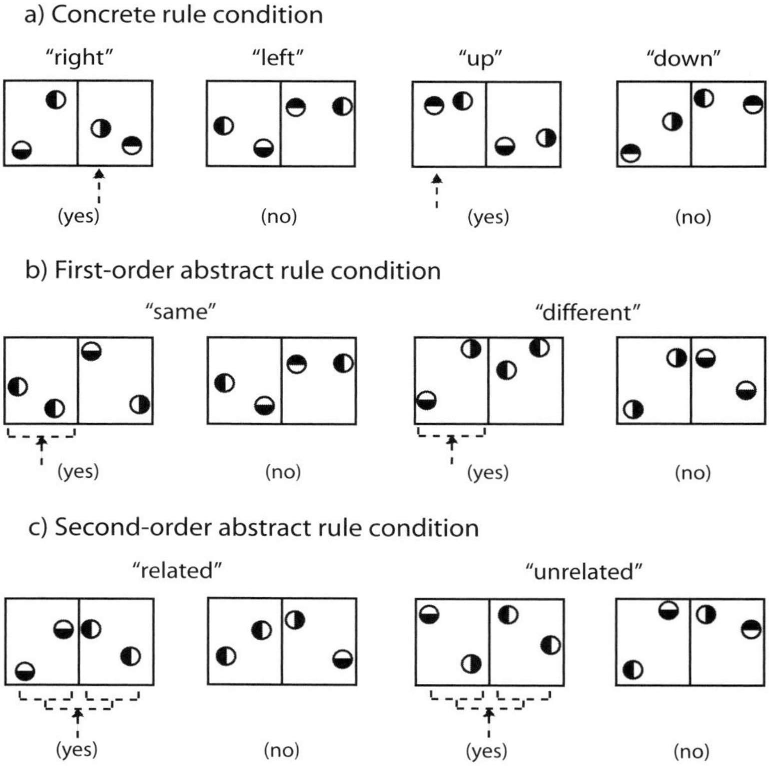

Figure 6–2 Following rules at different levels of abstraction: stimuli and targets for the three conditions. Rules are enclosed in quotation marks, and correct responses are shown in parentheses. Dashed arrows indicate the targets.

condition, significant activation was observed in left insula, posterior ventrolateral prefrontal cortex (VLPFC), and right supplementary motor cortex (BA 6 and 8). In the first-order abstraction condition, activation was limited to anterior ventrolateral prefrontal cortex (BA 11/47). Finally, in the second-order abstraction condition, right VLPFC (BA 47), left VLPFC (BA 45), and left RLPFC (BA 10) showed significant activation. This RLPFC activation, however, was specific to the second-order abstraction condition, and was not observed during rule reversal at the concrete or first-order abstraction rules (Fig. 6–5).

These results provide additional evidence that RLPFC is recruited when rules at the highest order of abstraction are used to guide behavior, in agreement with previous research (Christoff et al., 2001, 2003; Bunge et al., 2003; Sakai and Passingham, 2003). On the other hand, more posterior prefrontal regions were engaged during executive control at lower orders of abstraction and during concrete rules—a finding consistent with previous results (Dias et al., 1996,

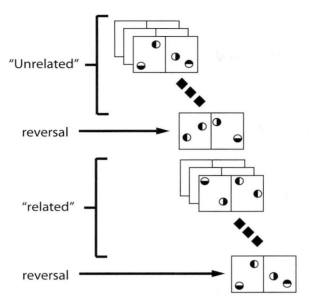

Figure 6–3 An example of rule reversal during the second-order abstract condition. Rule reversals during the experiment included the following possibilities: "right" to "left," "left" to "right," "up" to "down," and "down" to "up" (concrete condition); "same" to "different" and "different" to "same" (first-order abstract condition); "related" to "unrelated" and "unrelated" to "related" (second-order abstract condition).

1997; O'Reilly et al., 2002). One advantage of the study described here, however, is that it varied the level of abstraction in rule reversal at all three levels within each subject, thus allowing the regions recruited at different levels to be examined within the same data set. Within this study, the observed recruitment of different prefrontal subregions is strongly suggestive of organization topography based on levels of abstraction in mental representation.

A question that often arises when different levels of abstraction in executive processing are considered is whether such variation in abstraction is not the same as variation in difficulty of processing. A link between increasing level of abstraction and increasing complexity in processing, as indexed by reaction times and accuracy, is evident in the bulk of previous research (Christoff et al., 2001, 2003; Bunge et al., 2003; Sakai and Passingham, 2003). In fact, we have recently suggested that cognitive complexity may be one of the crucial factors in understanding the functions of higher-order regions, such as the anterior parts of prefrontal cortex (Christoff and Owen, 2006).

Even though this association between difficulty and level of abstraction has been addressed at the level of statistical analysis (Christoff et al., 2001, 2003),

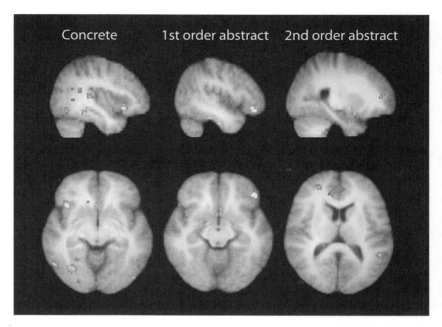

Figure 6–4 Group-averaged brain activations during rule reversal at different levels of abstraction. Ventrolateral (x, y, z = −44, 22, 0); orbitolateral (x, y, z = 48, 38, −12); and rostrolateral (x, y, z = −26, 48, 12). Prefrontal cortices showed significantly increased fMRI signal during the concrete, first-order abstract, and second-order abstract conditions, respectively ($p < 0.001$, uncorrected).

difficulty at the behavioral level almost invariably increases together with increasing level of abstraction. A similar simultaneous increase was also seen in this experiment, allowing for the argument that anterior prefrontal cortex recruitment was due to task difficulty, rather than the degree of abstractness. In the next section, we describe another study that directly aimed to dissociate the confounding effect of task difficulty and abstractness, while further testing the hypothesis for lateral prefrontal cortex organization according to abstraction in representation.

Maintaining a Cognitive Mindset at Different Levels of Abstraction during Problem-Solving

To keep difficulty constant while varying the level of abstraction during executive processing, we used a verbal problem-solving task (Fig. 6–6) (Christoff et al., manuscript under review b). In this task, participants unscrambled anagrams to form words that were either highly abstract (e.g., "appeal," "hope"), highly concrete (e.g., "desk," "bottle"), or in the medium range of concrete-

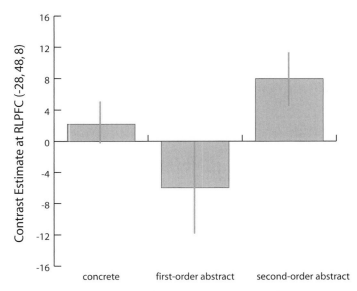

Figure 6–5 Condition-specific parameter estimates at the peak of activation in left rostrolateral prefrontal cortex (RLPFC) during rule reversal for concrete, first-order abstract, and second-order abstract conditions. The figure demonstrates significant recruitment of RLPFC specific to reversals of rules at second order of abstraction.

ness (e.g., "hero," "path"). All words (nouns) were selected from the MRC psycholinguistic database (Wilson, 1988), with abstraction ratings according to Paivio et al. (1968). The words were clustered into groups of abstract, medium, and concrete, and matched for frequency, number of letters, and number of syllables.

Subjects were instructed to press a button once they had identified each word and to say the unscrambled word aloud, which provided the measure of reaction time for each trial. Their voices were recorded to obtain an estimate of accuracy. To help the subjects enter a specific mindset (abstract, medium, or concrete), a 2-second instruction period was displayed at the beginning of each block, during which the word "Abstract," "Medium," or "Concrete" was presented at the top part of the screen. This instruction remained during the entire block, indicating the category for the solutions to the following anagrams. After the instruction period, a set of anagrams was displayed at the bottom of the screen, one at a time. A pilot study was carried out before the actual experiment, testing different scrambled versions for accuracy and response time. The results of this pilot study were used to select those combinations of scrambled letters that yielded comparable difficulty, as measured by accuracy and response time, across the different levels of abstraction.

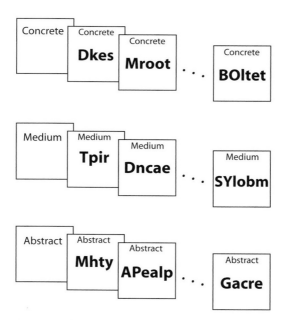

Figure 6–6 Verbal problem-solving task (anagram) design. Subjects were shown instructions about the condition (concrete, medium, or abstract) for 2 seconds, followed by eight anagram-solving trials lasting 4 seconds each. The instructions remained on the screen while participants attempted to solve the anagrams. Solutions to the concrete examples are "Desk," "Motor," and "Bottle"; to the medium examples are "Trip," "Dance," and "Symbol"; and to the abstract examples are "Myth," "Appeal," and "Grace."

Behavioral results from the fMRI experiment confirmed that reaction time and accuracy did not differ across different levels of abstraction (Fig. 6–7), allowing us to examine the regions of activation in the absence of difficulty variation. Each condition was compared with the other two conditions, resulting in three comparisons of interest. The observed activations (Fig. 6–8; see color insert) revealed a striking topography within lateral prefrontal cortex. RLPFC(BA 10/46) was the strongest region of activation in the prefrontal cortex when the abstract anagram solution was compared with the other two conditions. Right DLPFC (BA 46), on the other hand, was the strongest area of activation when the medium condition was compared with the other two. Finally, right VLPFC (BA 47/11) emerged as the most significant area of activation for concrete versus other conditions. These results provide the most conclusive evidence to date for lateral prefrontal cortex topography at different levels of abstractness.

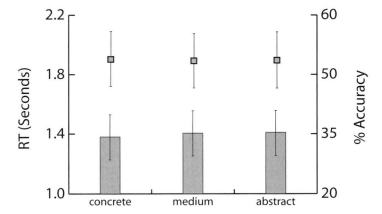

Figure 6–7 Difficulty did not differ across conditions for the anagram task. The mean reaction time (RT) for the abstract condition was 1380 msec; for the medium condition, 1405 msec; and for the concrete condition, 1407 msec. Mean accuracy for the abstract condition was 53.2%; for the medium condition, 52.7%; and for the concrete condition, 53.1%. The *bars* indicate standard error of the mean across subjects.

SUMMARY AND DISCUSSION

In the first half of this chapter, we briefly reviewed a number of theoretical considerations regarding the ontology of abstract entities as well as the issues involved in the mental representation of these nonphysical entities. In the second half, we described some experimental findings concerning the cortical representation of information at different levels of abstraction in nonhuman and human primates. We presented the results from two recent neuroimaging studies that support the hypothesis that the human lateral prefrontal cortex is organized according to working memory representations at different levels of abstraction.

In the first study, a rule-reversal task with three conditions at three levels of abstraction was used. Different areas in prefrontal cortex showed significant activation during executive control in each condition. The most anterior prefrontal region, RLPFC, was only activated during executive control at the highest level of abstraction. Posterior prefrontal cortices, on the other hand, were recruited for executive control at lower levels of abstraction. In the second study, we varied the levels of abstraction in mental mindset during a verbal problem-solving task in which anagram solutions were either highly concrete, highly abstract, or at a medium level of abstraction. To our knowledge, this is the first study that dissociates task difficulty from abstraction in mental representation. When the abstract condition was compared with the other two conditions, RLPFC was the only prefrontal subregion that showed

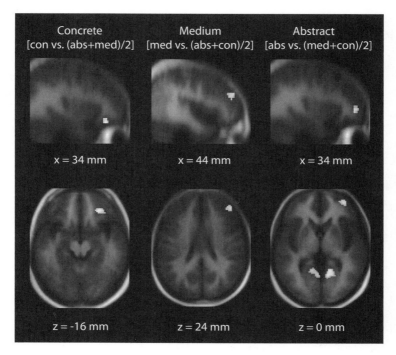

Figure 6–8 Group-average brain activations for anagram-solving at different levels of abstraction, each compared with the average activation for the other two conditions. Concrete blocks were associated with activation in ventro-lateral prefrontal cortex (x, y, z = 32, 36, −16). Medium blocks were associated with activation in right dorsolateral prefrontal cortex (x, y, z = 46, 42, 24). Abstract blocks were associated with activation in right rostrolateral prefrontal cortex (x, y, z = 36, 48, 4) [$p < 0.05$ corrected]. Abs, abstract; med, medium; con, concrete.

significant activation. Mental mindset at a medium level of abstraction during this task was associated with the strongest DLPFC recruitment, and concrete mindset was associated with VLPFC recruitment. These findings suggest an arcuate topography in the human lateral prefrontal cortex (Fig. 6–1), based on working memory representations at different gradients of abstraction.

The idea that lateral prefrontal cortex in primates is organized according to the content of working memory representations was first developed by Goldman-Rakic (1996). According to this notion, VLPFC is specialized for object representations in working memory, whereas DLPFC is specialized for spatial representations. The evidence for such modality-specific conceptualization of prefrontal function, however, is mixed (Owen, 1997), and on a number of occasions, it has been openly challenged by the more consistently observed process-specific separation between the ventral and dorsal parts of

lateral prefrontal cortex (Petrides, 1996; D'Esposito et al., 1998; Owen et al., 1999). The hereby proposed organization of prefrontal function, while focusing on the *content* of working memory representation, regards as important not its modality, but the level of abstractness of informational content. One of the main advantages of this account is that it includes all lateral prefrontal subregions—anterior prefrontal cortex (RLPFC) as well as ventral (VLPFC) and dorsal (DLPFC) regions—within the same conceptual framework.

Another account of lateral prefrontal cortex organization that encompasses all of these regions, however, was proposed a number of years ago (Christoff and Gabrieli, 2000), incorporating the ventral-dorsal process-based distinction (Petrides, 1996; D'Esposito et al., 1998; Owen et al., 1999) in conjunction with the mental operations known to recruit anterior prefrontal cortex. This was an exclusively process-based account and proved extremely successful in conceptualizing the results of subsequent studies. The question might arise then: What is a better way of understanding prefrontal organization—using a process-based or a representation-based account? It is our view that both are necessary and indeed complementary ways of conceptualizing prefrontal functions. Process-based accounts appear to be most useful in the context of incremental extraction of information from the environment, whereby the products of one mental process are used by another mental process. A good example of such a paradigm was developed and used by D'Esposito et al. (2000), in which the manipulation of working memory information is performed on the products of encoding. Other examples include paradigms from the reasoning (Christoff et al., 2001; Kroger et al., 2002) and problem-solving (Baker et al., 1996) literature. In most of these cases, incremental recruitment of prefrontal cortex regions in a posterior-to-anterior direction is observed as additional mental processes are added, possibly reflecting the interactions between adjacent prefrontal subregions (Fig. 6–9A).

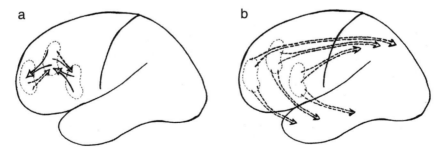

Figure 6–9 Examples of the hypothesized intrinsic (*A*) and extrinsic (*B*) interactions involving prefrontal subregions and their suggested topography based on patterns of connectivity found in studies in nonhuman primates (Pandya and Barnes, 1987.) The direction of arrows indicates the hypothesized direction of prefrontal attentional control.

Representation-based accounts, on the other hand, appear to be more useful in the context of attentional and cognitive control processes that require the maintenance of particular information in working memory for the purposes of biasing representations in regions outside of prefrontal cortex—as in the selective attention account proposed by Desimone and Duncan (1995). In these cases, recruitment of different prefrontal subregions may be observed in the absence of activation in other prefrontal regions, as in the results presented here from the anagram solution task. Thus, representation-based accounts of prefrontal function may be more useful in describing attentional control processes, presumably reflecting the interactions between prefrontal regions and other regions of the brain (Fig. 6–9B).

It is our belief that process and representation are flip sides of the same mental coin. Using fMRI forces us to treat relatively large brain regions as the basic unit of our analyses and theorizing. As such, "process" implies some interaction and information exchange between a region of interest and another brain region. On the other hand, "representation" implies a state of activation in a region of interest, without explicitly relating it to activation states in other brain regions. When a discussion is focused exclusively on a particular brain division, such as prefrontal cortex (as is the case in this chapter), the functions of particular prefrontal subregions may be best understood in terms of representational account (e.g., anterior prefrontal cortex supports working memory representations at high levels of abstraction). If the discussion is expanded to include areas outside prefrontal cortex, however, a process-based account may become relevant as well (e.g., anterior prefrontal cortex biases representations in anterior temporal cortex in support of the retrieval of semantic information at high levels of abstraction). To fully understand the organization of prefrontal function, it will be necessary to consider the functions of its subregions in terms of both process and representation—as well as the nature and systematicity of its intrinsic and extrinsic connections and interactions.

Another advantage of the hereby proposed account of prefrontal organization is that it is corroborated by findings from human neurodevelopment and patterns of brain connectivity in nonhuman primates. It has been suggested that, in human infants, maturation of prefrontal cortex starts from the most posterior part of prefrontal cortex and progresses toward the most anterior part (Diamond, 1991). These neurodevelopmental changes appear to be contemporaneous with the development of rule-learning abilities in preschoolers (Casey et al., 2000), who can first learn only concrete rules, and later can reason at increasingly higher levels of abstraction (Jacques and Zelazo, 2001; Bunge and Zelazo, 2006; see also Chapter 19). In addition, studies examining the connectivity patterns between prefrontal subregions and other brain areas have revealed a systematic topography whereby progressively more anterior prefrontal regions receive and send projections preferentially to regions of progressively higher levels of sensory integration (Pandya and Barnes, 1987). This pattern of connectivity supports the possibility that attentional

control processes may occur in parallel streams from more anterior prefrontal regions to areas of higher-order sensory integration (Fig. 6–9*B*).

Earlier in this chapter, we emphasized the process of selective attention that occurs ubiquitously in the discussions by philosophers and modern cognitive scientists alike. Berkeley's process of focusing attention on a particular feature, Lakoff and Johnson's "highlighting and hiding" in understanding abstract concepts through metaphor, and Barsalou's idea for the application of selective attention in the extraction of particular features of a generalized event sequence all represent accounts of the process of abstraction, prominently featuring this aspect of attention. At the same time, neuroscientific accounts of prefrontal functions have also strongly emphasized the process of selective attention (Desimone and Duncan, 1995; Everling et al., 2002) and attentional control processes in general (Cohen et al., 1996; Braver and Cohen, 2001) in understanding prefrontal functions. In view of the strong association between prefrontal functions and abstraction, the processes of selective attention will likely turn out to be crucial for our neuroscientific theories of abstraction. Although no such theory currently emphasizes this process, our discussion here suggests that this would be necessary to advance understanding of the way prefrontal cortex represents abstract information and implements the process of abstraction. It is with such advancement that we will ultimately be able to better understand not only the neural but also the corresponding cognitive processes that enable this most uniquely human phenomenon.

ACKNOWLEDGMENTS Support for the preparation of this chapter came from the Tula Foundation, the Natural Sciences and Engineering Research Council (NSERC) of Canada, and the Michael Smith Foundation for Health Research. The authors thank Rachelle Smith for help with data collection as well as helpful comments and suggestions at the chapter's conception. We are also greatly indebted to Alan Gordon for his extensive and thoughtful feedback and his invaluable help at the later manuscript preparation stage.

NOTE

1. The term "arcuate" is used here in its sense of "curved" or "formed in the shape of an arc."

REFERENCES

Aristotle (350 BCE/2002) Nichomachean ethics. New York: Oxford University Press.

Baker SC, Rogers RD, Owen AM, Frith CD, Dolan RJ, Frackowiak RSJ, Robbins TW (1996) Neural systems engaged by planning: a PET study of the Tower of London task. Neuropsychologia 34:515–526.

Barsalou LW (1999) Perceptual symbol systems. Behavioral and Brain Sciences 22:577–609; discussion 610–560.

Berkeley G (1734/1998) A treatise concerning the principles of human knowledge: introduction. Oxford, UK: Oxford University Press.

Braver TS, Bongiolatti SR (2002) The role of frontopolar cortex in subgoal processing during working memory. Neuroimage 15:523–536.

Braver TS, Cohen JD (2001) On the control of control: the role of dopamine in regulating prefrontal function and working memory. In: Attention and performance XVIII; Control of cognitive processes(Monsell S, Driver J, eds.), pp. 713–737. Cambridge: MIT Press.Buchel C, Holmes AP, Rees G, Friston KJ (1998) Characterizing stimulus-response functions using nonlinear regressors in parametric fMRI experiments. Neuroimage 8:140–148.

Bunge SA, Kahn I, Wallis JD, Miller EK, Wagner AD (2003) Neural circuits subserving the retrieval and maintenance of abstract rules. Journal of Neurophysiology 90: 3419–3428.

Bunge SA, Wendelken C, Badre D, Wagner AD (2005) Analogical reasoning and prefrontal cortex: evidence for separable retrieval and integration mechanisms. Cerebral Cortex 15:239–249.

Bunge SA, Zelazo PD (2006) A brain-based account of the development of rule use in childhood. Current Directions in Psychological Science 15:118–121.

Casey BJ, Giedd JN, Thomas KM (2000) Structural and functional brain development and its relation to cognitive development. Biological Psychology 54:241–257.

Christoff K (2003) Using and musing of abstract behavioural rules: peculiarities of prefrontal function in humans. Neuroimage 19. AbsTrak ID:18325.

Christoff K, Gabrieli JDE (2000) The frontopolar cortex and human cognition: evidence for a rostrocaudal hierarchical organization within the human prefrontal cortex. Psychobiology 28:168–186.

Christoff K, Keramatian K, Dove A, Owen AM (manuscript under review a) Executive processing at different levels of abstraction.

Christoff K, Keramatian K, Smith R, Maedler B (manuscript under review b) Prefrontal organization and levels of abstraction in working memory representation.

Christoff K, Owen AM (2006) Improving reverse neuroimaging inference: cognitive domain versus cognitive complexity. Trends in Cognitive Sciences 10:352–353.

Christoff K, Prabhakaran V, Dorfman J, Zhao Z, Kroger JK, Holyoak KJ, Gabrieli JDE (2001) Rostrolateral prefrontal cortex involvement in relational integration during reasoning. Neuroimage 14:1136–1149.

Christoff K, Ream JM, Gabrieli JD (2004) Neural basis of spontaneous thought processes. Cortex 40:623–630.

Christoff K, Ream JM, Geddes LPT, Gabrieli JDE (2003) Evaluating self-generated information: anterior prefrontal contributions to human cognition. Behavioral Neuroscience 117:1161–1168.

Cohen JD, Braver TS, O'Reilly RC (1996) A computational approach to prefrontal cortex, cognitive control and schizophrenia: recent developments and current challenges. Philosophical Transactions of the Royal Society of London B 351:1515–1527.

D'Esposito M, Aguirre GK, Zarahn E, Ballard D, Shin RK, Lease J (1998) Functional MRI studies of spatial and nonspatial working memory. Cognitive Brain Research 7:1–13.

D'Esposito M, Postle BR, Rypma B (2000) Prefrontal cortical contributions to working memory: evidence from event-related fMRI studies. Experimental Brain Research 133:3–11.

Desimone R, Duncan J (1995) Neural mechanisms of selective visual attention. Annual Reviews in Neuroscience 18:193–222.

Diamond A (1991) Neuropsychological insights into the meaning of object concept development. In: The epigenesis of mind: essays on biology and knowledge (Carey S, Gelman R, eds.), pp 67–110. Hillsdale, NJ: Lawrence Erlbaum Associates.

Dias R, Robbins TW, Roberts AC (1996) Dissociation in prefrontal cortex of affective and attentional shifts. Nature 380:69–72.

Dias R, Robbins TW, Roberts AC (1997) Dissociable forms of inhibitory control within prefrontal cortex with an analog of the Wisconsin Card Sort Test: restriction to novel situations and independence from 'on-line' processing. Journal of Neuroscience 17: 9285–9297.

Duncan J, Burgess P, Emslie H (1995) Fluid intelligence after frontal lobe lesions. Neuropsychologia 33:261–268.

Everling S, Tinsley CJ, Gaffan D, Duncan J (2002) Filtering of neural signals by focused attention in the monkey prefrontal cortex. Nature Neuroscience 5:671–676.

Gentner D, Holyoak KJ, Kokinov BN, eds. (2001) The analogical mind: perspectives from cognitive science. Cambridge: MIT Press.

Goldman-Rakic PS (1996) The prefrontal landscape: implications of functional architecture for understanding human mentation and the central executive. Philosophical Transactions of the Royal Society of London B 351:1445–1453.

Halford GS (1984) Can young children integrate premises in transitivity and serial order tasks? Cognitive Psychology 16:65–93.

Holloway RL (2002) Brief communication: how much larger is the relative volume of area 10 of the prefrontal cortex in humans? American Journal of Physical Anthropology 118:399–401.

Holyoak KJ, Kroger JK (1995) Forms of reasoning: insight into prefrontal functions? In: Structure and functions of the human prefrontal cortex (Grafman J, Holyoak KJ, Boller F, eds.), pp 253–263. New York: New York Academy of Sciences.

Hubel DH, Wiesel TN (1968) Receptive fields and functional architecture of monkey striate cortex. Journal of Physiology 195:215–243.

Jacques S, Zelazo PD (2001) The Flexible Item Selection Task (FIST): a measure of executive function in preschoolers. Developmental Neuropsychology 20:573–591.

Koechlin E, Basso G, Pietrini P, Panzer S, Grafman J (1999) The role of the anterior prefrontal cortex in human cognition. Nature 399:148–151.

Kroger JK, Sabb FW, Fales CL, Bookheimer SY, Cohen MS, Holyoak KJ (2002) Recruitment of anterior dorsolateral prefrontal cortex in human reasoning: a parametric study of relational complexity. Cerebral Cortex 12:477–485.

Lakoff G, Johnson M (1980a) The metaphorical structure of the human conceptual system. Cognitive Science 4:195–208.

Lakoff G, Johnson M (1980b) Metaphors we live by. Chicago: University of Chicago Press.

Lakoff G, Johnson M (1999) Philosophy in the flesh. New York: Basic Books.

Locke J (1690/1979) An essay concerning human understanding. New York: Oxford University Press.

Luria AR (1966) Higher cortical functions in man. London: Tavistock Publications.

Miller EK, Nieder A, Freedman DJ, Wallis JD (2003) Neural correlates of categories and concepts. Current Opinion in Neurobiology 13:198–203.

Milner B (1963) Effects of different brain lesions on card sorting. Archives of Neurology 9:90–100.

Milner B (1964) Some effects of frontal lobectomy in man. In: The frontal granular cortex and behavior (Warren JM, Akert K, eds.), pp 313–334. New York: McGraw-Hill.

Nieder A, Freedman DJ, Miller EK (2002) Representation of the quantity of visual items in the primate prefrontal cortex. Science 297:1708–1711.

O'Reilly RC, Noelle DC, Braver TS, Cohen JD (2002) Prefrontal cortex and dynamic categorization tasks: representational organization and neuromodulatory control. Cerebral Cortex 12:246–257.

Owen AM (1997) The functional organization of working memory processes within human lateral frontal cortex: the contribution of functional neuroimaging. European Journal of Neuroscience 9:1329–1339.

Owen AM, Herrod NJ, Menon DK, Clark JC, Downey SP, Carpenter TA, Minhas PS, Turkheimer FE, Williams EJ, Robbins TW, Sahakian BJ, Petrides M, Pickard JD (1999) Redefining the functional organization of working memory processes within human lateral prefrontal cortex. European Journal of Neuroscience 11:567–574.

Paivio A, Yuille JC, Madigan SA (1968) Concreteness, imagery, and meaningfulness values for 925 nouns. Journal of Experimental Psychology 76 (Supplement):1–25.

Pandya DN, Barnes CL (1987) Architecture and connections of the frontal lobe. In: The frontal lobes revisited (Perecman E, ed.), pp 41–72. New York: IRBN Press.

Petrides M (1996) Specialized systems for the processing of mnemonic information within the primate frontal cortex. Philosophical Transactions of the Royal Society of London B 351:1455–1461.

Plato (360 BCE/2003) The republic, 2nd edition. New York: Penguin Books.

Sakai K, Passingham RE (2003) Prefrontal interactions reflect future task operations. Nature Neuroscience 6:75–81.

Semendeferi K, Armstrong E, Schleicher A, Zilles K, Van Hoesen GW (2001) Prefrontal cortex in humans and apes: a comparative study of area 10. American Journal of Physical Anthropology 114:224–241.

Shallice T (1982) Specific impairments of planning. Philosophical Transactions of the Royal Society of London B 298:199–209.

Simoncelli EH, Heeger DJ (1998) A model of neuronal responses in visual area MT. Vision Research 38:743–761.

Smith R, Keramatian K, Smallwood J, Schooler J, Luus B, Christoff K (2006) Mind-wandering with and without awareness: an fMRI study of spontaneous thought processes. In: Proceedings of the 28th Annual Conference of the Cognitive Science Society (Sun R, ed.), pp 804–809. Vancouver: Lawrence Erlbaum Associates.

Thompson RKR, Oden DL, Boysen ST (1997) Language-naive chimpanzees (Pan troglodytes) judge relations between relations in a conceptual matching-to-sample task. Journal of Experimental Psychology: Animal Behavior Processes 23:31–43.

Wallis JD, Anderson KC, Miller EK (2001) Single neurons in prefrontal cortex encode abstract rules. Nature 411:953–956.

Wandell B (1995) Foundations of vision. Sunderland, MA: Sinauer Associates.

Wilson MD (1988) The MRC psycholinguistic database: machine readable dictionary, version 2. Behavioural Research Methods, Instruments and Computers 20:6–11.

II

RULE IMPLEMENTATION

7

Ventrolateral and Medial Frontal Contributions to Decision-Making and Action Selection

Matthew F. S. Rushworth, Paula L. Croxson,
Mark J. Buckley, and Mark E. Walton

The frontal cortex has a central role in the selection of actions, and in many circumstances, action selection is likely to be the consequence of activity distributed across a swathe of frontal lobe areas. Evidence from lesion and other interference techniques, such as transcranial magnetic stimulation (TMS), however, suggests that a useful distinction may be drawn between the roles of ventrolateral prefrontal cortex (PFv) and dorsomedial frontal cortex areas (Fig. 7–1), including the pre-supplementary motor area (pre-SMA) and the anterior cingulate cortex (ACC). The PFv region is centered on cytoarchitectonic region 47/12 (2002a) [see Fig. 7–5], but the lesions that are used to investigate this area often include adjacent lateral orbital areas 11 and 13 (PFv+o lesion) [for example, Bussey et al., 2001, 2002]. Cells in these areas have some similar responses to those in the PFv (Wallis et al., 2001). The pre-SMA is situated in an anterior division of area 6, whereas the ACC region under discussion in this chapter is in cytoarchitectonic areas 24c and 24c' (Matsuzaka et al., 1992; Luppino et al., 1993; Vogt, 1993).

A series of experiments have all suggested that the PFv has a central role in the selection of actions in response to external stimuli and according to learned arbitrary rules. However, it has been more difficult to describe how the contribution of the PFv differs from that made by premotor areas in more posterior parts of the frontal lobe. Recent results suggest that the PFv is particularly concerned with the selection of the behaviorally relevant stimulus information on which action selection will, in turn, be contingent, and the deployment of prospective coding strategies that facilitate rule learning. Once behavioral rules for action selection have been learned, it is often necessary to switch quickly between one set of rules and another as the context changes. The pre-SMA is known to be important at such times. The role of the ACC appears to be quite distinct. Both lesion investigations and neuroimaging implicate the ACC most

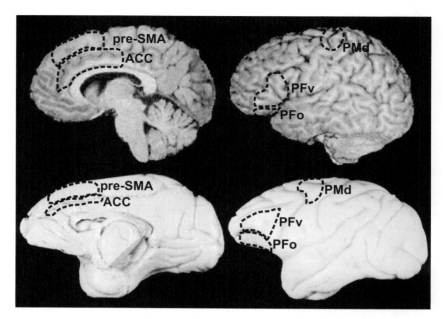

Figure 7–1 Medial (*left*) and lateral (*right*) views of magnetic resonance images of a human brain (*top*) and photographs of a macaque brain (*bottom*). The ventral and orbital prefrontal regions PFv and PFo, respectively, have a central role in learning conditional rules for response selection, perhaps because of their roles in identifying behaviorally relevant stimuli and guiding efficient learning strategies. More dorsal and medial areas, such as the anterior cingulate cortex (ACC), pre-supplementary motor area (pre-SMA), and dorsal premotor cortex (PMd), may also be active when conditional rules are used, but their functional contributions are distinct. Although PMd may use conditional rules to select actions, pre-SMA may be concerned with the selection of sets of responses rather than individual responses. The ACC is more concerned with representing the reinforcement value of actions and their reinforcement outcome associations than with representing the learned conditional associations of actions with sensory cues.

strongly when choices are made on the basis of the recent reward history rather than on the basis of learned conditional cue-action associations. The ACC may be important for representing the reinforcement values associated with actions rather than the stimulus conditional selection rules associated with actions. In both humans and macaques, the PFv is distinguished by a pattern of strong anatomical connection with the temporal lobe, whereas the ACC is unusual in being closely connected with reward processing areas and the motor system. Such differences in anatomical connectivity may underlie the different specializations of the areas.

VENTRAL PREFRONTAL CORTEX

Ventral Prefrontal Cortex and the Use of Conditional Rules for Action Selection

Discussions of prefrontal function have often focused on its role in working memory (Goldman-Rakic, 1996). This is consistent with the delay dependency of the deficits that are seen after some prefrontal lesions. For example, Funahashi and colleagues (1993) showed that macaques with lesions in the dorsolateral prefrontal cortex (PFdl) surrounding the principle sulcus were inaccurate when they made saccades in the absence of visible targets to locations that were held in memory. The same animals, however, were able to make visually instructed saccades in a relatively normal manner.

The deficits that follow PFv lesions are different, and are not delay-dependent in the same way (Rushworth and Owen, 1998). In one study, macaques were taught to select one of two colored shapes, A or B, at the bottom of a touch-screen monitor (Rushworth et al., 1997). The correct choice was conditional on the identity of a "sample" stimulus shown at the top of the screen at the beginning of the trial. If the macaque saw stimulus A as the sample at the beginning of the trial, then the rule was to select a matching copy of stimulus A when subsequently given a choice between it and stimulus B. Similarly, the macaques also learned to choose the matching stimulus B when the sample was stimulus B.

At the beginning of each trial, the macaques touched the sample stimulus to indicate that they had seen it. On "simultaneous" trials, the sample stayed on the screen even after it was touched, and it was still present at the time of the response choice. In the delay version of the task, the sample stimulus disappeared from the screen before the macaque could choose between the response options. After PFv lesions were made, the animals were first tested on the simultaneous version of the task, and their performance was found to be significantly impaired. After retraining, the animals with lesions eventually overcame their impairments on the simultaneous matching task. Notably, once the relearning of the simultaneous matching task was complete, the subsequent imposition of a delay between sample and choice periods did not cause them additional difficulty. Such a pattern of results suggests that the PFv lesion did not cause a delay-dependent deficit analogous to the one seen after PFdl lesions; the PFv lesion impaired the use of the matching rule that guided correct responding, but it did not selectively impair the retention in memory of which sample stimulus was presented at the beginning of each trial.

Although the ability to associate a sample stimulus with a matching stimulus when making a choice might seem like a trivial one, it is important to remember that from the macaque's perspective, using the matching rule is as arbitrary as using a nonmatching rule. The results of the experiment by Rushworth and colleagues (1997) suggest that it is the learning and use of the arbitrary rule for which the PFv is necessary. Once the rule is acquired, however,

memory for which sample stimulus has been recently shown may rely on distinct brain structures.

Several studies have confirmed that the learning of conditional rules that link stimuli to responses is a critical aspect of PFv function. Bussey and colleagues (2001) taught macaques to select joystick movements in response to the presentation of visual stimuli. Conditional rules linked the presentation of each stimulus to the retrieval of a particular response. The conclusion that the PFv was especially concerned with conditional rules was based on the finding that animals with lesions of the PFv and the adjacent lateral orbital prefrontal region (referred to as "PFv+o lesions") were impaired on the conditional visuomotor task, but could still learn visual discrimination problems well. In visual discrimination tasks, the correct choice is consistently associated with reinforcement, whereas the incorrect choice is never associated with reinforcement. In the conditional tasks, all of the responses are partially and equally well associated with reinforcement, and which one is correct varies from trial to trial in a manner that is conditional on the presence of the stimulus that is also presented.

Related accounts of the PFv have also emphasized its importance in mediating otherwise difficult associations (Petrides, 2005). Rather than emphasizing the conditional nature of the association, Petrides and others (Wagner et al., 2001) have emphasized the role of the PFv in the *active* nonautomatic retrieval of associations from memory. Active retrieval is needed when the association is arbitrary or learned, and activation of the representation does not occur automatically as the result of the arrival of matching sensory input in posterior cortex.

It has been argued that, when human participants follow instructions, they are essentially employing conditional rules linking certain stimuli, or more generally, any arbitrary antecedent, with subsequent action choices (Murray et al., 2000, 2002; Passingham et al., 2000; Wise and Murray, 2000). Petrides and Pandya (2002a) have identified a number of similarities between human and macaque PFv cytoarchitecture, and human PFv is active when human participants learn cue-conditional instructions for selecting actions (Toni et al., 2001; Bunge et al., 2003; Grol et al., 2006; see also Chapter 3).

Routes for Conditional Association: Interactions between Ventrolateral Prefrontal Cortex and Temporal Lobe

Conditional rule learning does not depend on PFv in isolation, but on its interaction with other brain areas, especially the temporal lobe. PFv is densely interconnected with the temporal lobe (Webster et al., 1994; Carmichael and Price, 1995; Petrides and Pandya, 2002a). Within PFv, area 12/47 is particularly well connected with visual association areas in the inferior temporal cortex, whereas the slightly more posterior area 45 may be more strongly connected with the auditory association cortex in the superior temporal lobe. The connections not only convey sensory information about visual and auditory

object identity to PFv but also provide a route by which PFv is able to exert a top-down influence over temporal lobe activity (Tomita et al., 1999).

The interaction between PFv and the temporal lobe during visual stimulus conditional learning can be examined by making a "crossed" disconnection lesion. A PFv+o lesion is made in one hemisphere and in the inferior temporal lobe cortex in the other hemisphere. Because most interareal connections are intrahemispheric, the crossed lesion prevents the possibility of direct, intra-hemispheric communication between PFv and the temporal lobe. Like PFv+o lesions, PFv+o-temporal disconnection lesions impair visual conditional tasks, but leave visual discrimination learning relatively intact (Parker and Gaffan, 1998; Bussey et al., 2002).

It is also possible to study frontotemporal interactions by directly trans-ecting the fibers that connect the two lobes. In the macaque, many of the direct connections between the visual association cortex in the inferior temporal lobe and PFv+o travel in a fiber bundle called the "uncinate fascicle" (Ungerleider et al., 1989; Schmahmann and Pandya, 2006). Connections with the auditory association cortex in the superior temporal gyrus, and perhaps more posterior parts of the inferior temporal cortex, run more dorsally in the extreme cap-sule (Petrides and Pandya, 1988, 2002b; Schmahmann and Pandya, 2006). Al-though the roles of the extreme capsule and auditory conditional associations have received little attention, a number of experiments have considered the effects of uncinate fascicle transection on visual conditional associations. As is the case with the disconnection lesions, the ability to follow rules that are con-ditional on visual stimuli is impaired if the uncinate fascicle is cut (Eacott and Gaffan, 1992; Gutnikov et al., 1997). Unlike the disconnection lesion, which disrupts all intrahemispheric communication between PFv+o and the inferior temporal lobe, uncinate fascicle transection only disrupts direct monosynaptic connections.

Macaques with uncinate fascicle transection are still able to use conditional rules to select actions if the rule is based on the presentation of reinforcement, as opposed to visual stimuli. Eacott and Gaffan (1992) gave macaques one of two free rewards at the beginning of each trial. If animals received a *free* reward A, they were taught to select action 1 to *earn* an additional reward A. If, on the other hand, the trial started with free delivery of reward B, then the condi-tional rule meant that animals were to select action 2 to earn an additional reward B. Surprisingly, macaques with uncinate fascicle transection were still able to perform this task, even though they were impaired at selecting actions in response to conditional visual instructions. The discrepancy can be un-derstood if the frontal lobe is not interacting with inferior temporal cortex in the case of reinforcement conditional action, but if the relevant information that the frontal lobe needs to access comes from elsewhere—perhaps an area such as the amygdala or the striatum, both of which are known to encode reinforcement information (Schultz, 2000; Yamada et al., 2004; Samejima et al., 2005; Paton et al., 2006).

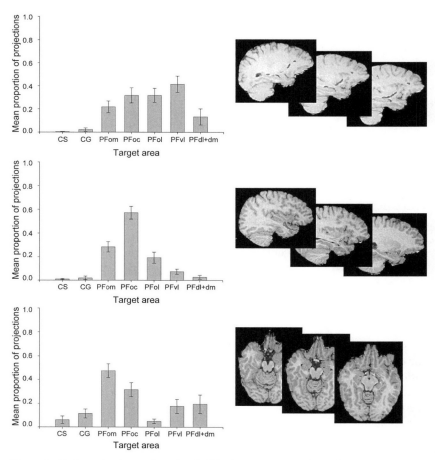

Figure 7–2 Quantitative results of probabilistic tractography from the human extreme capsule (*A*), uncinate fascicle (*B*), and amygdala (*C*) to the prefrontal regions. The probability of connection with each prefrontal region as a proportion of the total connectivity with all prefrontal regions is plotted on the y-axis. The majority of connections from the posterior and superior temporal lobe areas running in the extreme capsule are with areas ventral to the dorsal prefrontal cortex (PFdl+dm). High connection probabilities were found for the ventrolateral prefrontal areas (PFvl) and the lateral, central, and medial orbital regions (PFol, PFoc, and PFom, respectively). Connections from the anterior and inferior temporal lobe via the uncinate fascicle are more biased to orbital areas. The amygdala connections are most likely to be with even more medial regions, for example, PFom. The high diffusion levels in the corpus callosum distort connection estimates in the adjacent anterior cingulate cortex, but nevertheless, it is clear that there is still some evidence for connectivity between the amygdala and the cingulate gyral and sulcal regions (CG and CS, respectively). The *right* side of each part of the figure shows three sagittal sections depicting the estimated course taken by each connecting tract for a sample single participant. (Reprinted with permission from Croxon et al., *Journal of Neuroscience*, 25, 8854–8866. Copyright Society for Neuroscience, 2005.)

Frontostriatal connections take a course that differs from those running between the inferior temporal cortex and PFv+o. Outputs from the amygdala run ventral to the striatum, rather than in the more lateral parts of the uncinate fascicle affected by the transection (Schmahmann and Pandya, 2006). Indeed, anatomical tracing studies show that there is still evidence of connection between the frontal lobe and the amygdala, even after the uncinate fascicle has been cut (Ungerleider et al., 1989). Reinforcement conditional action selection may, therefore, depend on distinct inputs into the frontal lobe; it may even depend on additional frontal regions. Later in this chapter, it is argued that, in many situations, when action selection is guided not by well-defined conditional rules, but by the history of reinforcement associated with each action, then ACC, and not just PFv, is essential for selecting the correct action.

Diffusion weighted magnetic resonance imaging (DWI) and probabilistic tractography have recently been used to compare the trajectories of white matter fiber tracts, such as the uncinate fascicle, in vivo in the human and macaque. DWI provides information on the orientation of brain fiber pathways (Basser and Jones, 2002; Beaulieu, 2002). Such data can be analyzed with probabilistic tractography techniques that generate estimates on the likelihood of a pathway existing between two brain areas (Behrens et al., 2003b; Hagmann et al., 2003; Tournier et al., 2003). Using the method developed by Behrens et al. (2003a), Croxson and colleagues (2005) were able to show, in the macaque, that the extreme capsule was interconnected with more dorsal PFv regions (Fig. 7–2A), whereas the uncinate fascicle was interconnected with the more ventral PFv and the orbitofrontal cortex (Fig. 7–2B). Consistent with the tracer injection studies indicating that amygdala connections with the frontal lobe take a distinct course, the highest connectivity estimates for the amygdala were more medially displaced across a wider area of the orbital surface and extended onto the medial frontal cortex (Fig. 7–2C). A similar pattern was also observed in human participants. The extreme capsule and uncinate fascicle connection estimates within the human frontal lobe include the same regions that have been identified in human neuroimaging studies when conditional rules are used during action selection (Toni and Passingham, 1999; Toni et al., 1999, 2001; Walton et al., 2004; Crone et al., 2006; Grol et al., 2006).

STRATEGY USE AND ATTENTION SELECTION

Attention and Stimulus Selection during Conditional Rule Learning

A number of single-neuron recording studies have identified PFv activity related to the encoding of conditional rules linking stimuli and responses (Boussaoud and Wise, 1993a, b; Wilson et al., 1993; Asaad et al., 1998; White and Wise, 1999; Wallis et al., 2001; Wallis and Miller, 2003; see also Chapter 2). Another important aspect of PFv activity, however, concerns the encoding of the attended stimulus and its features. Many neurons in PFv exhibit distinct

activity patterns to repeated presentations of the same array of the same stimuli in the same positions when attention is directed to different stimuli within the array. Many neurons that have either form selectivity or spatial selectivity are only active when a stimulus with that form or location is the current focus of attention (Rainer et al., 1998). Only behaviorally relevant stimuli (Everling et al., 2002, 2006; Lebedev et al., 2004) or aspects of those stimuli, such as their color (Sakagami and Niki, 1994; Sakagami et al., 2001) or particular aspects of their form (Freedman et al., 2001; see also Chapter 17), appear to be represented.

When actions are chosen according to conditional rules, the instructing stimulus is often spatially removed from the location at which the action occurs. If a subject is learning how to use a conditional rule to select between actions, the first problem that must be confronted is identifying where within the stimulus array the relevant guiding information is present. It is particularly apparent when training animals that they are not always initially inclined to appreciate the behavioral relevance of stimuli that are spatially separated from the locus of action. It might even be argued that conditional learning tasks are more difficult to learn than discrimination learning tasks, not because of the conditional rule per se, but because the guiding stimulus and the behavioral response are at the same location in the latter case, but are separated in the former. In the conditional task, it is more difficult to associate the stimulus and the response, and it might be difficult to allocate attention to the stimulus, even when behavior is being directed to the location at which the response is made.

Two recent studies have examined whether attentional factors and the difficulty of associating the stimulus with the response—as opposed to the use of a conditional rule to actually select a response—are the determinants of the learning failures seen after prefrontal lesions (Browning et al., 2005; Rushworth et al., 2005). In one experiment, macaques were taught a visuospatial conditional task, and lesions were made in the PFv+o region (Rushworth et al., 2005). Depending on the identity of a stimulus, animals were instructed to touch a red response box on either the left or the right of a touch-screen monitor. In the "inside" condition, two copies of the guiding stimulus were presented inside each of the response boxes so that there was no spatial disjunction between the guiding stimulus and response locations, and no requirement to divide attention between the guiding stimulus and response locations (Fig. 7–3A). In the "far" condition, the guiding stimuli were spatially separated from the response location (Fig. 7–3B). A series of experiments confirmed that animals with PFv+o lesions were impaired, even in the "inside" condition, suggesting that the mere requirement to learn and employ a conditional rule, even in the absence of any attentional manipulation, is sufficient to cause an impairment after a PFv+o lesion (Fig. 7–3C, left). As the guiding stimulus was separated from the response, however, the deficit in the animals with PFv+o lesion became significantly worse (Fig. 7–3C, right). The results are consistent with the idea that PFv+o has a dual role in identifying

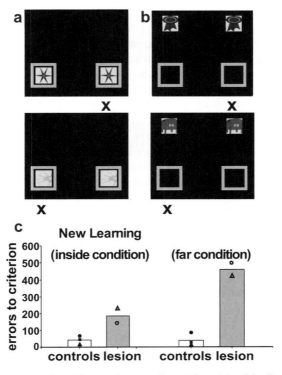

Figure 7–3 Two examples of the touch-screen layout for trials of the "inside" (*A*) and "far" (*B*) conditions in the study by Rushworth et al. (2005). In both cases, the monkeys made responses to either the left or the right response boxes, which were indicated by flashing red squares (colored grey in figure) in the lower left and right corners of the screen. Two copies of the same visual stimulus were shown on the screen on every trial. The visual stimuli instructed responses to either the box on the left or the box on the right. The correct response is to the right in each of the example problems shown at the *top*, whereas the correct response is to the left for each example problem shown at the *bottom*. Instructing visual stimuli were present in every trial. In "inside" trials (*A*), the instructing visual stimuli were placed inside the response box, but they were moved further away in "far" trials (*B*) *C*. Macaques with PFv+o lesions (*shaded bars*) made significantly more errors learning new "inside" condition problems (*left*) than did control animals (*open bars*). The deficit confirms that PFv+o lesions impair conditional action selection, even when there is no separation between the cue and the response and therefore no difficulty in identifying and attending to the behaviorally relevant conditional stimulus. The *right* side of the figure, however, shows that the PFv+o impairment is significantly worse when the cues and responses are separated so that it is more difficult to identify the behaviorally relevant information and to divide attention between the stimulus and action locations (Reprinted with permission from Rushworth et al., *Journal of Neuroscience*, 25, 11628–11636. Copyright Society for Neuroscience, 2005.)

behaviorally relevant stimulus information and using that information to guide choice and action selection.

In the other experiment, Browning and colleagues taught macaques to perform a visual stimulus discrimination learning task in which the stimuli were presented in the context of spatial scenes. In such situations, learning is significantly faster than when similar visual stimulus discriminations are learned in the absence of a spatial scene. The scenes probably do not act as conditional cues instructing a choice between the stimuli because a given stimulus pair is only ever presented in the context of one scene and one of the stimuli is always the correct choice, whereas the other is always the incorrect choice. It is believed that macaques make an association between the spatial context and the correct stimulus choice, and the context may reduce interference between discrimination problems. Macaques with either bilateral lesions of the entire prefrontal cortex or crossed prefrontal-inferotemporal lesions (unilateral lesions of one entire prefrontal cortex crossed and disconnected from the inferior temporal lobe cortex in the opposite hemisphere) are impaired in such tasks of stimulus-in-scene learning. They are, however, no worse than control animals at discrimination problems that are learned more slowly in the absence of any facilitating scene context (Parker and Gaffan, 1998; Gaffan et al., 2002; Browning et al., 2005) [Fig. 7–4A]. This result is important because it suggests that the prefrontal cortex is needed when an association between two parts of the visual array has to be learned, even when the association is not necessarily conditional. The animals in the scene-based task did not have to make different choices for a given discrimination problem depending on the context of different scenes, because a given problem was only ever presented in one scene context.

However, PFv+o is not the only region within the frontal lobe known to be critical for the employment of conditional rules. One of the first regions to be identified with conditional tasks was the periarcuate region (Halsband and Passingham, 1982; Petrides, 1982, 1986). Although the region surrounding the frontal eye fields anterior to the arcuate sulcus is needed for selecting spatial responses, the more posterior region in the vicinity of the dorsal premotor cortex (PMd) is critical for selecting limb movement responses (Halsband and Passingham, 1985). The distinct contribution made by PFv+o and PMd to the encoding of conditional action selection rules is not clear, but it is intriguing to note that rule encoding is actually more prevalent in neurons in PMd than in PFv (Wallis and Miller, 2003). It is possible that periarcuate regions, which are closely interconnected with neurons that play a direct role in the execution of eye and hand movements, are important for rule implementation (i.e., for using conditional rules to guide *response selection*). On the other hand, PFv may be more concerned with behaviorally relevant *stimulus selection,* identification of the stimulus on which the conditional rules will be contingent, and the process of *associating* the stimulus with the response. A number of comparisons have reported a bias toward stimulus encoding as opposed to response encoding in PFv as opposed to PMd (Boussaoud and Wise, 1993a, b; Wallis

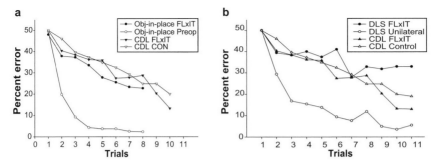

Figure 7–4 *A*. Control macaques make fewer errors learning visual discrimination problems when the stimuli are presented in the context of a background scene (Obj-in-place Preop) than when concurrent discrimination learning problems are simply presented in the absence of any scene (CDL CON). Although frontal temporal disconnection does not disrupt discrimination learning in the absence of scenes (CDL FLxIT), it does impair discrimination learning in the context of scenes (Obj-in-place FLxIT). (Reprinted with permission from Browning et al., *European Journal of Neuroscience*, 22 (12), 3281–3291. Copyright Blackwell Publishing, 2006.) *B*. Visual discrimination learning in control macaques is also facilitated when it is possible to employ a discrimination learning set because only a single problem is learned at a time (DLS Unilateral) as opposed to when several problems are learned concurrently (CDL control). This advantage is abolished after frontal temporal disconnection (DLS FLxIT versus CDL FLxIT). (Reprinted with permission from Browning et al., *Cerebral Cortex*, 17(4):859-64. Epub 2006 May 17. Copyright Oxford University Press, 2007.)

and Miller, 2003). A role for PFv in selecting behaviorally relevant stimulus information, on which action selection is then made contingent, is consistent with the strong connections of PFv with the temporal lobes in both humans and macaques. Some functional magnetic resonance imaging (fMRI) studies also emphasize the importance of the human PFv when task-relevant information must be selected (Brass and von Cramon, 2004; see also Chapter 9).

Strategy and Rule Learning

In addition to the selection of behaviorally relevant stimuli, PFv+o and adjacent lateral prefrontal cortex may also mediate the strategy that is used to learn the meaning of task rules. Bussey and colleagues (2001) reported that macaques spontaneously used a repeat-stay/change-shift strategy when they were learning a new set of conditional rules linking three stimuli to three actions. In other words, animals repeated their response if a stimulus was repeated from one trial to the next and the response used on the first trial had been successful, but they tended to change responses from trial to trial when the stimulus changed. When a response was unsuccessful, it was not attempted again if

the same stimulus appeared on the next trial. Both of these strategies were used significantly less after PFv+o lesions. Bussey and colleagues point out that these strategies may normally be important for fast and efficient learning of conditional rules, and it was noticeable that, although animals with PFv+o lesions were still able to learn task rules across several sessions, they were unable to learn them quickly within a session.

Such strategies may be important not only during conditional rule learning, but also during simpler types of learning, such as discrimination learning. Macaques learn discrimination problems more quickly when only one problem is presented at a time rather than when several problems are presented together within a block. This may be because monkeys can use repeat-stay strategies when learning a single discrimination problem, but the time between repetitions of a given problem when several others are learned concurrently may exceed the period over which the monkey can maintain a prospective code of what it should do on the next trial (Murray and Gaffan, 2006). Browning and colleagues (2007) have shown that disconnection of the entire prefrontal cortex from the inferior temporal cortex using the crossed lesion procedure abolished the normal advantage associated with single discrimination problem learning as opposed to concurrent discrimination problem learning (Fig. 7–4*B*).

Genovesio and colleagues (2005, 2006; see also Chapter 5) have recorded data from neurons in the lateral prefrontal cortex while monkeys select responses according to learned conditional rules linking them with stimuli or according to stimulus repeat-response stay and stimulus change-response shift strategies. They report that many prefrontal neurons selectively encode the use of strategies, such as repeat-stay and change-shift.

DORSOMEDIAL FRONTAL CORTEX

Changing between Rules and the Pre-Supplementary Motor Area

Rule-guided action selection depends on frontal areas beyond PFv—indeed, the role of periarcuate areas, such as PMd, in selecting responses has already been described. By combining careful fMRI with detailed attention to sulcal morphology, Amiez and colleagues (2006) demonstrated that the human PMd region active during response selection was located in and adjacent to the superior branch of the superior precentral sulcus. Lesions or the application of TMS at the same location disrupt response selection (Halsband and Freund, 1990; Schluter et al., 1998, 1999; Johansen-Berg et al., 2002; Rushworth et al., 2002).

More recently, the focus of research has moved to other motor association areas in the frontal lobe, such as the pre-SMA on the medial aspect of the superior frontal gyrus (Fig. 7–1). Originally, it was believed that this area was of little consequence for rule-guided action selection, because conditional tasks were unimpaired when lesions included this part of the macaque brain

(Chen et al., 1995). Several fMRI studies, however, have identified changes in activation of the human pre-SMA that are correlated with aspects of conditional tasks. Rather than being related to simple aspects of response selection, pre-SMA activity is most noticeable when participants change between sets of conditional rules—as, for example, in task-switching paradigms—or when it is possible to select responses according to more than one rule, for example, during response conflict paradigms (Brass and von Cramon, 2002; Rushworth et al., 2002; Garavan et al., 2003; Koechlin et al., 2003; Crone et al., 2006; see Chapters 3 and 9).

Lesion and interference studies also confirm that the pre-SMA is concerned with the selection of higher-order rules or response sets, even though it is not essential when a specific response must be selected according to a well-defined rule (Rushworth et al., 2004). In one study (Rushworth et al., 2002), human participants switched between two sets of conditional visuomotor rules that linked two stimuli to two different finger responses (either stimulus A response 1 and stimulus B response 2, or stimulus A response 2 and stimulus B response 1) [Fig. 7–5A]. Participants performed the task according to one superordinate rule set for several trials, and then a "switch" or "stay" cue appeared that instructed participants to either switch to the other rule set or to

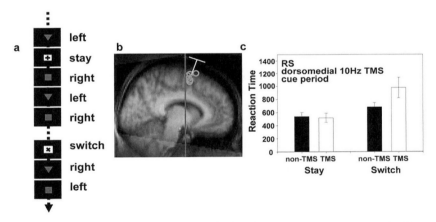

Figure 7–5 A. In the response switching (RS) task participants were presented with a series of task stimuli, red squares or triangles, and they responded by making right- and left-hand responses, respectively. Switch cues (white square with "X" at the center) instructed participants to change the response set, whereas stay cues (white square with "+" at the center) instructed participants to continue with the previous response set. B. Transcranial magnetic stimulation (TMS) over the pre-supplementary motor area (pre-SMA) disrupted performance on trials that followed a switch cue. C. It did not disrupt performance associated with a stay cue. RS, response switching. (Reprinted with permission from Rushworth et al., *Journal of Neurophysiology*, 87, 2577–2592. Copyright American Physiological Society, 2002.)

carry on with the same rule set. The application of TMS targeting the pre-SMA [Fig. 7–5B] disrupted performance most strongly if it was applied when participants were switching from one rule set to the other (Fig. 7–5C). TMS over PMd disrupted response performance whenever participants were attempting to select responses, regardless of whether they were doing so in the context of a task switch.

Lesions have a similar, although more permanent, effect relative to TMS. Husain and colleagues (2003) identified a patient with a small lesion circumscribed to the supplementary eye field, a region of the superior frontal gyrus close to the pre-SMA that is particularly concerned with the control of eye movements rather than limb movements (Fig. 7–6B). Husain and colleagues found that the patient could use arbitrary rules to guide the making of saccades to either the left or the right. The patient learned that the correct response was to saccade to a target on the left of a screen when one stimulus was

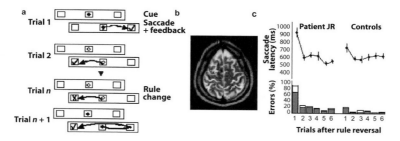

Figure 7–6 A patient with a lesion in the supplementary eye field region of the pre-supplementary motor area (pre-SMA) was tested on an oculomotor response-switching task that required saccades to targets on the left or right side of a screen, depending on the identify of a colored stimulus presented at the center of the screen. A. Two different rules linked the central stimuli to the responses made by the subject. At the beginning of the task, in trials 1 and 2, the subject performed correctly, and feedback, shown as a *tick* in the saccade target box on the *right* and the *left* in trials 1 and 2, respectively, informed the patient that the correct response has been made. The rule linking the stimuli to the responses was switched in trial *n*. The cross feedback at the saccade target box on the left informed the patient that the wrong movement has been made. The patient should respond according to the new rule in the subsequent trial, n + 1, but in this case, the subject made an initial incorrect saccade to the right, which was associated with incorrect feedback. The saccade was subsequently corrected, and an eye movement was made to the left. B. The yellow *arrow* indicates the position of the patient's lesion in the supplementary eye field. C. The patient (*left*) took longer to respond (*top*) and made more errors (*bottom*) on the trials that followed response switches than did control participants (*right*). *Open* and *shaded bars* on the *bottom* of the graph indicate corrected and uncorrected errors, respectively. (Reprinted with permission from Husain et al., *Nature Neuroscience*, 6, 117–118. Copyright Macmillan Publishers, Ltd., 2003.)

presented at the center of the screen, whereas the correct response was to saccade to the right when another stimulus was presented at the center of the
screen (Fig. 7–6A). Every so often, the rules linking cues to response direction
were switched so that the first and second cues now instructed saccades to the
right and left of the screen, respectively. It was just at these points that patient
performance was worse than that of control subjects (Fig. 7–6C). The TMS,
lesion, and fMRI data all emphasize the role of the pre-SMA and adjacent
cortex when participants are selecting between sets of rules rather than when
they are selecting a response according to a particular rule.

For some time, there has been an emphasis on action sequencing in discussions of the pre-SMA (Nakamura et al., 1998, 1999; Tanji, 2001). Although
action sequencing and task-switching may appear to be quite distinct processes, it is possible that the involvement of the pre-SMA in both is due to a
cognitive process that is common to both tasks. When people learn a long
sequence of actions that exceeds the span of short-term memory, they tend to
divide the sequence into shorter components ("chunks"). Just as the very first
movement of the sequence often has a long reaction time (Sternberg et al.,
1990), so does the first movement of a subsequent chunk within the sequence
(Kennerley et al., 2004) [Fig. 7–7A]. Longer reaction times at the beginning of
a sequence are believed to be due to the time taken to plan a set of consecutive
movements, not just the first movement. The same process of planning a set of
consecutive movements may also be occurring when long reaction times occur
at the start of a chunk later in the sequence. Just as the pre-SMA is important
when participants switch between one set of conditional action rules and
another, so it is important when participants switch between one set of rules
for sequencing actions and another. Kennerley and colleagues showed that

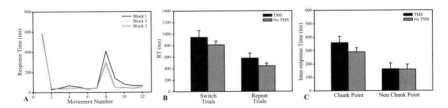

Figure 7–7 A. The first movement of a long sequence typically has a long response
time (RT), but often there is a further increase in the response time at a later point in
the sequence ("chunk point"). Although chunk points vary between participants, they
can be quite consistent across repetitions of the same sequence by the same participant.
Three repetitions are shown for this participant. Pre-supplementary motor area (pre-
SMA) transcranial magnetic stimulation (TMS) disrupts the initiation of a sequence
when the sequence is changed, as well as when it is repeated (B), and when it is applied
at the chunk point, but not when it is applied at the non-chunk point (C). RT, response
time. (Reprinted with permission from Kennerley et al., *Journal of Neurophysiology*,
91(2), 978–993. Copyright American Physiological Society, 2004.)

TMS over pre-SMA disrupts movement selection when it is applied at the time of the first action in the sequence (Fig. 7-7B) and when it is applied at the "chunk point," as participants switch from one chunk, or set, of movements to another (Fig. 7–7C). There is some suggestion from neurophysiology that pre-SMA neurons encode transitions between sequences of actions and chunks of action sequences. When macaques learn long sequences of actions composed of shorter, two-movement chunks, many of the pre-SMA neurons are active only for the first movement of each chunk (Nakamura et al., 1998). Additionally, many pre-SMA neurons are active when macaques switch from performing one sequence to performing another (Shima et al., 1996).

Changing between Rules and the Anterior Cingulate Cortex

It has sometimes been observed that more ventral parts of the medial frontal cortex, including the ACC, are active in neuroimaging studies of task-switching (Rushworth et al., 2002; Dosenbach et al., 2006; Liston et al., 2006). Competition between possible responses is higher on first switching from the old task set to the new task set because both the new response set and the old response set may be activated to similar degrees; response conflict may therefore be an integral component of task-switching. A number of studies have implicated the ACC in the detection of response conflict (Botvinick et al., 2004). Lesion studies, however, suggest that the ACC might not be as important as the pre-SMA for mediating changes in response sets and in situations of response conflict. It is not possible to examine the effects of ACC disruption with TMS, because it lies deep within the brain. Furthermore, its position, just ventral to the pre-SMA, means that, even if it were possible to apply TMS pulses of an intensity sufficient to disrupt ACC, the same pulses would be likely to disrupt the overlying pre-SMA as well. Macaques have, however, been trained on a task-switching paradigm, and the effects of ACC lesions have been examined (Rushworth et al., 2003). Animals were taught two competing sets of spatial-spatial conditional rules (left cue, respond top and right cue, respond bottom or left cue, respond bottom and right cue, respond top). Background visual patterns covering the entire touch-screen monitor on which the animals were responding instructed animals which rule set was in operation at any time. Although the ACC lesions caused a mild impairment in overall performance, it was difficult to identify any aspect of the impairment that was related to the process of task-switching per se. Single-cell recording studies have not investigated ACC activity during task-switching, but several studies have looked at ACC activity in situations that elicit more than one action, and response conflict occurs. An absence of modulation in relation to response conflict has been reported in single-unit recording studies of the ACC, whereas this modulation has been observed in pre-SMA (Stuphorn et al., 2000; Ito et al., 2003; Nakamura et al., 2005). Lesions of the superior frontal gyrus that encroach on the pre-SMA disrupt performance of tasks that elicit response conflict, just as they affect task-switching (Stuss et al., 2001;

Husain et al., 2003). In summary, paradigms that involve either response conflict or task-switching are associated with medial frontal cortical activity, but
the most critical region within the medial frontal cortex may be the pre-SMA
rather than the ACC.

Action Outcome Associations and the Anterior Cingulate Cortex

In situations that involve task-switching, response conflict, or both, participants are often concerned about whether the movements they are making are
appropriate. Thus, it is possible that they are monitoring the outcome of their
actions when they are task-switching. Along with conditional stimulus-action
associations, action-reinforcement outcome associations are critical determinants of the choices that humans and other animals make. As discussed earlier
in this chapter, reinforcement-guided action selection appears to depend on
different circuits than stimulus conditional action selection. An fMRI study
conducted by Walton and colleagues (2004) suggests that, although PFv is more
active when human participants employ conditional stimulus action associations, the ACC is more active when they monitor the outcomes of their own
voluntary choices.

Walton and colleagues taught their participants three sets of conditional
rules that could be used to link three shape stimuli with three button-press
responses (Fig. 7–8A). Participants performed the task according to a particular rule for several trials, until the presentation of a switch cue, similar to the
one used in the experiment by Rushworth and colleagues (2002) [see Fig. 7–5]
told them that the rule set was no longer valid. Activity in the period after the
switch cue was contrasted with activity recorded after a control event, a "stay"
cue that merely told subjects to continue performing the task the same way.
Unlike in the previous experiment, because there were three possible sets of
conditional rules, the switch cue did not tell subjects which rule was currently
in place (Fig. 7–8B). The subjects were able to work out which rule was
currently in place in different ways in the four task conditions that were used.
In the "generate and monitor" condition, participants had to guess which rule
set was valid after the switch cue. When participants encountered the first
shape stimulus after the switch cue, they were free to respond by pressing any
of the buttons. By monitoring the feedback that they received after the button
press, they could decide whether the response was correct for that shape and,
therefore, which set of rules was currently correct. Working out which rule set
is correct, therefore, involves two processes: (1) making a free choice, or decision, about which action to select and (2) monitoring the outcome of that
decision. The other three conditions, however, emphasized only the first or the
second of these processes in isolation ("generate" and "fixed and monitor") or
entailed neither process ("control"). Together, the four conditions constituted
a factorial design that made it possible to elucidate whether it was the type of
decision, free or externally determined, or the need for outcome monitoring
that was the cause of activation in the ACC (Fig. 7–8B).

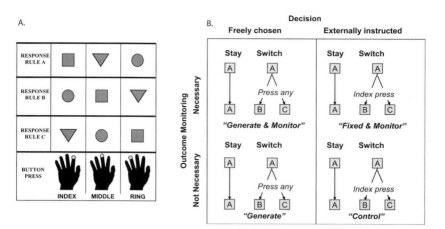

Figure 7–8 *A.* A representation of the three response rules linking stimulus shapes to finger-press actions during the task. *B.* The four conditions constituted a factorial design. The first factor was the type of decision that was made by the participants when they selected a candidate action after the cue informing them that the rule had changed. In the "generate and monitor" and "generate" conditions, the subjects had a free choice, but in the "fixed and monitor" and "control" conditions, the decision was externally determined. The second factor concerned the need to monitor the outcome of the decision. In the "generate and monitor" and "fixed and monitor" conditions, it was necessary to monitor the outcome of the decision, but the need to monitor outcomes was reduced in the "generate" and "control" conditions. Both factors were determinants of anterior cingulate cortex activity (see Fig. 9*B*). (Reprinted with permission from Walton et al., *Nature Neuroscience,* 7, 1259–1265. Copyright Macmillan Publishers, Ltd., 2004.)

In the "fixed and monitor" condition, participants were instructed always to attempt the same action first when the task sets changed. The element of outcome monitoring was still present in this condition, but the type of decision-making was altered; rather than the participant having a free choice, the decision about which finger to move was externally determined. In the "generate" condition, the opposite was true: The element of free choice in decision-making was retained, but the element of outcome monitoring was reduced. In this case, participants were asked to choose freely between the actions available, but were told that whatever action they selected would be the correct one. In the final, "control" condition, there was neither the need for a free choice when making the decision nor a need to monitor the outcome of the decision: Participants were told always to attempt the same action first whenever the switch cue told them that the rule set was changing. In this condition, participants were also told that whatever action was made would be the correct one (this was achieved by careful arrangement of which shape cues were presented after each switch event).

The ACC was the only frontal brain region that was more active after switching task sets in the "generate and monitor" condition than in the "fixed and monitor" condition (Fig. 7–9A). ACC activation was a function of the type of decision that was taken, free or externally determined. ACC activation was significantly higher in the conditions in which the decision was made freely ("generate and monitor" and "generate") as opposed to conditions in which the decision was externally determined ("fixed" and "control") [Figs. 7–8B and 7–9B]. However, ACC activity levels were also a function of the second task factor, outcome monitoring; ACC activity was significantly higher in the conditions in which it was necessary to monitor the outcomes of actions than in the conditions in which it was not necessary to do so (Figs. 7–8B and 7–9B). ACC activity was greatest when participants both made their decisions freely and had to monitor the outcomes of those decisions. ACC activity could not simply be attributed to the occurrence of errors because a similar pattern was also observed in trials in which the participant guessed correctly (Fig. 7–9C).

A distinct contrast that identified brain regions that are more active in the "fixed and monitor" condition than in the "generate and monitor" condition

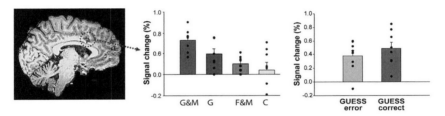

Figure 7–9 A. A dorsal anterior cingulate cortex (ACC) sulcal region was the only region to be more active in the "generate and monitor" (G&M) condition than in the "fixed and monitor" (F&M) condition. In the G&M condition, participants had a free decision about which action to select after the switch cue, and they had to monitor the outcome of that decision. In the F&M condition, participants were instructed always to attempt the same action when the task sets changed. The F&M condition retained the element of outcome monitoring, but the initial choice of which action to make was not voluntary. B. Signal change in the ACC was plotted in the G&M, F&M, and "generate" (G) conditions, when the element of free decision-making was retained but the element of outcome monitoring was reduced, and in the "control" condition (C) of the factorial design (Fig. 7–8B), when decision-making was externally determined rather than free and the need for outcome monitoring was reduced. ACC activation was a function of both of the experimentally manipulated factors; it was determined by both the type of decision (free versus externally determined; G&M and G versus F&M and C) and by the need for monitoring the outcome of the decision (G&M and F&M versus G and C). C. Activations in the G&M condition were not specific to trials in which participants made mistakes; there was a similar degree of signal change, even in the trials in which participants guessed correctly. (Reprinted with permission from Walton et al., *Nature Neuroscience, 7,* 1259–1265. Copyright Macmillan Publishers, Ltd., 2004).

revealed activity at the PFv/PFv+o boundary. The activation was located in the same region that had connections with the temporal lobe, via the uncinate fascicle and extreme capsule, in the DWI tractography study (Croxson et al., 2005) [Fig. 7–2]. The results suggest that the ACC and PFv may each play the preeminent role under complementary sets of conditions. Whereas the PFv is more active when monitoring to see if a predefined rule for action selection leads to the desired outcome, ACC is more active when choices are freely made, in the absence of instruction, and the outcome is used to guide future action choices.

The profiles of activity in individual neurons in lateral prefrontal cortex, including PFv, have been contrasted with those of the ACC (Matsumoto et al., 2003). The encoding of stimulus-action relationships is more prevalent and has an earlier onset in lateral prefrontal cortex than in ACC, whereas response-outcome encoding is more prevalent and has an earlier onset in ACC than in lateral prefrontal cortex. The effects of lesions in PFv and ACC have not been directly compared in the same tasks, but studies have examined whether ACC lesions impair outcome-guided action selection. ACC lesions in the macaque impair the reward-conditional tasks that are unimpaired by transection of the uncinate fascicle (Eacott and Gaffan, 1992; Hadland et al., 2003; also discussed earlier).

Action Values and the Anterior Cingulate Cortex

There is some ambiguity in reward-conditional tasks of the sort used by Hadland and colleagues (2003) as to whether the animal is using the visual appearance of one of the free rewards rather than the prospect of reward to guide action selection. To circumvent these ambiguities, Kennerley and colleagues (2006) taught macaques to perform an error-guided action-reversal task. The animals learned to make two different joystick movements: pull and turn. One movement was deemed the correct one for 25 successive trials, after which further instances of the same action were not rewarded. The only way that the macaque could tell that the reward contingencies had changed was by monitoring the outcomes of the actions and changing to the alternative whenever a given action no longer yielded a reward.

The first important result of the study was that control animals did not immediately switch to the alternative action on the very first trial after a previously successful action did not produce a reward (trials after an error are indicated as "E+1" trials in Fig. 7–10A). Instead, animals only gradually switched over to the alternative action. If a macaque switched to the correct action on the trial after an error, then it was more likely to make the correct action on the next trial ("EC+1" trials in Fig. 7–10A). As the macaque gradually accumulated more rewards by making the alternative action, it became more and more likely to continue making the alternative response. However, the increase in the probability of the alternative action was gradual. Even after much experience with a task, macaques do not naturally treat reinforcement

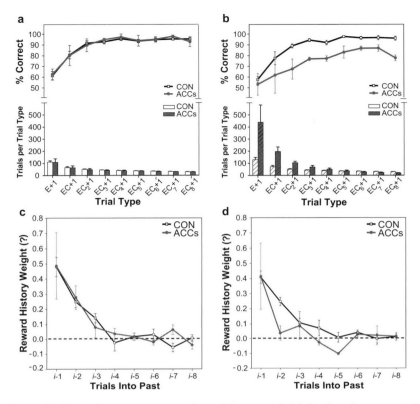

Figure 7–10 Performance on tests of sustaining rewarded behavior after an error in controls (CON) and after an anterior cingulate cortex sulcus (ACCs) lesion. Preoperative (A) and postoperative (B) performance is shown. Each line graph shows the mean percentage of trials of each type that were correct (± standard error of the mean) for each group. Control and ACCs lesion data are shown by the *black* and *gray lines*, respectively. The trial types are plotted across the x-axis and start on the *left*, with the trial immediately following an error (E + 1). The next data point corresponds to the trial after one error and then a correct response (EC + 1), the one after that corresponds to the trial after one error and then two correct responses (EC$_2$ + 1), and so on. Moving from left to right shows the animal's progress in acquiring more instances of positive reinforcement, after making the correct action, subsequent to an earlier error. The histogram at the *bottom* part of each graph indicates the number of instances of each trial type (± standard error of the mean). *White* and *gray bars* indicate control and ACCs lesion data, respectively, whereas *hatched bars* indicate data from the postoperative session. Estimates of the influence of the previous reward history on current choice in the preoperative (C) and postoperative (D) periods are also shown. Each point represents a group's mean regression coefficient value (± standard error of the mean) derived from multiple logistic regression analyses of choice on the current trial (i) against the outcomes (rewarded or unrewarded) on the previous eight trials for each animal. The influence of the previous trial ($i - 1$) is shown on the *left* side of each figure, the influence of two trials back ($i - 2$) is shown next, and so on until the trial that occurred eight trials previously ($i - 8$). Control and ACCs lesion data are shown by the *black* and *gray lines*, respectively. (Reprinted with permission from Kennerley et al., *Nature Neuroscience*, 9(7), 940–947. Copyright Macmillan Publishers, Ltd., 2006.)

change as an unambiguous instruction for one action or another in quite the same way as they treat sensory cues that have been linked to actions through conditional associations. In other words, the animals were guided by a sense of the action's value, which was based on its average reward history over the course of several trials; they were not simply guided by the most recent outcome that had followed the action. It is possible that something similar is occurring during other reversal learning tasks, but the necessary tests needed to check have not been performed.

The second important result was that, after the change in reward contingencies, animals with ACC lesions did not accumulate a revised sense of the alternative action's value at the same rate as the control animals, even if both groups responded to the occurrence of the first error in a similar manner (Fig. 7–10B). The conclusion that average action values were disrupted after an ACC lesion was supported by a logistic regression analysis that examined how well choices were predicted by the reward history associated with each action (Kennerley et al., 2006). Although the choices of control animals were influenced even by outcomes that had occurred five trials before, the choices of animals with ACC lesions were only influenced by the outcome of the previous trial (Fig. 7–10C and D). Amiez and colleagues (2006) have shown that neurons in the macaque ACC encode the average values of the different possible options that might be chosen, and the activity of posterior cingulate neurons is also sensitive to reward probability (McCoy and Platt, 2005).

Although the ACC has some connections with the anterior temporal lobe, its overall connection pattern is different from that of the PFv. In the macaque, several points in the ACC sulcus are directly interconnected with the ventral horn of the spinal cord (Dum and Strick, 1991, 1996), whereas PFv has more indirect access to the motor system (Dum and Strick, 2005; Miyachi et al., 2005). Adjacent ACC areas are interconnected with areas, such as the amygdala, caudate, and ventral striatum, which are important for the representation of reinforcement expectations and action outcome associations (Van Hoesen et al., 1993; Kunishio and Haber, 1994). When estimates of connection between the human ACC and various subcortical regions—based on DWI tractography (Croxson et al., 2005)—are compared, it is clear that human ACC is also more strongly interconnected with amygdala and parts of dorsal striatum and ventral striatum than it is with the temporal lobe via the uncinate fascicle and extreme capsule (Fig. 7–11). Thus, the role of PFv in identifying behaviorally relevant stimuli for guiding action selection and the role of ACC in representing action values are consistent with their anatomical connections in both the human and the macaque.

Conclusions

The frontal cortex has a central role in the selection of actions, both when the actions are selected on the basis of learned conditional associations with stimuli and when they are chosen on the basis of their reinforcement value and

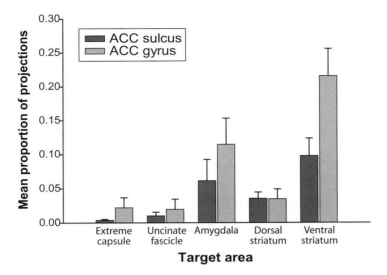

Figure 7–11 Quantitative results of probabilistic tractography from seed masks in the human extreme capsule, uncinate fascicle, amygdala, dorsal striatum, and ventral striatum to the anterior cingulate cortex (ACC) gyrus and ACC sulcus. The probability of connection with each prefrontal region as a proportion of the total connectivity with all prefrontal regions is plotted on the y-axis. The estimates of connection strength between the ACC and the amygdala, ventral striatum, and dorsal striatum are stronger than the estimates of ACC connectivity with the temporal lobe neocortex via the extreme capsule and the uncinate fascicle. (Adapted from Croxon et al., *Journal of Neuroscience,* 25, 8854–8866. Copyright Society for Neuroscience, 2005.)

associated reward expectancies. Lesion and interference studies suggest that the pre-SMA is critical when the rules for selecting responses are changed. Several lines of evidence, including neuroimaging, lesion investigation, and connectional anatomy, suggest that PFv and ACC are, respectively, more concerned with action selection on the basis of conditional associations and the representation of reinforcement values associated with actions. The particular contribution of PFv to conditional rule learning may concern the use of prospective coding strategies for efficient rule learning or the identification of behaviorally relevant stimuli that might then be associated with actions, rather than with the actual process of action retrieval. Exactly how these areas interact with one another and with other brain regions, such as the striatum, during the course of action selection remains to be determined.

ACKNOWLEDGMENTS Supported by the Medical Research Council and the Royal Society.

REFERENCES

Amiez C, Joseph JP, Procyk E (2006) Reward encoding in the monkey anterior cingulate cortex. Cerebral Cortex 16:1040–1055.

Amiez C, Kostopoulos P, Champod AS, Petrides M (2006) Local morphology predicts functional organization of the dorsal premotor region in the human brain. Journal of Neuroscience 26:2724–2731.

Asaad WF, Rainer G, Miller EK (1998) Neural activity in the primate prefrontal cortex during associative learning. Neuron 21:1399–1407.

Basser PJ, Jones DK (2002) Diffusion-tensor MRI: theory, experimental design and data Analysis—a technical review. NMR Biomedicine 15:456–467.

Beaulieu A (2002) A space for measuring mind and brain: interdisciplinarity and digital tools in the development of brain mapping and functional imaging, 1980–1990. Brain and Cognition 49:13–33.

Behrens TE, Johansen-Berg H, Woolrich MW, Smith SM, Wheeler-Kingshott CA, Boulby PA, Barker GJ, Sillery EL, Sheehan K, Ciccarelli O, Thompson AJ, Brady JM, Matthews PM (2003b) Non-invasive mapping of connections between human thalamus and cortex using diffusion imaging. Nature Neuroscience 6:750–757.

Behrens TE, Woolrich MW, Jenkinson M, Johansen-Berg H, Nunes RG, Clare S, Matthews PM, Brady JM, Smith SM (2003a) Characterization and propagation of uncertainty in diffusion-weighted MR imaging. Magnetic Resonance in Medicine 50:1077–1088.

Botvinick MM, Cohen JD, Carter CS (2004) Conflict monitoring and anterior cingulate cortex: an update. Trends in Cognitive Sciences 8:539–546.

Boussaoud D, Wise SP (1993a) Primate frontal cortex: neuronal activity following attentional versus intentional cues. Experimental Brain Research 95:15–27.

Boussaoud D, Wise SP (1993b) Primate frontal cortex: effects of stimulus and movement. Experimental Brain Research 95:28–40.

Brass M, von Cramon DY (2002) The role of the frontal cortex in task preparation. Cerebral Cortex 12:908–914.

Brass M, von Cramon DY (2004) Selection for cognitive control: a functional magnetic resonance imaging study on the selection of task-relevant information. Journal of Neuroscience 24:8847–8852.

Browning PG, Easton A, Buckley MJ, Gaffan D (2005) The role of prefrontal cortex in object-in-place learning in monkeys. European Journal of Neuroscience 22:3281–3291.

Browning PG, Easton A, Gaffan D (2007) Frontal-temporal disconnection abolishes object discrimination learning set in macaque monkeys. Cerebral Cortex 17:859–864.

Bunge SA, Kahn I, Wallis JD, Miller EK, Wagner AD (2003) Neural circuits subserving the retrieval and maintenance of abstract rules. Journal of Neurophysiology 90:3419–3428.

Bussey TJ, Wise SP, Murray EA (2001) The role of ventral and orbital prefrontal cortex in conditional visuomotor learning and strategy use in rhesus monkeys (*Macaca mulatta*). Behavioral Neuroscience 115:971–982.

Bussey TJ, Wise SP, Murray EA (2002) Interaction of ventral and orbital prefrontal cortex with inferotemporal cortex in conditional visuomotor learning. Behavioral Neuroscience 116:703–715.

Carmichael ST, Price JL (1995) Sensory and premotor connections of the orbital and medial prefrontal cortex of macaque monkeys. Journal of Comparative Neurology 363:642–664.

Chen Y, Thaler D, Nixon PD, Stern C, Passingham RE (1995) The functions of the medial premotor cortex (SMA), II. The timing and selection of learned movements. Experimental Brain Research 102:461–473.

Crone EA, Wendelken C, Donohue SE, Bunge SA (2006) Neural evidence for dissociable components of task-switching. Cerebral Cortex 16:475–486.

Croxson PL, Johansen-Berg H, Behrens TE, Robson MD, Pinsk MA, Gross CG, Richter W, Richter MC, Kastner S, Rushworth MF (2005) Quantitative investigation of connections of the prefrontal cortex in the human and macaque using probabilistic diffusion tractography. Journal of Neuroscience 25:8854–8866.

Dosenbach NU, Visscher KM, Palmer ED, Miezin FM, Wenger KK, Kang HC, Burgund ED, Grimes AL, Schlaggar BL, Petersen SE (2006) A core system for the implementation of task sets. Neuron 50:799–812.

Dum RP, Strick PL (1991) The origin of corticospinal projections from the premotor areas in the frontal lobe. Journal of Neuroscience 11:667–689.

Dum RP, Strick PL (1996) Spinal cord terminations of the medial wall motor areas in macaque monkeys. Journal of Neuroscience 16:6513–6525.

Dum RP, Strick PL (2005) Frontal lobe inputs to the digit representations of the motor areas on the lateral surface of the hemisphere. Journal of Neuroscience 25:1375–1386.

Eacott MJ, Gaffan D (1992) Inferotemporal-frontal disconnection: the uncinate fascicle and visual associative learning in monkeys. European Journal of Neuroscience 4:1320–1332.

Everling S, Tinsley CJ, Gaffan D, Duncan J (2002) Filtering of neural signals by focused attention in the monkey prefrontal cortex. Nature Neuroscience 5:671–676.

Everling S, Tinsley CJ, Gaffan D, Duncan J (2006) Selective representation of task-relevant objects and locations in the monkey prefrontal cortex. European Journal of Neuroscience 23:2197–2214.

Freedman DJ, Riesenhuber M, Poggio T, Miller EK (2001) Categorical representation of visual stimuli in the primate prefrontal cortex. Science 291:312–316.

Funahashi S, Bruce CJ, Goldman-Rakic PS (1993) Dorsolateral prefrontal lesions and oculomotor delayed response performance: Evidence for mnemonic 'scotomas.' Neuroscience 13:1479–1497.

Gaffan D, Easton A, Parker A (2002) Interaction of inferior temporal cortex with frontal cortex and basal forebrain: double dissociation in strategy implementation and associative learning. Journal of Neuroscience 22:7288–7296.

Garavan H, Ross TJ, Kaufman J, Stein EA (2003) A midline dissociation between error-processing and response-conflict monitoring. Neuroimage 20:1132–1139.

Genovesio A, Brasted PJ, Mitz AR, Wise SP (2005) Prefrontal cortex activity related to abstract response strategies. Neuron 47:307–320.

Genovesio A, Brasted PJ, Wise SP (2006) Representation of future and previous spatial goals by separate neural populations in prefrontal cortex. Journal of Neuroscience 26:7305–7316.

Goldman-Rakic PS (1996) The prefrontal landscape: implications of functional architecture for understanding human mentation and the central executive. Philosophical Transactions of the Royal Society of London B 351:1387–1527.

Grol MJ, de Lange FP, Verstraten FA, Passingham RE, Toni I (2006) Cerebral changes during performance of overlearned arbitrary visuomotor associations. Journal of Neuroscience 26:117–125.

Gutnikov S, Ma Y-Y, Gaffan D (1997) Temporo-frontal disconnection impairs visual-visual paired associate learning but not configural learning in Macaca monkeys. European Journal of Neuroscience 9:1524–1529.

Hadland KA, Rushworth MFS, Gaffan D, Passingham RE (2003) The anterior cingulate and reward-guided selection of actions. Journal of Neurophysiology 89:1161–1164.

Hagmann P, Thiran JP, Jonasson L, Vandergheynst P, Clarke S, Maeder P, Meuli R (2003) DTI mapping of human brain connectivity: statistical fiber tracking and virtual dissection. Neuroimage 19:545–554.

Halsband U, Passingham RE (1982) The role of premotor and parietal cortex in the direction of action. Brain Research 240:368–372.

Halsband U, Passingham RE (1985) Premotor cortex and the conditions for movement in monkeys (*Macaca fascicularis*). Behavioral Brain Research 18:269–277.

Halsband U, Freund H-J (1990) Premotor cortex and conditional motor learning in man. Brain 113:207–222.

Husain M, Parton A, Hodgson TL, Mort D, Rees G (2003) Self-control during response conflict by human supplementary eye field. Nature Neuroscience 6:117–118.

Ito S, Stuphorn V, Brown JW, Schall JD (2003) Performance monitoring by the anterior cingulate cortex during saccade countermanding. Science 302:120–122.

Johansen-Berg H, Rushworth MFS, Bogdanovic MD, Kischka U, Wimalaratna S, Matthews PM (2002) The role of ipsilateral premotor cortex in hand movement after stroke. Proceedings of the National Academy of Sciences U S A 99:14518–14523.

Kennerley SW, Sakai K, Rushworth MFS (2004) Organization of action sequences and the role of the pre-SMA. Journal of Neurophysiology 91:978–993.

Kennerley SW, Walton ME, Behrens TE, Buckley MJ, Rushworth MF (2006) Optimal decision making and the anterior cingulate cortex. Nature Neuroscience 9:940–947.

Koechlin E, Ody C, Kouneiher F (2003) The architecture of cognitive control in the human prefrontal cortex. Science 302:1181–1185.

Kunishio K, Haber SN (1994) Primate cingulostriatal projection: limbic striatal versus sensorimotor striatal input. Journal of Comparative Neurology 350:337–356.

Lebedev MA, Messinger A, Kralik JD, Wise SP (2004) Representation of attended versus remembered locations in prefrontal cortex. PLoS Biology 2:e365.

Liston C, Matalon S, Hare TA, Davidson MC, Casey BJ (2006) Anterior cingulate and posterior parietal cortices are sensitive to dissociable forms of conflict in a task-switching paradigm. Neuron 50:643–653.

Luppino G, Matelli M, Camarda R, Rizzolatti G (1993) Corticospinal connections of area F3 (SMA-proper) and area F6 (pre-SMA) in the macaque monkey. Journal of Comparative Neurology 338:114–140.

Matsumoto K, Suzuki W, Tanaka K (2003) Neuronal correlates of goal-based motor selection in the prefrontal cortex. Science 301:229–232.

Matsuzaka Y, Aizawa H, Tanji J (1992) A motor area rostral to the supplementary motor area (presupplementary motor area) in the monkey: neuronal activity during a learned motor task. Journal of Neurophysiology 68:653–662.

McCoy AN, Platt ML (2005) Risk-sensitive neurons in macaque posterior cingulate cortex. Nature Neuroscience 8:1220–1227.

Miyachi S, Lu X, Inoue S, Iwasaki T, Koike S, Nambu A, Takada M (2005) Organization of multisynaptic inputs from prefrontal cortex to primary motor cortex as revealed by retrograde transneuronal transport of rabies virus. Journal of Neuroscience 25:2547–2556.

Murray EA, Brasted PJ, Wise SP (2002) Arbitrary sensorimotor mapping and the life of primates. In: Neuropsychology of memory (Squire LR, Schacter DL, eds.), pp 339–348, 3rd edition. New York: Guilford Press.

Murray EA, Bussey TJ, Wise SP (2000) Role of prefrontal cortex in a network for arbitrary visuomotor mapping. Experimental Brain Research 133:114–129.

Murray EA, Gaffan D (2006) Prospective memory in the formation of learning sets by rhesus monkeys (*Macaca mulatta*). Journal of Experimental Psychology: Animal and Behavior Processes 32:87–90.

Nakamura K, Roesch MR, Olson CR (2005) Neuronal activity in macaque SEF and ACC during performance of tasks involving conflict. Journal of Neurophysiology 93:884–908.

Nakamura K, Sakai K, Hikosaka O (1998) Neuronal activity in the medial frontal cortex during learning of sequential procedures. Journal of Neurophysiology 80:2671–2687.

Nakamura K, Sakai K, Hikosaka O (1999) Effects of local inactivation of monkey medial frontal cortex in learning of sequential procedures. Journal of Neurophysiology 82:1063–1068.

Parker A, Gaffan D (1998) Memory after frontal/temporal disconnection in monkeys: conditional and non-conditional tasks, unilateral and bilateral frontal lesions. Neuropsychologia 36:259–271.

Passingham RE, Toni I, Rushworth MFS (2000) Specialisation within the prefrontal cortex: the ventral prefrontal cortex and associative learning. Experimental Brain Research 133:103–113.

Paton JJ, Belova MA, Morrison SE, Salzman CD (2006) The primate amygdala represents the positive and negative value of visual stimuli during learning. Nature 439:865–870.

Petrides M (1982) Motor conditional associative-learning after selective prefrontal lesions in the monkey. Behavioral Brain Research 5:407–413.

Petrides M (1986) The effect of periarcuate lesions in the monkey on performance of symmetrically and asymmetrically visual and auditory go, no-go tasks. Journal of Neuroscience 6:2054–2063.

Petrides M (2005) Lateral prefrontal cortex: architectonic and functional organization. Philosophical Transactions of the Royal Society of London 360:781–795.

Petrides M, Pandya DN (1988) Association fiber pathways to the frontal cortex from the superior temporal region in the rhesus monkey. Journal of Comparative Neurology 273:52–66.

Petrides M, Pandya DN (2002a) Comparative cytoarchitectonic analysis of the human and the macaque ventrolateral prefrontal cortex and corticocortical connection patterns in the monkey. European Journal of Neuroscience 16:291–310.

Petrides M, Pandya D (2002b) Association pathways of the prefrontal cortex and functional observations. In: Principles of frontal lobe function (Stuss DT, Knight RT, eds.), pp 31–50. New York: Oxford University Press.

Rainer G, Asaad WF, Miller EK (1998) Selective representation of relevant information by neurons in the primate prefrontal cortex. Nature 393:577–579.

Rushworth MF, Buckley MJ, Gough PM, Alexander IH, Kyriazis D, McDonald KR, Passingham RE (2005) Attentional selection and action selection in the ventral and orbital prefrontal cortex. Journal of Neuroscience 25:11628–11636.

Rushworth MFS, Hadland KA, Gaffan D, Passingham RE (2003) The effect of cingulate cortex lesions on task switching and working memory. Journal of Cognitive Neuroscience 15:338–353.

Rushworth MFS, Hadland KA, Paus T, Sipila PK (2002) Role of the human medial frontal cortex in task switching: a combined fMRI and TMS study. Journal of Neurophysiology 87:2577–2592.

Rushworth MFS, Nixon PD, Eacott MJ, Passingham RE (1997) Ventral prefrontal cortex is not essential for working memory. Journal of Neuroscience 17:4829–4838.

Rushworth MFS, Owen AM (1998) The functional organization of the lateral frontal cortex: conjecture or conjuncture in the electrophysiology literature? Trends in Cognitive Science 2:46–53.

Rushworth MFS, Walton ME, Kennerley SW, Bannerman DM (2004) Action sets and decisions in the medial frontal cortex. Trends in Cognitive Sciences 8:410–417.

Sakagami M, Niki H (1994) Encoding of behavioral significance of visual stimuli by primate prefrontal neurons: relation to relevant task conditions. Experimental Brain Research 97:423–436.

Sakagami M, Tsutsui K-i, Lauwereyns J, Koizumi M, Kobayashi S, Hikosaka O (2001) A code for behavioral inhibition on the basis of color, but not motion, in ventrolateral prefrontal cortex of macaque monkey. Journal of Neuroscience 21:4801–4808.

Samejima K, Ueda Y, Doya K, Kimura M (2005) Representation of action-specific reward values in the striatum. Science 310:1337–1340.

Schluter ND, Rushworth MFS, Mills KR, Passingham RE (1999) Signal-, set-, and movement-related activity in the human premotor cortex. Neuropsychologia 37:233–243.

Schluter ND, Rushworth MFS, Passingham RE, Mills KR (1998) Temporary interference in human lateral premotor cortex suggests dominance for the selection of movements: a study using transcranial magnetic stimulation. Brain 121 (Pt 5):785–799.

Schmahmann JD, Pandya DN (2006) Fiber pathways of the brain. Oxford: Oxford University Press.

Schultz W (2000) Multiple reward signals in the brain. Nature Reviews Neuroscience 1:199–207.

Shima K, Mushiake H, Saito N, Tanji J (1996) Role for cells in the presupplementary motor area in updating motor plans. Proceedings of the National Academy of Sciences U S A 93:8694–8698.

Sternberg S, Knoll RL, Turock DL (1990) Hierarchical control in the execution of action sequences: tests of two invariance properties. In: Attention and performance, XIII (Jeannerod M, ed.), pp 3–55. Hillsdale, New Jersey, Hove and London: Lawrence Erlbaum Associates.

Stuphorn V, Taylor TL, Schall JD (2000) Performance monitoring by the supplementary eye field. Nature 408:857–860.

Stuss DT, Floden D, Alexander MP, Levine B, Katz D (2001) Stroop performance in focal lesion patients: dissociation of processes and frontal lobe lesion location. Neuropsychologia 39:771–786.

Tanji J (2001) Sequential organization of multiple movements: involvement of cortical motor areas. Annual Review of Neuroscience 24:631–651.

Tomita H, Ohbayashi M, Nakahara K, Hasegawa I, Miyashita Y (1999) Top-down signal from prefrontal cortex in executive control of memory retrieval. Nature 401:699–703.

Toni I, Passingham RE (1999) Prefrontal-basal ganglia pathways are involved in the learning of visuomotor associations: a PET study. Experimental Brain Research 127:19–32.

Toni I, Rushworth MFS, Passingham RE (2001) Neural correlates of visuomotor associations: spatial rules compared with arbitrary rules. Experimental Brain Research 141:359–369.

Toni I, Schluter ND, Josephs O, Friston K, Passingham RE (1999) Signal-, set- and movement-related activity in the human brain: an event-related fMRI study. Cerebral Cortex 9:35–49.

Tournier JD, Calamante F, Gadian DG, Connelly A (2003) Diffusion-weighted magnetic resonance imaging fiber tracking using a front evolution algorithm. Neuroimage 20:276–288.

Ungerleider LG, Gaffan D, Pelak VS (1989) Projections from the inferior temporal cortex to prefrontal cortex via the uncinate fascicle in rhesus monkeys. Experimental Brain Research 76:473–484.

Van Hoesen GW, Morecraft RJ, Vogt BA (1993) Connections of the monkey cingulate cortex. In: Neurobiology of cingulate cortex and limbic thalamus: a comprehensive handbook (Vogt BA, Gabriel M, eds.), pp 249–284. Boston: Birkhauser.

Vogt BA (1993) Structural organization of cingulate cortex: areas, neurons, and somatodentritic transmitter receptors. In: Neurobiology of cingulate cortex and limbic thalamus: a comprehensive handbook (Vogt BA, Gabriel M, eds.), pp 19–70. Boston: Birkhauser.

Wagner AD, Pare-Blagoev EJ, Clark J, Poldrack RA (2001) Recovering meaning: left prefrontal cortex guides controlled semantic retrieval. Neuron 31:329–338.

Wallis JD, Anderson KC, Miller EK (2001) Single neurons in prefrontal cortex encode abstract rules. Nature 411:953–956.

Wallis JD, Miller EK (2003) From rule to response: neuronal processes in the premotor and prefrontal cortex. Journal of Neurophysiology 90:1790–1806.

Walton ME, Devlin JT, Rushworth MFS (2004) Interactions between decision making and performance monitoring within prefrontal cortex. Nature Neuroscience 7: 1259–1265.

Webster MJ, Bachevalier J, Ungerleider LG (1994) Connections of inferior temporal areas TEO and TE with parietal and frontal cortex in macaque monkeys. Cerebral Cortex 5:470–483.

White IM, Wise SP (1999) Rule-dependent neuronal activity in the prefrontal cortex. Experimental Brain Research 126:315–335.

Wilson FAW, Scalaidhe SPO, Goldman-Rakic PS (1993) Dissociation of object and spatial processing domains in primate prefrontal cortex. Science 260:1955–1957.

Wise SP, Murray EA (2000) Arbitrary associations between antecedents and actions. Trends in Neuroscience 23:271–276.

Yamada H, Matsumoto N, Kimura M (2004) Tonically active neurons in the primate caudate nucleus and putamen differentially encode instructed motivational outcomes of action. Journal of Neuroscience 24:3500–3510.

8

Differential Involvement of the Prefrontal, Premotor, and Primary Motor Cortices in Rule-Based Motor Behavior

Eiji Hoshi

Humans and nonhuman primates are capable of behaving in compliance with rules of behavior. A hallmark of rule-based behavior is flexible information processing across the sensory and motor domains following the behavioral rule. Depending on the behavioral rule, it is necessary to execute a different movement in response to a sensory signal (Fuster, 1997; Asaad et al., 1998; Miller and Cohen, 2001; Wallis et al., 2001; Bunge et al., 2005).

Of the structures in the brain, the frontal cortex appears to be the best place to achieve rule-based motor behavior for three reasons. (1) It collects exteroceptive sensory signals of all modalities, such as vision or hearing, and interoceptive signals, such as hunger or thirst (Jones and Powell, 1970; Goldman-Rakic, 1987; Pandya and Yeterian, 1996; Rolls, 1996; Fuster, 1997; Romanski et al., 1999; Cavada et al., 2000; Ongur and Price, 2000). (2) It is interconnected with the motor structures controlling effectors, such as the eyes and arms (Fries, 1984; Selemon and Goldman-Rakic, 1988; Dum and Strick, 1991; Barbas, 2000). (3) It contains a huge number of interconnections (Barbas and Pandya, 1989; Miyachi et al., 2005). These facts suggest that the frontal cortex plays a nodal role in achieving a behavioral goal by accessing and interconnecting both the sensory and motor domains (Goldman-Rakic et al., 1992; Passingham, 1993; Fuster, 1997, 2001).

This chapter focuses on the structural and functional networks in the frontal cortex that achieve rule-based motor behavior. Rather than reviewing a broad range of articles, I focus on several studies that are directly related to this topic (Lu et al., 1994; Hoshi et al., 1998; Hoshi et al., 2000; Miyachi et al., 2005; Hoshi and Tanji, 2006). Reaching movements are used as a model behavior because reaching is a basic action and the neuronal mechanisms underlying it have been studied intensively. Moreover, I discuss the functional roles of the lateral part of the frontal cortex because physiological studies show that it is crucial to both rule-based motor behavior (Wise et al., 1996; Wise et al., 1997; White and

Wise, 1999; Rizzolatti and Luppino, 2001; Tanji and Hoshi, 2001; Wallis et al., 2001) and reaching movements (Wise, 1985; Hoshi and Tanji, 2004).

In this chapter, I adopt the macaque monkey brain as a model system for three reasons. First, its anatomical networks have been studied in detail and its basic architecture is homologous to that of humans (Pandya and Yeterian, 1996; Petrides and Pandya, 1999). Second, it shows a remarkable ability to behave flexibly, conforming to behavioral rules (White and Wise, 1999; Wallis et al., 2001). Third, a variety of neuronal activities deemed to play crucial roles in rule-based motor behavior occur in the frontal cortex of the macaque monkey.

HIERARCHICAL ORGANIZATION OF THE REACHING MOVEMENT

A reaching movement brings the hand and arm to a target. To successfully reach an object, multiple sets of information must be processed and integrated. One way to organize this information is via a hierarchical system. Figure 8–1 illustrates three hierarchical levels in the process of planning and executing a reaching movement. At the first level, motor-related information regarding which arm to use is generated and the target location is selected. Neural computations at this level involve cognitive information processing because it is necessary to collect and integrate diverse sets of information and process it in conformity with the behavioral rule to select an appropriate target or effector. At the second level, the two sets of selected information (arm use and target location) are collected and integrated to plan the reaching movement.

This integration process is crucial to completing the reaching movement because of the need to handle fairly distinct types of motor-related informa-

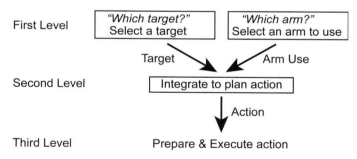

Figure 8–1 Hierarchical organization of the reaching movement. Three levels of information processing are summarized schematically. The first level gives rise to components of the reaching movement, such as arm use and target location. The second level integrates these components to plan the reaching movement. The third level prepares and executes the planned movement.

tion; although the arm is part of the participant's body, the target exists in extra-personal space. Once the reaching movement is planned, it can be prepared and executed by the neural elements at the third level. Based on this schema, neural processes at the second and third levels do not require a great deal of information processing based on the behavioral rule because the processes involved in integrating the selected arm and target location and in preparing and executing the movement are fairly straightforward.

ANATOMICAL ORGANIZATION OF THE LATERAL FRONTAL CORTEX

The lateral frontal cortex is not a homogenous entity, but one that consists of multiple distinct areas (Fig. 8–2). The most caudal part is the primary motor cortex, which corresponds to Brodmann area 4 (Brodmann, 1909). A somato-topic organization is evident: The area representing facial movement is located laterally, the trunk (or leg) area is located medially, and the area representing arm or shoulder movement (i.e., the body parts that are most involved in the reaching movement) is located in between. An area that corresponds to area

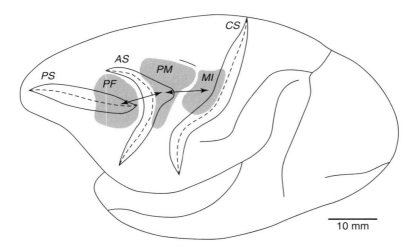

Figure 8–2 Connections of the prefrontal, premotor, and primary motor cortices. A lateral view of the cortex of the macaque monkey is illustrated. The rostral part points to the left. *Broken lines* indicate the fundi of the principal sulcus (PS), the arcuate sulcus (AS), and the central sulcus (CS). The *gray areas* indicate the cortical territories related to the rule-based motor behavior. The *bidirectional arrows* show the reciprocity of corticocortical connections. PF, prefrontal cortex; PM, premotor cortex; MI, primary motor cortex.

6 is located rostrally to the primary motor cortex and behind the depth of the arcuate sulcus. This is the premotor cortex. The broad territory of the prefrontal cortex is located rostrally to the arcuate sulcus. Studies show that its lateral part plays crucial roles in both the reaching movement and rule-based motor behavior (White and Wise, 1999; Hoshi et al., 2000; Wallis et al., 2001; Bunge et al., 2005).

A pioneering study by Lu et al. (1994) examined the corticocortical pathways from the prefrontal cortex to the arm region of the primary motor cortex. They injected distinct retrograde tracers into the lateral prefrontal cortex and the primary motor cortex. This enabled them to study the relationship between the premotor areas interconnected with the prefrontal cortex and the primary motor cortex. They found that the prefrontal cortex is linked with the rostral part of the premotor cortex, and that the caudal parts of the premotor cortex project to the primary motor cortex. Furthermore, they observed little direct overlap between them, except for the ventral part of the premotor cortex. However, because of the many connections between the rostral and caudal parts of the premotor cortex (Barbas and Pandya, 1987), their results suggest that the premotor cortex transfers information from the prefrontal cortex to the primary motor cortex.

More recently, using retrograde transneuronal transport, Miyachi et al. examined the multisynaptic projections from the prefrontal cortex to the arm region of the primary motor cortex (Miyachi et al., 2005). When they injected a strain of neurotropic rabies virus into the arm region of the primary motor cortex, the rabies virus was transported across synapses from postsynaptic neurons to the presynaptic neurons in a time-dependent manner. Consequently, they could identify the multisynaptic input to the injected region (i.e., primary motor cortex), and discovered that infected neurons first appeared in the caudal part of the premotor cortex, but not in the prefrontal cortex. Infected neurons were observed later in the lateral prefrontal cortex than in the premotor cortex.

These two reports provide evidence for the involvement of the lateral prefrontal cortex in arm movement and suggest that the premotor cortex plays an important role in conveying information from the prefrontal cortex to the primary motor cortex.

FUNCTIONAL ORGANIZATION OF THE LATERAL FRONTAL CORTEX

The previous section discussed an anatomical pathway from the prefrontal cortex to the primary motor cortex via the premotor cortex. Now, I turn to the functional involvement of these areas in rule-based motor behavior using a reaching movement as the behavioral model. I will discuss the distinct roles played by the three areas by introducing examples of neuronal activity recorded from monkeys performing behavioral tasks that required rule-based information processing to achieve a motor behavior goal.

The Prefrontal Cortex Is Involved in Selecting
a Reach Target Based on the Behavioral Rule

To examine how the prefrontal cortex is involved in motor selection, two monkeys were trained to select a reach target by integrating two successive visual signals in a rule-dependent manner (Hoshi et al., 2000) [Fig. 8–3]. In this task, a sample cue (triangle or circle) appeared at one of three locations

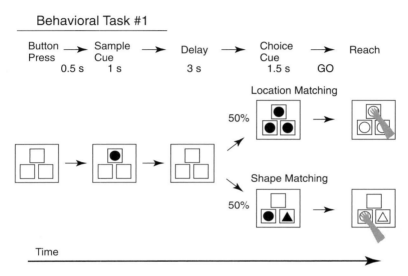

Figure 8–3 Behavioral task 1. The behavioral sequences of task 1 are depicted from left to right. When the monkey pressed a hold button for 0.5 s, a red sample cue, either a circle or a triangle, appeared in one of the three locations (top, left, or right). The sample cue disappeared 1 s later, and only the background remained visible for a 3-s delay period. After this delay, a red choice cue appeared. There were two different sets of cues; each required a different task to be performed. If the choice cue was either three triangles (after a triangle sample cue) or three circles (after a circle sample cue), the monkey was required to select the triangle or circle that was in the same location as the sample cue (location-matching rule; *center right*). On the other hand, if the choice cue was a triangle and a circle, the monkey had to select the object with the same shape as the sample cue (shape-matching rule; *bottom right*). If the participant continued to press the hold button for another 1.5 s, the color of the choice cue changed from red to green ("go" signal). If the animal touched the correct object, a drop of fruit juice was given as a reward. Because the two task rules (shape-matching and location-matching rules) were presented randomly, the monkeys had to remember both the shape and the location of the sample cue until the choice cue was presented. When the choice cue appeared, the monkey selected the correct target by combining the memorized information (provided by the sample cue) and the current information (provided by the choice cue).

(top, left, or right) for 1 s. After a 3-s delay period, during which the monkey was required to memorize both the shape and location of the sample cue, one of two choice cues appeared randomly. The first cue instructed the monkey to reach for a target that was in the same location as the sample cue (location-matching rule). The second cue instructed the monkey to reach for a target that was the same shape as the sample cue (shape-matching rule). The choice cue for location matching consisted of either three circles or three triangles. The choice cue for shape matching consisted of a pair of a circle and a triangle. When the color of the choice cue changed from red to green 1.5 s later ("go" signal), the monkey reached for the correct object to obtain a juice reward. In this task, after the choice cue appeared, the monkey was able to select the reach target by combining the two sets of information given by the sample and choice cues in a rule-dependent manner.

At the critical time corresponding to the presentation of the choice cue, three classes of neuronal activity were found in the lateral prefrontal cortex. The activity of neurons in the first class reflected past sensory information (the location or shape of the sample cue presented 3 s earlier). This selectivity began during the presentation of the sample cue and continued throughout the delay period.

The second class of activity was selective for the configuration of the choice cue. One group of neurons in this second class was selectively active when the configuration of the choice cue was a pair of a circle and triangle (i.e., when the behavioral task called for selecting a target based on the shape information) [shape-matching rule]. Another group of neurons in the second class was preferentially active when the choice cue consisted of three circles or three triangles (i.e., when the behavioral task called for selecting a target based on the location information) [location-matching rule].

Finally, activity of the third class reflected the location of the selected target. The neuron shown in Figure 8–4 was vigorously active when the monkey selected a target in the left location, regardless of the behavioral rule. The appearance of the third class of activity meant that the target-selection process was completed in the prefrontal cortex.

Figure 8–5 shows the population activities of the three classes of neuronal activity. Before the choice cue appeared, activity reflecting the sample cue (the first class of neurons) was dominant. The activity reached its peak soon after the appearance of the choice cue. Subsequently, this activity diminished quickly, while the choice cue was still present. In contrast, the second class of activity (reflecting the configuration of the choice cue) and the third class (reflecting the location of the selected target) developed shortly after the choice cue appeared. The population activity revealed that the sample cue-selective activity (the first class) reached its peak with the shortest latency after the choice cue appeared. Then the configuration-selective activity (the second class) reached its peak, followed by the activity reflecting the selected target location (the third class). Therefore, around the time when the choice cue was presented (i.e., when the monkey was actively engaged in selecting a reach target), the

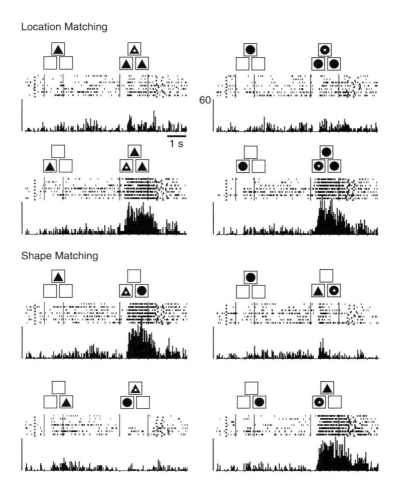

Figure 8–4 Reach target location selectivity for task 1. An example of a pre-frontal neuron whose activity was selective for the target location is shown. The *top two rows* illustrate neuronal activity for the location-matching rule. The *bottom two rows* show neuronal activity for the shape-matching rule. An *asterisk* centered in a *circle* or *triangle* shows the target to be touched in the response period. This neuron was most active when the target was on the left, regardless of the behavioral rule. In the raster displays, each row represents a trial, and *dots* denote discharges of this neuron. Discharges are summarized in the perievient histograms below each raster display. The ordinate of the histograms represents the discharge rate (spikes per second). (Adapted with permission from Hoshi et al., *Journal of Neurophysiology*, 83:2355–2373. Copyright American Physiological Society, 2000.)

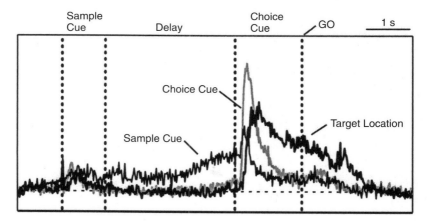

Figure 8–5 Population activity for task 1. Population histograms showing the time course of the three classes of activity. Data are aligned on the onset of the choice cue. The *thin black trace* is a population histogram of activity related to the sample cue. The *gray trace* is a population histogram of activity related to the choice cue configuration. The *thick black trace* is a population histogram of activity selective for the target location. The activity ratio on the ordinate is calculated by dividing the data in each bin by the control data (last 500 ms of an intertrial interval). Task periods are indicated at the *top*. (Adapted with permission from Hoshi et al., *Journal of Neurophysiology*, 83:2355–2373. Copyright American Physiological Society, 2000.)

representation of task-relevant information in the prefrontal cortex shifted quickly from the sample cue to the choice cue, and from the choice cue to the selected target location.

The existence of the three classes of activity reflecting the information essential to the task suggests that the lateral prefrontal cortex is critically involved in selecting a reach target based on the behavioral rule (Hoshi et al., 2000). Furthermore, the temporal relationships of the neuron population activity (Fig. 8–5) revealed that the information representation changed quickly from the sample and choice cues to the information on action (i.e., the target location). The changing representation of the task-relevant information seems to be a neural correlate for integrating multiple sets of information for generating novel information to guide a behavior in a rule-dependent manner (Tanji and Hoshi, 2001).

The Premotor Cortex Is Involved in Planning the Reaching Movement

The selected target information must be transformed into an actual reaching movement—a process that I refer to as "planning the reaching movement." As

discussed earlier, it is necessary to integrate distinct sets of information on the target location and arm use in planning this movement. To study the neuronal basis of this process, a new behavioral task was developed (Hoshi and Tanji, 2000, 2006).

In this task, two visual instruction cues were given successively, with an intervening delay (Fig. 8–6). One cue instructed the location of the target (right or left), and the other cue instructed which arm (right or left) to use. Subsequently, with the "go" signal (the disappearance of the fixation point), the participant was required to reach for the instructed target with the instructed arm. The order of the instructions on arm use and target location was reversed in a block of 20 trials. Therefore, after the first cue, it was necessary to collect and maintain information about the target location (if the first cue instructed target location) or arm use (if the first cue instructed arm use). After the second cue, the participant was able to combine the two successive instructions on target location and arm use. The task design enabled us to study the neuronal mechanisms underlying the second level of hierarchical organization for the reaching movement (Fig. 8–1).

Neurons in the premotor cortex showed three distinct patterns of activity during performance of this task (Hoshi and Tanji, 2000, 2006). Two groups of neuronal activity were observed after the appearance of the first cue. The first group of neurons responded to the appearance of the first cue instructing which arm to use, and its activity persisted until the second cue was presented. For example, the neuron shown in Figure 8–7A discharged selectively after the appearance of the right arm instruction. The second group of neurons became active after the appearance of the instruction on target location. The neuron shown in Figure 8–7B selectively discharged after the right target instruction was given, and like the first group, its activity persisted until the second cue was presented.

When the second cue appeared, the third group of neurons became active, although this activity did not reflect the instruction given by the second cue itself. Instead, the activity reflected a specific combination of the two instructions on arm use and target location, regardless of their order of presentation. The neuron shown in Figure 8–7C responded to the appearance of the second cue only when the combination of the two instructions on arm use and target location was right arm and left target. In other words, the third group of neurons reflected the forthcoming reaching movement by integrating the two distinct sets of motor information on arm use and target location.

The existence of the three groups of activity in the premotor cortex suggests that this area contributes to planning reaching movements by collecting and integrating distinct sets of information on target location and arm use. These processes are crucial for planning the reaching movement, and they correspond to the second-level processing in the hierarchical organization of the reaching movement (Fig. 8–1).

Behavioral Task #2

"Arm then Target" Instruction Order

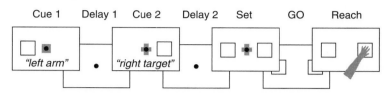

Cue 1   Delay 1   Cue 2   Delay 2   Set   GO   Reach

"left arm"   •   "right target"   •

"Target then Arm" Instruction Order

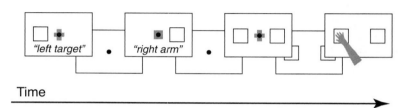

"left target"   •   "right arm"   •

Time

Figure 8–6 Behavioral task 2. The behavioral sequences of task 2 are depicted from left to right. The *top* shows a trial in which two instructions were given, namely, which arm to use ("arm") and which target to reach ("target"), in that order. The *bottom* shows a trial in which the two instructions were given in reverse order. The task commenced when a monkey placed one hand on each touch pad and gazed at a fixation point that appeared at the center of the touch-sensitive screen. If fixation continued for 1200 ms, the monkey was given the first instruction (first cue; 400-ms duration), which contained information about either the target location or which arm to use. A small, colored cue superimposed on the central fixation point indicated the type of instruction (i.e., whether it related to target location or arm use). A green square indicated an arm-use instruction, whereas a blue cross indicated a target-location instruction. At the same time, a white square appeared to the left or right of the fixation point and indicated laterality of arm use (for arm use-related instructions) or target location (for target-related instructions). If fixation continued for 1200 ms during the subsequent delay period (first delay), the second instruction (second cue; 400 ms) was given to complete the information required for the subsequent action. Thereafter, if fixation continued for 1200 ms during the second delay, squares appeared on each side of the fixation point, instructing the monkey to prepare to reach for the target when the fixation point disappeared ("go" signal). If the monkey subsequently reached for the target with the specified arm, it received a reward of fruit juice. The order of appearance of the target and arm instructions was alternated in a block of 20 trials, and laterality was randomized within each block. A series of five 250-Hz tones after a reward signaled reversal of instruction orders.

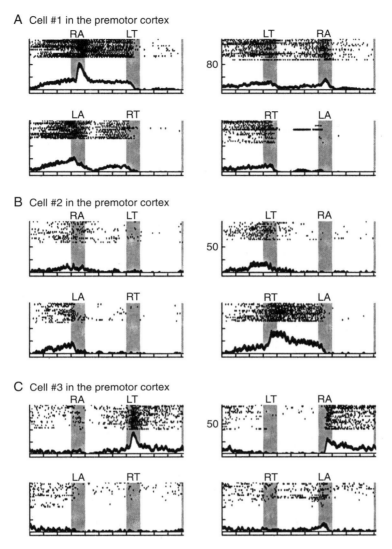

Figure 8–7 The three groups of premotor neuronal activity involved in planning the reaching movement (task 2). Neuronal activity is presented with raster displays and plots of spike density functions. *Gray areas* (from left to right) indicate when the first, second, and set cues were presented. *Tick marks* on the abscissa are at 400-ms intervals. The first and second instructions are shown on *top* of each panel. The spike density functions (smoothed by Gaussian kernel, $\sigma = 20$ ms, mean±standard error) are shown below each raster display. The ordinate represents the instantaneous firing rate, the degree of which is indicated. *A.* This neuron showed vigorous activity if the first cue, but not the second cue, instructed use of the right arm. *B.* This neuron showed vigorous activity if the first cue, but not the second cue, specified reaching for the right target. *C.* This neuron showed activity after the appearance of the second cue if the combination of the two instructions was right arm and left target. RA, right arm; LT, left target; LA, left arm; RT, right target. (Adapted with permission from Hoshi et al., *Journal of Neurophysiology,* 95:3596–3616. Copyright American Physiological Society, 2006.)

The Primary Motor Cortex Is Involved in Executing the Preplanned Reaching Movement

In the first (Fig. 8–3) and second (Fig. 8–6) experiments, neuronal activity was recorded from the primary motor cortex of the same monkeys performing the same task. In the first experiment (Fig. 8–3), neurons in the primary motor cortex did not respond to the appearance of the sample or choice cues. Furthermore, they were not active during the delay period between them. Instead, neurons in the primary motor cortex were highly active during actual execution of the reaching movement (Hoshi et al., 1998). In the second experiment (Fig. 8–6), the primary motor cortex neurons were again less active before movement execution. In addition, they mainly represented which arm to use, rather than which target to reach.

These findings suggest that the primary motor cortex is less involved in selecting the reach target or in planning the reaching movement, which is in great contrast to the findings in the prefrontal and premotor cortices. Anatomical studies show that the primary motor cortex sends output to segments in the spinal cord that govern the arm muscles (Dum and Strick, 1991; Rathelot and Strick, 2006). Together, these observations suggest that the primary motor cortex is involved mainly in controlling arm movements that were already selected and planned in the prefrontal and premotor cortices.

The Prefrontal Cortex Monitors Action during Execution of the Reaching Movement

In the first task (Fig. 8–3), neurons in the lateral prefrontal cortex were also active during execution of the reaching movement. However, the response profiles were very different from those in the primary motor cortex, which mainly reflected the arm movement itself. In contrast, the prefrontal cortex possessed two response properties that were extremely different from those of the primary motor cortex (Hoshi et al., 1998). (1) The activity of the prefrontal neurons reflected the identity of the target (i.e., the shape of the reach target). The neuron shown in Figure 8–8 was active when the reach target was a circle, but not when it was a triangle, although the target was in the same location. (2) The prefrontal neuronal activity was influenced by the behavioral rule. Some neurons were more active if the task called for the shape-matching rule rather than the location-matching rule, and vice versa. These two response properties (i.e., target shape selectivity and rule selectivity) in the lateral prefrontal cortex seem to play an important role in monitoring the behavioral rule or representing a goal or concept of the motor behavior.

SYNTHESIS: HIERARCHICAL ORGANIZATION OF THE FRONTAL CORTEX FOR RULE-BASED BEHAVIOR

Studies examining neuronal activity show that the prefrontal cortex possesses a variety of response profiles that play major roles in rule-based motor behavior

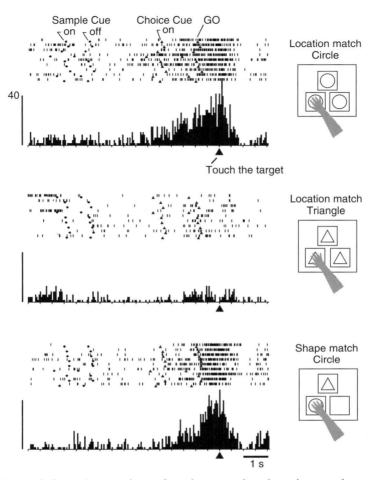

Figure 8–8 Discharges of a prefrontal neuron that showed target shape selectivity in task 1. In the raster displays, each row represents a trial, and *dots* denote discharges of this neuron. The first and second *circles* below each raster show when the sample cue was turned on and off, and the first and second *triangles* show when the choice cue and "go" signal appeared, respectively. Discharges are summarized in the perievent histograms below each raster display. The ordinate of the histograms represents the discharge rate (spikes per second). Each raster and histogram is aligned according to the time the animal touched the target. In the location-matching rule, this neuron was preferentially active if the reach target was a circle (*top*), but not a triangle (*center*). This neuron was similarly active in the shape-matching rule (*bottom*). The preferential activity for the circle target was also observed in other locations (i.e., in the top and right; not shown). (Adapted with permission from Hoshi et al., *Journal of Neurophysiology*, 80, 3392–3397. Copyright American Physiological Society, 1998.)

(White and Wise, 1999; Wallis et al., 2001). The prefrontal cortex contains a neuronal network that can execute complex information processing by conforming to the behavior rule (Hoshi et al., 2000; Miller, 2000). Furthermore, the prefrontal cortex monitors the action or represents a goal or concept of the motor behavior by representing the identity of the target and the behavioral rule (Hoshi et al., 1998). In contrast, the premotor cortex neurons collect a component of action, such as target location or arm use, and integrate them to achieve motor planning. Thus, once the prefrontal cortex selects an element of action (i.e., arm use or target location), the premotor cortex can subsequently retrieve that selected information to achieve motor planning. Because of the contributions of the premotor cortex, the prefrontal cortex (and other areas) can focus on the decision-making process to generate novel information concerning an action by integrating multiple sets of information (Tanji and Hoshi, 2001). The behavioral rule, encoded by neurons in prefrontal cortex, guides this decision.

In contrast to the prefrontal and premotor cortices, the primary motor cortex was minimally involved in target selection or motor planning and was instead involved in executing the already planned reaching movement (part of the third level shown in Fig. 8–1). Therefore, we can identify a hierarchical organization of the reaching movements and the corresponding structural and functional networks in the frontal cortex (Fig. 8–9). The illustrated schema of the hierarchical organization highlights a special role played by the prefrontal cortex in generating motor information by collecting multiple sets of information and integrating them while conforming to the rule of the behavior (first level; see Fig. 8–9). Once the motor information is generated, the pre-

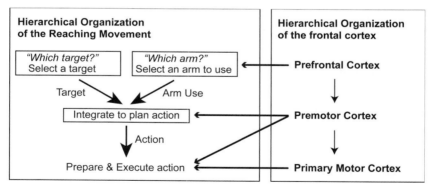

Figure 8–9 Hierarchical organization of the frontal cortex in the emerging process of the reaching movement. The *left* side shows the hierarchical organization of the reaching movement. The *right* side summarizes the hierarchical organization of the frontal cortex defined by anatomical studies. The *arrows* originating from the right panel and pointing to the organization in the left panel show the involvement of each cortical area in the neural processes depicted in the left panel.

motor cortex retrieves it and subsequently integrates it with other motor-related information to plan an action (second level; see Fig. 8–9). Finally, the primary motor and premotor cortices prepare and execute the planned action (third level; see Fig. 8–9).

In future research, it will be necessary to refine this schema by incorporating multiple cortical and subcortical structures. Furthermore, it is extremely important to test the extent to which we can generalize this schema to other behaviors, such as eye movements or sequential motor procedures. I am hopeful that this book will stimulate other studies in guiding the direction of future research.

ACKNOWLEDGMENTS This work was supported by a postdoctoral fellowship from the Japan Society for the Promotion of Science, a long-term fellowship from the International Human Frontier Science Program Organization, and a Center of Excellence (COE) program grant from the Ministry of Education, Culture, Sports, Science, and Technology of Japan. I sincerely thank Drs. K. Kurata and J. Tanji for their advice and encouragement.

REFERENCES

Asaad WF, Rainer G, Miller EK (1998) Neural activity in the primate prefrontal cortex during associative learning. Neuron 21:1399–1407.

Barbas H (2000) Connections underlying the synthesis of cognition, memory, and emotion in primate prefrontal cortices. Brain Research Bulletin 52:319–330.

Barbas H, Pandya DN (1987) Architecture and frontal cortical connections of the premotor cortex (area 6) in the rhesus monkey. Journal of Comparative Neurology 256:211–228.

Barbas H, Pandya DN (1989) Architecture and intrinsic connections of the prefrontal cortex in the rhesus monkey. Journal of Comparative Neurology 286:353–375.

Brodmann K (1909) Vergleichende Lokalisationslehre der Grohirnrinde. Leipzig: Barth.

Bunge SA, Wallis JD, Parker A, Brass M, Crone EA, Hoshi E, Sakai K (2005) Neural circuitry underlying rule use in humans and nonhuman primates. Journal of Neuroscience 25:10347–10350.

Cavada C, Company T, Tejedor J, Cruz-Rizzolo RJ, Reinoso-Suarez F (2000) The anatomical connections of the macaque monkey orbitofrontal cortex: a review. Cerebral Cortex 10:220–242.

Dum RP, Strick PL (1991) The origin of corticospinal projections from the premotor areas in the frontal lobe. Journal of Neuroscience 11:667–689.

Fries W (1984) Cortical projections to the superior colliculus in the macaque monkey: a retrograde study using horseradish peroxidase. Journal of Comparative Neurology 230:55–76.

Fuster JM (1997) The prefrontal cortex: anatomy, physiology, and neuropsychology of the frontal lobe. Philadelphia: Lippincott-Raven.

Fuster JM (2001) The prefrontal cortex—an update: time is of the essence. Neuron 30:319–333.

Goldman-Rakic PS (1987) Circuitry of the primate prefrontal cortex and regulation of behavior by representational memory. In: Handbook of physiology: the nervous system (Plum F, ed.), pp 373–417. Bethesda, MD: American Physiological Society.

Goldman-Rakic PS, Bates JF, Chafee MV (1992) The prefrontal cortex and internally generated motor acts. Current Opinion in Neurobiology 2:830–835.

Hoshi E, Shima K, Tanji J (1998) Task-dependent selectivity of movement-related neuronal activity in the primate prefrontal cortex. Journal of Neurophysiology 80: 3392–3397.

Hoshi E, Shima K, Tanji J (2000) Neuronal activity in the primate prefrontal cortex in the process of motor selection based on two behavioral rules. Journal of Neurophysiology 83:2355–2373.

Hoshi E, Tanji J (2000) Integration of target and body-part information in the premotor cortex when planning action. Nature 408:466–470.

Hoshi E, Tanji J (2004) Area-selective neuronal activity in the dorsolateral prefrontal cortex for information retrieval and action planning. Journal of Neurophysiology 91:2707–2722.

Hoshi E, Tanji J (2006) Differential involvement of neurons in the dorsal and ventral premotor cortex during processing of visual signals for action planning. Journal of Neurophysiology 95:3596–3616.

Jones EG, Powell TP (1970) An anatomical study of converging sensory pathways within the cerebral cortex of the monkey. Brain 93:793–820.

Lu MT, Preston JB, Strick PL (1994) Interconnections between the prefrontal cortex and the premotor areas in the frontal lobe. Journal of Comparative Neurology 341: 375–392.

Miller EK (2000) The prefrontal cortex and cognitive control. Nature Reviews Neuroscience 1:59–65.

Miller EK, Cohen JD (2001) An integrative theory of prefrontal cortex function. Annual Review of Neuroscience 24:167–202.

Miyachi S, Lu X, Inoue S, Iwasaki T, Koike S, Nambu A, Takada M (2005) Organization of multisynaptic inputs from prefrontal cortex to primary motor cortex as revealed by retrograde transneuronal transport of rabies virus. Journal of Neuroscience 25:2547–2556.

Ongur D, Price JL (2000) The organization of networks within the orbital and medial prefrontal cortex of rats, monkeys and humans. Cerebral Cortex 10:206–219.

Pandya DN, Yeterian EH (1996) Comparison of prefrontal architecture and connections. Philosophical Transactions of the Royal Society of London B 351:1423–1432.

Passingham RE (1993) The frontal lobes and voluntary action. Oxford, UK: Oxford University Press.

Petrides M, Pandya DN (1999) Dorsolateral prefrontal cortex: comparative cytoarchitectonic analysis in the human and the macaque brain and corticocortical connection patterns. European Journal of Neuroscience 11:1011–1036.

Rathelot JA, Strick PL (2006) Muscle representation in the macaque motor cortex: an anatomical perspective. Proceedings of the National Academy of Sciences U S A 103: 8257–8262.

Rizzolatti G, Luppino G (2001) The cortical motor system. Neuron 31:889–901.

Rolls ET (1996) The orbitofrontal cortex. Philosophical Transactions of the Royal Society of London B 351:1433–1443.

Romanski LM, Bates JF, Goldman-Rakic PS (1999) Auditory belt and parabelt projections to the prefrontal cortex in the rhesus monkey. Journal of Comparative Neurology 403:141–157.

Selemon LD, Goldman-Rakic PS (1988) Common cortical and subcortical targets of the dorsolateral prefrontal and posterior parietal cortices in the rhesus monkey:

evidence for a distributed neural network subserving spatially guided behavior. Journal of Neuroscience 8:4049–4068.

Tanji J, Hoshi E (2001) Behavioral planning in the prefrontal cortex. Current Opinion in Neurobiology 11:164–170.

Wallis JD, Anderson KC, Miller EK (2001) Single neurons in prefrontal cortex encode abstract rules. Nature 411:953–956.

White IM, Wise SP (1999) Rule-dependent neuronal activity in the prefrontal cortex. Experimental Brain Research 126:315–335.

Wise SP (1985) The primate premotor cortex: past, present, and preparatory. Annual Review of Neuroscience 8:1–19.

Wise SP, Boussaoud D, Johnson PB, Caminiti R (1997) Premotor and parietal cortex: corticocortical connectivity and combinatorial computations. Annual Review of Neuroscience 20:25–42.

Wise SP, Murray EA, Gerfen CR (1996) The frontal cortex-basal ganglia system in primates. Critical Reviews in Neurobiology 10:317–356.

9

The Role of the Posterior Frontolateral Cortex in Task-Related Control

Marcel Brass, Jan Derrfuss, and D. Yves von Cramon

Daily life requires a high degree of cognitive flexibility to adjust behavior to rapidly changing environmental demands. This flexible adjustment is driven by past experiences, current goals, and environmental factors. It is now widely accepted that the lateral prefrontal cortex plays a crucial role in such environmentally guided cognitive flexibility. More specifically, a number of brain imaging studies have claimed that cognitive control is primarily related to the so-called dorsolateral prefrontal cortex (DLPFC) or the mid-DLPFC (Banich et al., 2000; MacDonald et al., 2000; Petrides, 2000). This has been shown using a variety of different cognitive control paradigms, such as the task-switching paradigm and the Stroop task. However, closer inspection of the existing literature and new experimental findings reveals that the lateral prefrontal cortex can be further subdivided into functionally distinct regions (Koechlin et al., 2003; Bunge, 2004; Brass et al., 2005).

In the first part of this chapter, we will outline evidence from different approaches showing that an area posterior to the mid-DLPFC plays a crucial role in cognitive control. This region is located at the junction of the inferior frontal sulcus (IFS) and the inferior precentral sulcus and was therefore named the "inferior frontal junction area" (IFJ). First, we will outline the structural neuroanatomy of the posterior frontolateral cortex in general, with a strong focus on the IFJ. Then we will report a series of brain imaging studies in which we have shown that the IFJ is related to the updating of task representations. Moreover, we will provide data from comparisons of different cognitive control paradigms, indicating that these paradigms show a functional overlap in the IFJ. In the second part of the chapter, we will outline how the IFJ is functionally related to other prefrontal and parietal areas assumed to be involved in cognitive control. Finally, we will discuss the general implications of these findings for a functional parcellation of the prefrontal cortex.

THE NEGLECTED AREA IN THE POSTERIOR FRONTOLATERAL CORTEX

Before we outline the experimental evidence that suggests that the IFJ constitutes a functionally distinct region in the posterior frontolateral cortex, we would like to give a brief overview of the structural neuroanatomy of the posterior frontolateral cortex.

Structural Neuroanatomy of the Posterior Frontolateral Cortex

On the microanatomical level, the posterior frontolateral cortex includes the precentral gyrus and the caudal parts of the inferior, middle, and superior frontal gyri. Between the precentral gyrus and the inferior, middle, and superior frontal gyri lies the precentral sulcus. This sulcus is usually subdivided into the inferior precentral sulcus and the superior precentral sulcus. In this chapter, we will focus on the inferior precentral sulcus and the gyral regions directly adjacent to it (Fig. 9–1). This inferior part of the posterior frontolateral cortex shows a rather complex sulcal architecture. As a consequence, there have been different approaches to categorizing its sulcal morphology. One approach tends to view the inferior precentral sulcus as a unitary sulcus running in a dorsoventral direction (e.g., Ono et al., 1990). According to Ono et al., this sulcus very frequently has a junction with the IFS (88% in the left hemisphere and 92% in the right). Other schemes suggest that the inferior precentral sulcus is subdividable into a number of segments. For example, Germann and colleagues (2005) proposed that the inferior precentral sulcus consists of three sulcal segments. In particular, they suggested that the inferior precentral

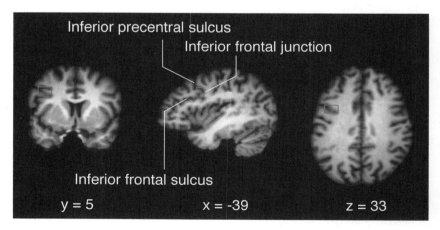

Figure 9–1 Lateral view of the human brain, showing the exact location of the inferior frontal junction, which is located at the junction of the inferior frontal sulcus and the inferior precentral sulcus. The x, y, and z values refer to Talairach coordinates.

sulcus possesses a segment running in a predominantly horizontal direction—the "horizontal extension"—and two segments running in a predominantly vertical direction—the dorsal and ventral segments of the inferior precentral sulcus.

Because it has been shown that sulci do not necessarily coincide with cytoarchitectonic borders (Amunts et al., 1999), a detailed description of the sulcal structure of this region is necessary, but not sufficient for understanding where activations of the IFJ really are located. Thus, to gain a better understanding of the possible structural correlate of the IFJ, the cytoarchitecture of the precentral sulcus must be investigated.

Based on our functional imaging studies (for an overview, see Brass et al., 2005), we have suggested that the approximate location of the IFJ in the stereotaxic system of Talairach and Tournoux (1988) can be described as follows: x-coordinates between ±30 and ±47,[1] y-coordinates between −1 and 10, and z-coordinates between 27 and 40 (Fig. 9–1). Thus, the focus of IFJ activations should be found in the precentral sulcus or in the most posterior part of the IFS, not on the gyral surface surrounding these sulci. Furthermore, given its posterior location in the lateral frontal lobe, the IFJ should not be regarded as part of the mid-DLPFC, which consists of Petrides and Pandya's (1994) areas 9, 9/46, and 46.

Following Talairach and Tournoux's (1988) projection of Brodmann's (1909) map onto their template brain, the IFJ includes parts of Brodmann areas 6, 9, and 44. However, the cortex on the posterior surface of the middle frontal gyrus has received different cytoarchitectonic labels by different researchers. Whereas it includes parts of areas 6 and 9 on Brodmann's map, it was labeled "area 8" by Petrides and Pandya (1994). Consequently, imaging studies have labeled activations within the limits of the IFJ inconsistently as belonging to one or a combination of these areas.

What is common to the maps of Brodmann and of Petrides and Pandya, however, is that the IFJ is located at the border between the agranular premotor cortex (area 6), dysgranular transitional cortex (area 44), and granular posterior prefrontal cortex (areas 9 and 8). However, none of these areas corresponds to the functionally defined IFJ in terms of location and size, motivating a reanalysis of the cytoarchitecture of the cortex in the precentral sulcus.

Interestingly, preliminary results from these cytoarchitectonic investigations conducted by Katrin Amunts (1999) suggest that there might be two areas submerged in the inferior precentral sulcus that were not charted on previous cytoarchitectonic maps. One of these areas is dysgranular; the other is agranular. Both are distinguishable from neighboring areas 6, 44, 45, 8, and 9 on the basis of their cytoarchitectonic features. Although it is currently not clear whether activations of the functionally defined IFJ are related to one of these areas, the close correspondence of their locations in terms of sulcal architecture points to the possibility that one of these areas might form a structural correlate of the functionally defined IFJ.

Given our current knowledge of these newly described areas, one can only speculate about their anatomical connectivity. Assuming that the premotor-prefrontal transitional cortex in the ventral frontal lobe in the macaque brain (Matelli et al., 1986; Barbas and Pandya, 1987; Pandya and Yeterian, 1996) and the human brain have similar connections, one would expect to find connections to the pre-supplementary motor area (pre-SMA), the prefrontal cortex, and the parietal cortex. Interestingly, in a conjunction analysis of three different cognitive control paradigms, we found—apart from an overlap in the IFJ—overlapping activations in the pre-SMA, the prefrontal cortex, and the parietal cortex (Derrfuss et al., 2004). Although these results provide some evidence for a close functional relationship of these areas, clearly, future studies using diffusion tensor imaging will be necessary to directly investigate the connectivity of the IFJ.

Using a Task-Switching Paradigm to Investigate Cognitive Flexibility

Task-switching paradigms have been widely used in the last decade to investigate flexible adjustment to changing environmental demands (Monsell, 2003). These paradigms require participants to alternate between two different tasks (Fig. 9–2). Behaviorally, switching between two tasks, compared with

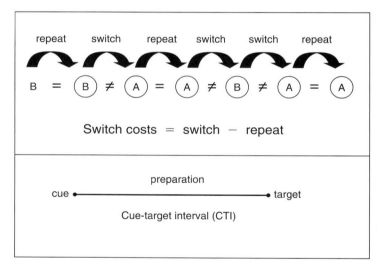

Figure 9–2 Schematic drawing of the task-switching paradigm. Participants have to alternate between two tasks. Usually, two types of trials are distinguished: trials where trial n−1 is different from trial n (switch trials) and trials where trial n−1 is identical to trial n (repeat trials). The *bottom* part of the figure illustrates a task-cuing trial. The experimental trial starts with a task cue that signals which task to execute. After a variable cue-target interval, the task stimulus (target) is presented.

repeating the same task, leads to prolonged reaction times and a higher error rate: the "switch cost" (Jersild, 1927; Allport et al., 1994; Rogers and Monsell, 1995). It has been argued that switch costs reflect cognitive processes needed to adjust to a new task, reflecting the prototypical cognitive control demand.

Recently, a number of brain imaging studies have investigated the neural mechanisms underlying this switch operation (Dove et al., 2000; Sohn et al., 2000; Brass and von Cramon, 2002, 2004; Dreher et al., 2002; Luks et al., 2002; Rushworth et al., 2002a; Braver et al., 2003; Ruge et al., 2005; Crone et al., 2006; Wylie et al., 2006). These studies have identified a number of different brain regions related to task-switching. From a functional perspective, this hetero-geneity of results is not surprising because it is known that even a simple operation, such as switching between different tasks, requires more than one cognitive operation (Meiran, 1996, Meiran et al., 2000; Rubinstein et al., 2001; Monsell, 2003). Hence, the first step in investigating the neural basis of cog-nitive control with a task-switching paradigm is to decompose complex op-erations into component processes. Behavioral data suggest that switch costs can be decomposed into at least two components: one that is related to the preparation of the upcoming task and one that is related to control processes involved in task execution.

In a series of experiments, we have tried to isolate the neural basis of what was assumed to be the most crucial process in task-switching, namely, the up-dating of task representations (Brass and von Cramon, 2002, 2004). By presen-ting a task cue before the task (Fig. 9–2), one can separate cue-related updating of task representations from task-related control processes (Meiran, 1996). However, with functional magnetic resonance imaging (fMRI), it is very dif-ficult to distinguish processes that are temporally separated by only a few hun-dred milliseconds. To bypass this problem, we implemented an experimental trick, randomly inserting trials where only a task cue, but no target, was pre-sented (Brass and von Cramon, 2002). In these trials, cue-related processing is not confounded with target-related processing because no target appears. When contrasting the cue-only condition with a lowÜlevel baseline, we found a number of prefrontal regions to be activated, including the mid-DLPFC and the IFJ. However, only two frontal brain regions showed a cue-related activa-tion correlated with the behavioral indicator of task preparation. One of these was located in the IFJ, and the other, in the pre-SMA.

Although this study succeeded in dissociating between preparation-related and execution-related control processes, the question arises as to whether the frontal activation reflects the coding of the cue or the updating of the relevant task representation. To address this question, we devised a new paradigm that manipulated the cue-task association (Bunge et al., 2003; Logan and Bunde-sen, 2003; Mayr and Kliegl, 2003; Brass and von Cramon, 2004). In this par-adigm, two different cues were assigned to each task. Furthermore, the cue alternation was implemented within a trial. In most of the trials, a first cue was followed by a second cue after a fixed cue-cue interval. With this manipula-tion, one can compare a switch in cue without a switch in task (two different

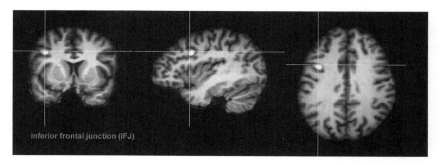

Figure 9–3 Activation in the inferior frontal junction for the updating of task representations (Brass and von Cramon, 2004a).

cues that indicate the same task) and a switch in both cue and task (two different cues that indicate different tasks). Although participants were required to encode the second cue in both conditions, updating task representations was only required in the condition in which the cue changed and simultaneously indicated a task change. When contrasting these two conditions, two frontal regions were found to be activated, the IFJ (Fig. 9–3; see color insert) and the right inferior frontal gyrus. Taken together, the data from these two studies indicate that the IFJ plays a crucial role in the updating of task representations. In this series of experiments, we were able to determine the functional role of the IFJ by using the task-switching paradigm. These findings raise an important question: If the IFJ plays such a crucial role in cognitive control, why hasn't it been reported in other experimental paradigms?

Role of the Inferior Frontal Junction Area in Different Cognitive Control Paradigms

A careful analysis of the literature reveals that the IFJ has actually been consistently reported in a number of other studies of cognitive control, across a wide range of experimental paradigms. However, in these studies, the area has been labeled inconsistently (e.g., Dove et al., 2000; Konishi et al., 2001; Monchi et al., 2001; Bunge et al., 2003). In the first event-related neuroimaging study on task-switching, Dove and colleagues (2000) found an activation in the posterior frontolateral cortex, but referred to it as the DLPFC. Konishi and colleagues (2001) carried out a study in which they showed that the posterior lateral prefrontal cortex was involved in the transition between different experimental tasks in a block design. They referred to this activation as the "dorsal extent of the inferior frontal gyrus." It is reasonable to assume that the transition between different experimental blocks crucially requires the updating of task representations. Monchi and colleagues (2001) found activation in the posterior frontolateral cortex in a Wisconsin Card Sorting study, referring to it as "premotor activation." Furthermore, Bunge and colleagues

(2003) demonstrated that a region, which they referred to as the "ventrolateral prefrontal cortex" (VLPFC), plays a role in rule representation. All of these studies describe activation within our definition of the IFJ and relate it to similar functional concepts, but due to different anatomical descriptions, the common neuroanatomical substrate was neglected.

Interestingly, even for very well-investigated paradigms, such as the Stroop task, which is assumed to involve task-related control processes (Milham et al., 2001; Monsell et al., 2001), the consistent finding of activation in the IFJ has been ignored. In a recent meta-analysis, Neumann and colleagues (2005) compared 15 Stroop studies taken from the Fox database BrainMap with a new meta-analytic algorithm. In the frontolateral cortex, two areas were consistently implicated: the IFJ and the mid-DLPFC. Furthermore, Derrfuss and colleagues (2005) carried out a meta-analysis on task-switching and set-shifting studies and identified an overlap in the IFJ. Therefore, it appears that the IFJ has been consistently activated by studies investigating cognitive control; however, this consistency has been overlooked.

Another way to address the commonality of activations across different paradigms is to carry out within-subject comparisons. In contrast to a meta-analytic investigation, this approach has the advantage of minimizing variance associated with different methods and subject populations. We have recently carried out a within-subject experiment to address the question of whether the IFJ plays a role in different paradigms of cognitive control (Derrfuss et al., 2004). We compared brain activation in a task-switching paradigm, a Stroop task, and a verbal n-back task. All three paradigms showed an activation overlap in the IFJ, as could be seen in the conjunction analysis of these tasks. Interestingly, this overlapping area was very consistent with the activation we found in our previous task-switching studies and the meta-analytic findings reported by both Neumann and colleagues (2005) and Derrfuss and colleagues (2005). Therefore, a close inspection of the existing literature using meta-analytic approaches and within-subject comparisons of different experimental paradigms provides overwhelming support for the assumption that the IFJ has a role in different paradigms of cognitive control (Fig. 9–4; see color insert).

COGNITIVE CONTROL AS AN INTERPLAY BETWEEN FRONTAL AND PARIETAL AREAS

We have argued so far that the IFJ plays a crucial role for the environmentally guided updating of task representations. However, the updating of task representations reflects only one aspect of the complex cognitive functions that are required to flexibly adjust our behavior to meet changing environmental demands. To obtain a complete picture of the functional role of the IFJ in cognitive control, one must assess the contribution of brain areas that are either neuroanatomically or functionally closely related to the IFJ. From a neuroanatomical perspective, the question arises as to how the function of the IFJ is related to that of the adjacent premotor cortex. Furthermore, one must

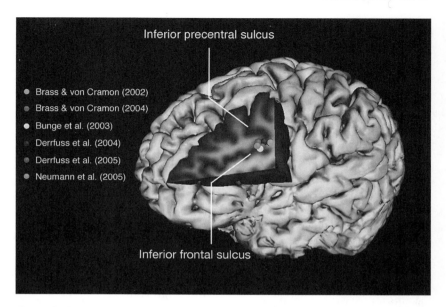

Figure 9–4 Peaks of activation from three experimental studies on task-switching and set-shifting (Brass and von Cramon, 2002, 2004a; Bunge et al., 2003): a within-subject comparison of three cognitive control paradigms (Derrfuss et al., 2004); a meta-analysis of the Stroop task (Neumann et al., 2005); and a meta-analysis of task-switching and set-shifting studies (Derrfuss et al., 2005).

distinguish between the cognitive control-related contribution of the mid-DLPFC and VLPFC and the role of the IFJ. From a functional perspective, it is crucial to address the fact that our behavior is guided by intentional processes that are primarily implemented in the frontomedial cortex. Additionally, the parietal cortex shows very reliable activations in cognitive control paradigms (e.g., Dove et al., 2000; Sohn et al., 2000; Brass and von Cramon, 2004), raising the question of how the frontolateral cortex interacts with the parietal cortex.

From Arbitrary Motor Mappings to Task Mappings

As outlined earlier, the IFJ is very close to the premotor cortex, which is believed to be involved in a number of cognitive functions, including motor control (Picard and Strick, 2001; Chouinard and Paus, 2006). The close proximity of the IFJ to the premotor cortex raises the crucial question of how the updating of task representations is related to motor control. One possibility is that task control is an abstraction from higher-order motor control: In motor control, an environmental stimulus determines the behavior in a given situation.

At least two types of visuomotor mappings have been distinguished: direct and arbitrary (Petrides, 1985; Wise and Murray, 2000). In direct visuomotor

mappings, the stimulus directly specifies the response. A good example of a direct visuomotor mapping is grasping an object. In arbitrary—or conditional—visuomotor mappings, the stimulus that specifies the response has an arbitrary relationship to the response (e.g., press the left key when a red stimulus appears). Arbitrary motor mappings require the application of an abstract rule, because there is no "natural" relationship between the stimulus and the appropriate response. The only major difference between such arbitrary stimulus-response (S-R) rules and task rules is the number of relevant S-R rules. Whereas task rules relate a set of S-R mappings to each cue, only one S-R rule is specified in arbitrary visuomotor mappings. From this perspective, motor control and task control might be functionally closely related.

This observation raises the possibility that there is also a tight relationship in functional organization between the premotor cortex and the adjacent dysgranular frontolateral cortex. Interestingly, the IFJ is located anterior to what is considered to be the premotor hand area. Godschalk et al. (1995) suggested that the premotor cortex follows, to some degree, a somatotopic organization similar to that of the primary motor cortex. If this organizational principle extends into the adjacent frontal cortex, the location of the IFJ might be related to the fact that participants respond with their hands. In fact, almost all experimental studies on task control use hands as the response modality. To investigate this possibility, we carried out a task-switching experiment in which participants had to respond with either their hands or their feet (Brass and von Cramon, submitted).

If the response modality is responsible for the location of cognitive control activation in the posterior frontolateral cortex, then this activation should differ for hand and foot responses. Because the foot area in the premotor cortex is located more dorsally than the hand area (Buccino et al., 2001), the action should shift in the dorsal direction when participants respond with their feet. However, the activation in the posterior frontolateral cortex was identical for hand and foot trials, indicating that the IFJ is activated, regardless of whether participants respond with their hands or their feet. Furthermore, a direct contrast of hand and foot trials yielded no frontal activation besides the primary motor hand and foot areas. These data suggest that the functional organization of the premotor cortex does not directly extend into the posterior frontolateral cortex.

Relating Rule-Guiding Information to Information to Which the Rule Applies

Another possible interpretation of how the premotor cortex and the posterior prefrontal cortex might be functionally related was provided recently by Adele Diamond (2006). She discussed the possibility that the posterior frontolateral cortex is involved whenever the information that guides behavior is not directly attached to the object on which participants act (see also Chapter 7). This argument is supported by developmental research (Diamond et al., 1999,

2003) and monkey research (Jarvik, 1956; Halsband and Passingham, 1982; Rushworth et al., 2005). If this argument holds true, the specificity of task rules lies in the fact that the task information is presented spatially segregated from the target. In accordance with this argument, in almost all task-switching experiments, the instruction that determines the relevant task is spatially separated from the stimulus on which participants have to act. From this perspective, the crucial difference between task rules and response rules would not be the number of S-R associations, but the separation of the rule-guiding information and the stimulus.

Dissociating the Inferior Frontal Junction Area from More Anterior Regions in the Frontolateral Cortex

In the anterior direction, the IFJ is close to what is usually called the "mid-DLPFC" and the "VLPFC." The mid-DLPFC has been implicated in cognitive control (MacDonald et al., 2000). This observation raises the question about the different contributions of the mid-DLPFC and IFJ in cognitive control. Koechlin and colleagues (2003) argued that activations in the posterior frontolateral cortex are related to the processing of the perceptual context in which stimuli occur, whereas activations more anterior in the frontolateral cortex reflect the temporal episode in which the stimulus is presented.

Our findings are, to some degree, consistent with the assumption that regions more anterior in the frontolateral cortex are involved in processing the temporal episode (Koechlin et al., 2003). We suggest that a region in the posterior IFS that is located anterior to the IFJ comes into play whenever the information in the environment does not unequivocally determine the relevant behavior. This is the case when environmental information has to be integrated with past events to determine what to do in a given situation. We have investigated the temporal integration of information in a cued task-switching paradigm adapted from a paradigm developed by Rushworth and colleagues (2002a). In our experiment, the task cue did not directly indicate the relevant task, but rather indicated whether to switch or repeat the task (Forstmann et al., 2005). Hence, participants were required to integrate the cue information with information from working memory, namely, which task they executed in the previous trial, to determine the relevant task set. In comparison with our previous studies with direct task cues (Brass and von Cramon, 2002, 2004a), this manipulation led to an anterior shift of activation along the IFS.

Another situation in which environmental information does not directly indicate the relevant behavior occurs when the context provides conflicting sources of information. Here, the relevant source of information must be selected. We have experimentally modeled such a situation by using bidimensional task cues (Brass and von Cramon, 2004b). As in the Stroop task, the task cues had a relevant and an irrelevant dimension. Although the relevant dimension indicated which task to execute, the irrelevant dimension could

indicate the same task, a different task, or no task at all. When contrasting the conditions in which both dimensions carried task information with the condition in which only the relevant dimension carried information, we again found activation in the posterior IFS.

Because these activations were located in the IFS, it is difficult to determine whether they belong to the DLPFC or VLPFC. Interestingly, the VLPFC has recently also been assumed to be related to task-related control processes (Bunge et al., 2005; Crone et al., 2006; Badre and Wager, 2006; see Chapter 16). More specifically, it has been argued that the VLPFC is implicated in rule representation (Bunge, 2005; Crone et al., 2006). Furthermore, Badre and colleagues (2005) showed that the mid-VLPFC (area 45) plays a fundamental role in the control of declarative memory retrieval. They argued that such processes are required to retrieve task-relevant information when conflicting information is present (Badre and Wager, 2006). This interpretation of the role of the mid-VLPFC in cognitive control is very consistent with our interpretation of posterior IFS activation outlined earlier. Both interpretations stress the relevance of selecting task-relevant information when conflicting sources of information are present.

In sum, these findings suggest that the posterior lateral prefrontal cortex is implicated whenever the information in the environment does not directly indicate which task to execute. Although the IFJ directly connects contextual information to the relevant behavioral options, the posterior IFS is needed whenever information from working memory has to be integrated or selected to determine the relevant task. Further research should show whether these activations in the posterior IFS belong to the domain of the mid-VLPFC— as suggested by the work of Badre (see Chapter 16) and Bunge et al. (2005)— or to the domain of the mid-DLPFC—as suggested by other authors (e.g., MacDonald et al., 2000).

Exogenous and Endogenous Components of Task Set Updating

So far, our discussion of the neural correlates of task-related control has primarily focused on the role of the frontolateral cortex. However, frontomedial brain regions have also been identified in a number of brain imaging studies of cognitive control (Rushworth et al., 2002a; Brass and von Cramon, 2004; Crone et al., 2006). In particular, pre-SMA activity has consistently been found when participants had to alternate between different task sets. Accordingly, Rushworth and colleagues (2004) argued that the pre-SMA might be involved in the selection of response sets. They provided fMRI and transcranial magnetic stimulation evidence for this hypothesis (Rushworth et al., 2002a). A similar conclusion was suggested by Crone and colleagues (2006). They dissociated the role of the pre-SMA and the frontolateral cortex in task-related control. Although they found the pre-SMA to be particularly involved in switching between sets of S-R rules, the frontolateral cortex was more involved in the representation of task rules, as outlined earlier.

One potential interpretation for these data (Brass and von Cramon, 2002; Rushworth et al., 2002a) might be that activation in the frontolateral cortex reflects the externally triggered component of task rule updating, whereas the pre-SMA might be related to internal components involved in updating the relevant sets of S-R rules. In the classical task-switching paradigm, both components are required. (1) The contextual information provided by the task cue must be related to a specific task rule. (2) The response set related to the task rule has to be internally activated. From this perspective, the functional distinction between the frontolateral and the frontomedial cortex in cognitive control would be similar to the distinction between externally triggered actions (lateral premotor cortex) and internal action generation (supplementary motor area) in motor control (Goldberg, 1985).

Intentional Selection of Task Sets

In almost all task-switching experiments, participants are explicitly told what to do in a given situation. Usually, a task cue or the task order determines the relevant task set (Monsell, 2003). However, from an ecological validity point of view, this is not very realistic. In everyday life, it is rarely the case that someone tells us what we have to do in a given context. Rather, we decide ourselves what to do, depending on our goals, past experiences, and contextual information. Only recently have experimental psychologists become interested in the intentional selection of task sets (Arrington and Logan, 2004). In such experimental paradigms, participants can choose for themselves which task to execute.

In a recent fMRI experiment, we set out to determine which brain areas are involved in the intentional selection of task sets (Forstmann et al., 2006). Participants could either choose between two or three task sets or were cued as to the relevant task set. Comparing the free selection of a task set with an externally triggered task set selection revealed activation in the rostral cingulate zone of the frontomedial cortex (Fig. 9–5). This activation was not modulated by the number of task sets from which participants could choose (two versus three degrees of freedom; see Figure 9–5). These findings suggest that the neural correlates of intentional task set selection differ from those of externally triggered task set selection. These findings lead us to question the assumption that the classical task-switching paradigm is very useful for investigating endogenous cognitive control processes.

The Frontal and Parietal Cortex in Cognitive Control

Research on cognitive control has primarily focused on the frontal cortex (Duncan and Owen, 2000; MacDonald et al., 2000; Miller and Cohen, 2001). This frontal bias is based on clinical neuropsychological findings indicating that patients with frontal lesions suffer from severe cognitive control deficits (Milner, 1963; Luria, 1966/1980; Stuss and Alexander, 2000). However, if one takes a closer look at the brain imaging literature on cognitive control, and in

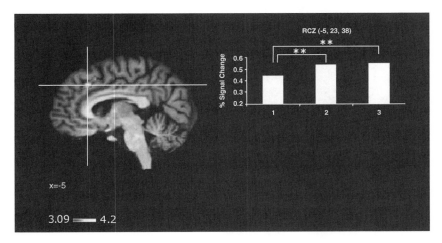

Figure 9–5 Activation in the rostral cingulate zone (RCZ) for the free selection of a task set compared with an externally triggered task set selection. On the *right* side, the signal change of the RCZ is plotted for the condition in which the relevant task set was predetermined (one degree of freedom), the condition in which participants could choose between two task sets (two degrees of freedom), and the condition in which participants could choose between three task sets (three degrees of freedom).

particular, task-switching, it becomes clear that almost all studies have identified parietal components in addition to frontal components. In some studies, the parietal component was even more dominant than the frontal component (Kimberg et al., 2000; Sohn et al., 2000).

Given the prevalence of parietal activations in these studies, it is very surprising that our understanding of parietal contributions to cognitive control and the interaction of parietal areas with frontal components is still very poor. One possible reason for this lack of a convincing conception of the interaction of the frontal cortex and the parietal cortex might be that these regions are involved in similar cognitive operations, but on different hierarchical levels. Recent single-unit research and lesion experiments in monkeys have suggested that the role of the frontal cortex is to bias processing in posterior brain regions (Tomita et al., 1999; Miller and Cohen, 2001). If the prefrontal cortex biases representations in the posterior cortices, as also suggested by combined electroencephalogram (EEG) and patient studies (e.g., Barcelo et al., 2000), activation in the frontal cortex should precede activation in the parietal cortex.

We have recently tested this prediction by combining results from an fMRI experiment and an event-related potential study (Brass et al., 2005b). The experimental paradigm was a task-switching experiment in which participants had to update the relevant task representations (Brass and von Cramon, 2004a). The fMRI data revealed a coactivation of the frontal and parietal areas for

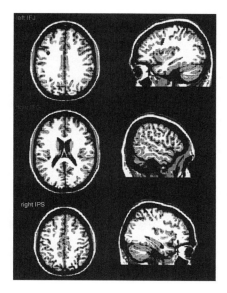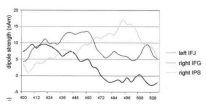

Figure 9–6 On the *left* side, the three dipoles are plotted on a representation of brain anatomy. On the *right* side, dipole strength is plotted for the left inferior frontal junction (IFJ), the right inferior frontal gyrus (IFG), and the right intraparietal sulcus (IPS).

this updating process. By using the loci of the fMRI experiment to perform a dipole modeling of the EEG data, we showed that the activation in the frontal cortex precedes that in the parietal cortex (Fig. 9–6; see color insert). This finding is consistent with previous EEG work on the relationship of frontal and parietal brain areas in cognitive control (Rushworth et al., 2002b) and suggests a hierarchical order of frontal and parietal areas. We assume that, in the case of contextually guided task preparation, the frontolateral cortex provides an abstract task representation that then biases concrete S-R associations in the parietal cortex. Although we have not explicitly tested the role of the pre-SMA in this experiment, a reasonable assumption would be that the pre-SMA is activated after the frontolateral cortex and before the parietal cortex, and is implicated in the updating of the response sets.

IMPLICATIONS FOR A FUNCTIONAL PARCELLATION OF THE FRONTAL CORTEX

A functional parcellation of the frontal cortex faces a number of problems that are inherent in the functional architecture of this region. In the frontal cortex, we deal with complex, multipurpose cognitive operations that are difficult to dissociate from one another experimentally. Therefore, careful experimentation is required to selectively engage various frontal cortex functions. At the

same time, a straight experimental approach introduces a strong bias toward interpreting activations in the context of specific experimental paradigms. Accordingly, most frontal regions have been associated with multiple functional interpretations, depending on the specific experimental context in which they were investigated (Cabeza and Nyberg, 2002). This leads to an apparent paradox. On the one hand, we have to rely on specific experimental paradigms to isolate component processes. On the other hand, we must integrate different paradigms, which might overlap on a functional level, to understand the common underlying functional principals of specific prefrontal areas.

In this chapter, we have outlined a research strategy for dealing with this apparent paradox. In a first step, a specific paradigm should be used to experimentally isolate a frontal area and provide information about its functional role. The ultimate goal of this experimental approach is to devise an experimental manipulation to which only the area of interest is sensitive, and not the underlying network. In a second step, a meta-analytic approach should be used to investigate the overlap of activation in the respective area for different experimental paradigms. Furthermore, the specific anatomical characteristics of the area should be specified to determine whether the functional characteristic maps onto specific structural properties. Finally, the relationship between this region and neuroanatomically and functionally related brain areas should be clarified to gain a better understanding of the broader network in which a specific brain area is embedded.

This research strategy combines the assets of cognitive experimental psychology and structural neuroanatomical research. It uses the greatest advantage of functional brain imaging, namely, that functional neuroanatomy provides a *tertium comparationis* to compare cognitive processes across phenomenologically different paradigms.

CONCLUSIONS

We have summarized empirical evidence that the IFJ plays a crucial role in cognitive control. This area, which has been widely neglected, plays a role in the contextually guided updating of task representations. We posit that this contextually guided task set updating can be seen as an abstraction from visuomotor response rules, which are represented in the premotor cortex. Furthermore, we have experimentally distinguished the IFJ from the neighboring IFS, by showing that the latter region is involved in the selection of task-relevant information and the integration of information over time. Moreover, we have discussed the relationship between the frontolateral and frontomedial cortex in task-related control. Although frontolateral regions seem to be involved in environmentally guided task control, areas in the frontomedial cortex are involved in internally guided cognitive control and the intentional updating of task representations. Finally, we have provided some electrophysiological evidence for the assumption that there is a hierarchical order of the frontal and parietal cortex in cognitive control.

ACKNOWLEDGMENTS This work was supported by the German Research Foundation.

NOTE

1. The medial border of the IFJ is the depth of the precentral sulcus, and this sulcal border should rarely be more medial than ±30.

REFERENCES

Allport DA, Styles EA, Hsieh S (1994) Shifting intentional set: exploring the dynamic control of tasks. In: Attention and performance (Umilta C, Moscovitch M, eds.), pp 421–452. Cambridge: MIT Press.

Amunts K, Schleicher A, Burgel U, Mohlberg H, Uylings HB, Zilles K (1999) Broca's region revisited: cytoarchitecture and intersubject variability. Journal of Comparative Neurology 412:319–341.

Arrington CM, Logan GD (2004) The cost of a voluntary task switch. Psychological Science 15:610–615.

Badre D, Poldrack RA, Pare-Blagoev EJ, Insler RZ, Wagner AD (2005) Dissociable controlled retrieval and generalized selection mechanisms in ventrolateral prefrontal cortex. Neuron 47:907–918.

Badre D, Wagner AD (2006) Computational and neurobiological mechanisms underlying cognitive flexibility. Proceedings of the National Academy of Sciences U S A 103:7186–7191.

Banich MT, Milham MP, Atchley RA, Cohen NJ, Webb A, Wszalek T, Kramer AF, Liang Z, Barad V, Gullett D, Shah C, Brown C (2000) The prefrontal regions play a predominant role in imposing an attentional 'set': evidence from fMRI. Brain Research: Cognitive Brain Research 10:1–9.

Barbas H, Pandya DN (1987) Architecture and frontal cortical connections of the premotor cortex (area 6) in the rhesus monkey. Journal of Comparative Neurology 256:211–228.

Barcelo F, Suwazono S, Knight RT (2000). Prefrontal modulation of visual processing in humans. Nature Neuroscience 3:399–403.

Brass M, Derrfuss J, Forstmann B, von Cramon DY (2005a) The role of the inferior frontal junction area in cognitive control. Trends in Cognitive Sciences 9:314–316.

Brass M, Ullsperger M, Knoesche TR, von Cramon DY, Phillips NA (2005b) Who comes first? The role of the prefrontal and parietal cortex in cognitive control. Journal of Cognitive Neuroscience 17:1367–1375.

Brass M, von Cramon DY (2002) The role of the frontal cortex in task preparation. Cerebral Cortex 12:908–914.

Brass M, von Cramon DY (2004a) Decomposing components of task preparation with functional magnetic resonance imaging. Journal of Cognitive Neuroscience 16:609–620.

Brass M, von Cramon DY (2004b) Selection for cognitive control: a functional magnetic resonance imaging study on the selection of task-relevant information. Journal of Neuroscience 24:8847–8852.

Braver TS, Reynolds JR, Donaldson DI (2003) Neural mechanisms of transient and sustained cognitive control during task switching. Neuron 39:713–726.

Brodmann K (1909) Vergleichende Lokalisationslehre der GroÔhirnrinde in ihren Prinzipien dargestellt auf Grund des Zellenbaues. Leipzig: Barth.

Buccino G, Binkofski F, Fink GR, Fadiga L, Fogassi L, Gallese V, Seitz RJ, Zilles K, Rizzolatti G, Freund HJ (2001) Action observation activates premotor and parietal areas in a somatotopic manner: an fMRI study. European Journal of Neuroscience 13:400–404.

Bunge SA (2004) How we use rules to select actions: a review of evidence from cognitive neuroscience. Cognitive, Affective, and Behavioral Neuroscience 4:564–579.

Bunge SA, Kahn I, Wallis JD, Miller EK, Wagner AD (2003) Neural circuits subserving the retrieval and maintenance of abstract rules. Journal of Neurophysiology 90: 3419–3428.

Bunge SA, Wallis JD, Parker A, Brass M, Crone EA, Hoshi E, Sakai K (2005) Neural circuitry underlying rule use in humans and nonhuman primates. Journal of Neuroscience 25:10347–10350.

Cabeza R, Nyberg L (2002) Seeing the forest through the trees: the cross-function approach to imaging cognition. In: The cognitive electrophysiology of mind and brain (Zani A, Proverbio AM, eds.), pp 41–68. San Diego: Academic Press.

Chouinard PA, Paus T (2006) The primary motor and premotor areas of the human cerebral cortex. Neuroscientist 12:143–152.

Crone EA, Wendelken C, Donohue SE, Bunge SA (2006) Neural evidence for dissociable components of task-switching. Cerebral Cortex 16:475–486.

Derrfuss J, Brass M, Neumann J, von Cramon DY (2005) Involvement of the inferior frontal junction in cognitive control: meta-analyses of switching and Stroop studies. Human Brain Mapping 25:22–34.

Derrfuss J, Brass M, von Cramon DY (2004) Cognitive control in the posterior frontolateral cortex: evidence from common activations in task coordination, interference control, and working memory. Neuroimage 23:604–612.

Diamond A (2006) Bootstrapping conceptual deduction using physical connection: rethinking frontal cortex. Trends in Cognitive Sciences 10:212–218.

Diamond A, Churchland A, Cruess L, Kirkham NZ (1999) Early developments in the ability to understand the relation between stimulus and reward. Developmental Psychology 35:1507–1517.

Diamond A, Lee EY, Hayden M (2003) Early success in using the relation between stimuli and rewards to deduce an abstract rule: perceived physical connection is key. Developmental Psychology 39:825–847.

Dove A, Pollmann S, Schubert T, Wiggins CJ, von Cramon DY (2000) Prefrontal cortex activation in task switching: an event-related fMRI study. Brain Research: Cognitive Brain Research 9:103–109.

Dreher JC, Koechlin E, Ali SO, Grafman J (2002) The roles of timing and task order during task switching. Neuroimage 17:95–109.

Duncan J, Owen AM (2000) Common regions of the human frontal lobe recruited by diverse cognitive demands. Trends in Neuroscience 23:475–483.

Forstmann BU, Brass M, Koch I, von Cramon DY (2005) Internally generated and directly cued task sets: an investigation with fMRI. Neuropsychologia 43:943–952.

Forstmann BU, Brass M, Koch I, von Cramon DY (2006) Voluntary selection of task sets revealed by functional magnetic resonance imaging. Journal of Cognitive Neuroscience 18:388–398.

Germann J, Robbins S, Halsband U, Petrides M (2005) Precentral sulcal complex of the human brain: morphology and statistical probability maps. Journal of Comparative Neurology 493:334–356.

Godschalk M, Mitz AR, van Duin B, van der Burg H (1995) Somatotopy of monkey premotor cortex examined with microstimulation. Neuroscience Research 23:269–279.

Goldberg G (1985) Supplementary motor area structure and function: review and hypothesis. Behavioral and Brain Sciences 8:567–616.

Halsband U, Passingham R (1982) The role of premotor and parietal cortex in the direction of action. Brain Research 240:368–372.

Jarvik ME (1956) Simple color discrimination in chimpanzees: effect of varying contiguity between cue and incentive. Journal of Comparative Physiological Psychology 49:492–495.

Jersild AT (1927) Mental set and shift. Archives of Psychology 89:1–81.

Kimberg DY, Aguirre GK, D'Esposito M (2000) Modulation of task-related neural activity in task-switching: an fMRI study. Brain Research: Cognitive Brain Research 10:189–196.

Koechlin E, Ody C, Kouneiher F (2003) The architecture of cognitive control in the human prefrontal cortex. Science 302:1181–1185.

Konishi S, Donaldson DI, Buckner RL (2001) Transient activation during block transition. Neuroimage 13:364–374.

Logan GD, Bundesen C (2003) Clever homunculus: is there an endogenous act of control in the explicit task-cuing procedure? Journal of Experimental Psychology: Human Perception and Performance 29:575–599.

Luks TL, Simpson GV, Feiwell RJ, Miller WL (2002) Evidence for anterior cingulate cortex involvement in monitoring preparatory attentional set. Neuroimage 17:792–802.

Luria AR (1966/1980) Higher cortical functions in man. New York: Consultants Bureau.

MacDonald AW III, Cohen JD, Stenger VA, Carter CS (2000) Dissociating the role of the dorsolateral prefrontal and anterior cingulate cortex in cognitive control. Science 288:1835–1838.

Matelli M, Camarda R, Glickstein M, Rizzolatti G (1986) Afferent and efferent projections of the inferior area 6 in the macaque monkey. Journal of Comparative Neurology 251:281–298.

Mayr U, Kliegl R (2003) Differential effects of cue changes and task changes on task-set selection costs. Journal of Experimental Psychology: Learning, Memory, and Cognition 29:362–372.

Meiran N (1996) Reconfiguration of processing mode prior to task performance. Journal of Experimental Psychology: Learning, Memory and Cognition 22:1423–1442.

Meiran N, Chorev Z, Sapir A (2000) Component processes in task switching. Cognitive Psychology 41:211–253.

Milham MP, Banich MT, Webb A, Barad V, Cohen NJ, Wszalek T, Kramer AF (2001) The relative involvement of anterior cingulate and prefrontal cortex in attentional control depends on nature of conflict. Brain Research: Cognitive Brain Research 12:467–473.

Miller EK, Cohen JD (2001) An integrative theory of prefrontal cortex function. Annual Review of Neuroscience 24:167–202.

Milner B (1963) Effects of different brain lesions on card sorting. Archives of Neurology 9:90–100.

Monchi O, Petrides M, Petre V, Worsley K, Dagher A (2001) Wisconsin Card Sorting revisited: distinct neural circuits participating in different stages of the task identified

by event-related functional magnetic resonance imaging. Journal of Neuroscience 21:7733–7741.

Monsell S (2003) Task switching. Trends in Cognitive Sciences 7:134–140.

Monsell S, Taylor TJ, Murphy K (2001) Naming the color of a word: is it responses or task sets that compete? Memory and Cognition 29:137–151.

Neumann J, Lohmann G, Derrfuss J, von Cramon DY (2005) Meta-analysis of functional imaging data using replicator dynamics. Human Brain Mapping 25:165–173.

Ono M, Kubik S, Abernathey CD (1990) Atlas of the cerebral sulci. Stuttgart: Georg Thieme Verlag.

Pandya DN, Yeterian EH (1996) Comparison of prefrontal architecture and connections. Philosophical Transactions of the Royal Society of London B 351:1423–1432.

Petrides M (1985) Deficits on conditional associative-learning tasks after frontal- and temporal-lobe lesions in man. Neuropsychologia 23:601–614.

Petrides M (2000) Mapping prefrontal cortical systems for the control of cognition. In: Brain mapping: the systems. (Toga AW, Mazziotta JC, eds.), pp 159–176: San Diego: Academic Press.

Petrides M, Pandya DN (1994) Comparative architectonic analysis of the human and the macaque frontal cortex. In: Handbook of neuropsychology (Boller F, Grafman J, eds.), pp 17–58. Amsterdam: Elsevier.

Picard N, Strick PL (2001) Imaging the premotor areas. Current Opinion in Neurobiology 11:663–672.

Rogers RD, Monsell S (1995) Costs of a predictable switch between simple cognitive tasks. Journal of Experimental Psychology 124:207–231.

Rubinstein JS, Meyer DE, Evans JE (2001) Executive control of cognitive processes in task switching. Journal of Experimental Psychology: Human Perception and Performance 27:763–797.

Ruge H, Brass M, Koch I, Rubin O, Meiran N, von Cramon DY (2005) Advance preparation and stimulus-induced interference in cued task switching: further insights from BOLD fMRI. Neuropsychologia 43:340–355.

Rushworth MF, Buckley MJ, Gough PM, Alexander IH, Kyriazis D, McDonald KR, Passingham RE (2005) Attentional selection and action selection in the ventral and orbital prefrontal cortex. Journal of Neuroscience 25:11628–11636.

Rushworth MF, Hadland KA, Paus T, Sipila PK (2002a) Role of the human medial frontal cortex in task switching: a combined fMRI and TMS study. Journal of Neurophysiology 87:2577–2592.

Rushworth MF, Passingham RE, Nobre AC (2002b) Components of switching intentional set. Journal of Cognitive Neuroscience 14:1139–1150.

Rushworth MF, Walton ME, Kennerley SW, Bannerman DM (2004) Action sets and decisions in the medial frontal cortex. Trends in Cognitive Sciences 8:410–417.

Sohn MH, Ursu S, Anderson JR, Stenger VA, Carter CS (2000) Inaugural article: the role of prefrontal cortex and posterior parietal cortex in task switching. Proceedings of the National Academy of Sciences U S A 97:13448–13453.

Stuss DT, Alexander MP (2000) Executive functions and the frontal lobes: a conceptual view. Psychological Research 63:289–298.

Talairach J, Tournoux P (1988) Co-planar stereotaxic atlas of the human brain. Stuttgart: Georg Thieme Verlag.

Tomita H, Ohbayashi M, Nakahara K, Hasegawa I, Miyashita Y (1999) Top-down signal from prefrontal cortex in executive control of memory retrieval. Nature 401: 699–703.

Wise SP, Murray EA (2000) Arbitrary associations between antecedents and actions. Trends in Neurosciences 23:271–276.

Wylie GR, Javitt DC, Foxe JJ (2006) Jumping the gun: is effective preparation contingent upon anticipatory activation in task-relevant neural circuitry? Cerebral Cortex 16:394–404.

10

Time Course of Executive Processes: Data from the Event-Related Optical Signal

Gabriele Gratton, Kathy A. Low, and Monica Fabiani

In our everyday experience, we commonly find ourselves in changing circumstances, such that actions that would have been appropriate until a short time ago are no longer so. In most cases, we adapt to these situations with ease. This observation implies that our information-processing system has the ability to modify itself very quickly, using new rules to react to the new context, and discarding old ones. Psychologists label the set of processes involved with this rapid adaptation to changing environmental contexts "executive function."

The flexibility inherent to executive processes implies that the brain has evolved mechanisms for comparing current environmental conditions with those occurring some time in the near past, which are used to make predictions about the near future, as well as mechanisms for setting behavioral rules and changing them. Necessarily, predictions about the near future are based on past events, of which the most informative are those that have occurred most recently. Hence, executive function is strictly associated with working memory (Baddeley and Hitch, 1974)—and the two concepts have evolved in parallel in the recent psychological literature.

Executive function, as it is commonly conceived, consists of two aspects: an evaluative aspect, related to forming, maintaining, and updating appropriate models of the environment (which may be carried out through various types of memory processes) and an action-oriented aspect, which is instead involved with the coordination of other cognitive functions, including perception, attention, and action. This coordination presumably takes place over time, and is reflected in future behavior, so that, when performed appropriately, it can lead to successful adaptation to changing task demands.

In this chapter, we apply a cognitive neuroscience perspective, specifically, a functional neuroimaging approach: We consider how data about brain activity may illuminate our view of executive function. Following several theorists (e.g., Baddeley and Hitch, 1974; Cowan, 1995), we use a framework for conceptualizing executive function that is based on a distinction between two

components: a domain-specific set of processes that differ for particular environmental dimensions to be monitored, and a domain-general set of processes,
a sort of general-purpose machinery that is used for a variety of different processes. We stress research not only on these components, but also on their relative roles and interactions. In particular, we consider two different modes of
operation of the executive function system: (1) a hierarchical, centralized mode
in which the domain-general system controls the operation of the domain-
specific systems; and (2) a distributed, parallel mode in which the selection of
appropriate stimulus-response dimensions and associations emerges from the
interactions between domain-specific systems. We present data from a brain
imaging technology possessing both temporal and spatial resolution, the event-
related optical signal (EROS) [Gratton et al., 1995a; Gratton and Fabiani, 2001],
supporting the coexistence of both modes of operation.

In the remainder of this chapter, we first consider the advantages and limitations of various imaging techniques in providing a spatiotemporal description of brain function. Then we review the basic literature on EROS, focusing in particular on the data that allow us to establish that this technique
can be used to provide brain images combining spatial resolution on the order
of several millimeters, with temporal resolution on the order of milliseconds.
Finally, we review some experimental data obtained with EROS that are relevant for executive function. The featured research includes studies of sensory
and working memory processes and attention, as well as preliminary results
from a set of studies of preparatory processes. As highlighted earlier, the data
suggest the existence of two types of preparatory activities in the brain: a general set, relatively similar across different preparation conditions, and a specific
set, which is more directly related to preparation for particular stimulus or
response modalities. These initial EROS studies lay the foundation for future
work on executive processes, including the representation and implementation
of behavioral rules.

BRAIN IMAGING TECHNIQUES: TRADEOFFS
BETWEEN SPATIAL AND TEMPORAL RESOLUTION

The last two decades have seen the rapid growth of brain imaging as a tool for
studying both normal and abnormal brain function. Brain imaging has two
major advantages: (1) It can be performed noninvasively and can therefore be
used extensively in humans, and (2) it has the potential to provide a dynamic
view of activity as it evolves within the brain. Ideally, brain imaging methods
should possess high spatial and temporal resolution as well as high sensitivity
and reliability. The most widely used techniques—functional magnetic resonance imaging (fMRI) and event-related brain potentials (ERPs)—trade off
between these characteristics because they emphasize spatial and temporal
information, respectively. For this reason, it has been proposed to combine
different techniques to achieve a more complete picture of brain activity (e.g.,
Barinaga, 1997). However, there are technical and methodological problems

associated with the combination of these techniques, and a generally accepted method of integration is still lacking.

An alternative approach is provided by methods that have high resolution in both the spatial and temporal domains. One technique that has been used with some success is magnetoencephalography (MEG) (e.g., Hari and Lounasmaa, 1989). However, the spatial resolution of MEG (where "spatial resolution" is defined as the ability to resolve the activity of two brain areas located in close proximity without cross-talk), although superior to that of ERPs, may still significantly limit the types of issues that can be addressed. In this chapter, we review the use of EROS (Gratton et al., 1995a; Gratton & Fabiani, 2001), a technology based on the measurement of localized fast changes in the optical properties of the brain, which are practically simultaneous with electrical activity.

EVENT-RELATED OPTICAL SIGNAL

Mechanisms Underlying Optical Changes in Active Neurons

It has long been known that the optical properties of isolated axons (e.g., Hill and Keynes, 1949; Cohen, 1973) and brain slices (Frostig et al., 1990) change with neuronal activity, concurrently with electrophysiological signals. Several recent studies have investigated the mechanisms underlying optical changes, and identified two major phenomena: changes in *birefringence* and changes in *scattering* (Foust and Rector, 2007).[1] Two possible mechanisms have been proposed to account for these phenomena: (1) The changes are associated with repolarization of molecules within the membrane due to changes in the transmembrane potential (Stepnosky et al., 1991), and/or (2) the changes are due to the movement of water associated with ion diffusion and transport, and to the consequent volume variations in intra- and extracellular space (Andrew and MacVicar, 1994).

Indeed, evidence has been presented for both mechanisms, and the most recent research suggests that changes in birefringence appear to be most closely associated with membrane phenomena, whereas changes in scattering appear to be most closely associated with volumetric effects (MacVicar and Hochman, 1991; Momose-Sato et al., 1998; Buchheim et al., 1999; Foust and Rector, 2007). Light polarization (required for birefringence measures) is lost rapidly in the head because of the relatively short free paths of photons in living tissue. Thus, noninvasive measures, as well as measures involving thick tissue preparations, are more likely to be related to scattering than to birefringence effects.

Optical Changes in the Human Brain

By the early 1990s, instruments capable of detecting changes in optical brain transparency had been developed sufficiently to be of practical use for non-invasive applications in humans. These machines were mostly designed to study

the variations in tissue coloration associated with changes in brain oxygen-ation (e.g., Jobsis, 1977; E. Gratton et al., 1990; Villringer and Chance, 1997). These instruments typically use near-infrared (NIR) light, which penetrates the tissue more deeply than visible light because of the low absorption of he-moglobin and water, the main absorbers in most human tissues, at wavelengths of 690–1000 nm.

For NIR light, the main factor limiting the penetration of photons into the tissue is scattering. The scatter is so pronounced that, within approximately 5 mm from the surface of the head, the movement of photons through tissue can be described as a random diffusion process (Ishimaru et al., 1978). Fur-ther, the scattering process makes it practically impossible to use sources and detectors located on opposite sides of the head to measure brain activity in the adult human. This makes it difficult or impossible to measure activity in struc-tures deeper than 3–4 cm from the surface of the head. Critically, sources and detectors located on the *same* side of the head, at a distance of a few (e.g., 2–6) centimeters from each other, can be used to infer optical properties related to the underlying tissue up to 3 cm deep, as illustrated in Figure 10–1 (see color insert). When measurements are taken at the scalp, physical separation be-tween the sources and detectors is critical to derive measures of intracranial structures, such as the cortex; otherwise, reflection from the surface of the scalp would dominate the image.

Techniques for Measuring Optical Signals

Some of the instruments used to derive these measurements employ sources that emit constant light (continuous-wave [CW] methods). In others, the light sources are modulated at radiofrequencies (frequency-domain [FD] methods). FD instruments allow investigators to measure not only the *amount* of light dif-fusing through a particular area of the brain and reaching the detectors (as in CW systems), but also the average *time* taken by photons to move between sources and detectors (photon delay). Because of the increase in photon path length induced by the diffusion process, this may take several nanoseconds and depends on the source-detector distance. Because intensity and photon delay are influ-enced differently by absorption and scattering effects, FD methods can provide simultaneous measures of the concentration of oxy- and deoxyhemoglobin (E. Gratton et al., 1990) and of brain phenomena related to neuronal activation.

The changes in tissue transparency are relatively small (on the order of 1%), and little light typically reaches the detectors; therefore, fast optical measures may have a relatively low signal-to-noise ratio (SNR) compared with other imaging methods. As such, averaging across trials or subjects is needed to reveal activity. However, recent advancements based on higher modulation frequencies (Maclin et al., in press) and frequency and spatial filtering methods (Wolf et al., 2000; Maclin et al., 2003) allow investigators to study conditions in which a relatively small number of trials (in some cases, fewer than 20) are used for the averaging.

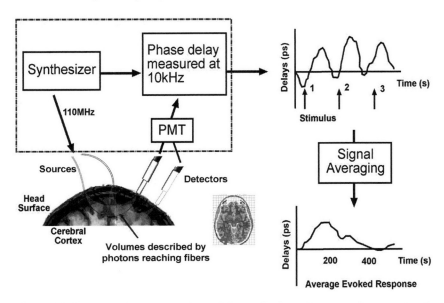

Figure 10–1 Schematic representation of the methods used to record event-related optical signal (EROS) data (frequency-domain [FD] method). *Top left.* The recording apparatus uses near-infrared light modulated at radiofrequencies (e.g., 110 MHz) to illuminate locations of the scalp (*bottom left*). The light propagates through the head in random fashion. Some of the light reaches detector fibers located a short distance (a few centimeters) from the sources. The average path followed by photons moving between sources and detectors can be described as a curved spindle volume (or a "banana") that reaches the cortex. This volume is the area relevant for the measurement from each source-detector pair. In a typical study, several source-detector pairs are used (up to 1024). Two types of measures can be taken at the detectors, intensity measures and delay measures. Intensity measures are variations in the amount of light reaching the detector as a function of activity. Delay measures are variations in the average time taken by photons to move between sources and detectors. The latter are used in the current chapter because they are more sensitive to events occurring inside the skull. *Right.* Schematic diagram of the averaging procedures used to derive the EROS. PMT= photomultiplier tube. (Reproduced with permission from Fabiani, Gratton & Corballis, *Journal of Biomedical Optics,* 1(4), 387–398. Copyright International Society for Optical Engineering, 1996).

Initial EROS Measurements

Using FD instrumentation, we were the first to report the noninvasive measurement of a fast optical signal in humans (EROS) [Gratton et al., 1995a] using a visual stimulation paradigm (pattern reversal). In this first study, we showed that stimulation of different quadrants of the visual field generated responses in occipital regions, with peak latencies between 50 and 100 ms. The surface distribution reflected the contralateral inverted representation of the visual field in

the underlying primary and secondary visual cortex. This fast optical signal was characterized by an increase in the delay (on the order of a few picoseconds) of the photon density wave passing through the occipital cortical regions. The response was simultaneous with the peak of the source-modeled, scalp-recorded electrical evoked potential (recorded in the same subjects) and colocalized with areas of activation measured using blood-oxygen level–dependent (BOLD) fMRI (also recorded in the same subjects) [Gratton et al., 1997b].

We followed up these initial reports with a number of other studies imaging the visual (Gratton, 1997; Gratton et al., 1998, 2000, 2001, 2006; Gratton and Fabiani, 2003), auditory (Rinne et al., 1999; Maclin et al., 2003; Fabiani et al., 2006), somatosensory (Maclin et al., 2004), and motor (Gratton et al., 1995b; De Soto et al., 2001) cortices. All of these studies showed EROS responses of a similar nature: *increases* of photon delay of a few picoseconds, simultaneous with concurrently recorded evoked potentials, and when measured, colocalized with BOLD fMRI responses. In work conducted over the last 2 years with FD instrumentation that uses up to 1024 channels and is capable of sampling nearly the entire cortical surface, the results have further generalized to the detection of neural activity from frontal and parietal areas during higher-level cognitive tasks (Agran et al., 2005; Low et al., 2006). Some of this research will be reviewed later in this chapter.

Fast Optical Signaling Studies from Other Laboratories

During the last 5 years, following up on our original work, several other laboratories have also reported the recording of fast optical signals in humans (e.g., Steinbrink et al., 2000; Wolf et al., 2000, 2002, 2003a, b; Franceschini and Boas, 2004; Lebid et al., 2004, 2005; Tse et al, 2006, in press) using visual, auditory, somatosensory, and motor modalities. Some of these investigators used CW instruments, which only afford measures of the intensity of light moving between sources and detectors (Steinbrink et al., 2000; Franceschini and Boas, 2004; Lebid et al., 2004, 2005). With this method, the scalp-recorded fast signal is typically characterized by a *reduction* in light intensity (1/1000–1/10,000 of the light normally reaching the detectors).

In two recent studies in which intensity and delay measures were both reported (Maclin et al., 2003; Gratton et al., 2006), we have also found that fast optical signals measured from the scalp in humans are typically characterized by the association of increases in photon delay and reductions in intensity. In contrast to this wealth of positive data, only one laboratory, to our knowledge, has reported an inability to detect the fast signal using FD methods (Syré et al., 2003), although the same group reported obtaining such signal with a CW method (Steinbrink et al., 2000; but see Steinbrink et al., 2005, for a criticism of this work).

In the 10 years since our original report, fast optical signals have also been described in live animals. Specifically, David Rector and his collaborators (1997) first reported the recording of fast optical signals from the hippocampus

of rats (characterized by a decrement in back-scattering[2]), and showed that this response is concurrent with evoked potentials from implanted electrodes. This study was followed by the demonstration of fast optical responses in other animal preparations, most recently from the barrel cortex of the rat (Rector et al., 2005). We have recently shown similar types of responses from the cat visual cortex (Tanner et al., 2006), using both CW and FD methods.

In addition to these basic results demonstrating the existence and generalizability of fast optical signals in humans, we have conducted a number of other studies showing three important aspects of the fast optical signal. (1) In studies investigating occipital, temporal, and other cortical regions, we have shown that the signal is graded in amplitude in a manner that is consistent with what is known about the activation of these areas from electrophysiological studies of mass activity (e.g., Gratton et al., 2001, 2006). (2) Fast optical signals are relatively well localized with sufficient spatial sampling, so that, at least in some cases, areas where the activity can be observed extend only a few millimeters (e.g., Gratton et al., 1997b; Gratton and Fabiani, 2003; Low et al., 2006). (3) Signals from deeper (up to 3 cm from the surface of the scalp) or more superficial cortical regions can be distinguished by comparing the fast optical signal measured from source-detector pairs that vary in source-detector distance (Gratton et al., 2000, 2006).

We have further shown that the amplitude of the fast optical signals (related to neuronal activity) can predict the amplitude of slow optical responses (related to hemodynamic phenomena) [Gratton et al., 2001; Fabiani et al., 2005], and BOLD fMRI responses (Gratton et al., 2005). These findings suggest the existence of a linear relationship between the amplitude of the neuronal response measured with EROS and that of the hemodynamic response measured with slow optical signals or BOLD fMRI.

Finally, in a series of recent studies, our laboratory and others have employed fast optical responses to address various issues in cognitive neuroscience, ranging from the localization and timing of attention and memory effects in the visual cortex (Gratton, 1997, Gratton et al., 1998; Fabiani et al., 2003) and auditory cortex (Fabiani et al., 2006; Tse et al., 2006, in press; Sable et al., 2006), to working memory effects in the frontal cortex (Low et al., 2006), the time course of preparatory processes (Agran et al., 2005), and whether parallel activation of multiple motor responses is possible (De Soto et al., 2001). These data are all consistent with the claim that fast optical signals can be used to derive images of brain activity combining sub-centimeter spatial resolution and millisecond-level temporal resolution.

EROS AND EXECUTIVE FUNCTION

During the last decade, it has been shown that EROS can be useful for studying the time course of brain activity associated with cognitive function, in general, and executive function, in particular. In the remainder of this chapter, we briefly review different lines of research that are relevant to the issue of

executive function as it unfolds during processing. In presenting this work, we follow a simplified view of executive function inspired by seminal cognitive models proposed by Broadbent (1957), Baddeley and Hitch (1974), Cowan (1995), and Engle (2002).

According to this view, executive function operates on information held in sensory buffer mechanisms, in which specific representations are selected for further processing through selective attention mechanisms. These mechanisms are, to some extent, based on current models of the contextual conditions, and their operation results in the coordination of processes to perform particular actions. Within this general framework, we focus on specific results that can be taken as examples of what could be achieved with a technology such as EROS, combining spatial and temporal information.

EROS and Sensory Memory

Theories of working memory typically postulate the existence of mechanisms for holding information that may occur outside the control of attention (e.g., Baddeley and Hitch, 1974; Cowan 1995). When needed, this information may be accessed at a later time (within a few hundred milliseconds or a few seconds) for further processing. Sensory memory mechanisms are typically considered to have high fidelity, although they are very short-lived, highly sensitive to inter-ference, or both. Because sensory memory may occur outside attentional control (and perhaps awareness), brain imaging methods, and ERPs in particular, have been useful for its study, by making it possible to measure aspects of these very transient processes. The goal of the optical imaging studies reviewed here was to determine whether EROS could be used to dissociate various ERP components associated with sensory memory, and to better localize these components.

Components of the ERP Associated with Sensory Memory and Their Possible Optical Counterparts

A large number of ERP studies have investigated auditory sensory memory by focusing on a particular component, mismatch negativity (MMN) [see Ritter et al., 1995, for a review]. This component is elicited by stimuli that differ from prior stimuli along one or more dimensions, even if the stimuli are not at-tended to. It has a peak latency of 100–200 ms after stimulus presentation, and it is believed to have its primary generator in secondary auditory cortex, with an additional generator in frontal cortex (Näätänen, 2000). It is postulated that the MMN may reflect aspects of preattentive processing of potentially important information (i.e., information that may need to capture attention) as it indexes the detection of changes within a steady context, even during sleep or anesthesia (Näätänen, 2000).

Another early ERP component that has been associated with auditory sensory memory is the N1, or N100 (Näätänen and Picton, 1987). This is a short-latency component (peaking approximately 100 ms after stimulus onset) whose ampli-tude is influenced, among other things, by the occurrence of stimuli immedi-

ately preceding the eliciting stimulus, as well as by attention manipulations. It differs from the MMN because physical dissimilarity between the eliciting stimulus and the prior stimuli is not critical for its elicitation.

Both the MMN and the N1 are considered evidence for the existence of memory buffers that retain stimulus information over time (albeit with different characteristics), even for unattended stimuli. However, in part because of the low spatial resolution of ERPs, and because these two components overlap somewhat in both time and scalp distribution, it is often difficult to confidently attribute the variance observed in a particular study to one or the other. This limitation may hinder the interpretation of the results. In fact, it is often unclear whether a particular effect can be uniquely attributed to the N1 or the MMN because they are considered to underlie different types of sensory memory buffers (but see Jaaskelainen et al., 2004).

We used EROS to separate these two components (Rinne et al., 1999), and showed that they are actually generated in slightly different regions of the superior temporal gyrus. In more recent studies, we showed that EROS can separate N100 effects related to stimulus repetition from MMN effects related to stimulus deviance—effects that are also dissociated in young and old adults (Fabiani et al., 2006). Penney and his collaborators (Tse et al., 2006, in press) conducted a series of studies using EROS to separate possible contributions of superior temporal and inferior frontal areas to the scalp-recorded MMN. These studies showed that the frontal and temporal components of the MMN were dissociable. Dissociations between these two components of the MMN have also been reported in studies combining ERPs and fMRI (e.g., Optiz et al., 2002), and these dissociations are consistent with those observed with EROS.

Visual sensory memory has been investigated much less than auditory sensory memory. However, in a series of studies involving ERPs, we showed that memory for early visual representations can be studied using a divided-field paradigm (Gratton et al., 1997a, Gratton, 1998). Corresponding EROS data, in this case, indicate that memory effects can already be evident at the level of the first response recorded in medial (probably primary) visual cortex (latency: approximately 80 ms) [Gratton et al., 1998; Fabiani et al., 2003].

In summary, EROS data suggest that auditory and visual sensory memory buffers may be supported by mechanisms occurring early in the visual and auditory cortical pathways. Whether these mechanisms are inherent to the sensory areas investigated, or are, in fact, based on feedback coming from higher-order areas (such as those involved in executive processes), is a matter for future investigation. The current data do extend those obtained with ERPs by providing better separation of individual brain responses and better localization of the cortical areas involved.

EROS and Selective Attention

The concept of selective attention is closely related to that of executive function, so much so that executive function is sometimes considered as the ability

to control attention (Engle, 2002). Selective attention can be defined as a differential response of the information-processing system to important compared with irrelevant stimuli. A question that has elicited substantial research relates to the earliest level of the information-processing system at which selective attention operates (e.g., Johnston and Dark, 1986). In cognitive neuroscientific terms, this question can be rephrased as the first area along a sensory pathway, or the first neuronal response (over time) that is influenced by selective attention. Considerable research on this issue has been carried out in the case of visual spatial selective attention: The question here is typically whether the initial response in primary visual cortex is influenced by attention.

In humans, this question has been investigated primarily with two methods: ERPs and fMRI. The results obtained with these two methods are partially contradictory. The fMRI work (e.g., Brefczynski and DeYoe, 1999) has, for the most part, suggested that activity in primary visual cortex distinguishes between attended and unattended stimuli. In contrast, ERP evidence collected by Hillyard and his collaborators (Martinez et al., 1999, 2001) suggested that the initial response in primary visual cortex is not affected by attention, although the same group found that subsequent responses in primary visual cortex are. In fact, Martinez and colleagues concluded that the fMRI differences in primary visual cortex between attended and unattended stimuli are due to re-afferent (top-down) activity from other cortical areas rather than to the initial response related to information coming from the thalamus (lateral geniculate nucleus). A limitation of this work is that it is in part dependent on a relatively low-spatial resolution technique (ERP)—although this group reported rather sophisticated methods, based on source modeling, for distinguishing between responses from primary visual cortex and responses from other areas (Martinez et al., 1999, 2001).

Because of its spatiotemporal properties, we used EROS in a visual selective attention paradigm to test the relative effects of attention on primary and secondary visual areas (Gratton, 1997). The results of this study supported the findings of Hillyard's group: Areas in medial occipital cortex (presumably, primary visual cortex) showed similar short-latency (80 ms) responses for attended and unattended stimuli, whereas attention effects were only visible at early latencies in more lateral areas (presumably, secondary visual cortex).

EROS in Studies of Working Memory and Executive Function

As discussed earlier, working memory is a concept that is strongly related to that of executive function. Further, there is a long tradition of studies of working memory conducted with brain imaging methods. This work has emphasized the role of prefrontal and parietal regions in working memory paradigms (e.g., Cohen et al., 1997; Corbetta et al., 1998). In our laboratory, we have conducted a few studies on working memory based on EROS. We were

particularly interested in determining whether EROS could be useful in investigating various aspects of the frontoparietal network (FPN) often associated with working memory and executive function. Specifically, our question was whether EROS could further our understanding of the specific function of these cortical regions, as well as their interactions. Note that the temporal resolution of EROS should be particularly useful for investigating how these interactions play out over time. In fact, timing information, coupled with spatial resolution, provides modeling constraints that can be exploited statistically (e.g., if area X is activated *before* area Y, then X may influence Y, but not vice versa) [Rykhlevskaia et al., 2006a]. We have conducted various studies aimed at determining whether EROS can help provide initial answers to the following questions:

1. Is there a functional specialization of the activity within the FPN? Specifically, is there a functional specialization dependent on the type of material involved and the type of task required?
2. Is there evidence of interactions among different areas? How do these interactions play out over time? Do they involve coordination of activity among areas, including reciprocal inhibition phenomena? Are these interactions mediated by the anatomical connection between areas?
3. Is there a hierarchy between processes, with some related to general-purpose activities and others more domain-specific? Do the general-purpose activities operate earlier than the domain-specific mechanisms, consistent with the idea that the former control the latter?

To address these types of issues with EROS, it is important to first determine that this method can, in fact, be used to study the time course of activity in frontal cortical regions, even with a relatively small number of trials (i.e., fewer than 50 per condition per subject). As such, we (Low et al., 2006) investigated the time course of frontal activity during an auditory oddball paradigm, in which two classes of stimuli are presented—one rare (occurring 20% of the time, and yielding approximately 50 trials per subject) and one frequent (Donchin, 1981). In different blocks of trials, these stimuli were attended or unattended. We found that the right middle frontal gyrus was engaged by rare stimuli when they were attended to, but not by unattended stimuli, approximately 300 ms after stimulus presentation. This latency corresponds to that of the frontal area P3 (sometimes labeled P3a) [e.g., Katayama and Polich, 1998], which can be recorded using ERPs in the same paradigm and under the same experimental conditions. Activity in the right middle frontal gyrus has also been recorded in fMRI studies of the oddball paradigm (e.g., Kirino et al., 2000), although these studies have also often reported a response in left prefrontal regions. In summary, these data support the idea that EROS can be effectively used to study activity in the FPN, even with a limited number of trials.

EROS and Specialization within the Frontoparietal Network

In a second study, we recorded EROS from frontal regions in a paradigm commonly employed to study working memory, the n-back task (Leaver et al., submitted). This task has been employed extensively in brain imaging research; studies typically reveal activation of the middle and inferior frontal regions (Buckner and Peterson, 1996; Cabeza et al., 1997; Fletcher, 1997). We were interested in determining whether EROS could detect this activity and establish the timing of its occurrence. We were also interested in determining whether EROS could help characterize the frontal responses, regionally and/or temporally, as a function of the type of material to be memorized and the memory load. Therefore, two versions of this task were used, one based on verbal information and one based on spatial information; for each version of the task, we varied the memory load by contrasting a two-back to a one-back condition. Finally, we were interested in determining whether individual differences in brain connectivity may have an effect on the functional organization of working memory and its relationship to behavior. For this reason, we compared young adults with old adults, because the latter may be expected to have a lower level of brain connectivity. More importantly, we further compared old adults who had either a large or a small anterior corpus callosum (CC), the major white matter structure connecting the left and right frontal lobes. This is an individual difference that could be more directly related to the brain connections essential to working memory function.

Results indicate that areas in the left middle frontal gyrus were active with a latency of approximately 250 ms for the verbal version of the task, and homologous right regions were active for the spatial task. Further, regions in the inferior and middle frontal gyrus of the right hemisphere were activated in the one-back condition and inhibited in the two-back condition. Conversely, analogous regions of the left hemisphere were activated in the two-back condition and inhibited in the one-back condition. Both of these left-right lateralizations (verbal versus spatial and two-back versus one-back) were significantly less pronounced in old adults with small anterior CCs than in those with large CCs or in young adults.[3] The old adults with small CCs also showed impaired performance, particularly in the most difficult task conditions.

In interpreting these results, we considered that the one- and two-back conditions differ as follows: The one-back condition requires the use of the most recently activated representation, whereas the two-back condition requires *ignoring* this information and instead accessing representations of previously presented items. Thus, the two-back condition requires the retrieval of information in the presence of interference. As noted in Chapter 16, the left inferior frontal gyrus appears to be particularly important for retrieval of information under these conditions (Jonides et al., 1998; Badre and Wagner, 2002, 2005). Activation of the right inferior frontal gyrus during retrieval of information in the *absence* of interference has been instead shown in other brain imaging studies (for a review, see Nolde et al., 1998). These findings are

consistent with those of our experiment. Thus, it is possible that the relative activation of these two areas may be related to which information is relevant for a particular condition. Perhaps the right hemisphere is less capable of discriminating between information acquired over time than the left hemisphere. We will come back to this interpretation of the function of these areas later in this chapter, when we discuss effects observed during task-switching.

In conclusion, the EROS, aging, and structural CC data obtained in the n-back task point to the importance of brain connectivity in working memory function. These data indicate that anatomical variations (especially those of structures connecting the relevant areas) may contribute to changes in both brain activity and performance. Further, they stress how working memory function requires the appropriate and timely integration of different cortical regions.

EROS and Coordination of Activity in Different Brain Regions

Inherent to the concept of executive function is the idea that different brain regions are coordinated with each other in performing particular cognitive operations. Within a brain imaging framework, the concept of coordination between regions is associated with that of functional connectivity. Functional connectivity is typically defined as the correlation over time of activity in different areas (Friston, 1993a). This concept is distinguished from that of effective connectivity, which implies causality in the relationship between brain areas (Friston, 1993b); causality is, of course, much more difficult to prove than correlation. As was highlighted in the previous section, another related concept is that of anatomical connectivity, which is related to the anatomical connections between different brain regions.

Within the framework of executive function, functional connectivity may be considered a dynamic operation that varies according to the context in which the operation occurs. Further, it can be considered that functional connectivity evolves over time, and that activity in a particular area is associated with excitation (or inhibition) of another area with some lag.

This type of relationship can be best demonstrated with a technique possessing high spatial and temporal resolution. Both are important: If a technique lacks spatial resolution, it would be impossible to determine whether a correlation between the activity observed at two different locations is real or a consequence of the spatial cross-talk between the measurements; if a technique lacks temporal resolution, it is impossible to determine the order of activation of different areas—thus limiting the types of conclusions that can be drawn from the data. Of course, all brain imaging techniques possess some degree of both spatial and temporal resolution, allowing for various implementations of this approach (see, for instance, Friston et al., 1993 a,b).

In a recent study (Rykhlevskaia et al., 2006a), we have provided two examples demonstrating that EROS can be particularly useful for studying functional connectivity, specifically, to demonstrate lagged correlations between different areas. In the first example, we used data from visual cortex to show how EROS

can be used to study the propagation of activity between different occipital areas after visual stimulation.

The second example, which is more relevant to the purposes of the current chapter, was focused on task-switching (i.e., the requirement of updating rules that are currently relevant for the task and discarding rules that may have been valid a short time earlier). The goal of this experiment was to demonstrate that task-switching involves the appropriate coordination of activity of different cortical regions—a coordination that may be affected by the strength of the anatomical connections between homologous areas. Here, we measured brain activity elicited by cues signaling whether upcoming stimuli in a spatial Stroop task (DeSoto et al., 2001) should be processed according to a verbal or a spatial dimension. Both young and old adults participated in a study in which EROS was measured from frontal areas. As in the n-back study described earlier, structural magnetic resonance images were also collected and used to derive estimates of the size of the anterior portion of the CC. This provided a measure of the anatomical connectivity between left and right prefrontal areas in these subjects.

The analysis focused on the relationship between two homologous regions of the prefrontal cortex (BA 9), which were activated selectively for the verbal (left hemisphere) and spatial (right hemisphere) cues. These areas closely corresponded with the spatial and verbal areas observed in the n-back task described earlier. Activation in these regions peaked approximately 300 ms after cue onset, and was more pronounced during trials requiring a change (switch) in task rules. We employed a new technique, based on confirmatory factor analysis (a structural equation modeling technique), for modeling the pattern of cross-correlations between these two regions accounting for different lags.

The results indicated that each hemisphere tended to be negatively correlated with activity in the opposite hemisphere, with a lag of approximately 200–250 ms. We interpreted this negative correlation as evidence for competition (or reciprocal inhibition) between homologous areas in the two hemispheres involved in the selection of the appropriate rules to be used on a particular trial: When a cue signaled that a verbal rule was to be used, the spatial rule was inhibited, and vice versa.

Further, the results indicated that this negative correlation was modulated by the size of the anterior one-third of the CC: It was most evident in subjects with a large CC. Further, we found that CC size was also inversely related to the cost of switching between verbal and spatial rules, thus indicating that the anatomical connectivity (or lack thereof) had behavioral consequences (Gratton et al., submitted). The size of the anterior CC was also reduced with age, although CC size was a better predictor of both differences in functional connectivity and behavioral effects than age per se. All of these phenomena held true when CC size was adjusted by total brain size. In Chapter 4, it is shown how a higher-level brain region—the anterior prefrontal cortex—interacts with verbal versus spatial regions to prepare to perform a task. Our data

suggest a second mechanism for ensuring that the currently relevant task set is followed, namely, interactions (in the form of reciprocal inhibition) between the verbal and spatial regions themselves.

The concept that attentional control may be mediated by the reciprocal inhibition of different attention nodes is present in recent models of attention (e.g., Miller and Cohen, 2001; see also Herd et al., 2006). These authors also consider the middle frontal gyrus a critical structure for attentional control. Note that, by using the spatial versus verbal dimension, we have been able to physically segregate nodes related to attentional control in different hemispheres. This facilitates the investigation of reciprocal inhibition mechanisms. Further, this study suggests that attentional control may be impaired through a reduction of reciprocal inhibition, mediated by changes in anatomical connectivity. However, in the current case, reciprocal inhibition was only evident through a spatiotemporal cross-correlational analysis, which itself requires a technique combining spatial and temporal resolution.

In summary, these findings indicate that a combination of structural information and functional connectivity data obtained with EROS can be particularly useful for studying the interactions that occur across brain areas when context conditions require cognitive adjustments—i.e., when executive function is deployed.

EROS and General Versus Specific Processes

Flexible adaptation to changing task demands is essential for successful behavior in a complex environment—and is a critical feature of executive function. An important question concerns the general organization of the processes underlying adaptation. One possibility is that these adaptation processes may be executed through a *hierarchical* system, involving both general-purpose mechanisms, related to the control of attention (presumably, related to the FPN described earlier), as well as more specific mechanisms, dependent on the particular dimensions that need to be tracked. We may hypothesize that activation of the general-purpose areas should *precede* activation of the more task-specific areas. Alternatively, adaptation may depend on a *distributed* process, so that a centralized control mechanism is not required. Interaction between different areas may still be important (e.g., exhibiting reciprocal inhibition, as shown in the previous section), but this interaction may not reflect a particular hierarchy. Finally, it is possible that the two systems may coexist, and that their engagement depends on task demands, strategic alternatives, and individual differences. To characterize these two modes of operation, it may be useful to compare the activation patterns observed when different types of environmental dimensions need to be tracked.

To investigate the brain regions involved in dynamically switching between task instructions, we have conducted a series of four additional experiments using EROS (Low et al., 2006). We used a cueing paradigm in which a precue provides specific instructions about the rule to be used on a given trial

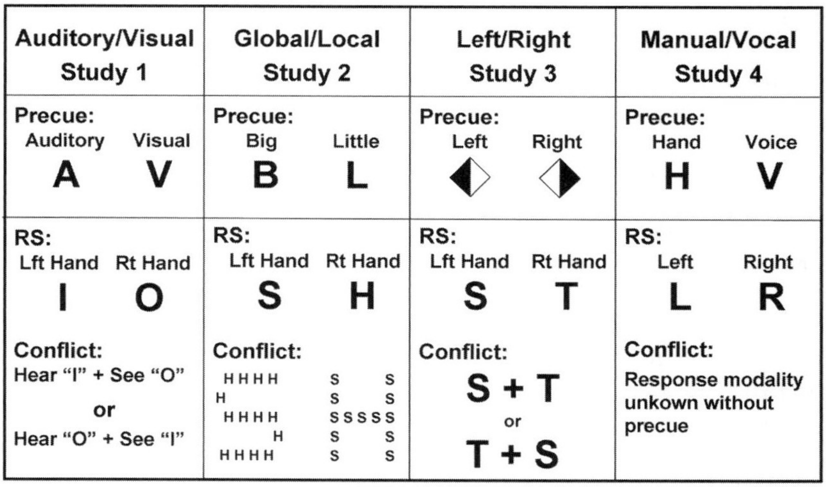

Auditory/Visual Study 1		Global/Local Study 2		Left/Right Study 3		Manual/Vocal Study 4	
Precue: Auditory	Visual	**Precue:** Big	Little	**Precue:** Left	Right	**Precue:** Hand	Voice
A	**V**	**B**	**L**	◆▷	◁▶	**H**	**V**
RS: Lft Hand	Rt Hand	**RS:** Lft Hand	Rt Hand	**RS:** Lft Hand	Rt Hand	**RS:** Left	Right
I	**O**	**S**	**H**	**S**	**T**	**L**	**R**
Conflict: Hear "I" + See "O" or Hear "O" + See "I"		**Conflict:** H H H H S S H S S H H H H S S S S S H S S H H H H S S		**Conflict:** **S + T** or **T + S**		**Conflict:** **Response modality unkown without precue**	

Figure 10–2 Schematic representation of the paradigms used in the task-switching studies. For all paradigms, the response stimulus (RS) could be responded to according to different stimulus dimensions (study 1–3) or response dimensions (study 4). The relevant dimension was determined by a pre-cue presented 2 s before the RS. The pre-cue was randomized across trials, thus generating conditions in which the same rule was used on consecutive trials (no-switch conditions) and conditions in which the rule changed (switch conditions). Each column in the figure refers to a different study; each row refers to a different event (stimulus or response).

(Fig. 10–2). In different experiments, we varied the stimulus dimension to be attended from trial to trial (auditory versus visual, local versus global, or left versus right visual field) or the response to be emitted (verbal versus manual). The EROS data were then sorted, based on whether the current trial contained the same task demand as the previous trial (no-switch) or a different task demand (switch).

The data from the pre-cueing paradigm reveal both general and specific activations associated with task-switching. The term "general" is used to indicate activities that are relatively similar across different modalities and tasks. The "specific" activities are proper to each task and appear to represent early activation of brain regions that are involved in upcoming tasks related to the imperative (response) stimuli. A possible interpretation of these activities is that setting up appropriate preparatory processes may involve activation of the same cortical regions that will later be used in the upcoming reaction time task. This type of activation appears consistent with attention effects reported in the brain imaging literature (see Kastner et al., 1999; Hopfinger et al., 2000; see also Corbetta et al., 1991). An important observation is that activity in these areas typically shows two peaks: one shortly after the cue (within the first 200 ms) and one occurring at much longer latencies (typically, approximately

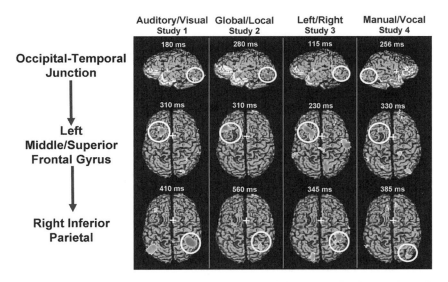

Figure 10–3 Statistical parametric maps (*Z* scores) of the event-related optical signal (EROS) response elicited by pre-cues during the pre-cueing paradigm computed across subjects. All maps represent activity related to cues signaling a switch in the rule to be used for processing the upcoming imperative stimuli, relative to no-switch cues. EROS allows investigators to compute maps at several multiple latencies from stimulations. Presented here are latencies that were most representative for each of the three regions of activation (lateral occipital, prefrontal, and parietal).

600 ms after the cue). We will come back later to a possible interpretation of this double peak.

The areas activated in task-general processing appear to be consistent with those included in the FPN (Corbetta et al., 1995; Cohen et al., 1997), and typically correlate with executive function. However, the data collected in the different experiments allow us to describe these activities, their mutual relationship, and their relationship with subsequent behavior, in greater detail. A complex picture appears to emerge. A cursory summary of the results (see Fig. 10–3; see color insert) suggests that general preparatory processes include activities in roughly three regions and intervals:

1. Early (latency = 200 ± 50 ms) activity in the lateral occipitotemporal boundary. This activity is often most evident in the left hemisphere, but it appears in the right hemisphere for motor tasks. It may be correlated across subjects with the subsequent middle frontal gyrus activity, as discussed later. Currently, we have no evidence that the activity in this area is predictive of subsequent behavior.
2. Intermediate (latency = 350 ± 100 ms) activity in the middle frontal gyrus. This activity is typically positive in the left hemisphere and

negative in the right hemisphere. Positivity in the right hemisphere may be evident for no-switch trials. The left hemisphere activity is well correlated with subsequent activity in more posterior parietal regions (discussed later). It is also moderately correlated with subsequent behavior: Subjects showing greater activity in the left middle frontal gyrus also show better overall accuracy and a reduced difference between error rates on switch compared to no-switch trials, suggesting that this activity may be correlated with the adoption of particular strategies. This correlation with subsequent behavior is not evident for right hemisphere activity.

3. Late (latency $= 450 \pm 100$ ms) activity in the inferior parietal lobule (or regions around the intraparietal sulcus). This activity is bilateral, although, in some cases, it appears most evident in the right hemisphere. The parietal activity is correlated with subsequent behavior. Specifically, it appears that the right hemisphere activity is predictive of overall accuracy, whereas the left hemisphere activity is more correlated with a reduction in switch costs (in particular, for reaction time).

These data lend themselves to some theoretical speculations. The presence of activation in a task-general network (FPN) appears to support to the hierarchical hypotheses of the organization of these processes (rather than to the distributed hypothesis). However, an important issue to consider is the relative order of activation of the general and specific processes. The hierarchical theory would lead to the prediction that the general processes should usually occur before the specific processes. In fact, the data suggest a different picture: Activity in the domain-specific regions occurs at two points in time, one relatively early (i.e., before activation of the FPN) and one relatively late (i.e., after activation of the FPN). Whereas the second peak is consistent with the predictions made by the hierarchical hypothesis, the early peak appears to be consistent with the distributed hypothesis. It should be noted that, at least in one study (Gratton et al., submitted), the amplitude of the late peak, but not of the early one, appears to predict the absence of behavioral switch costs. This may suggest that the second activation may be more important for preparatory processes than the first one. However, the data provide some support for the idea that executive control results from the interplay between two modes of operation: (1) a distributed mode in which activation of domain-specific elements does not require prior activation of domain-general elements, and (2) a hierarchical mode in which the domain-general elements are activated first, followed by activation of the domain-specific elements.

The data also appear informative with respect to the organization of the FPN, and suggest two basic organizational principles: (1) There is an anterior-to-posterior organization within this system; prefrontal regions are more involved in working with memory representations (which include representations of stimuli, the meaning of the cues and tasks), whereas parietal regions are more involved with the representation of stimulus-response associations.

This finding is consistent with views about the organization of the FPN discussed in other chapters of this book (e.g., Chapters 2, 3, 4, 6, and 12). This view is also consistent with previous accounts based on lesion, single-unit, and imaging studies (Corbetta et al., 1995; Cohen et al., 1997; Miller and Cohen, 2001). (2) Although homologous regions in the left and right hemisphere may support relatively analogous information-processing roles, there is a left-to-right organization, with the left hemisphere more capable of subtle distinctions (and therefore possessing a greater degree of functional resolution) and the right hemisphere having a coarser level of representation (and therefore possessing a smaller degree of functional resolution, but being capable of more rapid processing).

Within the pre-cueing task-switching paradigm, we then assume that the left prefrontal cortex is particularly involved when a switch is required, whereas the right prefrontal cortex is inhibited (with respect to the pre-cue baseline) in this case. The opposite occurs during no-switch trials. The reason for this is that the no-switch trials require reactivation of recently presented representations. No particular temporal-order resolution is required in this case, because the strongest representation is the one that is used—thus, the right middle frontal region is perfectly adequate for this process. The left prefrontal cortex is instead required on switch trials, because a previous representation is required in this case—whereas the last representation needs to be inhibited. This finding is consistent with the results obtained with EROS in the n-back task (Leaver et al., submitted; see Chapter 10), showing activation of the right middle and inferior frontal gyrus for the one-back condition, and of the left middle and inferior frontal gyrus for the two-back condition. Note that, within this view, the left middle frontal gyrus assumes a key role in preparatory processes, allowing more fine-tuned preparation to occur. This may occur because this area is capable of better discrimination between task rules and the temporal order of information than its homologous region in the right hemisphere. This would allow it to operate in the presence of interfering information (see Chapter 16; see also Badre and Wagner, 2002, 2005). Left hemisphere activity is therefore more correlated with fine-tuned preparation than activity in the right hemisphere.

According to this framework, the elicitation of appropriate task representations needs to be transformed into specific stimulus-response associations. For this to occur, activation of parietal regions, which are more directly related to the instantiation of stimulus-response associations, appears be important (see Chapters 11 and 16). Again, a left-right difference is noticeable: Whereas the activation of the right inferior parietal lobule leads to a generic increase in accuracy (for both switch and no-switch trials), indicating an overall change in the criteria set for response activation, the left hemisphere activity is more specific to the switch condition only, representing, presumably, changes that are context-dependent and possess a greater level of tuning.

This framework is, of course, tentative and requires further work, but it may be used to make predictions about other paradigms. The data and speculations

described in this section provide examples of how the use of a spatiotemporal analysis could help to dissect preparatory processes and executive function.

The data also help us to make a few methodological points. First, correlations across subjects between brain activity at various locations as well as with behavior may prove very useful for increasing our understanding of executive function and brain function in general. Note that these correlations should not be interpreted as indicative of causal relations. Rather, they imply that individual differences in brain function at a particular location and latency are associated with individual differences in brain activity at other locations or latencies as well as behavior. A way to describe these types of relationships is that they may indicate that processing modes, or strategies varying across individuals, are associated with both particular patterns of brain activity and particular patterns of behavior. For instance, subjects who show a large difference between switch and no-switch trials in right parietal regions may also show greater accuracy in general. In other words, a particular pattern of brain activity is typical of subjects who exhibit a particular pattern of behavior.

Second, the data indicate that fast optical imaging can be used to study these types of individual differences in processing strategies. These types of correlations are commonly used in other brain imaging studies. However, until recently, this approach had not been successfully applied to fast optical imaging data. The relatively low SNR afforded by this technique has led some people to suggest that the fast optical signal could only be used as an aggregate across subjects. However, the data reported here indicate that this is not the case. The fact that individual differences in fast optical measures lead to consistent and interpretable effects suggests that these measures can be powerful tools in the study of brain-behavior relationships.

SUMMARY AND DISCUSSION

We have briefly reviewed EROS as a technology that could be useful in the study of executive function. An advantage of EROS with respect to the most currently used brain imaging technologies (ERPs and fMRI) is the combination of sub-centimeter spatial resolution with millisecond-level temporal resolution. Currently, its major limitations are its limited penetration (approximately 3 cm from the surface of the head) and relatively low signal-to-noise ratio.

Why is the combination of spatial and temporal information important in studying executive function? We have argued here that executive function implies the coordinated and presumably sequential activation and inhibition of different cortical regions. We have presented some examples of data that we have recently obtained in different paradigms (in particular, from various versions of the task-switching pre-cueing paradigm), indicating that executive function does, in fact, imply the occurrence of an ordered sequence of regional activations and inhibitions. These findings are consistent with fMRI data demonstrating that several brain areas are activated during these types of tasks and with data from ERPs showing a sequence of different components that are also

regularly observed in these tasks. Specifically, we found two types of prepa-ratory processes: (1) a set of general activities that occur in regular fashion in different versions of the pre-cueing paradigm, and (2) another set of more specific activities that depend on the particular nature of the preparatory pro-cesses involved. The first set includes the commonly observed FPN, whereas the second includes cortical areas that are likely to be involved in subsequent processing of the imperative stimulus.

We also reviewed data indicating how a technique combining spatial and temporal resolution, such as EROS, can provide useful data about the func-tional connectivity between different areas. Importantly, the temporal reso-lution of EROS allows us also to study the order of events in the brain (e.g., the ordering of activity in domain-general and domain-specific regions). This type of information can be useful for generating causal hypotheses about the relationship between the activities observed in different areas, and can provide support for different theories about executive function operation mode. For instance, our data support the coexistence of a hierarchical and a distributed mode of operation. Further, some of our data suggest a relationship between individual differences in functional connectivity and those existing in anatom-ical connectivity (e.g., in the size of the anterior portion of the CC). Although the type of analysis presented here was most appropriate for interhemispheric connectivity, we are currently investigating its extension to intrahemispheric connectivity. This may involve the use of diffusion tensor imaging, a relatively recent magnetic resonance imaging technology that permits visualization of white matter tracts (Rykhlevskaia et al., 2006b).

Of course, as with any other brain imaging method, EROS alone is in-sufficient to provide a complete picture of the brain processes underlying executive function. (1) EROS does not provide information about structures deep in the brain. (2) Causality in the links between different cortical areas, and even between cortical activity and behavior, can be hypothesized, but not proven by EROS data alone. Other data, such as information from neuropsy-chological, pharmacological, or transcranial magnetic stimulation studies, may provide this type of information. (3) Anatomical information, which can be very useful in the study of executive function, is not readily available through EROS, and as such, EROS is best combined with anatomical MRI data. In summary, EROS can effectively complement other brain imaging tech-nologies in the study of executive function.

ACKNOWLEDGMENTS The work presented in this paper was supported by NIMH grant MH080182 to G. Gratton, by NIA grant AG21887 to M. Fabiani, and by funds provided by DARPA to G. Gratton and M. Fabiani.

NOTES

1. "Birefringence" is a property of material to change the angle of polarization of polarized incident light; "scattering" refers to a randomization of the direction of movement of photons due to diffraction and reflection.

2. "Back-scattering" is the portion of scattered photons that are reflected back by tissue to a location at or near their source.

3. Anterior corpus callosum size was not correlated with overall brain volume, but tended to decrease with age.

REFERENCES

Agran J, Low KA, Leaver E, Fabiani M, Gratton G (2005) Switching between input modalities: an event-related optical signal (EROS) study (abstract). Journal of Cognitive Neuroscience (Supplement):89.

Andrew RD, MacVicar BA (1994) Imaging cell volume changes and neuronal excitation in the hippocampal slice. Neuroscience 62:371–383.

Baddeley AD, Hitch GJ (1974) Working memory. In: The psychology of learning and motivation (Bower GH, ed.), pp. 47–90, volume 8. New York: Academic Press.

Badre D, Wagner AD (2002) Semantic retrieval, mnemonic control, and prefrontal cortex. Behavioral and Cognitive Neuroscience Reviews 1:206–218.

Badre D, Wagner AD (2005) Frontal lobe mechanisms that resolve proactive interference. Cerebral Cortex 15:2003–2012.

Barinaga M (1997) New imaging methods provide a better view into the brain [news]. Science 276:1974–1976.

Brefczynski JA, DeYoe EA (1999) A physiological correlate of the 'spotlight' of visual attention. Nature Neuroscience 2:370–374.

Broadbent DE (1957) A mathematical model for human attention and immediate memory. Psychological Review 64:205–215.

Buchheim K, Schuchmann S, Siegmund H, Gabriel HJ, Heinemann U, Meierkord H (1999) Intrinsic optical signal measurements reveal characteristic features during different forms of spontaneous neuronal hyperactivity associated with ECS shrinkage in vitro. European Journal of Neuroscience 11:1877–1882.

Buckner RL, Petersen SE (1996) What does neuroimaging tell us about the role of prefrontal cortex in memory retrieval? Seminars in Neuroscience 8:47–55.

Cabeza R, Kapur S, Craik FIM, McIntosh AR, Houlse S, Tulving E (1997) Functional neuroanatomy of recall and recognition: a PET study of episodic memory. Journal of Cognitive Neuroscience 9:254–265.

Cohen LB (1973) Changes in neuron structure during action potential propagation and synaptic transmission. Physiological Reviews 53:373–418.

Cohen JD, Perlstein WM, Braver TS, Nystrom LE, Noll DC, Jonides J, Smith EE (1997) Temporal dynamics of brain activation during a working memory task. Nature 386:604–608.

Corbetta M, Akbudak E, Conturo T, Snyder A, Ollinher J, Drury H, Lineweber M, Petersen S, Raichle M, Van Essen D, Shulman G (1998) A common network for functional areas for attention and eye movements. Neuron 21:761–773.

Corbetta M, Miezin FM, Dobmeyer S, Shulman GL, Petersen SE (1991) Selective and divided attention during visual discriminations of shape color and speed: functional anatomy by positron emission tomography. Journal of Neuroscience 11:2383–2402.

Corbetta M, Shulman GL, Miezin FM, Petersen SE (1995) Superior parietal cortex activation during spatial attention shifts and visual feature conjunction. Science 270: 802–805.

Cowan N (1995) Attention and memory: an integrated framework. New York: Oxford University Press.

DeSoto MC, Fabiani M, Geary DC, Gratton G (2001) When in doubt do it both ways: brain evidence of the simultaneous activation of conflicting responses in a spatial Stroop task. Journal of Cognitive Neuroscience 13:523–536.

Donchin E (1981) Surprise! Surprise? Psychophysiology 18:493–513.

Engle RW (2002) Working memory capacity as executive attention. Current Directions in Psychological Science 11:19–23.

Fabiani, M. Brumback, C. R., Pearson, M.A., Gordon, B. A., Lee, Y., Barre, M., O'Dell, J., Maclin, E.L., Elavsky, S., Konopack, J.F., McAuley, E., Kramer, A.F., & Gratton, G. (2005). Neurovascular coupling in young and old adults assessed with neuronal (EROS) and hemodynamic (NIRS) optical imaging measures. Journal of Cognitive Neuroscience Supplement, 34.

Fabiani, M., Ho, J., Stinard, A., & Gratton, G. (2003). Multiple visual memory phenomena in a memory search task. Psychophysiology 40: 472–485.

Fabiani M, Low KA, Wee E, Sable JJ, Gratton G (2006) Reduced suppression or labile memory? Mechanisms of inefficient filtering of irrelevant information in older adults. Journal of Cognitive Neuroscience 18:637–650.

Fletcher PC, Frith CD, Rugg MD (1997) The functional neuroanatomy of episodic memory. Trends in Neurosciences 20:213–218.

Foust AJ, Rector DM (2007) Optically teasing apart neural swelling and depolarization. Neuroscience 145:887–899.

Franceschini MA, Boas DA (2004) Noninvasive measurement of neuronal activity with near-infrared optical imaging. Neuroimage 21:372–386.

Friston KJ, Frith CD, Frackowiak RSJ (1993a) Time-dependent changes in effective connectivity measured with PET. Human Brain Mapping 1:69–80.

Friston KJ, Frith CD, Liddle PF, Frackowiak RSJ (1993b) Functional connectivity: the principal component analysis of large (PET) data sets. Journal of Cerebral Blood Flow and Metabolism 13:5–14.

Frostig RD, Lieke EE, Ts'o DY, Grinvald A (1990) Cortical functional architecture and local coupling between neuronal activity and the microcirculation revealed by in vivo high-resolution optical imaging of intrinsic signals. Proceedings of the National Academy of Sciences U S A 87:6082–6086.

Gratton G (1997) Attention and probability effects in the human occipital cortex: An optical imaging study. Neuroreport 8:1749–1753.

Gratton G (1998) The contralateral organization of visual memory: a theoretical concept and a research tool. Psychophysiology 35:638–647.

Gratton G, Brumback CR, Gordon BA, Pearson MA, Low KA, Fabiani M (2006) Effects of measurement method, wavelength, and source-detector distance on the fast optical signal. Neuroimage 32:1576–1590.

Gratton G, Corballis PM, Cho E, Fabiani M, Hood D (1995a) Shades of gray matter: noninvasive optical images of human brain responses during visual stimulation. Psychophysiology 32:505–509.

Gratton G, Corballis PM, Jain S (1997a) Hemispheric organization of visual memories. Journal of Cognitive Neuroscience 9:92–104.

Gratton G, Fabiani M (2003) The event-related optical signal (EROS) in visual cortex: replicability, consistency, localization, and resolution. Psychophysiology 40:561–571.

Gratton G, Fabiani M (2001) Shedding light on brain function: the event-related optical signal. Trends in Cognitive Science 5:357–363.

Gratton G, Fabiani M (2005) Comparison of optical (NIRS and EROS) and fMRI measures in young adults and old adults varying in fitness levels (abstract). Journal of Cognitive Neuroscience (Supplement):34.

Gratton G, Fabiani M, Corballis PM, Hood DC, Goodman-Wood MR, Hirsch J, Kim K, Friedman D, Gratton E (1997b) Fast and localized event-related optical signals (EROS) in the human occipital cortex: comparisons with the visual evoked potential and fMRI. Neuroimage 6:168–180.

Gratton G, Fabiani M, Friedman D, Franceschini MA, Fantini S, Gratton E (1995b) Rapid changes of optical parameters in the human brain during a tapping task. Journal of Cognitive Neuroscience 7:446–456.

Gratton G, Fabiani M, Goodman-Wood MR, DeSoto MC (1998) Memory-driven processing in human medial occipital cortex: an event-related optical signal (EROS) study. Psychophysiology 35:348–351.

Gratton G, Goodman-Wood MR, Fabiani M (2001) Comparison of neuronal and hemodynamic measures of the brain response to visual stimulation: an optical imaging study. Human Brain Mapping 13:13–25.

Gratton G, Low KA, Maclin EL, Brumback CR, Gordon BA, Fabiani M (2006) Time course of activation of human occipital cortex measured with the event-related optical signal (EROS). In: Biomedical optics 2006 technical digest. Washington, DC: Optical Society of America: MD4.

Gratton E, Mantulin WW, van de Ven MJ, Fishkin JB, Maris MB, Chance B (1990) The possibility of a near-infrared optical imaging system using frequency-domain methods. Proceedings of III International Conference for Peace through Mind, Hamamatsu City, Japan, 1990. Brain Science, pp 183–189.

Gratton G, Rykhlevskaia E, Wee E, Leaver E, Fabiani M (submitted) White matter matters: corpus callosum size is related to inter-hemispheric functional connectivity and task-switching effects in aging.

Gratton G, Sarno AJ, Maclin E, Corballis P, Fabiani M (2000) Toward non-invasive 3-D imaging of the time course of cortical activity: investigation of the depth of the event-related optical signal (EROS). Neuroimage 11:491–504.

Hari R, Lounasmaa OV (1989) Recording and interpretation of cerebral magnetic fields. Science 244:432–436.

Herd SA, Banich MT, O'Reilly RC (2006) Neural mechanisms of cognitive control: an integrative model of Stroop task performance and fMRI data. Journal of Cognitive Neuroscience 18:22–32.

Hill DK, Keynes RD (1949) Opacity changes in stimulated nerve. Journal of Physiology 108:278–281.

Hopfinger JB, Buonocore MH, Mangun GR (2000) The neural mechanisms of top-down attentional control. Nature Neuroscience 3:284–291.

Ishimaru A (1978) Diffusion of a pulse in densely distributed scatterers. Journal of the Optical Society of America 68:1045–1050.

Jaaskelainen IP, Ahveninen J, Bonmassar G, Dale AM, Ilmoniemi RJ, Levanen S, Lin FH, May P, Melcher J, Stufflebeam S, Tiitinen H, Belliveau JW (2004) Human posterior auditory cortex gates novel sounds to consciousness. Proceedings of the National Academy of Sciences U S A101:6809–6814.

Jobsis FF (1977) Noninvasive infrared monitoring of cerebral and myocardial oxygen sufficiency and circulatory parameters. Science 198:1264–1267.

Johnston WA, Dark VJ (1986) Selective attention. Annual Review of Psychology 37:43–75.

Jonides J, Smith EE, Marshuetz C, Koeppe R, Reuter-Lorenz P (1998) Inhibition on verbal working memory revealed by brain activation. Proceedings of the National Academy of Sciences U S A 95:8410–8413.

Kastner S, Pinsk MA, De Weerd P, Desimone R, Ungerleider LG (1999) Increased activity in human visual cortex during directed attention in the absence of visual stimulation. Neuron 22:751–761.

Katayama J, Polich J (1998) Stimulus context determines P3a and P3b. Psychophysiology 35:23–33.

Kirino E, Belger A, Goldman-Rakic P, McCarthy G (2000) Prefrontal activation evoked by infrequent target and novel stimuli in a visual target detection task: an event-related functional magnetic resonance imaging study. Journal of Neuroscience 20: 6612–6618.

Leaver E, Rykhlevskaia EI, Wee E, Gratton G, Fabiani M (submitted) Corpus callosum size is related to age-related decline in working memory.

Lebid S, O'Neill RO, Markham C, Ward T, Coyle S (2004) Functional brain signals: a photon counting system for brain activity monitoring. IEE Conference Proceedings of the Irish Signals and Systems Conference (ISSC), Queen's University, Belfast, NI 469–474.

Lebid S, O'Neill RO, Markham C, Ward T, Coyle S (2005) Multi-timescale measurements of brain responses in visual cortex during stimulation using time-resolved spectroscopy. Proceedings—SPIE The International Society for Optical Engineering 5826:606–617.

Low KA, Leaver E, Agran J, Rowley T, Fabiani M, Gratton G (2006) When the rules change: the event-related optical signal (EROS) shows the timing of task-general and task-specific brain regions involved in preparation. (Abstract) Journal of Cognitive Neuroscience (Supplement): 200.

Low KA, Leaver E, Kramer AF, Fabiani M Gratton G (2006) Fast optical imaging of frontal cortex during active and passive oddball tasks. Psychophysiology 43:127–136.

Maclin E, Gratton G, Fabiani M (2003) Optimum filtering for EROS measurements. Psychophysiology 40:542–547.

Maclin EL, Low KA, Fabiani M, Gratton G (in press) Improving the signal-to-noise ratio of event related optical signals (EROS) by manipulating wavelength and modulation frequency. Special issue of IEEE EMBM.

Maclin EL, Low KA, Sable JJ, Fabiani M, Gratton G (2004) The event related optical signal (EROS) to electrical stimulation of the median nerve. Neuroimage 21:1798–1804.

MacVicar BA, Hochman D (1991) Imaging of synaptically evoked intrinsic optical signals in hippocampal slices. Journal of Neuroscience 11:1458–1469.

Martinez A, Anllo-Vento L, Sereno MI, Frank LR, Buxton RB, Dubowitz DJ, Wong EC, Hinrichs H, Heinze HJ, Hillyard SA (1999) Involvement of striate and extrastriate visual cortical areas in spatial attention. Nature Neuroscience 2:364–369.

Martinez A, DiRusso F, Anllo-Vento L, Sereno MI, Buxton RB, Hillyard SA (2001) Putting spatial attention on the map: timing and localization of stimulus selection processes in striate and extrastriate visual areas. Vision Research 41:1437–1457.

Miller EK, Cohen JD (2001) An integrative theory of prefrontal cortex function. Annual Review of Neuroscience 24:167–202.

Momose-Sato Y, Sato K, Hirota A, Kamino K (1998) GABA-induced intrinsic light-scattering changes associated with voltage-sensitive dye signals in embryonic brain stem slices: coupling of depolarization and cell shrinkage. Journal of Neurophysiology 79:2208–2217.

Näätänen R (2000) Mismatch negativity (MMN): perspectives for application. International Journal of Psychophysiology 37:3–10.

Näätänen R, Picton T (1987) The N1 wave of the human electric and magnetic response to sound: a review and an analysis of the component structure. Psychophysiology 24:375–425.

Nolde SF, Johnson MK, Raye CL (1998) The role of prefrontal cortex during tests of episodic memory. Trends in Cognitive Science 2:399–406.

Opitz B, Rinne T, Mecklinger A, von Cramon DY, Schroger E (2002) Differential contribution of frontal and temporal cortices to auditory change detection: fMRI and ERP results. Neuroimage 15:167–174.

Rector (2006) In: Biomedical optics 2006 technical digest. Washington, DC: Optical Society of America.

Rector DM, Carter KM, Volegov PL, George JS (2005) Spatio-temporal mapping of rat whisker barrels with fast scattered light signals. Neuroimage 26:619–627.

Rector DM, Poe GR, Kristensen MP, Harper RM (1997) Light scattering changes follow evoked potentials from hippocampal Schaeffer collateral stimulation. Journal of Neurophysiology 78:1707–1713.

Rinne T, Gratton G, Fabiani M, Cowan N, Maclin E, Stinard A, Sinkkonen J, Alho K, Näätänen R (1999) Scalp-recorded optical signals make sound processing from the auditory cortex visible. Neuroimage 10:620–624.

Ritter W, Deacon D, Gomes H, Javitt DC, Vaughan HG Jr (1995) The mismatch negativity of event-related potentials as a probe of transient auditory memory: a review. Ear and Hearing 16:52–67.

Rykhlevskaia E, Fabiani M, Gratton G (2006a) Lagged covariance structure models for studying functional connectivity in the brain. Neuroimage 30:1203–1218.

Rykhlevskaia EI, Gordon B, Brumback C, Gratton G, Fabiani M (2006b) A method for incorporating diffusion tensor imaging into models of effective connectivity. (Abstract) Journal of Cognitive Neuroscience (Supplement): 22

Sable JJ, Low KA, Whalen CJ, Maclin EL, Fabiani M, Gratton G (2006) Optical Imaging of Perceptual Grouping in Human Auditory Cortex. European Journal of Neuroscience 25: 298–306.

Steinbrink J, Kempf FCD, Villringer A, Obrig H (2005) The fast optical signal: robust or elusive when non-invasively measured in the human adult? Neuroimage 26:996–1008.

Steinbrink J, Kohl M, Obrig H, Curio G, Syré F, Thomas F, Wabnitz H, Rinneberg H, Villringer A (2000) Somatosensory evoked fast optical intensity changes detected non-invasively in the adult human head. Neuroscience Letters 291:105–108.

Stepnoski RA, LaPorta A, Raccuia-Behling F, Blonder GE, Slusher RE, Kleinfeld D (1991) Noninvasive detection of changes in membrane potential in cultured neurons by light scattering. Proceedings of the National Academy of Sciences U S A 88:9382–9386.

Syré F, Obrig H, Steinbrink J, Kohl M, Wenzel R, Villringer A (2003) Are VEP correlated fast optical signals detectable in the human adult by non-invasive nearinfrared spectroscopy (NIRS)? Advances in Experimental Medicine and Biology 530: 421–431.

Tanner K, Beitel E, D'Amico E, Mantulin WW, Gratton E (2006) Effects of vasodilation on intrinsic optical signals in the mammalian brain: a phantom study. Journal of Biomedical Optics 11: 064020 (10 pages).

Tse C-Y, Penney TB (in press) Optical imaging of cortical activity elicited by unat-
    tended temporal deviants. Special issue of IEEE EMB Magazine on Optical imaging.
Tse C-Y, Tien K-R, Penney TB (2006) Event-related optical imaging reveals the tem-
    poral dynamics of right temporal and frontal cortex activation in pre-attentive
    change detection. Neuroimage 29:314–320.
Villringer A, Chance B (1997) Non-invasive optical spectroscopy and imaging of
    human brain function. Trends in Neuroscience 20:435–442.
Wolf M, Wolf U, Choi JH, Gupta R, Safonova LP, Paunescu LA, Michalos A, Gratton E
    (2002) Functional frequency-domain near-infrared spectroscopy detects fast neu-
    ronal signals in the motor cortex. Neuroimage 17:1868–1875.
Wolf M, Wolf U, Choi JH, Gupta R, Safonova LP, Paunescu LA, Michalos A, Gratton E
    (2003a) Detection of the fast neuronal signal on the motor cortex using functional
    frequency domain near infrared spectroscopy. Advances in Experimental Medicine
    and Biology 510:193–197.
Wolf M, Wolf U, Choi JH, Toronov V, Paunescu LA, Michalos A, Gratton E (2003b)
    Fast cerebral functional signal in the 100 ms range detected in the visual cortex by
    frequency-domain near-infrared spectrophotometry. Psychophysiology 40:521–
    528.
Wolf U, Wolf M, Toronov V, Michalos A, Paunescu LA, Gratton E (2000) Detecting
    cerebral functional slow and fast signals by frequency-domain near-infrared spec-
    troscopy using two different sensors. Paper presented at OSA Meeting in Optical
    Spectroscopy and Imaging and Photon Migration, Miami, April 2–5, 2000).

III

TASK-SWITCHING

11

Task-Switching in Human and Nonhuman Primates: Understanding Rule Encoding and Control from Behavior to Single Neurons

Gijsbert Stoet and Lawrence Snyder

Task-switching paradigms are a favorite choice for studying how humans represent and apply rules. These paradigms consist of trials of two different task contexts, each with its own rules, between which subjects frequently switch. Measuring the difficulty subjects have when switching between tasks taps into a fundamental property of executive control, that is, the capacity to respond to stimuli according to task context.

Although any biological organism can have a fixed response to sensory inputs, it is nontrivial to process identical inputs in different ways, depending on the task context. Task-switching paradigms are designed to study how subjects respond in the face of changing task contexts. In the last decade, more than 400 studies using this paradigm have been published (for an overview, see Monsell, 2003). Most of these studies are about human task-switching. However, unfortunately, there are limits to what we can learn from humans. We can look at behavior, and at regional brain metabolism, but it is very difficult to study the individual neuronal level using invasive techniques. In this chapter, we use rhesus monkeys as a model system to look at executive control at the neuronal level. A large number of studies have done something similar in the frontal lobes (e.g., see Chapters 9, 10, 11, and 13). We concentrate on the parietal lobe, and show that parietal neurons play a critical role in executive control. The idea that the parietal lobe might play a role in executive control is surprising, but not altogether unanticipated. After all, the posterior parietal cortex (PPC) is an association area, and thus a likely candidate for integrating different cortical processes. A number of brain imaging studies have focused on executive functions in the parietal cortex (e.g., Sohn et al., 2000; Rushworth et al., 2001; Gurd et al., 2002; Sylvester et al., 2003), and several recent studies in monkeys demonstrated the integration between top-down and bottom-up information (e.g., Chafee and Goldman-Rakic, 2000). We hypothesize that the complex set of general functions necessary for controlling mental functions is

distributed over a large area of the brain, rather than being limited to just one region or lobe of the brain.

Before we address any of the questions regarding neural activity, we will first ask whether monkeys and humans behave similarly in their deployment of executive processes. This is an interesting question because executive control in a human appears to be quite sophisticated. A rhesus monkey might not have available the full range of human executive functions and therefore might perform quite differently from a human in a task-switching paradigm. Therefore, we will first ask whether it is the case that humans have evolved to be particularly good at processing information in different ways and in rapidly switching their processing in response to changes in the task context. We will show that this is not the case; what humans are good at, compared with monkeys, is not switching between two tasks, but rather, locking on to a single task.

THE TASK-SWITCHING PARADIGM

In a task-switching paradigm, subjects perform interleaved trials of two or more different tasks in rapid succession. There are different types of task-switching paradigms. In uncued task-switching paradigms, subjects know through an instruction when to perform what task. For example, in the alternating-runs paradigm of Rogers and Monsell (1995), subjects know that they have to switch tasks every two trials. A disadvantage of this paradigm is that it is impossible to determine when subjects start to prepare for an upcoming task switch. This problem is solved in cued task-switching paradigms, in which each trial begins with the presentation of a task instruction cue. This cue indicates the rule that must be applied to the subsequent imperative stimulus. For example, in a switch paradigm in which the imperative stimulus is a number, one cue might instruct the subject to determine whether the number is even, whereas another cue might instruct the subject to determine whether the number is greater than 5. With randomly interleaved tasks in a cued task-switching paradigm, subjects cannot reliably prepare the upcoming task until the task cue has been presented. If the purpose of an experiment is to measure neural correlates of task preparation or rule application, it is an advantage to be able to determine exactly when the preparation process starts.

Finally, a very different type of task-switching paradigm is the Wisconsin Card Sorting Task (WCST), in which subjects sort cards according to a rule that is based on either the color or the symbols on the cards. After a fixed number of consecutive successful trials, the experimenter changes the sorting rule. This change results in sorting errors, and the subject must use error feedback to learn the new rule. One measure of executive control in this test is the number of trials required for a subject to learn a new rule. Perseveration on the old rule is taken as an indication of executive impairment, and is seen in various frontal brain syndromes (Sullivan et al., 1993). Although the WCST has been used for decades to diagnose cognitive impairment, computerized variations have been used in studying executive control and rule representation in animals

(Dias et al., 1996; Mansouri and Tanaka, 2002; Rushworth et al., 2002; Everling and DeSouza, 2005). The WCST has a similar problem to the alternating-runs paradigm. Because rule switches are unannounced and have to be discovered by the subjects themselves, the time at which the subject switches from preparing one task to preparing another task is ambiguous. Thus, although the WCST is useful for studying how long it takes subjects to discover a change in the task, the processes that underlie switching to apply a new set of task rules are more difficult to pin down.

Task-switching paradigms provide two independent measures of task-switching performance: switch costs and incongruity costs. The subject's ability to switch from one task to another is quantified by subtracting the performance (e.g., response time) in task-repetition trials from the performance in task-switching trials. The subject's ability to ignore distracting, irrelevant information is assessed by subtracting the performance in trials using a stimulus that instructs the same response on each task (an example of a congruent stimulus in the aforementioned example task is the digit "7," which is both odd and greater than 5) from performance in trials using a stimulus that instructs different responses (an incongruent stimulus) [e.g., the digit "3," which is odd, but not greater than 5]. To compare monkey and human behavior in task-switching, we needed to develop a version of the task that could be performed by both species. Instead of using letters and numbers, as is common in human task-switching experiments, we used shapes or colors, rather than verbal instructions, to cue the two different tasks, and we made the tasks themselves concrete (based on simple, observable properties of the stimuli).

Two monkeys (*Macaca mulatta*) [M1 and M2] and seven human volunteers (H1–H7) were compared using the same experimental setup. At the beginning of each trial, subjects were informed by a yellow or blue screen, or by an upright or inverted triangle, which of two tasks was to be performed. After a short preparatory delay, an imperative stimulus appeared. For half of the subjects, this stimulus was a square; for the other half of the subjects, this stimulus was a line. In task A, the subjects had to judge whether the color of the imperative stimulus (the square or the line) was closer to red or to green. In task B, subjects M1 and H1–H4 had to judge whether the inside of the square was more or less bright than the outer border of the square, and subjects M2 and H5–H7 had to judge whether the line orientation was horizontal or vertical (Fig. 11–1; see color insert). Subjects pressed a left or right response button to indicate their judgment.

Stimuli were presented on a touch-sensitive video screen located just in front of the subject. Subjects began each trial by holding a home key, and then responded to the imperative stimulus by moving to touch one of two white squares positioned at the left and right bottom portions of the screen. Target color was randomly chosen from a large number of different shades of red and green (e.g., pink, orange, cyan). For square stimuli (the first half of the subjects), the luminances of the border and inside regions were similarly chosen from a wide range of possible values. The different combinations of color and luminance contrasts yielded 104 different target stimuli. For lines (the second

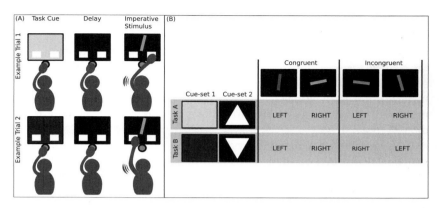

Figure 11–1 Experimental paradigm and stimulus response associations. *A.* Two example trials. The monkey (or human) sits behind a touch-sensitive screen and the hand is positioned in resting position on the orange home key. Each trial started with a 250-ms task cue indicating which of two task rules to apply to the subsequent stimulus. The task was cued by either a color (*blue* or *yellow*) or a shape (*upright* or *inverted triangle*). After a 190- to 485-ms delay period, the imperative stimulus, a *colored, oriented bar,* appeared. Depending on the task rule, either the color or the orientation of the stimulus was relevant. In the color discrimination task (example trial 1), or task A, *red* stimuli required a left button press and *green* stimuli required a right button press. In the orientation discrimination task (example trial 2), or task B, *vertical bars* required a left button press and *horizontal bars* required a right button press. Liquid rewards followed correct responses for monkeys. *B.* Stimulus-response combinations. One of two possible cues was used to indicate task A or task B. A single set of imperative stimuli was used in both tasks. Congruent stimuli were mapped to the same response button in both tasks, whereas incongruent stimuli were mapped to opposite buttons.

half of the subjects), orientation was graded, but limited to within 10 degrees of horizontal or vertical. The large range of color and luminance, or color and orientation, was chosen to encourage the use of general rules rather than a memory-based strategy for solving the tasks. A memory-based strategy might, for example, involve memorizing every possible cue-response pair, along with its correct response. In this undesirable scenario, animals might perform the task using associative recall, rather than performing one of two different discrimination tasks. The use of two different stimulus shapes (lines or squares), two different sets of task cues (triangles or screen color), and two different second tasks (orientation or luminance gradient) were all intended to help to establish the generality of our results.

Animals were first trained on a single task. Once proficient, they were trained on a second task. When they learned the second task, they were switched back to the first task, which had to be relearned. This process of switching continued, with switches occurring ever more frequently, until the two tasks were completely and randomly interleaved.

Each trial started when the subject put its dominant hand on the home key (Fig. 11–1A). The response buttons appeared immediately and remained on until the end of the trial. Next, the task cue appeared (250 ms), followed by a blank screen (500–600 ms). Then the imperative stimulus appeared and remained on-screen until the subject released the home key. The subject then had 2000 ms to move to within approximately 6 cm of the left or right response button. The behavioral reaction time (RT) was measured as the interval between onset of the imperative stimulus and release of the home key. Monkeys were rewarded for correct responses with a drop of water; humans were not rewarded. Incorrect trials for both species were followed by a visual error signal and a 1-s time-out period.

We recorded eye movements in monkeys using the scleral search coil technique. The data show that monkeys typically kept their eyes at the center of the screen and made a saccade to the response button shortly before moving their arm.

For the monkeys and for three of the seven humans, the task cue was present for only the first 200 ms of the task preparation interval. This was intended to encourage the subjects to actively process the task cue before receiving the imperative stimulus. An analysis of the data obtained with variable preparatory intervals demonstrated that this was, in fact, the case (Stoet and Snyder, 2003). For the first four humans tested, the task cue remained on-screen throughout the task preparation interval, making the task slightly easier. In these first four human subjects, the intertrial interval (ITI) was shorter than that used with the monkeys and with the final three humans (250 ms versus 345 ms). The shorter ITI compensated for the quicker responses to target stimuli in the monkey subjects. See Meiran (1996) for a discussion of the effects of ITIs on human switch costs. The second set of humans served as a control for the differences in timing between the animals and the first set of humans. The results were identical, and we mainly report data from the first set of humans (H1–H4).

COMPARISON OF MONKEY AND HUMAN TASK-SWITCHING

We first compared the behavioral performance of monkeys and humans during task-switching. To use monkey task-switching as a model system to study human cognition processing, it is not necessary that monkeys perform identically to humans. However, it is crucial to have a good understanding of any differences that might exist.

We assessed switch costs after monkeys and humans were trained to comparable success rates. We analyzed RTs using analysis of variance with the factors "switch" and "congruency." For this data analysis, we excluded all error trials and trials that immediately followed an error trial. We analyzed the percentage of errors (PE) with chi-square tests. When computed across all trials, performance was similar for the two species (Fig. 11–2A). Monkeys were generally faster than humans (mean RT = 325 ms versus 440 ms), although RT in the two

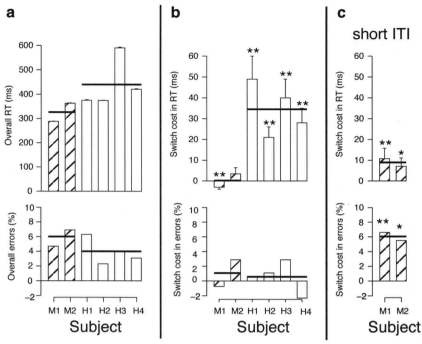

Figure 11–2 Humans show switch costs, but monkeys do not. *A.* Overall performance by monkeys (M1 and M2) [*cross-hatched bars*] and human subjects (H1–H4) [*open bars*]. Monkeys showed a faster reaction time (RT) [*top*], but had similar accuracy, as measured by percentage of errors (PE) [*bottom*]. *Horizontal lines* show species means. *Error bars* show standard error of the mean for RT. *B.* Switch costs in RT (mean RT on switch trials minus mean RT in repetition trials, ± standard error of the mean) and PE (PE on switch trials minus PE in repetition trials) in monkeys and humans. Only humans showed significant switch costs in RT (assessed using analysis of variance, **$p < 0.01$, *$p < 0.05$). Neither humans nor monkeys showed significant costs in PE. This indicates that monkeys, unlike humans, are able to switch their cognitive focus to a new task without cost. Human data are taken from the final day of testing. *C.* Switch costs appeared in monkeys when short intertrial intervals (ITI) were used (170 ms).

fastest humans was comparable to that of the slower monkey. On average, humans were slightly more accurate than monkeys (mean PE = 3.9% versus 5.8%).

Despite their similarity in overall RT and error rate, humans and monkeys show a striking difference in their ability to switch from one task to another. Human RTs were significantly slowed in the trial immediately after a task switch (Fig. 11–2*B*). Switch costs in response times were large and highly significant for each of the four human subjects ($p < 0.01$). Costs ranged from 21 to 49 ms and had a mean value of 35 ms. Results were similar in the second set of subjects (costs ranged from 20 to 49 ms, with a mean switch cost of 31 ms in RT). In contrast, neither monkey showed a significant switch cost, in either RT

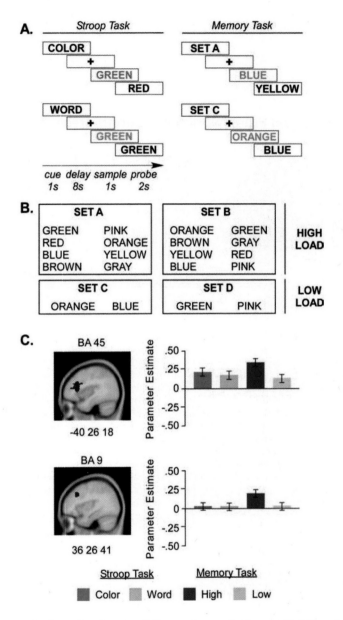

Figure 3–7. Retrieving and maintaining different rule types for future action (Donohue et al., under review). A . In the second rules study, participants memorized various set sizes of color pairings. B. On a given trial, a cue would indicate the type of rule to be followed. The delay was followed by a sample and a probe, and participants responded to the sample-probe pairing based on the instructional cue. C. During the Delay period, left ventrolateral prefrontal cortex (BA 45) was significantly activated for every condition. D. Right dorsolateral prefrontal cortex (BA 9), however, was specifically activated for the High-load condition.

Theoretical Framework for Action Representation

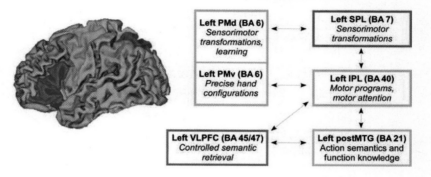

Figure 3–8. A theoretical framework for brain regions involved in action representation. Left ventrolateral prefrontal cortex (VLPFC) [BA 44/45/47] is involved in the controlled retrieval of semantics and rules (Wagner et al., 2001; Bunge et al., 2003). Left posterior middle temporal gyrus (postMTG) [BA 21] is involved in representing rules and action semantics (Bunge et al., 2003; Donohue et al., 2005; Souza and Bunge, under review). Ventral premotor cortex (PMv) [BA 6] is involved in precise hand grips required for object-related interactions (Kellenbach et al., 2003). Dorsal premotor cortex (PMd) [BA 6] is involved in sensorimotor learning and transformations (Petrides, 1997). Inferior parietal lobule (IPL) [BA 40] is involved in motor programs (Chao and Martin, 2000; Kellenbach et al., 2003) and motor attention (Rushworth et al., 2001, 2003). Superior parietal lobule (SPL) [BA 7] is involved in goal-directed sensorimotor transformations (Fogassi and Luppino, 2005). Left hemisphere fiducial rendering is from Caret 5.5 (Van Essen et al., 2001, 2002; http://brainmap.wustl.edu/caret). Regional demarcations are imprecise, and are meant for illustrative purposes only; the region encompassing the premotor cortex includes the primary motor cortex.

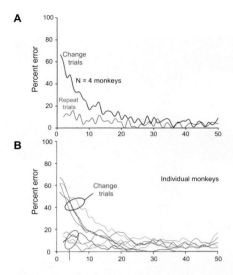

Figure 5–1. Conditional motor task. A. Performance rate for repeat (red) and change (blue) trials during the learning of the task. The curves show the grand means for four monkeys, each for data sets including 40 three-choice conditional motor problems. B. Individual scores for the same four monkeys, with each monkey color-matched for the repeat and change trials, bounded by the ovals in the early stages of learning.

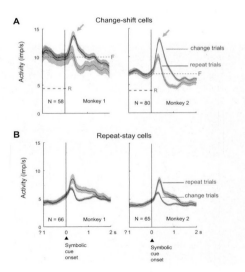

Figure 5–6. Population averages for neurons with selectivity for either the Change-shift strategy (A) or the Repeat-stay strategy (B), for two monkeys (left versus right column). The red curves show mean discharge rates for repeat trials; the blue curves show comparable data for change trials. The shading surrounding each curve shows activity rates ± 1 standard error of the mean. F, mean activity level for repeat trials during the fixation period; R, mean activity level during the fixation period for Repeat-stay cells.

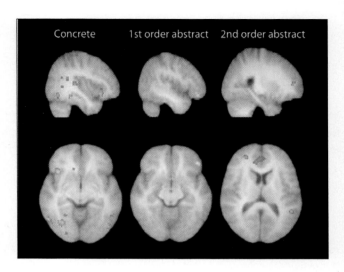

Figure 6–4. Group-averaged brain activations during rule reversal at different levels of abstraction. Ventrolateral (x, y, z = −44, 22, 0); orbitolateral (x, y, z = 48, 38, −12); and rostrolateral (x, y, z = −26, 48, 12). Prefrontal cortices showed significantly increased fMRI signal during the concrete, first-order abstract, and second-order abstract conditions, respectively (p < 0.001, uncorrected).

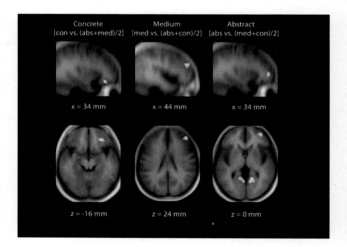

Figure 6–8. Group-average brain activations for anagram-solving at different levels of abstraction, each compared with the average activation for the other two conditions. Concrete blocks were associated with activation in ventrolateral prefrontal cortex (x, y, z = 32, 36, −16). Medium blocks were associated with activation in right dorsolateral prefrontal cortex (x, y, z = 46, 42, 24). Abstract blocks were associated with activation in right rostrolateral prefrontal cortex (x, y, z = 36, 48, 4) [p < 0.05 corrected]. Abs, abstract; med, medium; con, concrete.

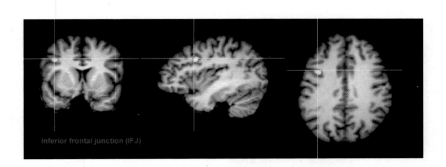

Figure 9–3. Activation in the inferior frontal junction for the updating of task representations (Brass and von Cramon, 2004a).

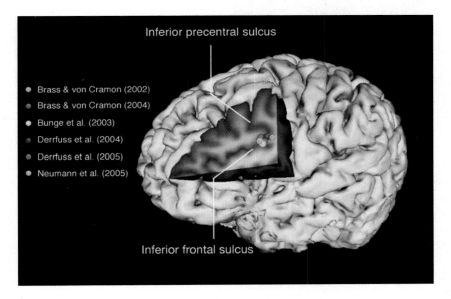

Figure 9–4. Peaks of activation from three experimental studies on task-switching and set-shifting (Brass and von Cramon, 2002, 2004a; Bunge et al., 2003): a within-subject comparison of three cognitive control paradigms (Derrfuss et al., 2004); a meta-analysis of the Stroop task (Neumann et al., 2005); and a meta-analysis of task-switching and set-shifting studies (Derrfuss et al., 2005).

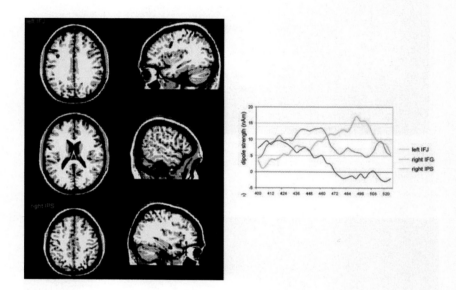

Figure 9–6. On the left side, the three dipoles are plotted on a representation of brain anatomy. On the right side, dipole strength is plotted for the left inferior frontal junction (IFJ), the right inferior frontal gyrus (IFG), and the right intraparietal sulcus (IPS).

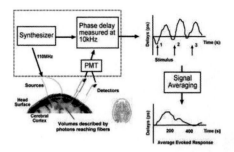

Figure 10–1. Schematic representation of the methods used to record event-related optical signal (EROS) data (frequency-domain [FD] method). Top left. The recording apparatus uses near-infrared light modulated at radiofrequencies (e.g., 110 MHz) to illuminate locations of the scalp (bottom left). The light propagates through the head in random fashion. Some of the light reaches detector fibers located a short distance (a few centimeters) from the sources. The average path followed by photons moving between sources and detectors can be described as a curved spindle volume (or a "banana") that reaches the cortex. This volume is the area relevant for the measurement from each source-detector pair. In a typical study, several source-detector pairs are used (up to 1024). Two types of measures can be taken at the detectors, intensity measures and delay measures. Intensity measures are variations in the amount of light reaching the detector as a function of activity. Delay measures are variations in the average time taken by photons to move between sources and detectors. The latter are used in the current chapter because they are more sensitive to events occurring inside the skull. Right. Schematic diagram of the averaging procedures used to derive the EROS. PMT= photo multiplier tube.(Reproduced with permission from Fabiani, Gratton & Corballis, Journal of Biomedical Optics, 1(4), 387–398. Copyright International Society for Optical Engineering, 1996.)

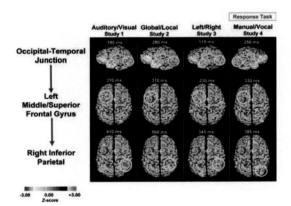

Figure 10–3. Statistical parametric maps (Z scores) of the event-related optical signal (EROS) response elicited by pre-cues during the pre-cueing paradigm computed across subjects. All maps represent activity related to cues signaling a switch in the rule to be used for processing the upcoming imperative stimuli, relative to no-switch cues. EROS allows investigators to compute maps at several multiple latencies from stimulations. Presented here are latencies that were most representative for each of the three regions of activation (lateral occipital, prefrontal, and parietal).

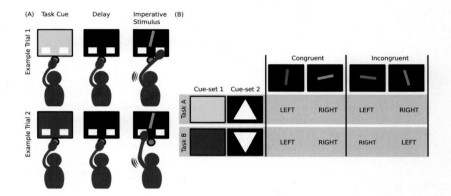

Figure 11–1. Experimental paradigm and stimulus response associations. A. Two example trials. The monkey (or human) sits behind a touch-sensitive screen and the hand is positioned in resting position on the orange home key. Each trial started with a 250-ms task cue indicating which of two task rules to apply to the subsequent stimulus. The task was cued by either a color (blue or yellow) or a shape (upright or inverted triangle). After a 190- to 485-ms delay period, the imperative stimulus, a colored, oriented bar, appeared. Depending on the task rule, either the color or the orientation of the stimulus was relevant. In the color discrimination task (example trial 1), or task A, red stimuli required a left button press and green stimuli required a right button press. In the orientation discrimination task (example trial 2), or task B, vertical bars required a left button press and horizontal bars required a right button press. Liquid rewards followed correct responses for monkeys. B. Stimulus-response combinations. One of two possible cues was used to indicate task A or task B. A single set of imperative stimuli was used in both tasks. Congruent stimuli were mapped to the same response button in both tasks, whereas incongruent stimuli were mapped to opposite buttons.

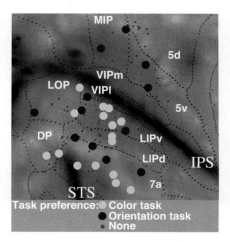

Figure 11–3. Map of flattened cortex showing the recording sites in monkey 2, derived from a magnetic resonance image that was processed using the software packages Caret and SureFit (Van Essen et al., 2001) [retrieved in 2004 from http://brainmap.wustl.edu/caret]. Broad black lines indicate fundi of sulci. The top of the panel is medial and anterior; the bottom of the panel is lateral and posterior. Yellow and blue dots indicate locations of cells that fire preferentially in connection with task A or task B rules, respectively. Small red dots indicate recording locations of the remaining cells. Areal boundaries, although drawn as sharp lines, reflect the maximum likelihood based on a probability map and are therefore only approximate (Lewis and Van Essen, 2000).

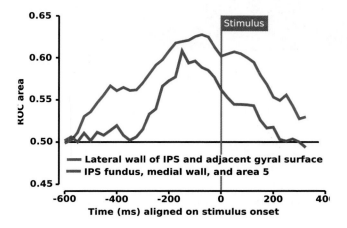

Figure 11–5. The time course of receiver operating characteristic (ROC) values for significant task cells shows that task-selective activity in the lateral intraparietal sulcus (IPS) and adjacent gyral surface (including areas LIPd, LIPv, 7a, LOP, and DP) [red trace] starts earlier, reaches a higher value, and is maintained for longer than task-selective activity in the IPS fundus, medial wall, and area 5 (green trace).

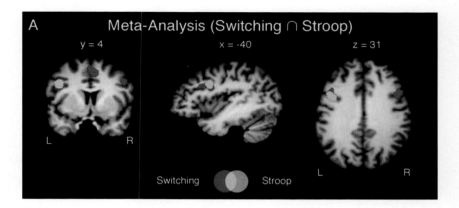

Figure 12–3. Meta-analysis conducted by Derrfuss et al. (2005), demonstrating the involvement of inferior frontal junction across different studies that commonly shared a strong demand for top-down task control.

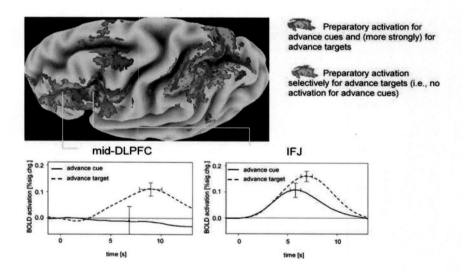

Figure 12–4. Two different patterns of preparatory brain activation associated with advance task cues, advance-target stimuli, or both. Remarkably, neither IFJ nor any other region was selectively (or even more strongly) activated for advance task cues. Conversely, a number of areas, such as mid-dorsolateral prefrontal cortex, were selectively activated by advance targets.

A

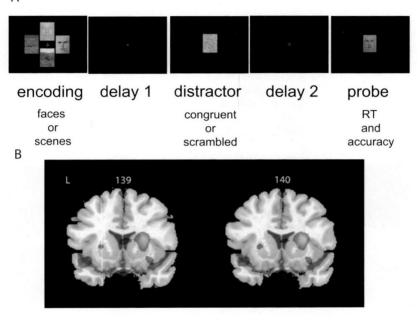

encoding   delay 1   distractor   delay 2   probe

faces   congruent   RT
or   or   and
scenes   scrambled   accuracy

B

Figure 14–4. A. Sequence of trial events in the paradigm used to assess which brain regions mediate the dopaminergic modulation of cognitive flexibility and cognitive stability. See text for a description of the task. B. Brain activity (contrast values) reflecting a significant interaction effect between impulsive personality (high versus low), drug (bromocriptine versus placebo), and trial-type (switch versus nonswitch). RT, response time.

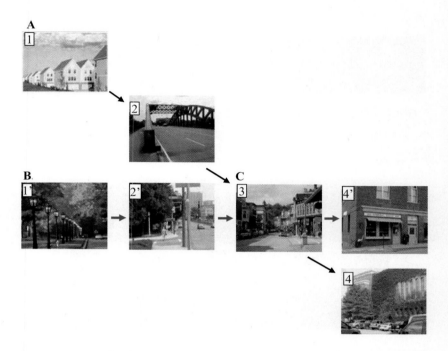

Figure 15–1. A sample relational network composed of two overlapping episodes (A and B), the first associated with a trip to work from home (A), and the second with a trip to the store from a friend's house (B). Each episode is construed as a sequence of elements that represent the conjunction of an event and the place where it occurred. C is an element that contains the same features in both episodes.

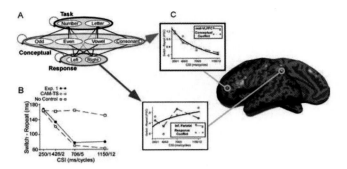

Figure 16–4. A. The model contains three reciprocally connected layers of units representing the task, conceptual, and response components of the explicit cueing task. B. Simulated switch costs and preparation costs track empirically derived behavioral responses very well. However, when control during the preparation period was turned off, there was no decline in switch costs with increased preparation. C. The switch versus repeat contrast revealed activation in left ventrolateral prefrontal cortex (VLPFC) [opercularis and triangularis], supplementary motor area (SMA), and parietal cortex. Responses across preparation intervals in mid-VLPFC matched the model's predicted conceptual conflict signal. This mid-VLPFC responses dissociated from the response in parietal cortex that appeared to match the predicted response conflict signal from the model. CSI, cue-to-stimulus interval; iPSC, integrated percent signal change. (Adapted from Badre and Wagner, Proceedings of the National Academy of Sciences, 103, 7186–7191. Copyright PNAS, 2006.)

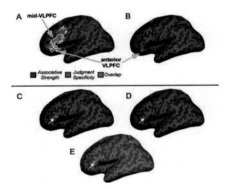

Figure 16–5. A. Overlap of judgment specificity (red) and associative strength (blue) manipulations on inflated canonical surface. Overlap in mid-ventrolateral prefrontal cortex (mid-VLPFC) to posterior VLPFC (purple). B. Contrast of weak–associative strength, two-target trials with strong–associative strength, four-target trials reveals activation in anterior VLPFC (Wagner et al., 2001; Badre et al., 2005). C–E. Inflated surface renderings demonstrate the high convergence in mid-VLPFC in response to selection demands across independent data sets, including "selection component" activation (Badre et al., 2005) [C], negative recent > negative nonrecent contrast (Badre and Wagner, 2005) [D], and switch minus repeat at the shortest cue-to-stimulus interval of 250 ms (Badre and Wagner, 2006) [E]. Note that the reference arrow is in the same position in each map.

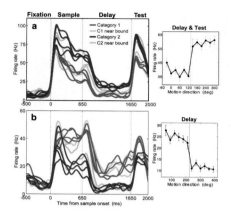

Figure 17–8. Examples of two category-selective lateral intraparietal (LIP) neurons. Average activity to the 12 sample directions for two LIP neurons is shown. The red and blue traces correspond to directions in the two categories (red [solid], category 1 or C1; blue [dashed], category 2 or C2), and pale traces indicate the directions closest to (15 degrees) the boundary. The three vertical dotted lines indicate (left to right) the timing of the sample onset, the sample offset, and the test stimulus onset. The neuron in A was recorded with the original category boundary. The neuron in B was recorded after the monkey had been retrained on the new categories. The plots at the right of each peristimulus time histogram show activity (mean ± standard error of the mean) for the 12 directions during the late delay and test epochs (A) and the delay epoch (B). C1, C2.

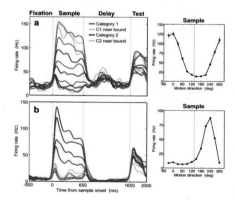

Figure 17–10. Examples of two direction-selective middle temporal (MT) neurons. A and B. Peristimulus time histograms show the average activity to the 12 sample stimulus directions for two single MT neurons. The red (solid) and blue (dashed) traces correspond to directions in the two categories. The pale red and blue traces indicate those directions that were close to (15 degrees) the category boundary. The three vertical dotted lines indicate (left to right) the timing of the sample onset, the sample offset, and the test stimulus onset. The plots at the right of each peri-stimulus time histogram (PSTH) show the average firing rate to the 12 directions during the sample epoch. Error bars indicate the standard error of the mean.

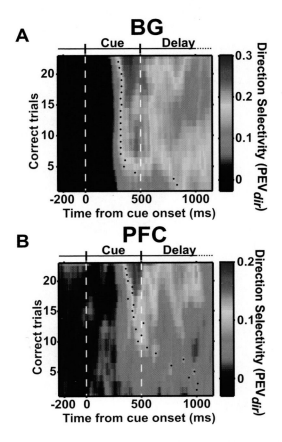

Figure 18–5. A and B. Selectivity for the direction of eye movement associated with the presented cue. Selectivity was measured as the percent of explained variance by direction (PEVdir), and is shown in the color gradient across time for both the basal ganglia (BG) [A], and prefrontal cortex (PFC) [B] . Black dots show the time of rise, as measured by the time to half-peak.

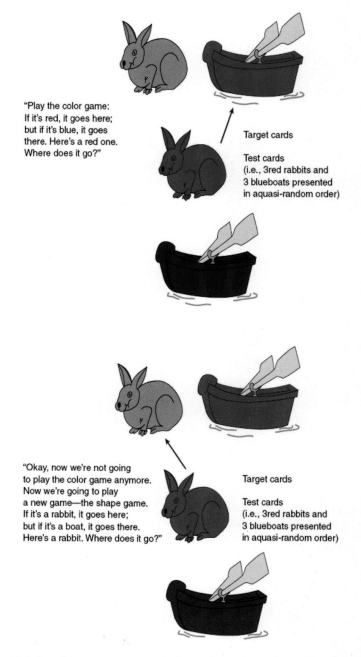

"Play the color game:
If it's red, it goes here;
but if it's blue, it goes
there. Here's a red one.
Where does it go?"

Target cards

Test cards
(i.e., 3red rabbits and
3 blueboats presented
in aquasi-random order)

"Okay, now we're not going
to play the color game anymore.
Now we're going to play
a new game—the shape game.
If it's a rabbit, it goes here;
but if it's a boat, it goes there.
Here's a rabbit. Where does it go?"

Target cards

Test cards
(i.e., 3red rabbits and
3 blueboats presented
in aquasi-random order)

Figure 19–1. Sample target and test cards in the standard version of the Dimensional Change Card Sort (DCCS). (Reprinted with permission from Zelazo, Nature Protocols, 1, 297–301. Nature Publishing Group, 2006).

(mean cost $= 0.2$ ms) or PE (mean cost $= 1\%$). Monkey 1 had a small, but significant ($p < 0.01$), negative switch cost in the original experiments, but we were unable to reproduce this effect on subsequent testing; therefore, we believe it to be a false-positive finding.

Switch costs may arise in at least two ways: (1) There may be task inertia, that is, a lingering representation of the previous task set that inhibits the installation of a new task set (Allport et al., 1994). (2) The installation of a new task set, that is, the reconfiguration of neural circuits to perform a new task, may remain incomplete until a stimulus for that task is actually received. Both mechanisms are believed to contribute to human switch costs (Allport et al., 1994; Meiran, 1996). Evidence for the role of task inertia is provided by the decrease in human switch costs with increasing preparation time, as if the effect of the previous task wears off over time (Meiran, 1996). However, even with long preparation or ITIs (e.g., 1.6 s), human switch costs are not completely abolished (Meiran, 1996). The persistence of residual switch costs, even after the representation of the previous task has had ample time to wear off, suggests that the installation of the new task remains incomplete until a new stimulus actually arrives (Rogers and Monsell, 1995; Meiran, 1996).

The absence of residual switch costs in monkeys suggests that, in monkeys, unlike in humans, neural circuits can be completely reconfigured to perform a new task before the arrival of the first stimulus. Thus, the second of the two mechanisms just described for generating switch costs in humans does not seem to operate in highly trained monkeys. To test whether the first mechanism for switch costs operates in monkeys, that is, whether lingering representations of previous tasks might conflict with the installation of a new task, we compared blocks of trials using short (170 ms) versus long (345 ms) ITIs. We found significant switch costs in both monkeys in the short ITI blocks (11 ms and 7 ms in RT; 6.6% and 5.5% in PE, all measures different from zero at $p < 0.05$) [Fig. 11–2C]. Thus, in the monkey, small switch costs may arise as a result of a conflict between a lingering representation of a previous task and the installation of a new task. In contrast to the case in humans, however, this lingering representation decays very quickly, so that, at an ITI of 345 ms, the effect is no longer present in the monkey.

Task-switching paradigms require not only the ability to switch from one task to another, but also the ability to focus on the task currently at hand. Part of focusing on the task at hand is the ability to attend only to those stimulus features that are relevant, and to ignore those that are irrelevant. Incongruency costs measure the extent to which a subject fails in this ability. As illustrated in Figure 11–2, both animals showed clear incongruency costs in RT (9 ms and 36 ms, both significant at $p < 0.01$) as well as in PE (5.7% and 9.9%, both significant at $p < 0.01$). In contrast, human subjects did not show a significant effect in either RT (mean value -4 ms) or PE (mean value 3%). Consistent results were found with a shortened ITI in monkeys: Incongruency costs in both RT (33 ms and 28 ms) and PE (9.2% and 11.8%) were both highly significant.

The higher incongruency costs in monkeys suggest one possible reason that monkeys, unlike humans, do not show switch costs: They are not as focused on the relevant features of the task in the first place. There are several other potential explanations for why the monkeys do not show persistent switch costs. For example, animals might use an approach that circumvents the need to change strategies between the two tasks. One way to do this would be to memorize every possible cue-target response triplet. We intentionally used a wide range of target stimuli to promote the use of a rule-based rather than memory-based strategy. However, it is nonetheless conceivable that monkeys memorized all 208 combinations and employ a memory-based strategy to solve the task. To distinguish between these two strategies, we used a probe task that introduced 11 novel stimuli to monkey M2, interspersed with the practiced target stimuli. The novel stimuli were created using various combinations of a previously unseen line orientation (20 or 45 degrees from either the horizontal or vertical axis), a new color (blue-gray), or a new line thickness (1.1 degree). Combinations of novel features were chosen such that the task-relevant stimulus dimension was unambiguous in the task context, even though some features of the novel stimuli were ambiguous (e.g., blue-gray color, 45-degree orientation). For example, a novel stimulus consisting of a 45-degree red line in the context of task A would instruct the animal to move left. Each novel stimulus was presented only once, after the animal was extremely well practiced on two tasks using the standard stimuli. If the monkey learned specific cue-target-response combinations rather than general rules, then it should have performed at chance levels on the novel stimuli. Instead, performance was correct for 10 of the 11 novel stimuli (90% success rate). This is significantly greater than chance (chi square $[1] = 7.4$, $p < 0.01$), indicating that the animal had learned to apply general rules and was not using a memory-based strategy to solve the task.

NEURAL ENCODING OF TASK RULES

The task-switching paradigm provides an opportunity to study the neural instantiation of rules, despite the fact that monkeys do not show persistent switch costs. Behavioral evidence demonstrates that monkeys prepare each task in advance, processing whichever rule has been cued in advance of seeing the imperative stimulus: Monkeys perform faster and more accurately in the task-switching paradigm when there are longer delays between the task cue and the imperative stimulus (Stoet and Snyder, 2003). By comparing neural activity during the preparation periods of two different tasks, we can therefore determine whether and how a particular neuronal population encodes task rules. The particular advantage of the task-switching paradigm for this purpose is that, by comparing activity during the preparation period for the two tasks before the appearance of the imperative stimulus, everything but the rule itself is completely controlled for. Thus, any differential activity that occurs during the preparatory period for the two tasks can be unambiguously assigned to

the processing of the rules themselves. In this section, we apply this method to investigate neurons in the monkey PPC.

We recorded data from 378 isolated neurons in and around the right intraparietal sulcus (IPS) of the right PPC of two animals. We tested for task-rule selectivity by comparing the final 150 or 250 ms of delay-period activity in trials starting with yellow versus blue task cues (Student's t-test). Twenty-nine percent of neurons ($n = 111$) showed a significant difference in activity, depending on which task was being prepared.

We projected each recording site location onto an anatomical magnetic resonance image of the cortex to determine which cortical areas the neurons belonged to (see Fig. 11–3; see color insert). Neurons that were selective for one particular task rule over the other (henceforth called task-positive, or TASK$^+$, cells) were located primarily on the lateral bank of the IPS and the adjacent gyral surface (including areas LIPd, LIPv, 7a, LOP, and DP). Taking into account that we sampled these areas more densely than more medial areas (i.e., IPS fundus, medial wall, and area 5), the frequency of task rule-selective neurons was still more than twice as high in the lateral areas (35%, $n = 95$ of 274) compared with the medial areas (15%, $n = 16$ of 104, chi-square test, $p < 0.001$).

Each of the two tasks was equally well represented in the population of recorded neurons, and there was no statistically significant clustering of neurons preferring a single task within a particular area (tested by comparing proportions of neurons of each rule type per area with chi-square tests). Visual inspection of Figure 11–3 suggests a clustering of neurons selective for task A (color task rule) in monkey 2 in areas 7a, DP, LIPd, and LIPv, but this did not reach statistical significance and was not replicated in monkey 1.

Different spike rates in the two task rule conditions could reflect a difference in preparation for the upcoming task, but could also reflect a difference in the sensory features of the two cues. For example, a given neuron might be sensitive to cue color (i.e., yellow versus blue) rather than to the task rule indicated by the color of the cue. Further, differences in spike rates could combine effects of task rule and cue features. To separate these two effects, we performed an additional experiment to determine whether task rule selectivity was independent of the sensory features of the cue.

We tested an entirely new set of 192 neurons in the same two monkeys using either a color cue (yellow or blue) or a shape cue (upright or inverted triangles) to instruct the task rule (Fig. 11–1B). Figure 11–4 shows two examples of TASK$^+$ neurons in area 7a tested with this design. Four hundred milliseconds after cue onset, firing became markedly larger for task B trials compared with task A trials. This was true whether the task rule was conveyed by a color cue or by a shape cue. Differences in rule-selective activity developed slowly, but were maintained throughout the remainder of the delay period. In one of the two neurons (Fig. 11–4, bottom), this difference persisted for more than 300 ms after the imperative stimulus appeared.

We analyzed whether neural responses during the delay period were different in the two task rule conditions. We applied a 2×2 analysis of variance

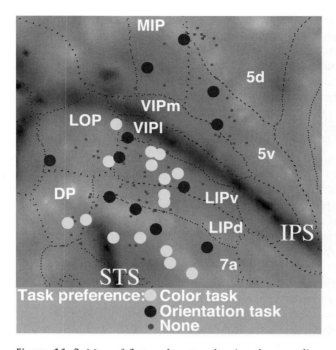

Figure 11–3 Map of flattened cortex showing the recording sites in monkey 2, derived from a magnetic resonance image that was processed using the software packages Caret and SureFit (Van Essen et al., 2001) [retrieved in 2004 from http://brainmap.wustl.edu/caret]. *Broad black lines* indicate fundi of sulci. The *top* of the panel is medial and anterior; the *bottom* of the panel is lateral and posterior. *Yellow* and *blue dots* indicate locations of cells that fire preferentially in connection with task A or task B rules, respectively. *Small red dots* indicate recording locations of the remaining cells. Areal boundaries, although drawn as sharp lines, reflect the maximum likelihood based on a probability map and are therefore only approximate (Lewis and Van Essen, 2000).

(ANOVA) with the factors "task rule" (task A or task B) and "task instruction cue set" (colors or shapes) to each neuron's responses during the late delay period. The results indicated that 32% of neurons (42 of 132) in the lateral wall of the IPS and the adjacent gyral surface had a main effect of task rule, which provides an independent replication of the findings based on one cue set (35% TASK$^+$ cells). Of these, two-thirds ($n = 29$) showed a main effect of task rule without an interaction with task instruction cue set (colors versus shapes). This indicates that most TASK$^+$ neurons reflect the task rule,

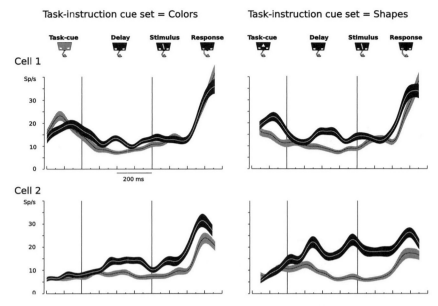

Figure 11–4 Examples of two task rule–selective cells in area 7a. *Thick black* and *gray traces* represent neuronal responses (mean ± 1 standard error of the mean) to color cues (*left*) and shape cues (*right*) instructing task A and task B, respectively. The *top panels* show a cell (364 trials) preferring task B. Delay activity was consistently higher for task B (for this animal, the orientation task trials), irrespective of the task instruction cue set. The *bottom panels* show a cell (384 trials) with a main effect of task (preferring task B) as well as an interaction between task and cue. The interaction is evident in the larger task-selective response in the *bottom right panel.* Sp/s, spikes per second.

independent of the way in which the rule was instructed. Outside of these regions (i.e., in the IPS fundus, medial wall, and area 5), effects were similar, albeit weaker: Only 20% of neurons showed a main effect of task rule, and in more than half of these neurons, there was an interaction between task rule and task instruction cue set.

To quantify the strength of the encoding of task rules, we examined the magnitude of the task effect using a receiver operating characteristic (ROC) analysis (Metz, 1978). This analysis measures how well an ideal observer could identify which task rule was in effect, based solely on the firing rate from a single trial. For neurons in the lateral wall of the IPS and the adjacent gyral surface, the area under the ROC curve was greater than 0.60 or less than 0.40 for 28.5% of neurons. The area under the ROC curve was greater than 0.60 or less than 0.40 for only 13.5% of neurons in more medial areas. The time course of the mean ROC area is shown for both sets of areas (Fig. 11–5; see color insert). Compared with the effect in the medial areas, task effects in the lateral

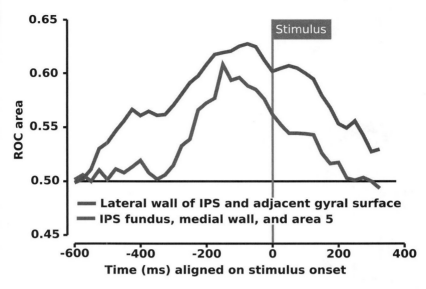

Figure 11–5 The time course of receiver operating characteristic (ROC) values for significant task cells shows that task-selective activity in the lateral intraparietal sulcus (IPS) and adjacent gyral surface (including areas LIPd, LIPv, 7a, LOP, and DP) [*upper trace*] starts earlier, reaches a higher value, and is maintained for longer than task-selective activity in the IPS fundus, medial wall, and area 5 (*lower trace*).

areas begin sooner, are stronger, and are sustained well after the presentation of the imperative stimulus. In contrast, the encoding of task information in the more medial areas starts later, is weaker, and is prominent only during the delay interval itself.

To determine how the presentation of the imperative stimulus affects task selectivity, we compared task selectivity immediately before and after stimulus presentation. Task encoding was very similar among neurons in the lateral bank of the IPS and adjacent gyral surface: 27% of these neurons showed a main effect of task rule in the period after the imperative stimulus compared with 29% in the late delay period. ROC analysis showed a strong correlation between task selectivity in these two intervals. Thus, these neurons continue to encode the particular task that is being performed, even after the imperative stimulus appears. This is exactly what we might expect if these neurons play a role in processing sensory information from the imperative stimulus in the context of the particular task at hand.

We have so far demonstrated that many neurons in the PPC reflect information about the task, both before and after the appearance of the imperative stimulus. In the next section, we describe the special role that TASK$^+$ neurons play in the processing of congruent and incongruent stimuli.

ENCODING OF CONGRUENCY

In our task-switching paradigm, incongruent stimuli are ambiguous because they are associated with different responses, depending on the task context. From the subject's perspective, only knowledge about the task can resolve the response ambiguity of incongruent stimuli. In comparison, congruent stimuli are associated with the same response alternative in both tasks. Thus, given this difference in the relevance of the task context in the congruent and incongruent conditions, the processing of congruent and incongruent stimuli is likely to differ. Imaging studies of human subjects performing task-switching and other paradigms with incongruent stimuli have concluded that stimulus incongruity leads to heightened neural activity in the PPC (Bench et al., 1993; Carter et al., 1995; Taylor et al., 1997; Peterson et al., 1999; Adleman et al., 2002), as well as in a number of frontal areas (e.g., Schlag-Rey et al., 1997; Olson and Gettner, 2002; Munoz and Everling, 2004; Nakamura et al., 2005).

In the following analyses, we first address whether neurons in the PPC show different activity after congruent versus incongruent stimuli. Then we analyze whether $TASK^+$ and task-negative ($TASK^-$) neurons differ in their responses to congruent and incongruent stimuli.

The analyses are applied to the same neuronal data as used in the previous section. For each neuron, we determined whether spike rate reflected stimulus incongruity in the period 25–225 ms after stimulus onset. We calculated the fraction of neurons that were significantly more active after an incongruent stimulus compared with a congruent stimulus. We found that this fraction was not significantly different from chance (3.7%), and was similar to the fraction of significantly less active neurons (3.9%). At the population level, mean activity was exactly the same for incongruent and congruent stimuli (15.7 ± 0.7 spikes per second [sp/s] in both conditions). Similar results were obtained when we considered other time intervals (i.e., 50–250 ms, 100–300 ms, and 50–350 ms after onset of the imperative stimulus). Altogether, we observed neither an increase nor a decrease in firing rate after the presentation of an incongruent versus a congruent stimulus, either at the single-neuron level or at the population level, in the PPC.

Next, we tested for an effect of congruence on neuronal latency. We used a particular property of neurons in the PPC, that is, spatial tuning, to quantify neural latency. Neuronal activity in the PPC is often correlated with some spatial aspect of the task, for example, the distance of a stimulus or motor response from a particular location in space. Spatially tuned neurons are common in the PPC (Andersen et al., 1985; Colby and Goldberg, 1999; Snyder et al., 2000). Tuned spatial responses that occur around the time of a motor response may reflect the generation of a motor command (Mountcastle et al., 1975), or they may reflect an efference copy of a command that has been generated elsewhere (von Holst and Mittelstaedt, 1950). If the spatially tuned activity substantially precedes the motor output, then it may reflect a sustained sensory response

(Duhamel et al., 1992), a neural correlate of covert attentional processes (Bush-nell et al., 1981), a neural correlate of motor intention (Snyder et al., 1997, 2000), or a decision variable related to the value of either a particular stimulus or a particular response (Platt and Glimcher, 1999; Sugrue et al., 2004).

There are a number of different ways in which congruency could affect the latency of a spatially tuned response component. Consider the interval that elapses between the first appearance of response-related activity in a particular brain area, and the time at which a motor response is initiated. It seems natural to think that this "neuronal-behavioral response latency" should be unaffected by factors such as congruence. However, other results are possible. For example, in the face of conflict (e.g., incongruent stimuli), the downstream mechanisms may require a higher level of certainty before a response is initiated, thereby increasing the neuronal-behavioral response latency on incongruent compared with congruent trials. As another example, when performing a sequence of effortful motor responses in which easy and difficult trials are mixed together, one might delay responses in easy trials to maintain a consistent rhythm across all trials. Most generally, neurons that show a consistent temporal relationship between activation and a particular motor response across a wide range of conditions are more likely to represent motor variables. Neurons whose temporal relationship between activation and a particular motor response depends on task condition are more likely to represent a cognitive (decision) variable. We found that parietal neurons that lacked task information (TASK$^-$ cells) fell into the former category, whereas TASK$^+$ cells fell into the latter category.

To perform this analysis, we considered only the subset of neurons with significant spatial tuning. We selected these neurons by comparing whether the spike rate in an interval starting 200 ms before home key release and lasting until 100 ms after home key release was significantly different for trials in which the animal moved to the right versus the left response button (Student's t-test, alpha level of 5%). We found that the firing rates of 62% of neurons (233 of 378) were significantly different for leftward and rightward responses.

We then determined the latency of neuronal responses in the congruent and incongruent trials. In Figure 11–6, we show an example neuron with higher firing for reaches to the left compared with the right (solid versus dashed traces). In this neuron, the divergence in firing rate occurred 41 ms sooner for congruent trials than for incongruent trials (dark gray versus light gray traces). Unfortunately, neuronal latency is difficult to measure accurately, because in these neurons (in contrast to, for example, the response of a V1 neuron to a visual transient), the change in activity is initially quite slow. As a result, small differences in instantaneous activity can lead to large differences in measured latency. In contrast, the rise time to half-maximum activity was well correlated with response latency, and was much more robust. For the example neuron, the rise time to half-maximum activity was 55 ms.

Even when using rise time to half-maximum activity, the data from individual neurons were often noisy. Therefore, we determined the neural latency

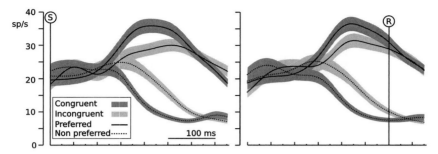

Figure 11–6 Neuron showing delayed spatial response latencies due to stimulus in-congruity. Average spike rate and standard error are displayed, aligned on the onset of the imperative stimulus (S) [*left*], or on the onset of the response (R) [*right*]. The cell was spatially responsive, and fired more vigorously when the monkey reached for the left response button than for the right button. Hence, the preferred direction was to the left. The latency of this directional specificity occurs when the curves for the preferred (*solid lines*) and nonpreferred directions (*dashed lines*) diverge. Note that the divergence and the half-maximum amplitude occur earlier in the congruent condition (*dark gray*) than in the incongruent condition (*light gray*). Sp/s, spikes per second.

of the entire population of spatially tuned neurons. For each tuned neuron, we first performed a millisecond-by-millisecond subtraction of firing rate when the response was made in the preferred minus the nonpreferred direction. For example, in Figure 11–6, we subtracted the dashed lines from the correspond-ing solid lines. The resulting data isolate the directional component of the re-sponse. We then averaged the data across neurons and smoothed it using a low-pass filter (-3 dB point of 9 Hz). This analysis (Fig. 11–7A) revealed that modulation resulting from directional preference appeared sooner in con-gruent trials (dark gray) than in incongruent trials (light gray). There was also a slight (19%, $p > 0.1$) reduction in the maximum amplitude of direction-related activity, which came approximately 350 ms after the onset of the im-perative stimulus.

The neural latencies were 90 ms in congruent trials and 113 ms in incon-gruent trials (Fig. 11–7A). The activity is unlikely to reflect an efference copy of the saccade command or a visual reafference response, because the neuronal activity precedes the corresponding mean saccadic latencies (202 ms and 217 ms, respectively) by more than 100 ms. The difference between congruent and incongruent neural response latencies approached, but did not reach, statistical significance ($p < 0.08$, Monte Carlo test). Nevertheless, this differ-ence was highly statistically significant when a more robust measure of timing was used: Half-maximum activity was achieved 196 ms and 224 ms after stimulus onset for congruent and incongruent stimuli, respectively ($p < 0.0003$, Monte Carlo test). The latency differences identified by the two methods were similar (23 ms and 28 ms), although variability was substantially less for the latter measurement.

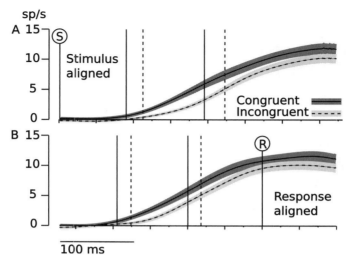

Figure 11–7 The timing of the directional response of the population of spatially tuned neurons from both animals. For each cell, the
trials were sorted by the direction of the reach. Responses on null
direction reaches were subtracted from responses on preferred direction reaches. The data were then averaged across cells and plotted as a
function of time. The *vertical lines* indicate the onset of directional
tuning and the time to half-maximum activity. *A.* Data aligned on the
onset of the imperative stimulus (S). The population response to congruent stimuli starts earlier (90 ms after stimulus onset) [*left solid line*]
than the response to incongruent stimuli (113 ms after stimulus
onset) [*left dashed line*]. The difference in timing is similarly reflected
in the time to half-maximum activity (196 ms for congruent stimuli
[*right solid line*] and 224 ms for incongruent stimuli [*right dashed
line*]). *B.* Data aligned on the onset of the arm response (R). The
population response to congruent stimuli starts earlier (197 ms before
response onset) [*left solid line*] than the response to incongruent
stimuli (178 ms before response onset) [*left dashed line*]; henceforth,
onset before the alignment point will be indicated by a minus sign. The
difference in timing is similarly reflected in the time to half-maximum
activity (−101 ms for congruent stimuli [*right solid line*] and −83 ms
for incongruent stimuli [*right dashed line*]). Sp/s,spikes per second.

We used two different alignments. First, we aligned individual trials on the
onset of the imperative stimulus, emphasizing differences in the perceptual
and cognitive components of processing (Fig. 11–7*A*). Next, we aligned on the
onset of the button release, emphasizing differences in cognitive and motor
components of processing (Fig. 11–7*B*). Even when aligned on the response
onset, both the divergence time and half-maximum time occurred sooner in

the congruent compared with the incongruent condition (by 19 ms, $p < 0.08$; by 18 ms, $p < 0.001$, respectively).

To examine this result further, and to explore the possibility that neurons that maintain task information may play a different role in stimulus-response mapping than neurons that do not maintain task information, we analyzed neurons with and without task information separately ($TASK^+$ and $TASK^-$ neurons).

We repeated the same analysis that we performed on the population of all spatially tuned neurons on the separate subpopulations of $TASK^+$ and $TASK^-$ neurons. Effects in neurons preferring task A ($n = 37$) and task B ($n = 40$) were similar, and therefore these two subpopulations of neurons were pooled.

We expected that, in a neuron population representing a motor variable (including an efference copy signal), the neuronal congruency effect would match the behavioral congruency effect. We found that this was true for $TASK^-$ cells, but not for $TASK^+$ cells. Incongruent stimuli resulted in a 15-ms slowing of the time to the half-maximum neuronal response in $TASK^-$ neurons (Fig. 11–8A) [215 ms versus 230 ms] and a 49-ms slowing in $TASK^+$ neurons (Fig. 11–8C) [164 ms versus 213 ms]. Although these congruency costs were statistically significant in both neuronal populations ($p < 0.007$ and $p < 0.0004$, respectively, Monte Carlo test), only the effect in the $TASK^-$ cells matched the behavioral (arm movement) effect (10–16 ms).

The marked difference in the timing of $TASK^-$ and $TASK^+$ neuronal responses can be better appreciated when the data are aligned to the time of the motor response (arm movement). With this alignment (Fig. 11–8B), it can be seen that $TASK^-$ cell activity was time-locked to the arm movement, with the time to half-maximum response differing by only 5 ms in congruent compared with incongruent trials. In contrast, $TASK^+$ cell activity was independent of the motor response, with a 32-ms difference in time to half-maximum activity in congruent compared with incongruent trials (Fig. 11–8D) [$p < 0.01$, Monte Carlo test].

Thus, the activity of $TASK^-$ cells, but not $TASK^+$ cells, appears to reflect a motor variable. However, animals moved not only their arms to the response button, but also their eyes. Might the activity of $TASK^-$ cells reflect arm movement responses and the activity of $TASK^+$ cells reflect eye movement responses? We were able to rule out this intriguing possibility. Eye movements were typically initiated approximately 150 ms before the arm movement. However, these eye movement responses were time-locked to the arm movement responses. Relative to the onset of the arm movement, mean saccade latencies differed by no more than 3 ms (black and gray arrows in Figs. 11–8B and 11–8D). Therefore, the timing of $TASK^+$ neurons cannot be explained by the timing of either saccades or arm movements.

These results clearly dissociate the activity of $TASK^+$ neurons from both sensory variables (Fig. 11–8C) and motor variables (Fig. 11–8D). These dissociations indicate that an independently defined subset of parietal neurons "solves" the stimulus-response mapping problem sooner in congruent

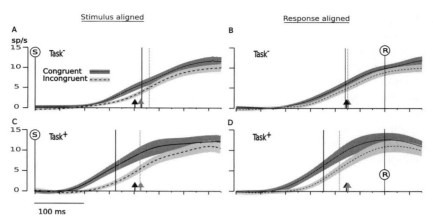

Figure 11–8 Onset of neural directional response (preferred minus nonpreferred direction) as a function of task selectivity and imperative stimulus congruency (spatially tuned neurons only). *A.* The difference in the time to half-maximum activity for congruent trials (215 ms) [*solid vertical line*] and incongruent trials (230 ms) [*dashed vertical line*] is similar to the behavioral response latency difference. *B.* Same data as in *A,* but aligned on the arm response onset. The latency difference between congruent (−80 ms) and incongruent (−75 ms) is 5 ms. The eyes began to move to the target approximately 150 ms before the arm began to move. The average saccade response times are indicated by black (*congruent*) and gray (*incongruent*) *arrows. C.* Similar to *A,* but for the task-positive (Task$^+$) cells. In contrast to the task-negative (Task$^-$) cells, there is a large latency difference in the time to half-maximum activity between congruent (164 ms) and incongruent trials (213 ms). *D,* Similar to *B,* but for the TASK$^+$ cells. The latency difference between congruent (−123 ms) and incongruent (−91 ms) trial is 32 ms. S, stimulus; R, response; sp/s, spikes per second.

compared with incongruent trials, even when the data are aligned on the motor response.

In summary, analyses of the effects of congruency suggest that TASK$^+$ neurons play a substantially different role than TASK$^-$ neurons in sensory-to-motor transformations. TASK$^-$ neurons in the PPC appear to reflect motor variables. TASK$^+$ cells, unlike TASK$^-$ cells, are influenced by task context, and the observation that TASK$^+$ cells respond so differently from TASK$^-$ cells under incongruent compared with congruent conditions (Fig. 11–8*B* versus 11–8*D*), supports the idea that TASK$^+$ cells do not merely reflect sensory or motor variables, but instead are involved in applying task rules during sensorimotor processing.

GENERAL DISCUSSION

We studied rule representation and rule-based processing of stimuli in monkeys using a task-switching paradigm. The animals were able to interleave

two tasks quite well, with speed and accuracy comparable to those of human subjects. Surprisingly, however, the monkeys did not show switch costs, which are a hallmark of human performance in these types of paradigms. We went on to record data from neurons in the PPC to study the neural mechanisms underlying task-switching and rule representation in the monkey. Our most important findings from these recordings are that parietal neurons encode information about abstract task rules, and play a role in disambiguating response-ambiguous stimuli.

Comparison of Human and Monkey Behavior

Overall, task-switching performance is similar in monkeys and humans, although monkeys are somewhat faster than humans (Fig. 11–2). We do not take the faster RTs in monkeys versus humans as evidence of superior behavioral performance. For example, physical differences in the conduction pathways of the smaller brain (Ringo and Doty, 1994) or mechanical factors in the musculature could partially explain the differences in speed.

Monkeys show no difficulty in switching their attention from one task to another (little or no residual switch costs) [Fig. 11–2]. However, their ability to focus on the task at hand is comparatively poor: Their performance is significantly affected by irrelevant stimulus features (high incongruency costs). The opposite is true for humans, who have difficulty switching, but little difficulty maintaining attention on the appropriate stimulus features.

We considered the possibility that monkeys, unlike humans, memorized all separate cue-target-response combinations, and then used a memory-based strategy. The use of a memory-based strategy might explain the absence of switch costs, because in this case, the animals would not actually be switching between two different rules. Two pieces of evidence refute this idea: (1) We found small switch costs when ITIs were very short, suggesting that monkeys treat the two tasks differently. (2) An animal successfully responded to 11 completely novel stimuli, which would not be possible if it used a memory-based strategy.

It is also possible that the varying amounts of practice might explain the difference in human and monkey switch costs. The humans in our study performed only 3000 trials, whereas monkeys performed tens or hundreds of thousands of trials. However, a recent study from our laboratory demonstrates that switch costs are retained in humans after more than 30,000 practice trials (Stoet and Snyder, in press).

The existence of persistent switch costs and lower incongruency costs in humans compared with monkeys could be two manifestations of a single process. Humans appear to be able to "lock in" a particular task, thereby minimizing incongruency costs, but paying the price of having to take time to "unlock" the mapping when the task switches. We experience this "unlocking" as a persistent switch cost. In comparison, monkeys cannot lock in a particular task and therefore are distracted by irrelevant stimulus dimensions, resulting

in incongruency costs. However, because they do not lock in a task in the same way a human does, they do not experience persistent switch costs.

Both humans and monkeys show nonpersistent switch costs, that is, costs that appear only with short preparation times. Nonpersistent switch costs may therefore reflect an independent process by which both humans and monkeys instantiate a particular stimulus-response mapping. This independent process supports the ability to switch between tasks rapidly, but neither protects against task incongruency nor incurs persistent switch costs.

A general theory of task-switching should offer an explanation for species-specific effects. It seems unlikely that humans suffer from an undesirable cost in task-switching that monkeys completely avoid. We hypothesize that human switch costs reflect an evolutionarily advantageous cognitive mechanism that helps to maintain focused attention on a particular task for long periods.

Of course, as in many comparative studies, we cannot rule out the possibility that our results were influenced by some minor difference in procedures. For example, animals, but not humans, were rewarded with drops of water for each correct response. As another example, only the humans were provided with a verbal description of the task (although one human was intentionally left to work out the task in the same way that the animals did, and her performance was similar to those of the other humans).

The finding that monkeys do not show persistent switch costs is interesting, but also somewhat disappointing, because this absence means that monkeys cannot be used to investigate the neural basis of persistent switch costs in humans. However, there are many aspects of task-switching that humans and monkeys share, and for these processes, monkeys make excellent models. In particular, the macaque monkey is a good model for the ability to switch between tasks (because monkeys, like humans, can learn to switch between tasks quite well); a good model for the ability to prepare tasks in advance; a good model for task incongruency; a good model for nonpersistent switch costs; and a good model for looking at task representations.

Representation and Application of Rules in the Monkey Posterior Cortex

We have presented evidence that a subset of neurons (TASK$^+$) in the PPC, concentrated in the lateral bank of the IPS and on the adjacent angular gyrus, responds selectively to cues for different task rules.

The encoding of information about task rules is often called "cognitive set." We propose that true cognitive set signals should exist completely independent of sensory signals. This definition distinguishes true cognitive set signals, such as those reported in the prefrontal and premotor cortices (Konishi et al., 2002; Nakahara et al., 2002; Wallis and Miller, 2003) from signals that reflect sensory information, but are modulated by nonsensory variables (e.g., spatial attention or other task contingencies) [Britten et al., 1996; Treue and Maunsell,

1996; Snyder et al., 1997; Colby and Goldberg, 1999; Bisley and Goldberg, 2003].

Until recently, it appeared that task-related signals in the parietal cortex fell into the latter category and not the former, encoding task-relevant sensory information, not abstract signals related to task preparation (Assad, 2003). The current results from the parietal cortex, in contrast, clearly demonstrate the encoding of task-rule information in advance of receiving stimulus information. The task-switching paradigm separates out the presentation of the instruction of which rule is to be used from the presentation of the stimulus to which that rule is to be applied. This separation is extremely useful, allowing us not only to identify those cells involved in task coding (TASK$^+$ cells), but also to study sensorimotor processing in these cells.

To study the effect of task-rule information on stimulus processing, we compared trials using congruent stimuli (stimuli that require the same response in the two tasks) with trials using incongruent stimuli (stimuli that require different responses in the two tasks).

This comparison allows for a simple test of neural responses to incongruency, and has been explored in human imaging studies. Brain imaging studies of the human PPC reveal an increased blood-oxygen level–dependent signal after incongruent stimuli (Bench et al., 1993; Carter et al., 1995; Taylor et al., 1997; Peterson et al., 1999; Adleman et al., 2002). We did not observe increased neural activity in our population of recorded neurons. There are many reasons why the results from functional magnetic resonance imaging (fMRI) and neurophysiology experiments might differ. First, the human studies used a linguistic task (Stroop task), whereas our study used a nonverbal task. It is possible, for example, that the involvement of the parietal cortex in conflict depends on the type of task (e.g., verbal versus nonverbal). Second, the PPC may be used differently in humans and monkeys. Given that the human PPC is larger and more developed in humans, it is likely that the human PPC fulfills many functions not available to monkeys. Finally, unit recording and fMRI results may not be directly comparable. For example, Logothetis et al. (2001) simultaneously recorded blood-oxygen level–dependent signals and microelectrode recordings, and concluded that fMRI reflects input and intracortical processing rather than spiking output.

We found a surprising result when comparing the neuronal response during congruent and incongruent trials. Because incongruent stimuli are associated with longer behavioral RTs than congruent stimuli, it was not surprising to find that incongruent stimuli were also associated with longer neuronal latencies. In TASK$^-$ cells, incongruity had similar effects on behavioral and neuronal latency differences (15 ms and 10 to 16 ms, respectively). This can be seen graphically by the fact that, when aligned on response onset, the neuronal responses of TASK$^-$ cells are indistinguishable (Fig. 11–8B). In contrast, TASK$^+$ cells showed a neuronal effect of incongruity that was much larger than the behavioral effect (49 ms versus 10 to 16 ms, respectively): TASK$^+$ cell responses

do not overlap one another when aligned on the time of the motor response (Fig. 11–8D). Furthermore, by comparing the upper and lower halves of Figure 11–8, it can be appreciated that TASK$^+$ cells encode the animal's upcoming choice of where to move sooner than TASK$^-$ cells, especially in congruent trials.

These results have important implications. The finding that TASK$^+$ neurons encode the animal's choice of where to move substantially sooner than TASK$^-$ neurons supports the idea that TASK$^+$ neurons play an important role in the task-switching paradigm, and that this role is distinct from that played by TASK$^-$ neurons (Stoet and Snyder, 2004). TASK$^+$ cells are likely to help map sensory stimuli onto motor responses, given a particular task context, whereas TASK$^-$ cells represent the outcome of the mapping. Our results dissociate TASK$^+$ cell responses from both sensory inputs and motor outputs. This suggests that TASK$^+$ cells play an intermediate role, helping to map sensory stimuli onto motor responses. In contrast, TASK$^-$ cell responses are well correlated with the motor response. This suggests that TASK$^-$ cells represent the outcome of the sensory-to-motor mapping. This interpretation is consistent with the idea that TASK$^-$ cells carry either a motor command signal (Mountcastle et al., 1975) or an efference copy signal (von Holst and Mittelstaedt, 1950).

Furthermore, by isolating the responses of TASK$^+$ and TASK$^-$ cell populations, we are able to see that monkeys do not always respond as soon as parietal neurons encode a decision. Based on the neuronal recording, we would have expected that responses in the congruent trials would be approximately 50 ms faster than in incongruent trials, but that is not what we observed. Instead, button presses in difficult (congruent) trials are delayed relative to button presses in easy (congruent) trials. What could explain the finding that TASK$^+$ cells encode the correct response in congruent trials nearly 50 ms sooner than in incongruent trials, and yet the behavioral cost of stimulus incongruity is only 10 to 16 ms? Put differently, why don't monkeys respond still faster to congruent stimuli, given that their parietal cortices encode the correct response so quickly? The parietal cortex may not be the only brain area that performs this sensory-to-motor computation. It is possible that parallel pathways are involved, with different latencies in the different pathways in congruent and incongruent trials. In the absence of conflict (congruent trials), TASK$^+$ cells in the parietal cortex may compute an answer first. However, in the presence of conflict (incongruent trials), it may be that another area (e.g., the frontal cortex) computes a response more quickly than the parietal cortex. As a result, behavioral RTs would be determined by TASK$^+$ cell latencies in congruent trials, but not in incongruent trials.

The Role of Language

The implications of this study go beyond understanding task-specific processing in simple cognitive tasks. Rule representation and rule-dependent stimulus processing is a hallmark of human cognition, and characterizing the

neural underpinnings of a nonverbal task-switching paradigm may help us to approach the more complex context-dependent processing that occurs in human cognition. Like the incongruent stimuli of the current study, particular words and phrases have multiple possible meanings that are disambiguated by context. For example, the meaning of a linguistic expression depends on the meaning of the words that immediately precede or follow it (Gerrig and Murphy, 1992; Strohner and Stoet, 1999). It is intriguing to try to identify the origins of human language skills in the abilities of present-day nonhuman primates (Gardner and Gardner, 1969; Premack, 1971; Ujhelyi, 1996), and to determine whether these origins might involve the PPC and its role in context-specific processing (Gurd et al., 2002). This is a very important question, albeit far from being answered. A more fundamental question is whether human language skills can help us to understand basic differences in understanding human and animal rule-guided behavior.

Humans can learn a new rule in seconds, simply by following verbal instructions, and this constitutes a fascinating and fundamental difference between humans and monkeys. Arguably, it is the nature of language that makes efficient representation and quick communication possible, and language is unique in doing so. Any attempt to communicate a rule other than with words either would not be as efficient or would involve some of the symbolic characteristics unique to language. Therefore, it is not too far-fetched to assume that language is a key component in understanding the differences between human and animal rule-based behavior and cognition. Unfortunately, very little is known about the role of language in explaining differences between human and animal rule use. We would like to mention three of the most important questions that must be answered to improve our understanding of this issue.

First, there is the question of how the process of acquisition of verbal and nonverbal rules differs in humans. It is possible, for example, that humans process nonverbal rules by first conceptualizing them in a verbal format. Given that humans are able to act on rules before they are able to express them verbally, however, this seems unlikely (Bechara et al., 1997). Conversely, verbal rules might first be converted into a nonverbal currency before they can actually be applied in a task. Finally, verbal and nonverbal rules may be handled in completely different ways in the human.

Closely related to the issue of rule acquisition and application is the issue of rule representation. Does language play a role in rule representation only as a tool during the acquisition of the rule, or is language an essential component of the representation itself? It is possible that representations of rules differ depending on how they are acquired; one can imagine that identical rules, conveyed directly through language or learned through some nonverbal mechanism (e.g., trial-and-error, imitation), might be represented in different parts of the brain.

Finally, does the lack of verbal language skills in monkeys imply that they represent rules differently? The answer may depend on the particular rule—on

its complexity, for example—or on its amenity to being expressed by language. The null hypothesis is that simple rules are represented and implemented similarly in the two species. However, introspection suggests that language is incredibly important to human cognition, whereas monkeys show no evidence of any similar abilities. Furthermore, human cortices are functionally lateralized, and this lateralization appears to be related, at least in part, to verbal abilities. This suggests that verbal abilities have had a large effect on our cortical architecture. It is intriguing to consider that human language abilities may relate to the ability, which monkeys lack, to lock in to a particular task.

We believe that monkeys provide an essential model system, if not for directly understanding human cognition, then at least for developing the tools and hypotheses needed to approach the issue in humans. We believe that the current findings demonstrate that task-switching paradigms provide an excellent entry point for this work.

ACKNOWLEDGMENTS This study was supported by the NIH (NEI and Silvio Conte Center), the McDonnell Center for the Study of Higher Brain function, the EJLB Foundation, and the Otto-Hahn Fellowship of the Max Planck Society.

REFERENCES

Adleman NE, Menon V, Blasey CM, White CD, Warsofsky IS, Glover GH, Reiss AL (2002) A developmental fMRI study of the Stroop Color-Word task. Neuroimage 16:61–75.

Allport DA, Styles EA, Hsieh S (1994) Shifting intentional set: exploring the dynamic control of tasks. In: Attention and performance XV (Umilta C, Moscovitch M, eds.), pp 421–452. Cambridge: MIT Press.

Andersen RA, Essick GK, Siegel RM (1985) Encoding of spatial location by posterior parietal neurons. Science 230:456–458.

Assad JA (2003) Neural coding of behavioral relevance in parietal cortex. Current Opinion in Neurobiology 13:194–197.

Bechara A, Damasio H, Tranel D, Damasio AR (1997) Deciding advantageously before knowing the advantageous strategy. Science 275:1293–1295.

Bench CJ, Frith CD, Grasby PM, Friston KJ, Paulesu E, Frackowiak RS, Dolan RJ (1993) Investigations of the functional anatomy of attention using the Stroop test. Neuropsychologia 31:907–922.

Bisley JW, Goldberg ME (2003) Neuronal activity in the lateral intraparietal area and spatial attention. Science 299:81–86.

Britten KH, Newsome WT, Shadlen MN, Celebrini S, Movshon JA (1996) A relationship between behavioral choice and the visual responses of neurons in macaque MT. Visual Neuroscience 13:87–100.

Bushnell MC, Goldberg ME, Robinson DL (1981) Behavioral enhancement of visual responses in monkey cerebral cortex, I: Modulation in posterior parietal cortex related to selective visual attention. Journal of Neurophysiology 46:755–772.

Carter CS, Mintun M, Cohen JD (1995) Interference and facilitation effects during selective attention: An $H_2^{15}O$ PET study of Stroop task performance. Neuroimage 2:264–272.

Chafee MV, Goldman-Rakic PS (2000) Inactivation of parietal and prefrontal cortex reveals interdependence of neural activity during memory-guided saccades. Journal of Neurophysiology 83:1550–1566.

Colby CL, Goldberg ME (1999) Space and attention in parietal cortex. Annual Review of Neuroscience 22:319–349.

Dias R, Robbins TW, Roberts AC (1996) Primate analogue of the Wisconsin card sorting test: effects of excitotoxic lesions of the prefrontal cortex in the marmoset. Behavioral Neuroscience 110:872–886.

Duhamel JR, Colby CL, Goldberg ME (1992) The updating of the representation of visual space in parietal cortex by intended eye movements. Science 255:90–92.

Everling S, DeSouza JF (2005) Rule-dependent activity for prosaccades and antisaccades in the primate prefrontal cortex. Journal of Cognitive Neuroscience 17:1483–1496.

Gardner RA, Gardner BT (1969) Teaching sign language to a chimpanzee. Science 165:664–672.

Gerrig RJ, Murphy GL (1992) Contextual influences on the comprehension of complex concepts. Language and Cognitive Processes 7:205–230.

Gurd JM, Amunts K, Weiss PH, Zafiris O, Zilles K, Marshall JC, Fink GR (2002) Posterior parietal cortex is implicated in continuous switching between verbal fluency tasks: an fMRI study with clinical implications. Brain 125:1024–1038.

Konishi S, Hayashi T, Uchida I, Kikyo H, Takahashi E, Miyashita Y (2002) Hemispheric asymmetry in human lateral prefrontal cortex during cognitive set shifting. Proceedings of the National Academy of Sciences U S A 99:7803–7808.

Lewis JW, Van Essen DC (2000) Mapping of architectonic subdivisions in the macaque monkey, with emphasis on parieto-occipital cortex. Journal of Comparative Neurology 428:79–111.

Logothetis N, Pauls J, Augath M, Trinath T, Oeltermann A (2001) Neurophysiological investigation of the basis of the fMRI signal. Nature 412:128–130.

Mansouri F, Tanaka K (2002) Behavioral evidence for working memory of sensory dimensions in macaque monkeys. Behavioral Brain Research 136:415–426.

Meiran N (1996) Reconfiguration of processing mode prior to task performance. Journal of Experimental Psychology: Learning, Memory and Cognition 22:1423–1442.

Metz CE (1978) Basic principle of ROC analysis. Seminars in Nuclear Medicine 8:283–298.

Monsell S (2003) Task switching. Trends in Cognitive Sciences 7:134–140.

Mountcastle VB, Lynch JC, Georgopoulos A, Sakata H, Acuna C (1975) Posterior parietal association cortex of the monkey: command functions for operations within extrapersonal space. Journal of Neurophysiology 38:871–908.

Munoz DP, Everling S (2004) Look away: the anti-saccade task and the voluntary control of eye movement. Nature Reviews Neuroscience 5:218–228.

Nakahara K, Hayashi T, Konishi S, Miyashita Y (2002) Functional MRI of macaque monkeys performing a cognitive set-shifting task. Science 295:1532–1536.

Nakamura K, Roesch MR, Olson CR (2005) Neuronal activity in macaque SEF and ACC during performance of tasks involving conflict. Journal of Neurophysiology 93:884–908.

Olson CR, Gettner SN (2002) Neuronal activity related to rule and conflict in macaque supplementary eye field. Physiology and Behavior 77:664–670.

Peterson BS, Skudlarski P, Gatenby JC, Zhang H, Anderson AW, Gore JC (1999) An fMRI study of Stroop word-color interference: evidence for cingulate subregions subserving multiple distributed attentional systems. Biological Psychiatry 45:1237–1258.

Platt ML, Glimcher PW (1999) Neural correlates of decision variables in parietal cortex. Nature 400:233–238.

Premack D (1971) Language in chimpanzee? Science 172:808–822.

Ringo JL, Doty RW (1994) Time is of the essence: a conjecture that hemispheric-specialization arises from interhemispheric conduction delay. Cerebral Cortex 4: 331–343.

Rogers RD, Monsell S (1995) Cost of a predictable switch between simple cognitive tasks. Journal of Experimental Psychology: Human Perception and Performance 124: 207–231.

Rushworth MFS, Passingham RE, Nobre AC (2002) Components of switching intentional set. Journal of Cognitive Neuroscience 14:1139–1150.

Rushworth MFS, Paus T, Sipila PK (2001) Attention systems and the organization of the human parietal cortex. Journal of Neuroscience 21:5262–5271.

Schlag-Rey M, Amador N, Sanchez H, Schlag J (1997) Antisaccade performance predicted by neuronal activity in the supplementary eye field. Nature 390:398–401.

Snyder LH, Batista AP, Andersen RA (1997) Coding of intention in the posterior parietal cortex. Nature 386:167–170.

Snyder LH, Batista AP, Andersen RA (2000) Intention-related activity in the posterior parietal cortex: a review. Vision Research 40:1433–1441.

Sohn M, Ursu S, Anderson JR, Stenger VA, Carter CS (2000) The role of prefrontal cortex and posterior parietal cortex in task switching. Proceedings of the National Academy of Sciences U S A 97:13448–13453.

Stoet G, Snyder LH (2003) Task preparation in macaque monkeys (*Macaca mulatta*). Animal Cognition 6:121–130.

Stoet G, Snyder LH (2004) Single neurons in posterior parietal cortex (PPC) of monkeys encode cognitive sets. Neuron 42:1003–1012.

Stoet G, Snyder LH (in press) Extensive practice does not eliminate human switch costs. Cognitive, Affective, and Behavioral Neuroscience.

Strohner H, Stoet G (1999) Cognitive compositionality: an activation and evaluation hypothesis. In: Cultural, psychological and typological issues in cognitive linguistics: current issues in linguistic theory (Hiraga MK. Sinha C, Wilcox S, eds.), pp. 195–208. Amsterdam: John Benjamins.

Sugrue LP, Corrado GS, Newsome WT (2004) Matching behaviour and the representation of value in the parietal cortex. Science 304:1782–1787.

Sullivan EV, Mathalon DH, Zipursky RB, Kersteen-Tucker Z, Knight RT, Pfefferbaum A (1993) Factors of the Wisconsin Card Sorting Test as measures of frontal-lobe function in schizophrenia and in chronic alcoholism. Psychiatry Research 46:175–199.

Sylvester CC, Wager TD, Lacey SC, Hernandez L, Nichols TE, Smith EE, Jonides J (2003) Switching attention and resolving interference: fMRI measures of executive functions. Neuropsychologia 41:357–370.

Taylor SF, Kornblum S, Lauber EJ, Minoshima S, Koeppe RA (1997) Isolation of specific interference processing in the Stroop task: PET activation studies. Neuroimage 6:81–92.

Treue S, Maunsell JH (1996) Attentional modulation of visual motion processing in cortical areas MT and MST. Nature 382:539–541.

Ujhelyi M (1996) Is there any intermediate stage between animal communication and language? Journal of Theoretical Biology 180:71–76.

Van Essen DC, Dickson J, Harwell J, Hanlon D, Anderson CH, Drury HA (2001) An integrated software system for surface-based analyses of cerebral cortex. Journal of the American Medical Informatics Association 8:443–459.

von Holst E, Mittelstaedt H (1950) Das Reafferenzprinzip. Naturwissenschaften 37:464–476.

Wallis JD, Miller EK (2003) From rule to response: neuronal processes in the premotor and prefrontal cortex. Journal of Neurophysiology 90:1790–1806.

12

Neural Mechanisms of Cognitive Control in Cued Task-Switching: Rules, Representations, and Preparation

Hannes Ruge and Todd S. Braver

A hallmark of human cognition is its flexibility. We are able to pursue multiple goals or tasks simultaneously, but can also prioritize these in accord with both our internal states and the continually changing nature of the external environment. Moreover, we are able to switch rapidly from one primary task to another, which can have a dramatic effect on the way in which we interact with the environment, even when that environment remains constant (Norman and Shallice, 1986; Miller and Cohen, 2001). This ability suggests that task-related information must be actively represented in a way that can bias perception and action.

The task-switching paradigm has become one of the most widely used tools for studying cognitive flexibility and the nature of task-related representations (Monsell, 2003). Typically, experiments are set up in such a way that participants are exposed to multivalent target stimuli that imply multiple behavioral opportunities (e.g., a letter-digit target pair affording either vowel-consonant or odd-even classification). However, only a single option is to be selected at a given moment, depending on which task is currently set to a higher priority. Task priority is typically specified by the experimenter, either through a pre-experimentally defined sequence (e.g., AABB . . .) or through an explicit task cue that varies randomly from trial to trial. Thus, in the sense that appropriate behavior is made *conditional* on (experimentally defined) changing task priorities, task-switching implies a form of high-level, *rule-guided* control. Rule-guided control provides a means of selecting relevant perceptual dimensions and response parameters based on signals relating to task priority. Moreover, such control is critical for preventing behavior from being erratically driven in a bottom-up fashion by the most salient, but not necessarily most appropriate, stimulus affordances.

In this chapter, we specifically focus on the cognitive and neural mechanisms that subserve the different types of *preparatory* task control that can be

engaged in such multitasking situations. Numerous previous studies have sought to specify the preparatory mechanisms involved when a specific task can be prioritized in preparation for processing task-ambiguous target stimuli (for a review, see Monsell, 2003), often based on explicit task cues indicating the currently relevant task (e.g., Sudevan and Taylor, 1987; Meiran, 1996; Brass and von Cramon, 2002). Surprisingly little (if anything) is known about the reverse preparatory condition, in which it is possible to consider the multiple behavioral opportunities afforded by task-ambiguous target stimuli before a final task decision can be made based on an unambiguous task cue (for exceptions in the behavioral literature, see Shaffer, 1965, 1966; Gotler and Meiran, 2003). To close this gap in the literature, we have recently begun to systematically compare the mechanisms of preparatory control involved in these two situations in a series of behavioral and brain imaging studies.

As described later, this seemingly straightforward comparison of two preparatory conditions (that we term "advance-cue" versus "advance-target") during multitasking has proven highly informative, but also reveals a number of tricky theoretical issues regarding the nature of the underlying functional and neural architecture of task control. Specifically, we examine three key issues in this chapter. (1) We examine whether cue-based task prioritization should be conceptualized as a distinct function in terms of both cognitive architecture and brain localization, or if not, what kind of alternative theoretical views are possible. (2) We argue that a comprehensive account of task control must consider the distinction between *attentional* control mechanisms guiding action selection based on perceptual stimulus representations versus *intentional* control mechanisms guiding action selection based on action goal representations. (3) We discuss the possibility that top-down control might not be limited to the biasing of action selection processes, but that certain phenomena can be better explained by assuming an additional control point at the interface between action selection and concrete motor planning—especially when behavior relies on novel and arbitrary task rules. Finally, we begin an attempt to determine the extent to which the two preparatory mechanisms can be considered "voluntary."

Our theoretical views of these issues draw heavily on the results of behavioral and imaging studies of task-switching that we have recently conducted (Ruge and Braver, in preparation; Ruge et al., submitted). We describe these findings briefly, and discuss their theoretical implications in relation to a broad range of other empirical and conceptual approaches. In particular, we hope to convey a novel perspective on task-switching phenomena that we believe opens up important new future directions for research and understanding.

SELECTIVE REVIEW OF THE TASK-SWITCHING LITERATURE

Before we turn to the theoretical issues mentioned earlier, we set the stage by briefly summarizing one of the most frequently discussed issues in the extant task-switching literature. As the label "task-switching" suggests, most studies

have been interested in the processes that enable task priority *changes* from one trial to the next (Monsell, 2003; Wager et al., 2004). One key assumption, probably inspired by early neuropsychological observations of so-called "perseverative behavior" (Milner, 1963; Stuss and Benson, 1984), is that there is a default tendency to repeat the previously performed task, and that this tendency has to be overcome if a different task must be implemented. Indeed, behavioral task-switching studies have consistently shown that task-switch trials are more demanding than task-repeat trials, as indicated by behavioral switch costs (i.e., performance differences between the two types of trials). However, the theoretical interpretation of this observation remains a focus of heated debate.

One account suggests that, after a task priority change, implementation of the new task can occur only after an active reconfiguration of relevant processing routines, akin to a mental "gear shift" (Meiran, 1996; Monsell, 2003). If this were true, the implementation of a new task should benefit from additional time for preparatory "task set" reconfiguration, resulting in a reduction of switch costs. Many studies have used the *cued* task-switching procedure, in which a random task cue indicates which of (typically) two alternative tasks to prioritize in each trial. This procedure allows for a well-controlled examination of task preparation effects, by presenting the cue at various time intervals before a task-ambiguous target stimulus. Typically, switch costs are reduced when the preparatory (cue-target) interval is longer. This finding is consistent with the idea that task set reconfiguration can be at least partially completed before target stimuli are presented (Rogers and Monsell, 1995; Meiran, 1996).

In contrast, this finding is often believed to be less compatible with an alternative explanation of switch costs, here referred to as the "competition-resolution account" (e.g., Allport and Wylie, 2000). According to this view, a new task set is not established during the preparatory interval. Rather, the new task set is believed to emerge during the course of task implementation (i.e., during target processing) as the result of the successful resolution of competing processing tendencies associated with: (1) the current task cue, and (2) the current stimulus affordances, which are biased toward the more recently performed task (this bias facilitates performance in repeat trials, but interferes with performance in switch trials). However, a number of authors have recently pointed out that the preparation-related reduction of switch costs is, in fact, equally consistent with the competition-resolution account as it is with the reconfiguration account. Under the competition-resolution account, a prior task cue confers a temporal advantage to the processing tendencies associated with the cue, which provides protection against the activation of misleading processing tendencies triggered by subsequently presented targets (Goschke, 2000; Gilbert and Shallice, 2002; Yeung and Monsell, 2003).

A potentially more conclusive approach for distinguishing between these two theoretical accounts is to isolate and selectively analyze neural activity occurring during the preparation interval (Ruge et al., 2005; Badre and Wagner,

2006). According to the reconfiguration account, preparatory activation should be increased in switch trials compared with repeat trials, reflecting the additional effort to reconfigure the task set. In contrast, the competition-resolution account would predict equal preparatory activation levels for switch and repeat trials, because target-induced competition is absent at this point. The pattern of results across studies and methods is, however, rather inconsistent. In support of the competition-resolution account, event-related functional magnetic resonance imaging (fMRI) studies of cued task-switching usually do not report reliable preparatory activation differences between switch and repeat trials. Moreover, when the cue-target interval is short (which should produce stronger target-induced interference, according to the competition-resolution account), blood-oxygen level–dependent (BOLD) activation is typically increased for switch trials versus repeat trials (Dove et al., 2000; Brass and von Cramon, 2004; Ruge et al., 2005; Badre and Wagner, 2006). In contrast, and in support of the task set reconfiguration account, event-related electroencephalogram (EEG) studies do consistently report preparatory activation differences between switch and repeat trials (Rushworth et al., 2002; Kieffaber and Hetrick, 2005; Nicholson et al., 2005). These discrepancies between the types of methods have not yet been resolved, and may require more systematic comparison of fMRI and EEG studies.

In particular, four key issues still need to be addressed: (1) There may be systematic procedural differences in the studies conducted across the two methods (e.g., different lengths of the cue-target interval or the response-cue interval). (2) The fMRI and EEG studies may be picking up on different aspects of neural activation (e.g., synchronous or oscillatory effects between brain regions that affect EEG more than fMRI). (3) Event-related potential activation may be more strongly dominated by repetition priming effects that occur at the time of the cue. Such repetition effects are typically confounded with task-switch effects (see Logan and Bundesen, 2004), and might originate and propagate from brain regions typically ignored in fMRI studies of executive control, such as occipital cortex. (4) An fMRI study may be less sensitive when effects occur in a temporally variable manner. For example, Braver et al. (2003) showed that, in a subset of trials presumably associated with the highest degree of task preparation (because reaction times were the fastest), a switch-related enhancement of preparatory BOLD activation was, in fact, observed in posterior parietal cortex. The reason might be that only in these trials were preparatory processes implemented quickly and reliably during the preparation interval.

NEW PERSPECTIVES

In this chapter, our goal is to step back from this debate and examine a number of alternative approaches and conceptualizations that might be important for characterizing cue-based and target-based processes in task-switching. First, regarding cue-based processes, we start from the assumption that performance

during multitasking conditions requires determination of the current task priority before task implementation, regardless of whether a *new* task needs to be implemented in a given trial, and whether task switches involve task set reconfiguration processes (see Rubinstein et al., 2001). In other words, presentation of a task cue provides a clear signal regarding which task has highest priority, regardless of whether that task also had high priority in a previous trial. Thus, instead of focusing on the potential functional differences between switch and repeat trials, our aim is to scrutinize in more detail the nature of cue-based task prioritization as a common feature of both trial types. Second, we adopt a perspective on target-based processes that goes beyond the dichotomy between cue-based top-down control (i.e., strictly facilitative) and target-induced bottom-up processes (i.e., primarily interfering). Instead, we characterize target-based preparatory processes in terms of their potentially active role in generating task-related opportunities implied by the current stimulus affordances. Figure 12–1 depicts the experimental setup we used and the methodological issues one faces when preparatory BOLD activation is to be isolated.

Task Prioritization

How can we operationalize the functional characteristics of task prioritization? One approach is to ask under what circumstances prioritization is *necessary*. Prioritization is obviously required in situations in which stimuli afford multiple tasks (multivalent stimuli). One straightforward experimental manipulation, therefore, is to compare multivalent stimuli with univalent stimuli, which afford only a single task and thus do not require task prioritization (Rubin and Meiran, 2005; Rubin et al., submitted). Similarly, one could compare mixed-task blocks with single-task blocks, again, assuming that task prioritization becomes unnecessary when the same single task is implemented over and over again (Braver et al., 2003; Rubin and Meiran, 2005; Rubin et al., submitted).

However, one potential caveat to both approaches is that, even in apparently unambiguous situations, participants might still need to prioritize, because even with only one available task, there is always the possibility of not carrying it out (except in the case of highly automatized behaviors that tend to be initiated in an obligatory and ballistic fashion). Indeed, a study by Rubin et al. (submitted) showed that, although prefrontal and parietal areas exhibited enhanced event-related activation for mixed-task block trials as well as for multivalent target stimuli, the same areas were still substantially activated above baseline for single-task block trials and for univalent stimuli. However, results obtained by Braver et al. (2003) suggest that mixed-task blocks and single-task blocks might not differ so much in terms of the transient processes engaged on a trial-by-trial basis, but that task-mixing is accompanied by a specific sustained processing mode maintained across an entire experimental block.

Alternatively, instead of studying the circumstances under which task prioritization is *necessary,* one can manipulate the conditions under which it is

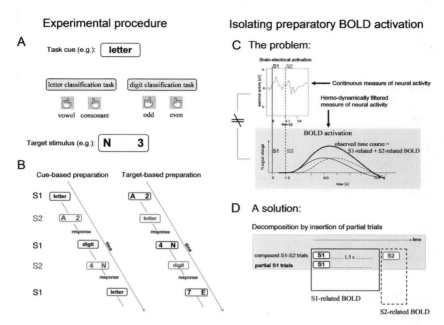

Figure 12–1 The basic task design that was used in our own studies presented in this chapter (*A* and *B*). The analysis of functional magnetic resonance imaging data collected in such S1-S2 designs needs to take into account temporal overlap between event-related blood-oxygen level–dependent (BOLD) responses associated with consecutive S1 and S2 events appearing in a fixed order (*C* and *D*). *A.* Participants were made familiar pre-experimentally with the task rules for letter classification and digit classification. In each trial, a task cue (e.g., letter) indicated which task to implement in the presence of a task-ambiguous target stimulus (e.g., "N 3"). *B.* The order of the cue and target presentation was varied across two blocked conditions, either cue-target or target-cue. The main goal was to compare preparatory BOLD activation associated with advance cues versus advance targets. *C.* Unlike brain electrical event-related responses, which directly reflect the time course of neural activity associated with consecutive events, the BOLD response reflects a hemodynamically filtered measure of the underlying neural activity that causes massive signal overlap. *D.* To reconstruct the BOLD components associated with S1 and S2 events occurring within a single trial, we used a deconvolution technique based on the insertion of partial S1-only trials (Ollinger et al., 2001; Serences, 2004).

possible. Generally speaking, priority information needs to be available, and in the cued task-switching paradigm, it is the task cue that is supposed to convey it.[1] In contrast—and this constitutes the key experimental innovation we introduced—advance task-ambiguous target stimuli demand a priority decision, but do not (by definition) provide the kind of priority information from which task selection could occur. Thus, we hypothesized that brain areas involved in task prioritization should be activated by advance task cues, but not by advance-target stimuli (Fig. 12–2).

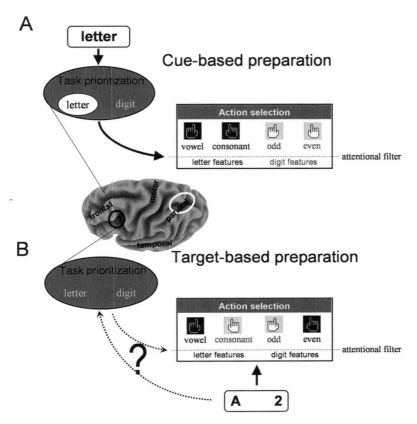

Figure 12–2 Hypotheses regarding the involvement of a putative task prioritization mechanism localized within posterior lateral prefrontal cortex. *A*. Presentation of advance task cues is supposed to enable task prioritization based on a prefrontal representation of abstract task demands that can bias lower-level action selection processes so that they will operate preferentially on target input that matches the currently task-relevant perceptual dimension. *B*. According to our initial hypothesis, target stimuli would not engage the prioritization mechanism because they are, by definition, task-ambiguous and thus do not convey information that would significantly affect a priority decision.

Hierarchical Model

In fact, such a prediction is very much in line with rather traditional, but still popular and highly intuitive, hierarchical models of executive control that postulate that regions within lateral prefrontal cortex (PFC): (1) represent task demands or task goals in a relatively abstract form, and (2) sit at the top of a task-processing hierarchy by providing the top-down information needed to resolve competing processing tendencies developing in parallel on lower

hierarchy levels in other parts of the brain, such as posterior parietal cortex (e.g., Norman and Shallice, 1986; Cohen et al., 1990). A number of previous studies have been conducted in an effort to isolate cue-related preparatory activation, but these studies did not include a direct comparison with target-based preparation. In such studies, one frontal cortex region in particular has been most consistently identified in paradigms with advance task cues, namely, the posterior part of inferior frontal sulcus (Brass and von Cramon, 2002; Bunge et al., 2003; Sakai and Passingham, 2003; Ruge et al., 2005). The same region, sometimes referred to as "inferior frontal junction" (IFJ) [Derrfuss et al., 2005], also exhibits elevated activation under high task-interference conditions, suggesting that its functional role is not restricted to cue-based task preparation per se. More generally, it appears to process task information in such a way as to exert top-down task control when required. See Figure 12–3 (see color insert) for the results of a recent meta-analysis (Koechlin et al., 2003; Derrfuss et al., 2005; Ruge et al., 2005).

Although these observations are consistent with a cue-specific task prioritization function of IFJ, it remains to be answered whether advance task cues are necessary or merely sufficient to engage the presumed high-level task representations. If lateral PFC areas, such as IFJ, were also activated by advance targets, thus demonstrating that advance task cues are not a *necessary* condition, the standard hierarchical model would be called into question. Indeed, when we conducted the direct comparison of cue-related and target-related preparatory activation (Ruge et al., submitted), we found results that called into question the original interpretation that IFJ implements a cue-specific task prioritization mechanism. Specifically, we found that neither IFJ nor any other

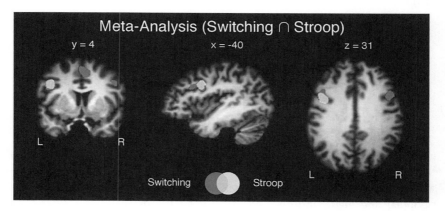

Figure 12–3 Meta-analysis conducted by Derrfuss et al. (2005), demonstrating the involvement of inferior frontal junction across different studies that commonly shared a strong demand for top-down task control.

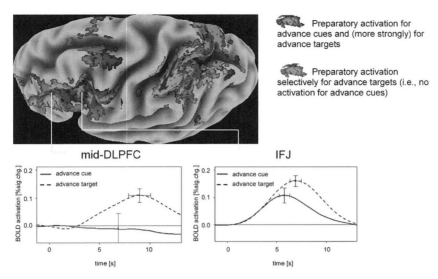

Figure 12–4 Two different patterns of preparatory brain activation associated with advance task cues, advance-target stimuli, or both. Remarkably, neither IFJ nor any other region was selectively (or even more strongly) activated for advance task cues. Conversely, a number of areas, such as mid-dorsolateral prefrontal cortex, were selectively activated by advance targets. mid-DLPFC, mid-dorsolateral prefrontal cortex; IFJ, inferior frontal junction.

brain region was selectively activated for advance cues. Instead, all regions that were activated by advance cues (including IFJ) were equally or even more strongly activated for advance-target stimuli (Fig. 12–4; see color insert). This surprising result seems to prompt a reconceptualization of the standard hierarchical account of task prioritization. Next, we provide two possible explanations that attempt such a reconceptualization.

Nonhierarchical Model I: Cumulative Prioritization

A good starting point is the computational model by Gilbert and Shallice (2002) depicted in Figure 12–5. One important difference between this model and related previous computational models (e.g., Cohen et al., 1990) is that task-ambiguous target stimulus input can fully activate the processing pathways for both tasks (word-reading and color-naming) in parallel up to the level of abstract task demands. In this sense, the model can be considered nonhierarchical,[2] and it seems to be suited to accommodate our brain activation results.

According to such an interpretation, abstract task demands (assumed to be represented within IFJ) are activated directly and equally well by both cues and

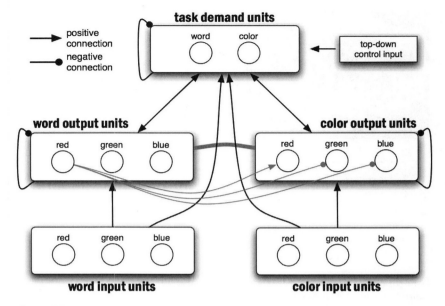

Figure 12–5 Computational task-switching model by Gilbert and Shallice (2002), in a modified graphical representation. The novel contribution of this model is that target stimulus input is allowed to activate abstract task demand units (word-reading and color-naming), thereby activating its own task-related processing pathways.

targets, with cue-associated task information being relayed via the task demand layer in exactly the same fashion as target information. From this perspective, there is no true functional difference between a situation in which multiple task demands are activated in parallel by multivalent targets and a situation in which a single task demand is activated by an unambiguous task cue. Accordingly, task prioritization is not a distinct functional (and neuroanatomical) entity specifically associated with task cues, but instead, it emerges cumulatively, with the representation of task demands settling into a unique and stable state as soon as sufficient evidence has been accumulated for a single task. This happens immediately after an advance task cue, but it requires additional information when the representation of task demands remains in an undecided state after advance multivalent targets. Thus, according to this alternative "cumulative prioritization" account, task control is a continuously evolving process, with no privileged route of access to task demand representations.

Interpreted in this way, our imaging results can also potentially arbitrate a debate within the behavioral task-switching literature concerning the processing level at which stimulus-induced task competition occurs (Hübner et al., 2004). Although there is now ample evidence that target stimuli are not merely passive objects of top-down cue-based control biasing (e.g., Allport and

Wylie, 2000; Waszak et al., 2003; Yeung and Monsell, 2003), it has been unclear whether targets activate task-related processing pathways at the level of abstract task demands (presumably represented within lateral PFC), or instead, at the lower level of specific stimulus-response (S-R) associations (presumably represented within posterior parietal cortex). Under the assumption that IFJ represents abstract task demands, our results clearly favor the former interpretation.

Nonhierarchical Model II: Compound Cue-Target-Response Mappings

The cumulative prioritization model is a nonhierarchical account of task control, in the sense that it abandons the idea of a *cue-specific* task prioritization module. However, it still assumes a control hierarchy in the sense that higher-order abstract task demands are used to modulate the activation strength of lower-order representations: the actual S-R mapping rules. Alternatively, it is possible to entirely abandon the idea that a representation of abstract task demands is involved in task control. Instead, IFJ could directly code the actual task rules by integrating task cues and target categories into compound S-R mappings using conjunctions, such as, "if the cue indicates letter AND the target is a vowel, then press the right button OR if the cue indicates letter AND the target is a consonant, then press the left button." From this perspective, IFJ is activated by both advance cues and advance targets because they both provide information that can be used to partially instantiate the same compound mapping rule. This view of IFJ-mediated task control is reminiscent of Logan and Bundesen's (2003, 2004) account of cue-repetition effects, which led them to the conclusion that ". . . the explicit task cuing procedure is not a viable method for investigating executive control." (Logan and Bundesen, 2004, p. 839). An alternative, and in our view, more adequate conceptualization would be that the employment of compound mapping rules in cued task-switching genuinely constitutes an "executive control" function. The reasoning is that the tasks are typically novel and only weakly practiced. Therefore, compound S-R mappings may have to be computed in an online, possibly verbally coded fashion (Goschke, 2000), within working memory. Maintaining compound S-R mappings in working memory (when necessary) might be critical because the components of the conjunction might be presented in a temporally separated fashion and thereby might require a mechanism capable of cross-temporal integration to complete the conjunction. Indeed, these conjunctive working memory representations may be the instantiation of what is meant by the term "rule-like" when describing the mechanisms of task control (Bunge, 2004).

Target-Specific Preparatory Processes

Regardless of which of these models one prefers, they share one common feature. In these models, control over action selection is assumed to be exerted

via "attentional" mechanisms that guide the transformation from perceptual stimulus representations into response options according to pre-experimentally instructed S-R mapping rules. Furthermore, both cue-based and target-based preparatory mechanisms are presumed to share this attentional (i.e., S-R) pathway. Yet, we would like to suggest that this model, as intuitive as it may be, is not complete. Instead, we argue that a more comprehensive account of *target-based* preparatory control must take into consideration two additional levels of processing.

First, a viable model must incorporate an *intentional* control path, where behavioral options are selected in accordance with potentially obtainable action goals suggested by the current state of the environment (Meiran, 2000b; Waszak et al., 2005). Importantly, we make a clear distinction between "intention," referring to the encoding of action goals (i.e., the anticipated action effects), and "volition," referring to the actual commitment to implement a planned action based on cost-benefit considerations.

Second, such a model needs to take into account the fact that the generation of future behavioral options based on abstract mapping rules (S-R or goal-response associations)—hereafter referred to as "action selection"—is not identical to the planning of concrete motor responses based thereon. We will argue that the interface between abstract action selection and concrete motor planning is controlled by an additional rule type related to the consideration of subjective cost-benefit tradeoffs.

Intentional Control of Action Selection

Within the task-switching context, Meiran (2000a, b) was the first to propose that concrete target stimuli might not only activate action selection processes based on perceptual stimulus representations, but also trigger additional action selection processes based on representations of action goals, which are themselves supposed to be independent of cue-based control biases. This conclusion was derived from the observation that cue-based preparation reduces subsequent target-induced competition on a perceptual level, but fails when competition among action goals is present.

Additional support for these conclusions comes from brain imaging studies. One study compared task-switching conditions in which the competing tasks comprised overlapping goal-response associations (referred to as "response meanings" in that study) against a control condition in which there was no overlap. The overlap condition was associated with increased activity in mid-dorsolateral PFC (mid-DLPFC), suggesting that this might be the prefrontal region that contributes to intention-based conflict resolution (Brass et al., 2003). Yet another task-switching study that specifically focused on cue-based preparation did *not* observe activity in mid-DLPFC (Ruge et al., 2005). This pattern of results suggests that intentional control is only weakly (if at all) engaged during cue-based preparation, again supporting the earlier performance-based conclusions.

To summarize the findings so far, there is evidence that intentional processes are associated with concrete target stimuli (but not task cues), and that specifically, mid-DLPFC is implicated in intentional control. Still missing in this picture is evidence showing that target-based intentional processes can be engaged in preparation. If this were true, we would expect preparatory activation in mid-DLPFC after advance-target stimuli. Our recent study (Ruge et al., submitted) replicated the absence of mid-DLPFC activity during the preparatory period for the advance-cue condition. At the same time, we found, as hypothesized, that preparation after advance targets was associated with robust activity in this brain area. Moreover, as shown in Figure 12–4, the comparison of cue-related and target-related preparatory activation reveals that the distinct neuronal signatures of attentional control (preparatory activation for both advance cues and advance targets) versus intentional control (preparatory activation selectively for advance targets) are not limited to IFJ and mid-DLPFC, respectively. Rather, the same two activation patterns are found in a number of other brain regions (parietal cortex along IPS, dorsal premotor cortex, and medial frontal cortex), thereby forming two widely distributed, but segregated control networks.

Although the empirical results, both behavioral and imaging, do quite convincingly converge onto a dual-path (attention-intention) model, it still seems important to discuss the somewhat unusual notion that intentional control can be externally triggered by target stimuli. In fact, a popular view in the literature is that intentional control becomes relevant specifically when action selection is *not* fully determined by the current stimulus input, but instead needs to be based on *internally* generated future action goals (e.g., Frith et al., 1991; Jahanshahi and Dirnberger, 1999).[3] Yet, from a general theoretical standpoint, we do not see any good reason why intentional processes should not also be triggered externally (i.e., activated by the appearance of stimuli that are associated with particular action goals). For instance, to give a real-world example, the fasten-your-seat-belt alarm ringing in your car suggests the action goal of silencing it (by fastening your seat belt).[4]

Based on the notion that intention is associated with the "internal" generation of action goals, many studies of intentional control have used free selection tasks. The respective brain imaging studies have typically identified mid-DPLFC as one key brain region (besides medial frontal cortex) involved in the internal intention generation process (e.g., Frith et al., 1991; Jahanshahi and Dirnberger, 1999). Mid-DLPFC is exactly the region we reported to be involved in externally triggered target-based intentional control. This suggests that this brain region might be engaged during both internally guided and externally guided intention. Indeed, a recent fMRI study conducted by Lau et al. (2004) *directly* compared the two situations and found that mid-DLPFC is engaged, regardless of whether action selection is externally or internally guided. In contrast, it was medial frontal cortex that seemed to be specifically associated with internal action selection.

The perspective of externally guided intention becomes particularly clear in the light of the "mirror neuron" literature (Rizzolatti and Craighero, 2004; Arbib, 2005). The central notion of this work is that there exists a special class of neurons that codes actions according to their anticipated observable effects (i.e., action goals) [see also Hommel et al., 2001]. This interpretation is based on the intriguing finding that such neurons are active not only when an action is about to be performed, but also when the same action is observed being performed by another individual (i.e., when the effects of another person's actions are perceived). This data pattern demonstrates that intention (i.e., activation of action goals) can easily be triggered *externally* by adequate stimulus input. Brain imaging studies seeking to identify the human equivalent of the monkey mirror neuron system have revealed a set of brain areas that overlap remarkably well with the brain regions we have found to be selectively engaged during target-based preparation, including the anterior part of intraparietal sulcus, and Broca's area (BA 44), which is supposed to be the human homolog of the monkey's mirror neuron area F5 within ventral premotor cortex (e.g., Buccino et al., 2001; Grezes et al., 2003; Manthey et al., 2003; Hamilton and Grafton, 2006; for a review, see Rizzolatti and Craighero, 2004). Mid-DLPFC does not seem to be as consistently implicated in human activation studies. However, cortical connectivity studies in monkeys suggest that mid-DLPFC has a strong projection to the anterior intra-parietal sulcus (aIPS), and also, to a lesser degree, with ventral premotor area F5 (Rizzolatti and Luppino, 2001).

Action Selection Versus Motor Planning

So far, our discussion of target-based preparation has dealt with the distinction between attentional and intentional action selection processes that generate response options based on either abstract S-R rules or abstract goal-response rules, respectively. In this section, we argue that the examination of target-based preparation is also useful for elucidating the putative role of mechanisms that regulate the transfer from an "action selection" stage into a final "motor planning" stage. The conceptual distinction between these two processing levels becomes especially useful in task situations for which motoric response codes are *not* automatically activated via associative shortcuts that are either pre-experimentally overlearned (e.g., word-reading in the Stroop task) or otherwise predisposed, for instance, by their spatial compatibility (e.g., Simon task). When, instead, novel and relatively unpracticed tasks are involved, we postulate that the transfer from action selection into motor planning processes is under a more flexible control regime.

The idea is that action selection processes first generate abstract behavioral options that may or may not be translated into concrete motor plans. Such flexibility in motor planning is of particular relevance in the context of multivalent advance-target stimuli that can present in one of two opposing types. On one hand, advance targets can be *congruent* (i.e., different tasks require the same response; for example, the target "A 7," if both vowels and odd digits

require a left-button response). In this case, it would be of great use to engage in advance motor planning to prepare a single motor response, which could then be executed right away, as soon as the subsequent cue gives the "go" signal. On the other hand, for *incongruent* advance targets (i.e., different tasks require different responses, such as "A 8" in the example discussed earlier), such advance motor planning would have costs as well as benefits because the preparation of motor plans would lead to competition between mutually incompatible responses that could create interference before and during response execution. Thus, in contrast to congruent trials, for incongruent trials, the cost of the extra effort required for preparation of motor responses may outweigh the potential benefits to be gained in response time (Fig. 12–6).

The presence of such a cost-benefit tradeoff related to motor planning makes it clear that different preparation strategies are possible. It is therefore of interest to determine how actual participants decide to optimize the interface between action selection and motor planning. A first strategy would be always to defer the start of motor planning until the cue is presented to effectively prevent interference in case of incongruent targets, yet, at the cost of

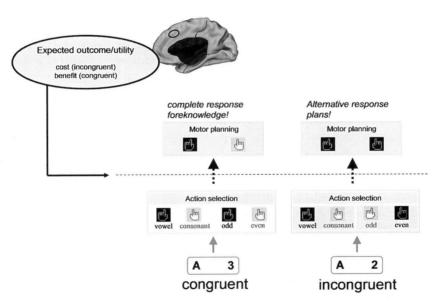

Figure 12–6 Model assumptions about the involvement of strategic control at the interface between action selection and motor planning processes. The core assumption is that this interface is regulated by the subjective evaluation of expected utility (implemented by medial frontal cortex) associated with preparation based on congruent versus incongruent advance-target stimuli.

suboptimal preparedness in case of congruent targets. A second strategy would be always to start motor planning right away after advance-target presentation, to be optimally prepared in case of congruent targets, yet, at the cost of risking motor interference in case of incongruent targets. Of course, a third, mixture strategy is also possible, in which the decision to engage in preparatory motor planning occurs flexibly on a trial-by-trial basis, depending on whether the current target is recognized as congruent or incongruent.

We examined this issue in our recent study of advance-target preparation (Ruge et al., submitted). We found evidence that different individuals seemed to adopt different strategies (Fig. 12–7). This interpretation is most strikingly evidenced by the observation that one group of participants ("congruency-sensitive") exhibited a large speeding up in reaction time for advance congruent targets compared with incongruent targets. Yet, in the other group of participants ("congruency-insensitive"), performance in congruent and incongruent targets was almost identical, in terms of reaction time. We also examined brain activation patterns as a function of this behavioral group difference, and observed a complex pattern (Fig. 12–7). We found that group differences in preparatory brain activity were observed in all advance-target trials, not just congruent ones. This suggests that participants were not adopting the mixture strategy of engaging in preparatory motor planning on a trial-by-trial basis, depending on whether the current target is congruent (engage) or incongruent (do not engage). Instead, we observed that the congruency-sensitive group had increased preparatory activity in medial frontal regions (along with other regions) compared with the congruency-insensitive group, even in incongruent trials.

These results suggest that participants in the congruency-sensitive group adopted a global strategy (i.e., maintained across all individual trials) to generally engage in advance motor planning, irrespective of the status of congruency. This interpretation was also supported by the observation that, during the final response planning and execution phase after the cue, brain activation in the congruency-sensitive group was reduced for congruent targets and increased for incongruent targets in posterior parietal cortex and dorsal premotor cortex—notably, in the caudal part that has been postulated to represent more concrete motor codes, as opposed to the more abstract, "cognitive" representation of motor plans represented in the rostral portion (Picard and Strick, 2001). This activity pattern is exactly what would be expected of the congruency-sensitive participants if they: (1) benefited in congruent trials from an already prepared single motor response ready for execution (less planning effort, reduced activation), and (2) faced a disadvantage in incongruent trials because of the concurrently prepared competing motor response (more effort to eliminate erroneous response tendencies, enhanced activation).

To conclude, these results tentatively suggest that the interface between action selection and motor planning processes is under voluntary control—for two reasons: (1) Motor planning seems to be an *optional* strategy adopted by only a subset of participants, instead of being the inevitable result of

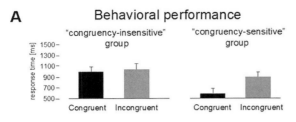

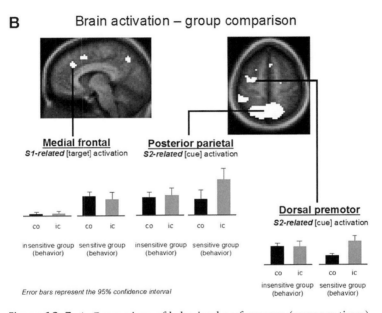

Figure 12–7 *A.* Comparison of behavioral performance (response times) for congruent and incongruent advance targets. A distributional analysis of congruency effects suggested a subdivision into two groups of subjects, either showing a strong speed-up for advance congruent targets or showing no difference between congruent and incongruent advance targets. *B.* Three different patterns of brain activation that followed the group difference, defined according to the presence or absence of a behavioral congruency effect. co, congruent; ic, incongruent.

automatic priming processes taking place in each and every participant. (2) This presumed strategy difference was accompanied by selective medial frontal cortex activation for the congruency-sensitive group. As noted earlier, medial frontal cortex is a brain region that has long been associated with the initiation and perpetuation of voluntary motor behavior (Barris and Schuman, 1953; Paus, 2001; Rushworth et al., 2004). In the next and final section, we elaborate on the idea that only some components of task preparation might be volitional.

Voluntary Control?

A putative hallmark of executive control is its presumed voluntary nature. Although volition is certainly the most fascinating aspect of higher-order brain function, it is also an enigmatic and elusive one. As we have mentioned earlier, in the context of free selection tasks, we draw a clear conceptual line between intention and volition. On one hand, the notion of intention is used to refer to the activation of action goals (i.e., anticipated action effects) and action selection processes based thereon (e.g., Hommel et al., 2001). On the other hand, the notion of volition is used to refer to the actual initiation and perpetuation of behavior based on the assessment of expected subjective outcome or utility in terms of cost-benefit tradeoffs (e.g., Rushworth et al., 2004). Thus, we distinguish between anticipated action *effects* and action *outcomes*. We use the term "effect" to refer to an expected perceptual or conceptual state produced by an action, and the term "outcome" to refer to the subjective value (in terms of reward components) associated with that expected state. Thus, volitional processes may be more directly motivational (i.e., "hot"), whereas intentional processes are more coldly cognitive.

Maybe the most intuitive observable property of voluntary control is its optional engagement. Based on this criterion, we suggested in the preceding section that target-based preparation involves a volitional component operating at the interface between action selection and motor planning processes. However, a potential weakness of this conclusion is that it relies on a post hoc interpretation of naturally occurring interindividual differences. It would therefore be desirable to employ procedures that enable tighter experimental control over volitional processes. A number of reasonable experimental approaches have been suggested in the context of cue-based preparation, two of which we discuss in more detail below.

Measuring Volition I: Optional Engagement of Preparatory Processes

The first experimental approach to measuring volition is based on the presumption that participants are, in principle, free *not* to use the task cue.[5] In this case, they would exhibit "utilization behavior" (Lhermitte, 1983; Shallice et al., 1989) driven by the currently most salient stimulus affordances. DeJong (2000) followed this line of reasoning to explain the often limited effectiveness of cue-based preparation by postulating that participants would occasionally fail to initiate cue-based preparation. Based on a distributional analysis of within-subject response times, DeJong demonstrated that participants are optimally prepared in a subset of trials (i.e., show no switch costs), but completely unprepared (i.e., show switch costs equivalent to having no preparation time) in another subset of trials. The all-or-none character of task preparation suggests that it is optional, and therefore under voluntary engagement. If, instead, preparation was achieved via automatic cue-based priming processes, the degree of preparedness (measured via the amount of residual switch cost) should have followed a unimodal distribution across trials.

Measuring Volition II: Conscious Accessibility of Preparatory Processing

The second experimental approach to measuring volition was pursued by Meiran et al. (2002), who allowed participants to have full control over their level of preparedness by self-determining how long to process an advance cue. Thus, preparation time was self-paced, and target stimuli appeared on the screen only after a readiness response was given. The rationale for this procedure was the assumption that voluntary control operates in a *conscious* mode. Participants should therefore be able to estimate their own state of preparedness. Based on this assumption, one can make inferences based on the relationship between preparation time and target response time. To derive precise predictions for this relationship, we need to apply somewhat complex reasoning. First of all, in a perfect world, self-pacing would allow each participant to be optimally prepared in every trial, resulting in zero variability of the actual state of preparedness, which would also imply a zero correlation between preparation time and response time.

Assuming a more realistic model, subjective estimates of the true state of preparedness should be subject to both interindividual and intraindividual variability. *Interindividually,* different participants might systematically adopt different criteria for when they feel sufficiently well prepared. This implies that more liberal (i.e., impulsive) participants would indicate their readiness sooner, leaving them less well prepared. Conversely, more conservative participants would indicate their readiness later, which leaves them better prepared. Thus, a negative correlation between average preparation time and average response time would be expected (i.e., participants with *slower* average readiness response times would tend to have a more conservative criterion and thus better preparedness, which would lead them to have to *faster* average response times).

Similarly, as a source of *intraindividual* variability, participants would be assumed to exhibit a certain estimation error around their subjective criterion, which implies that, in some trials, they underestimate their preparedness (thus indicating their readiness later than necessary, thereby being better prepared), whereas in other trials, they overestimate it (thus indicating their readiness too early, thereby being less well prepared). In effect, as for the correlation across participants, a negative relationship between trial-by-trial preparation times and response times would be expected (e.g., slower preparation times within individuals would occur in trials with better preparedness than at criterion, which should lead to faster response times).

Surprisingly, and in direct contradiction to the conclusions derived from DeJong's distributional analysis, Meiran et al. (2002) did not find the predicted negative relationship between preparation time and response time (even though there was substantial inter- and intraindividual variability).[6] Thus, they arrived at the conclusion that the internal state of preparedness is not consciously accessible; therefore, participants are unable to come up with a reasonable estimate.

Voluntary Control during Cue-Based and Target-Based Preparation

We recently attempted to replicate and extend the results of Meiran et al. (2002) by comparing preparation time effects in advance-cue as well as advance-target conditions (Ruge and Braver, in preparation). In the advance-cue condition, we also did not find negative correlations between preparation time and response time. However, in the advance-target condition, we observed strong negative correlations both inter- and intraindividually (Fig. 12–8).

Our results, therefore, suggest that target-based preparation is consciously accessible, whereas cue-based preparation may not be. Thus, if conscious accessibility is taken as a criterion for the engagement of voluntary control, target-based preparation would meet this criterion. This conclusion is also in line with our earlier interpretation of interindividual differences regarding congruency-related effects in performance and brain activation. In that study, even under standard conditions of a fixed-duration preparatory interval, we attributed the effects of individual differences to the optional character of voluntarily initiated motor planning processes during target-based preparation (discussed earlier). A second finding from the self-paced study is also important in supporting the brain imaging results. We found that the negative correlation between preparation time and response time was present in both congruent and incongruent target trials. This confirms our earlier conclusion that the initiation of motor planning processes is the result of a global strategy applied in all trials, rather than a mixture strategy applied only after determining whether a target stimulus is congruent or incongruent. Nevertheless, the shallower slope of the regression line in the incongruent condition supports the hypothesis that preparation was somewhat less effective in this condition, presumably due to induced response competition effects induced by motor planning.

Two Modes of Voluntary Control

The results described earlier, obtained across a variety of studies, can be summarized as follows. If voluntary control is defined by its optional engagement, then both cue-based and target-based preparation should be classified as voluntary. In contrast, under the assumption that voluntarily controlled processes are consciously accessible, our recent self-pacing results suggest that cue-based preparation should not be categorized as voluntary. To explain this discrepancy, we tentatively suggest a distinction between two modes of voluntary control: a "semiautomatic" mode, employed during cue-based preparation, and a "fully controlled" mode, employed during target-based preparation. Which of these two modes is active in a given situation depends on whether participants are merely consciously aware of the initiation of preparatory processes (as might occur for advance cues) or whether they are also consciously monitoring the unfolding of preparatory information processing after its initial activation (as might occur for advance targets). Accordingly, we

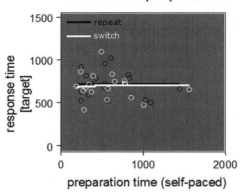

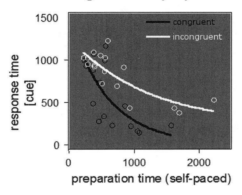

Figure 12–8 Relationship between self-paced preparation time and response times (across subjects). For the advance-cue condition, there was no noticeable relationship—either when the advance cue implied a task switch (Spearman rho = −0.08) or when it implied a task repetition (Spearman rho = −0.09). For the advance-target condition, instead, there was a strong negative relationship (longer preparation times, faster response times) for both advance congruent targets (Spearman rho = −071, $p < 0.002$) and advance incongruent targets (Spearman rho = −0.67, $p < 0.004$).

suggest that self-paced preparation time can provide a reasonable measure of voluntary processes only in the fully controlled mode.

Fully Controlled Mode during Target-Based Preparation

How can we explain why only target-based preparation (more specifically, the advance motor planning component), but not cue-based preparation, is

consciously monitored under the proposed regime of fully engaged voluntary control? A possible answer to this question is that target-based motor planning is only a small step shy of actual response execution and is therefore associated with a high risk of erroneous behavior. In contrast, cue-based preparatory processes are relatively far removed from the final execution of motor responses (at least in the way in which these cue-based processes have been operationalized in the laboratory).

Such reasoning naturally relates to theoretical concepts developed in the context of error processing and performance monitoring that point to the central role played by medial frontal cortex (Ridderinkhof et al., 2004). Not surprisingly, this is the same region whose activation pattern we found to be reflective of whether a given participant was engaging in target-based preparatory motor planning (discussed earlier). The specific contribution of medial frontal cortex in the context of target-based preparation seems to be to compute and represent the expected outcome or utility in terms of benefits (speeding response time) and costs (extra effort, potential response competition in incongruent trials), when engaging in concrete preparatory motor planning. Depending on subjective evaluation criteria, which we postulate to be computed in medial frontal cortex, an individual may or may not feel motivated to engage in advance motor planning.

Semiautomatic Control Mode during Cue-Based Preparation

What is the reasoning behind the notion of semiautomatic voluntary control operating during cue-based preparation? The rationale is that the preparatory benefit associated with advance task cues may rely on processes that subconsciously operate on task-related representations. Yet, whether such processes can unfold may depend on the status of a voluntarily controlled initiating signal. Thus, in the self-paced situation, participants would be able to consciously indicate whether they started active preparation, but they would be unable to give a reasonable estimate of the progress they make during the unfolding of this process. As such, preparation in the cue-based condition should be considered semiautomatic, because only the initiation, and not the unfolding and duration, of preparatory processes is under voluntary control.

A computational model that we designed recently helps to clarify the role of a voluntary gating signal in cue-based task preparation (Reynolds et al., 2006). In this modeling study, the success of cue-based preparation relies on an optional all-or-none (dopaminergic) gating signal that controls whether task information conveyed by advance cues would gain access to a PFC-based representation of abstract task demands. Importantly, the gating signal need only occur briefly, as long as it coincides with the presentation of the cue. This gating signal then initiates the encoding and activation of cue-related task information into PFC. As a consequence of this activation, the current task demand representation settles into a self-maintained stable activity pattern that persists across time. Thus, it could be that only the initial gating mechanism operates consciously, whereas the actual preparation of the subsequent task

might rely on the subconscious maintenance of a PFC representation. This PFC representation may, in turn, also subconsciously bias task-appropriate S-R transformation processes in posterior cortical regions (e.g., posterior parietal cortex).[7]

CONCLUSIONS

In our recent studies, the comparison of cue-based and target-based preparatory conditions have proven highly potent in generating a wealth of interesting, and often unexpected, empirical phenomena and novel theoretical insights. Consequently, the conceptualization of rule-based control evolved and expanded throughout this chapter, often leading to questions about what seemed intuitive from the standard perspective of cue-based (preparatory) task control.

We started from a highly intuitive, strictly hierarchical model that assumes that high-level task prioritization rules are employed to disambiguate action selection processes that occur at a lower level of the task hierarchy, and that are activated by task-ambiguous target stimuli. One of the key assumptions of such a model is that task prioritization rules (represented within lateral PFC) would become engaged to fulfill their function of task disambiguation only under conditions in which unambiguous task decisions are possible (i.e., after advance task cues, but not after advance-target stimuli). The failure to find brain regions (particularly IFJ area) exhibiting cue-specific preparatory activation does not confirm this initial hypothesis, and prompts a re-evaluation of the nature of PFC representations underlying task control. Two fundamentally different models seem possible, one of which retains a notion of semi-hierarchical task rules, whereas the other implies a nonhierarchical representational scheme. In particular, a critical question regarding the function of IFJ is whether this region exerts "attentional" control based on representations of either (1) abstract templates of task-relevant stimulus dimensions employed to activate and configure lower-level S-R transformation processes or (2) compound S-R mapping rules composed of conjunctions between stimulus categories and task cues. Further research will be needed to adjudicate between these two possibilities (see Ruge et al., submitted, for a more detailed argument in favor of the compound mapping account).

Beyond shedding some new light on the functional characteristics of brain areas commonly found to be involved in cue-based attentional control, the use and comparison of the advance-target condition also demonstrated the relevance of preparatory processes occurring via an additional "intentional" control path originating from dorsolateral PFC regions specifically engaged when action selection can be based on concrete action goals. Similar to the discussion about the representational code underlying attentional control, it remains unclear whether intentional control is based on representations of (1) abstract templates of task-relevant action goals employed for activating and configuring lower-level goal-response transformation processes or (2) the actual goal-response mapping rules.

Finally, we started to explore the question of whether there is a meaningful distinction between different forms of preparation in terms of the extent to which they involve strategic or voluntary control. Although, once again, seemingly counterintuitive, our results and those of others suggest that it is not cue-based preparation, but instead, target-based preparation that is more dominantly guided by volitional strategy. More specifically, it seems that subjective estimates of cost-benefit tradeoffs represent another type of rule that guides the task preparation process. These representations appear to be housed within medial frontal cortex, and help to determine whether concrete motor planning processes will be engaged during preparation. A future challenge will be to design experiments that more systematically manipulate and dissociate the factors that determine subjective cost-benefit tradeoffs, along with the attentional and intentional control processes that enable effective task preparation.

ACKNOWLEDGMENTS This research was supported by R01 Grant MH066078.

NOTES

1. Task prioritization can also be based on subjective task preferences (e.g., Forstmann et al., 2006) or memorized task sequences, as is the case in the alternating-runs paradigm (e.g., Rogers and Monsell, 1995).

2. Despite its nonhierarchical nature, the model seems to contain a "hidden" hierarchy (which is not explicitly modeled) by assuming that cue-associated task information is mediated via a privileged route that provides "top-down control input" into lower-level task demand units to disambiguate competing activation there. Again, the lack of cue-selective prefrontal activation in our study argues against such a conceptualization.

3. In contrast to the distinction we made earlier, in this context, the terms "intention" and "volition" are typically used synonymously.

4. In many experimental settings, it is difficult to determine whether an observable motor response was planned under the influence of attentional control (stimulus-response associations), intentional control (goal-response associations), or both. For instance, both the stimulus-response rule "if the alarm rings, fasten your seat belt" and the goal-response rule "to silence the alarm [the goal], fasten your seat belt" do imply the same response on hearing the alarm. Thus, just from observing the overt response (fastening the seat belt), it is not possible to infer the type of rule it was based on.

5. A conceptually different approach was pursued by Forstmann et al. (2006), who allowed subjects to freely choose which task to implement next.

6. Instead, readiness response time and target response time were positively correlated. According to Meiran et al. (2002), this somewhat paradoxical pattern suggests that readiness response time, rather than reflecting an estimate of the internal state of preparedness, merely reflects random fluctuations of the currently adopted speed-accuracy criterion. This criterion then "spills over" into the subsequent period of target processing, thus implicating that a relatively fast (slow) readiness response is likely to be followed also by a relatively fast (slow) target response.

7. Although such an interpretation might seem unintuitive for prefrontal cortex functioning, it would not be the first example of prefrontal cortex operating in an un-

conscious mode. For instance, it has been demonstrated that mid-dorsolateral prefrontal cortex can acquire novel action selection rules without subjects being able to report these rules (Berns et al., 1997).

REFERENCES

Allport A, Wylie G (2000) Task-switching, stimulus-response bindings, and negative priming. In: Attention and performance, XVIII: Control of cognitive processes (Monsell S, Driver JS, eds.), pp 35–70. Cambridge: MIT Press.

Arbib MA (2005) From monkey-like action recognition to human language: an evolutionary framework for neurolinguistics. Behavioral and Brain Sciences 28:105–124; discussion 125–167.

Badre D, Wagner AD (2006) Computational and neurobiological mechanisms underlying cognitive flexibility. Proceedings of the National Academy of Sciences U S A 103:7186–7191.

Barris RW, Schuman HR (1953) Bilateral anterior cingulate gyrus lesions: syndrome of the anterior cingulate gyri. Neurology 3:44–52.

Berns GS, Cohen JD, Mintun MA (1997) Brain regions responsive to novelty in the absence of awareness. Science 276:1272–1275.

Brass M, Ruge H, Meiran N, Koch I, Rubin O, Prinz W, von Cramon DY (2003) When the same response has different meanings: recoding the response meaning in the lateral prefrontal cortex. Neuroimage 20:1026–1031.

Brass M, von Cramon DY (2002) The role of the frontal cortex in task preparation. Cerebral Cortex 12:908–914.

Brass M, von Cramon DY (2004) Decomposing components of task preparation with functional magnetic resonance imaging. Journal of Cognitive Neuroscience 16:609–620.

Braver TS, Reynolds JR, Donaldson DI (2003) Neural mechanisms of transient and sustained cognitive control during task switching. Neuron 39:713–726.

Buccino G, Binkofski F, Fink GR, Fadiga L, Fogassi L, Gallese V, Seitz RJ, Zilles K, Rizzolatti G, Freund HJ (2001) Action observation activates premotor and parietal areas in a somatotopic manner: an fMRI study. European Journal of Neuroscience 13:400–404.

Bunge SA (2004) How we use rules to select actions: a review of evidence from cognitive neuroscience. Cognitive, Affective, and Behavioral Neuroscience 4:564–579.

Bunge SA, Kahn I, Wallis JD, Miller EK, Wagner AD (2003) Neural circuits subserving the retrieval and maintenance of abstract rules. Journal of Neurophysiology 90:3419–3428.

Cohen JD, Dunbar K, McClelland JL (1990) On the control of automatic processes: a parallel distributed processing account of the Stroop effect. Psychological Review 97:332–361.

DeJong R (2000) An intention-activation account of residual switch costs. In: Control of cognitive processes: attention and performance, XVIII (Monsell S, Driver J, eds.), pp 357–376. Cambridge: MIT Press.

Derrfuss J, Brass M, Neumann J, von Cramon DY (2005) Involvement of the inferior frontal junction in cognitive control: meta-analyses of switching and Stroop studies. Human Brain Mapping 25:22–34.

Dove A, Pollmann S, Schubert T, Wiggins CJ, von Cramon DY (2000) Prefrontal cortex activation in task switching: an event-related fMRI study. Cognitive Brain Research 9:103–109.

Forstmann BU, Brass M, Koch I, von Cramon DY (2006) Voluntary selection of task sets revealed by functional magnetic resonance imaging. Journal of Cognitive Neuroscience 18:388–398.

Frith CD, Friston K, Liddle PF, Frackowiak RS (1991) Willed action and the prefrontal cortex in man: a study with PET. Proceedings: Biological Sciences 244:241–246.

Gilbert SJ, Shallice T (2002) Task switching: a PDP model. Cognitive Psychology 44: 297–337.

Goschke T (2000) Involuntary persistence and intentional reconfiguration in task-set switching. In: Control of cognitive processes: attention and performance, XVIII (Monsell S, Driver J, eds.), pp 331–355. Cambridge: MIT Press.

Gotler, A., & Meiran, N. (2003, September). *Implicit strategic preparation towards conflict situation: Evidence from implicit sequence learning of congruence conditions in the task switching paradigm.* Paper presented at the XIII Meeting of The European Society for Cognitive Psychology, Granada, Spain.

Grezes J, Armony JL, Rowe J, Passingham RE (2003) Activations related to 'mirror' and 'canonical' neurones in the human brain: an fMRI study. Neuroimage 18:928–937.

Haider H, Frensch PA, Joram D (2005) Are strategy shifts caused by data-driven processes or by voluntary processes? Consciousness and Cognition 14:495–519.

Hamilton AF, Grafton ST (2006) Goal representation in human anterior intraparietal sulcus. Journal of Neuroscience 26:1133–1137.

Hommel B, Musseler J, Aschersleben G, Prinz W (2001) The theory of event coding (TEC): a framework for perception and action planning. Behavioral and Brain Sciences 24:849–878; discussion 878–937.

Hübner M, Kluwe RH, Luna-Rodriguez A, Peters A (2004) Task preparation and stimulus-evoked competition. Acta Psychologica 115:211–234.

Jahanshahi M, Dirnberger G (1999) The left dorsolateral prefrontal cortex and random generation of responses: studies with transcranial magnetic stimulation. Neuropsychologia 37:181–190.

Kieffaber PD, Hetrick WP (2005) Event-related potential correlates of task switching and switch costs. Psychophysiology 42:56–71.

Koechlin E, Ody C, Kouneiher F (2003) The architecture of cognitive control in the human prefrontal cortex. Science 302:1181–1185.

Lau HC, Rogers RD, Ramnani N, Passingham RE (2004) Willed action and attention to the selection of action. Neuroimage 21:1407–1415.

Lhermitte F (1983) 'Utilization behaviour' and its relation to lesions of the frontal lobes. Brain 106 (Pt 2):237–255.

Logan GD, Bundesen C (2003) Clever homunculus: is there an endogenous act of control in the explicit task cuing procedure? Journal of Experimental Psychology: Human Perception and Performance 29:575–599.

Logan GD, Bundesen C (2004) Very clever homunculus: compound stimulus strategies for the explicit task-cuing procedure. Psychonomic Bulletin and Review 11: 832–840.

Manthey S, Schubotz RI, von Cramon DY (2003) Premotor cortex in observing erroneous action: an fMRI study. Brain Research: Cognitive Brain Research 15:296–307.

Meiran N (1996) Reconfiguration of processing mode prior to task performance. Journal of Experimental Psychology: Learning, Memory, and Cognition 22:1423–1442.

Meiran N (2000a) Modeling cognitive control in task-switching. Psychological Research 63:234–249.

Meiran N (2000b) Reconfiguration of stimulus task-sets and response task-sets during task-switching. In: Control of cognitive processes: attention and performance XVIII (Monsell S, Driver J, eds.), pp 377–400. Cambridge: MIT Press.

Meiran N, Hommel B, Bibi U, Lev I (2002) Consciousness and control in task switching. Consciousness and Cognition 11:10–33.

Miller EK, Cohen JD (2001) An integrative theory of prefrontal cortex function. Annual Review of Neuroscience 24:167–202.

Milner B (1963) Effects of different brain lesions on card sorting. Archives of Neurology 9:90–100.

Monsell S (2003) Task switching. Trends in Cognitive Sciences 7:134–140.

Nicholson R, Karayanidis F, Poboka D, Heathcote A, Michie PT (2005) Electrophysiological correlates of anticipatory task-switching processes. Psychophysiology 42: 540–554.

Norman DA, Shallice T (1986) Attention to action: willed and automatic control of behavior. In: Consciousness and self-regulation (Davidson RJ, Schwartz GE, Shapiro D, eds.), pp 1–18: New York: Plenum Press.

Ollinger JM, Shulman GL, Corbetta M (2001) Separating processes within a trial in event-related functional MRI, I. Neuroimage 13:210–217.

Paus T (2001) Primate anterior cingulate cortex: where motor control, drive and cognition interface. Nature Reviews Neuroscience 2:417–424.

Picard N, Strick PL (2001) Imaging the premotor areas. Current Opinion in Neurobiology11:663–672.

Reynolds JR, Braver TS, Brown JW, van der Stigchel S (2006) Computational and neural mechanisms of task switching. Neurocomputing 69:1332–1336.

Ridderinkhof KR, Ullsperger M, Crone EA, Nieuwenhuis S (2004) The role of the medial frontal cortex in cognitive control. Science 306:443–447.

Rizzolatti G, Craighero L (2004) The mirror-neuron system. Annual Review of Neuroscience 27:169–192.

Rizzolatti G, Luppino G (2001) The cortical motor system. Neuron 31:889–901.

Rogers RD, Monsell S (1995) Costs of a predictable switch between simple cognitive tasks. Journal of Experimental Psychology: General 124:207–231.

Rubin O, Brass M, Koch I, Ruge H, Meiran N (submitted) Anterior and posterior executive control mechanisms resolve stimulus ambiguity: an fMRI investigation of task switching.

Rubin O, Meiran N (2005) On the origins of the task mixing cost in the cuing task-switching paradigm. Journal of Experimental Psychology: Learning, Memory, and Cognition 31:1477–1491.

Rubinstein JS, Meyer DE, Evans JE (2001) Executive control of cognitive processes in task switching. Journal of Experimental Psychology: Human Perception and Performance 27:763–797.

Ruge H, Braver TS (in preparation) Two modes of voluntary control: insights from the self-paced preparation paradigm.

Ruge H, Braver TS, Meiran N (submitted) Attentional, intentional, and volitional aspects of preparatory task control in the human brain.

Ruge H, Brass M, Koch I, Rubin O, Meiran N, von Cramon DY (2005) Advance preparation and stimulus-induced interference in cued task switching: further insights from BOLD fMRI. Neuropsychologia 43:340–355.

Rushworth MF, Passingham RE, Nobre AC (2002) Components of switching intentional set. Journal of Cognitive Neuroscience 14:1139–1150.

Rushworth MF, Walton ME, Kennerley SW, Bannerman DM (2004) Action sets and decisions in the medial frontal cortex. Trends in Cognitive Sciences 8:410–417.

Sakai K, Passingham RE (2003) Prefrontal interactions reflect future task operations. Nature Neuroscience 6:75–81.

Serences JT (2004) A comparison of methods for characterizing the event-related BOLD timeseries in rapid fMRI. Neuroimage 21:1690–1700.

Shaffer LH (1965) Choice reaction with variable S-R mapping. Journal of Experimental Psychology 70:284–288.

Shaffer LH (1966) Some effects of partial advance information on choice reaction with fixed or variable S-R mapping. Journal of Experimental Psychology 72:541–545.

Shallice T, Burgess PW, Schon F, Baxter DM (1989) The origins of utilization behaviour. Brain 112 (Pt 6):1587–1598.

Stuss DT, Benson DF (1984) Neuropsychological studies of the frontal lobes. Psychological Bulletin 95:3–28.

Sudevan P, Taylor DA (1987) The cuing and priming of cognitive operations. Journal of Experimental Psychology: Human Perception and Performance 13:89–103.

Wager TD, Jonides J, Reading S (2004) Neuroimaging studies of shifting attention: a meta-analysis. Neuroimage 22:1679–1693.

Waszak F, Hommel B, Allport A (2003) Task-switching and long-term priming: role of episodic stimulus-task bindings in task-shift costs. Cognitive Psychology 46:361–413.

Waszak F, Wascher E, Keller P, Koch I, Aschersleben G, Rosenbaum DA, Prinz W (2005) Intention-based and stimulus-based mechanisms in action selection. Experimental Brain Research162:346–356.

Yeung N, Monsell S (2003) The effects of recent practice on task switching. Journal of Experimental Psychology: Human Perception and Performance 29:919–936.

13

Dopaminergic and Serotonergic Modulation of Two Distinct Forms of Flexible Cognitive Control: Attentional Set-Shifting and Reversal Learning

Angela C. Roberts

The ability to shift an attentional set and the ability to reverse a stimulus-reward association are two examples of cognitive flexibility that have been shown to depend on the prefrontal cortex (PFC) in a number of different animal species, including humans, monkeys, and rodents (Milner, 1963; Jones and Mishkin, 1972; Owen et al., 1991; Dias et al., 1996a, b; Birrell and Brown, 2000; McAlonan and Brown, 2003). These abilities are dependent on distinct regions of the PFC because lesions of the orbitofrontal cortex (OFC) disrupt reversal learning, but not attentional set-shifting (Dias et al., 1996b, 1997; McAlonan and Brown, 2003), and lesions of the lateral PFC in humans and monkeys (and of the medial PFC in rats) impair attentional set-shifting, but not reversal learning (Owen et al., 1991; Dias et al., 1996a, b; Birrell and Brown, 2000; McAlonan and Brown, 2003). These abilities have also been shown to be differentially sensitive to manipulations of dopamine and serotonin (5-hydroxytryptamine) [5-HT] within the PFC. As a consequence, they have begun to provide us with considerable insight into the critical role of these widespread neurochemical systems in cognitive control processes. This chapter will consider attentional set-shifting and reversal learning, with respect to the different types of control processes that contribute to them and the distinct neural networks that underlie them, and review the role of dopamine and serotonin in their regulation.

COGNITIVE PROCESSES AND NEURONAL NETWORKS UNDERLYING BEHAVIORAL FLEXIBILITY

Attentional Set-Shifting

Behavioral Considerations

An important aspect of complex behavior is the ability to develop an "attentional set." We learn to attend to the sensory features and motor responses that are relevant to performing a task and ignore the features and responses that are irrelevant. When certain features and responses retain their relevance across tasks, then an "attentional set" may develop that biases our perception and responses and increases our speed of learning new tasks as long as those features and responses remain relevant. Such an "attentional set" is an example of an abstract rule. However, flexible behavior depends on being able to shift rapidly between different attentional sets or abstract rules, as demands dictate. Traditionally, attentional set-shifting ability was measured in humans in the clinic using the Wisconsin Card Sort Test (WCST). This required subjects to learn to sort a pack a cards according to a particular dimension, (e.g., color, shape, or number), based on feedback from the experimenter. Subsequently, the subject had to shift from sorting the cards according to one dimension (e.g., shapes), to sorting them according to another (e.g., color) [Nelson, 1976].

More recent studies developed a visual discrimination task that not only provided a componential analysis of attentional set-shifting ability, but also enabled this ability to be tested in both humans and other animals using the same task. It is based on intradimensional and extradimensional transfer tests (Slamecka, 1968) used to investigate selective attention in humans (Eimas, 1966) and other animals (Shepp and Schrier, 1969; Durlach and Mackintosh, 1986). The test comprises a series of visual discriminations, each involving a pair of two-dimensional compound stimuli (e.g., white lines superimposed over blue shapes) presented to a subject on a touch-sensitive computer screen. The subjects have to learn that one of the exemplars from a specific dimension is associated with reward (e.g., a specific white line) [Roberts et al., 1988]. On any one trial, a particular shape exemplar may be paired with one or the other of the line exemplars, and may be presented on the left or right side of the screen. By presenting novel compound stimuli for each discrimination that vary along the same two perceptual dimensions, it is possible to measure two aspects of cognitive control. (1) We can measure the ability to acquire and maintain an attentional set, such that behavioral control is transferred from one pair of exemplars to another within the same perceptual dimension (e.g., from one pair of blue shapes to another) [intradimensional shift] (IDS). (2) We can measure the ability to shift an attentional set from one perceptual dimension to another (e.g., from a pair of blue shapes to a pair of white lines) [extradimensional shift] (EDS).

This test differs from other task-switching paradigms (e.g., see Chapter 11) in that its emphasis is on learning. Thus, the subject has to learn which of an array of stimuli in the environment is relevant to the task, acquire a higher-order rule or response strategy that facilitates successful performance across the series of discriminations, and subsequently, at the EDS stage of the test, learn to abandon one response strategy in favor of a new strategy. In contrast, in other task-switching paradigms, the learning component is minimized. Subjects are required to switch between the use of one or the other of two previously acquired higher-order rules to perform a discrimination task, with the appropriate rule to be used being cued in advance of the trial (e.g., Rogers et al., 1998; Stoet and Snyder, 2003). In addition, in many such paradigms, reconfiguration of stimulus-response mappings is also required at the time of the switch from one higher-order rule to another, thus confounding these two processes.

Neuronal Networks Underlying Attentional Set-Shifting

A recent functional magnetic resonance imaging (fMRI) study (Hampshire and Owen, 2006) sought to fractionate the specific components of attentional set-shifting using a task design that the authors argued overcame some of the confounding factors that were present in earlier human imaging studies of set-shifting (Konishi et al., 1998b; Rogers et al., 2000; Nagahama et al., 2001). The compound stimuli presented to subjects were composed of two dimensions—buildings and faces—superimposed on one another, and subjects learned to select an exemplar from one or the other of these dimensions across a series of discriminations. By comparing neural activity between different switching conditions, it was revealed that the ventrolateral PFC was differentially activated when attention was switched between stimulus dimensions. This finding was consistent with some of the earlier imaging studies (Nagahama et al., 2001). It is also consistent with the selective deficit in switching attention between abstract dimensions in New World monkeys with lesions of the lateral PFC (Dias et al., 1996b). These lesions include an area reported to be comparable to ventrolateral area 12/47 in rhesus monkeys and humans (Burman et al., 2006). In rats, an impaired ability to switch attentional sets is associated with lesions of the medial PFC (Birrell and Brown, 2000). This region shares similar anatomical patterns of connectivity with the medial PFC in primates (Ongur and Price, 2000), but has also been proposed to share some functional homology with dorsolateral regions of the primate PFC (Brown and Bowman, 2002; Uylings et al., 2003). Now, given its proposed role in set-shifting, it would also appear to share some homology with the primate ventrolateral PFC. However, until the contribution of the primate medial PFC to set-shifting is investigated, the true extent of any homology between the rat medial PFC and the primate ventrolateral PFC remains unclear.

Interestingly, the ability of the ventrolateral PFC to contribute to attentional set-shifting does not appear to depend on its interaction with the underlying striatum. In an earlier positron emission tomography study (Rogers et al.,

2000), activations in the PFC related to attentional set-shifting were not accompanied by corresponding activations in the striatum, even though other types of response shifting in that same study (i.e., reversal learning) did induce striatal activation. A more recent study designed specifically to address this issue also found no striatal activation when switching between abstract rules (Cools et al., 2004), a finding supported by the intact rule-shifting performance of patients with striatal damage (Cools et al 2006). However, it should be noted that the damage in this study was restricted to the putamen, sparing the head of the caudate.

The ventrolateral PFC, besides being activated during shifting of higher-order attentional sets, is also activated in a variety of other, relatively simple paradigms, including go/no-go (Konishi et al., 1998a, 1999) and discrimination reversal tasks (Cools et al., 2002)—tasks that all have in common the reconfiguration of stimulus-response mappings. Consequently, it has been argued by a number of authors that the ventrolateral PFC region in humans may have a general adaptive function, being involved whenever behavioral change is required (Aron et al., 2004; Cools et al., 2004). However, an alternative explanation lies in the finding that this region has also been implicated in the development and maintenance of an attentional set, and not just in set-shifting.

In many theories of cognitive control, the mechanisms by which currently relevant representations are maintained must act in concert with those involved in updating such representations in response to newly relevant information (Braver and Cohen, 2000; Botvinick et al., 2001). If the representations are too stable and fully protected from irrelevant distractors, then newly relevant information may be ignored, resulting in cognitive inflexibility. In contrast, if salient cues are able to enter the network too easily, then currently relevant representations do not become stable, resulting in distractibility. Evidence from electrophysiological and lesion studies have emphasized a role for the ventrolateral PFC in the attentional selection of behaviorally relevant stimuli (Sakagami and Niki, 1994; Rushworth et al., 2005) and behaviorally relevant dimensions of stimuli (Corbetta et al., 1991; Brass and von Cramon, 2004). In addition, the ventrolateral PFC has been implicated in the learning of abstract rules, including delayed matching and nonmatching-to-sample. Although electrophysiological studies have identified such rule-learning activity in dorsolateral, ventrolateral, and orbitofrontal regions (Wallis et al., 2001a), findings from lesion studies have directly implicated the ventrolateral region in the process by which such rules guide response selection (Kowalska et al., 1991; Malkova et al., 2000; Wallis et al., 2001b). Indeed, activations in this region during selective attention to behaviorally relevant dimensions coincide with enhanced activations in the region of the posterior sensory cortex involved in the processing of the particular sensory dimension being attended to (Corbetta et al., 1991). Because it appears that the specific sensory regions processing the incoming information do not appear to be involved in rule-learning per se (see Chapters 2 and 18), this enhanced activation in the posterior sensory regions probably reflects enhanced processing of the specific

exemplars within a dimension. Thus, the ventrolateral PFC appears to be involved in the learning and maintenance of higher-order rules. If so, another explanation for why this region is activated in functional neuroimaging studies using simple tasks of go/no-go and discrimination reversal is that such studies have required subjects to perform multiple discriminations, very likely resulting in the development of higher-order rules or sets to perform the tasks (e.g., "if it's not this stimulus, it's the other").

Summary

An important component of flexible behavior is the ability to switch between attentional sets. Findings from multiple studies and methodologies have implicated the PFC in mediating this ability, particularly the ventrolateral region. However, flexible behavior requires flexibility at multiple levels of behavioral control, not just at the level of higher-order rules or sets. One task that has been used to study lower-level flexibility is the discrimination reversal task. This task requires subjects—having learned to respond to one of two particular objects or stimuli to gain reward—to switch to responding to the other, previously unrewarded, or incorrect, stimulus. Unlike attentional set-shifting, in which the switch occurs between higher-order rules or strategies, the switch in reversal learning is at the level of responses to concrete stimuli. The next section considers the neuronal networks that are believed to underlie this capacity.

Discrimination Reversal

Prefrontal Mechanisms Underlying Reversal Learning

At the heart of all discrimination reversal tasks is the requirement to inhibit responding to a previously rewarded stimulus. However, beyond this core requirement, there is considerable variation in how the task is administered. This, in turn, may have quite profound effects on the precise psychological mechanisms underlying the task and thus the regions of the brain contributing to its performance. This is particularly the case with respect to spatial reversal tasks, in which the cues that subjects are using to guide responses are often ambiguous, being either egocentric-based or allocentric-based. If the cue is egocentric-based, then the underlying associative processing may be biased toward action-outcome associations that depend on distinct neural circuitry to that of cue-outcome associations. For example, in rats, the former are disrupted by medial prefrontal lesions (Balleine and Dickinson, 1998), whereas the latter are disrupted by orbitofrontal lesions (Gallagher et al., 1999). It should be noted, however, that the neural circuitry specifically involved in linking allocentric cues with outcome has not been investigated. For purposes of clarity, this chapter will focus on the reversal of specific sensory discriminations involving either visual or olfactory cues.

Consistent across all species tested, including humans, monkeys and rats, is the importance of the OFC in switching responses between one of two cues in

a sensory discrimination task (Butter, 1969; Iversen and Mishkin, 1970; Rolls et al., 1994; Dias et al., 1996b; Schoenbaum et al., 2002; Chudasama and Robbins, 2003; Fellows and Farah, 2003; Kringelbach and Rolls, 2003; McAlonan and Brown, 2003; Hornak et al., 2004; Izquierdo et al., 2004). Also consistent with this is the activation of orbitofrontal regions in fMRI studies of reversal learning in humans, regardless of whether the reward is juice (O'Doherty et al., 2003), happy faces (Kringelbach and Rolls, 2003), money (O'Doherty et al., 2001), or a "correct" feedback signal (Hampshire and Owen, 2006). This is also regardless of whether the reversal task is presented in isolation (Kringelbach and Rolls, 2003; O'Doherty et al., 2003) or is embedded in an attentional set-shifting task (Hampshire and Owen, 2006).

Despite this considerable agreement across both human and animal studies, certain inconsistencies in the literature should be highlighted. First, different studies report that OFC lesions either disrupt reversal learning over repeated reversals or disrupt performance on only the first one or two reversals (Dias et al., 1997; Schoenbaum et al., 2002; McAlonan and Brown, 2003; Izquierdo et al., 2004). There are no consistent differences between these studies that could easily explain the differential effects. Second, fMRI studies in humans show activations in the lateral, but not medial, regions of the OFC that are specifically related to the reversal of the response. In contrast, neuropsychological studies in rhesus monkeys show that object reversal learning is profoundly disrupted after ablations of the medial regions of the OFC that spare the more lateral regions (Izquierdo et al., 2004). One explanation may lie in the finding that the same medial region of the OFC that impairs reversal learning is also involved in representing object-outcome associations (Izquierdo et al., 2004; but see recent findings by Kazama and Bachevalier, 2006), and also perhaps object-object associations that may also be relevant to some reversal tasks (see Roberts, 2006, for a discussion of the different associations that may underlie discrimination learning in monkeys). Thus, activation in more medial regions of the OFC may not be identified in an imaging study that is attempting to identify regions specifically involved in the process of response switching per se. Instead, the involvement of the medial OFC in reversal learning may be related to its ability to represent multiple associations involving the same visual stimulus. Certainly, such a function would be expected to be an important contributor to reversal learning. This is because, after a reversal, the association between the stimulus and reward is not extinguished, but instead, that particular stimulus acquires a second meaning (i.e., no reward) that becomes available along with the first meaning (i.e., reward) [for a review of evidence that the original association remains intact, see Rescorla et al., 2001; Delamater et al., 2004). Consistent with the hypothesis that the OFC represents multiple associations is the finding by Schoenbaum and colleagues that, during the reversal of an odor discrimination, neurons in the rat OFC that were selectively activated by the presence of the previously rewarded stimulus do not reverse their activity. Instead, their selectivity disappears and a different population of neurons acquires activity in response to the previously unrewarded stimulus (Schoenbaum et al., 1998, 1999).

In contrast to the proposed role for the medial OFC in reversal learning, the activation within the lateral OFC that is seen in human imaging studies—and is specifically related to the switch in response away from the previously rewarded stimulus—is more likely to be related to the change in behavior itself, to the detection of a change in the contingencies, or to this region's involvement in processing negative feedback (for further discussion of this issue, see O'Doherty et al., 2003; Kringelbach and Rolls, 2004; Frank and Claus, 2006; Roberts, 2006). That this region is involved in reversal learning is supported by early studies in rhesus monkeys that reported marked deficits in reversal learning after ablations of the inferior convexity region (including the lateral OFC), although the deficit was shorter-lived than that seen after ablations of the medial OFC (Iversen and Mishkin, 1970).

Subcortical Mechanisms Underlying Reversal Learning

Which other neural structures interact with the OFC in the control of discrimination reversals remains unclear. Original studies by Divac and colleagues using radiofrequency lesions implicated the ventromedial caudate nucleus in rhesus monkeys in the learning of object discrimination reversals (Divac et al., 1967). This was reported to be consistent with the known projections of the OFC into this ventromedial region. However, due to the incidental damage to fibers of passage that can accompany radiofrequency lesions, a recent study has been undertaken in marmosets to reassess the role of the primate striatum in visual discrimination reversal learning. The results confirm that a lesion of the striatal regions in the marmoset that receive innervation from the OFC, including the medial caudate nucleus and nucleus accumbens, produce a marked deficit in reversal learning (Clarke et al., 2006a). This deficit is comparable to that seen in rats when performing a reversal of an odor discrimination after lesions of the ventromedial striatum (Ferry et al., 2000). The nucleus accumbens has also been implicated in visual discrimination reversal learning in humans (Cools et al., 2007). However, its specific contribution is unclear because the only deficits in reversal learning associated with a lesion of the nucleus accumbens in rats or monkeys have been spatial in nature, and in the rat, the deficit was not confined to the reversal stage (Annett et al., 1989; Stern and Passingham, 1995). Lesions of the nucleus accumbens on the reversal of either a visual (Stern and Passingham, 1995) or an odor (Schoenbaum and Setlow, 2003) discrimination were without effect, although in the latter, effects on response latency support the role of the nucleus accumbens in incentive learning. Thus, the reversal deficits in marmosets with striatal lesions are more likely due to cell loss in the medial caudate nucleus.

Another region to have been implicated in discrimination reversal learning is the amygdala, based on ablation studies in rhesus monkeys that demonstrated marked impairments across a series of object discrimination reversals (Jones and Mishkin, 1972). Apparently consistent with this were the findings from Schoenbaum and colleagues that, after a unilateral lesion of the OFC, neurons in the ipsilateral amygdala lost the ability to rapidly reverse the

activity related to the conditioned stimulus- that accompanied the reversal of an odor discrimination (Saddoris et al., 2005). Moreover, excitotoxic lesions of the amygdala were shown to impair the first reversal, but not subsequent reversals, of the odor discrimination task (Schoenbaum et al., 2003). In contrast, excitotoxic lesions of the amygdala in rhesus monkeys (Izquierdo and Murray, 2007; Izquierdo et al., 2003) and marmosets (Clarke et al., 2006a) are without affect on discrimination reversal learning.

One likely explanation for these discrepant results may lie in differences between studies in the nature of the underlying associations in discrimination reversal learning. Although the amygdala is important in associating sensory cues with the incentive value of reward, such associations are not the only associations to be formed when an animal learns to select one of two objects to obtain food reward. Alternative associations include those between the object and the sensory properties of the food reward, as distinct from its incentive properties (Gaffan and Harrison, 1987; Baxter et al., 2000; Roberts, 2006). It has been proposed that these stimulus-stimulus associations may depend on adjacent structures within the temporal lobes, such as the perirhinal cortex (Murray and Richmond, 2001), and it may be this region that the OFC interacts with in the performance of the types of visual discrimination reversals used in studies with rhesus monkeys (Izquierdo et al., 2004). Moreover, there is also evidence that the hippocampus may contribute to such learning (Murray et al., 1998). In contrast, where initial learning of the discrimination is dependent on the amygdala, the OFC may well interact with the amygdala in the execution of a reversal of that discrimination. For example, in Pavlovian conditioning, when an animal learns that one of two visual cues is associated with food reward, conditioned orienting to that cue (Hatfield et al., 1996) and accompanying increases in blood pressure and heart rate (Braesicke et al., 2005) are dependent on an intact amygdala. An excitotoxic lesion of the OFC in marmosets impairs the reversal of both the conditioned orienting and the conditioned autonomic responses after reversal of the reward contingencies in an appetitive Pavlovian discrimination task (Reekie et al., 2006). Thus, it is likely that reversal learning in this context will depend, at some level, on interactions between the OFC and the amygdala. What remains to be determined is whether the medial caudate nucleus, as opposed to the nucleus accumbens, is also involved in this type of Pavlovian reversal learning task because the nucleus accumbens has been implicated in the expression of some Pavlovian conditioned responses (Cardinal et al., 2002).

Summary

To summarize, behavioral flexibility is controlled at multiple levels. The different levels appear to be controlled by very different neuronal networks. Attentional set-shifting appears to be under the control of the PFC, especially the ventrolateral region, but the contribution from the striatum appears to be minimal. This is consistent with neurophysiological studies also emphasizing the PFC over the striatum in high-level control (see Chapters 2, 14, and 18).

The PFC also contributes to the low-level control required by discrimination reversals, but in this case, the contribution is from the orbitofrontal region. In addition, subcortical structures, such as the striatum and amygdala, also contribute to the process. The next section reviews the neuropharmacological modulation of these processes.

NEUROPHARMACOLOGICAL CONTRIBUTIONS TO BEHAVIORAL FLEXIBILITY

Neuromodulation of Attentional Set-Shifting

Selective Contributions of Prefrontal Dopamine to the Acquisition and Shifting of Attentional Sets

Recognition that dopamine plays a central role in cognition is reflected in the prominence that dopamine is given in the many neurocomputational models seeking to identify the specific processing within and between the PFC and basal ganglia that underlies cognitive flexibility (Servan-Schreiber et al., 1998a, b; Braver and Cohen, 1999, 2000; Cohen et al., 2002; Frank, 2005; Frank and Claus, 2006). This prominence stems from the landmark study of Brozoski and colleagues (Brozoski et al., 1979) demonstrating that 6-hydroxydopamine (6-OHDA)-induced dopamine lesions of the dorsolateral PFC in rhesus monkeys markedly impaired performance on a spatial delayed response task. This deficit was almost as profound as that seen after ablation of the PFC itself. Further work revealed the selective contribution of dopamine D1 receptors to spatial delayed response performance (Sawaguchi and Goldman-Rakic, 1991) and also identified a critical role for dopamine in regulating the level of persistent firing of prefrontal neurons that are engaged specifically during the delay period of such tasks (Sawaguchi et al., 1990). However, only more recently have the effects of dopamine on prefrontal functions, other than those related specifically to spatial working memory, been investigated, and it is these that will be the focus of this discussion.

As discussed earlier, the ability to switch attentional sets was known to depend on an intact PFC (Milner, 1963). In addition, this ability was impaired in a number of patient groups in which dysregulation of cortical dopamine was implicated, including Parkinson's disease (Taylor et al., 1986; Canavan et al., 1989; Downes et al., 1989) and progressive supranuclear palsy (Pillon et al., 1986; Robbins et al., 1994). Thus, the contribution of prefrontal dopamine to attentional set-shifting was investigated (Roberts et al., 1994). Marmosets were trained to perform a series of visual discriminations in which, for any one individual, the exemplars from one particular perceptual dimension were consistently associated with reward. Having acquired this rule before surgery, marmosets with 6-OHDA-induced depletions of prefrontal dopamine (and to a lesser extent, norepinephrine) performed equivalently to control animals on a series of discriminations requiring intradimensional shifts. However, on learning a new discrimination requiring a shift of attentional set

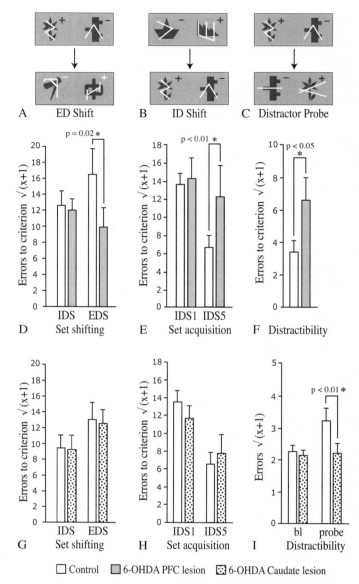

A ED Shift

B ID Shift

C Distractor Probe

D Set shifting

E Set acquisition

F Distractibility

G Set shifting

H Set acquisition

I Distractibility

□ Control   ■ 6-OHDA PFC lesion   ▦ 6-OHDA Caudate lesion

Figure 13–1 The effects of 6-hydroxydopamine (6-OHDA) lesions of the prefrontal cortex (PFC) and caudate nucleus on the acquisition and shifting of attentional sets. An example of a discrimination requiring a shift of attentional set (i.e., extradimensional shift [EDS]), from shapes to lines, is depicted in A. *Bottom.* A visual discrimination in which a line exemplar is associated with reward and exemplars from the shape dimension that had been relevant previously (*top*) are irrelevant. The mean number of errors to meet the criteria for these two types of discrimination (i.e., intradimensional shift [IDS] and EDS) in animals with 6-OHDA lesions of the PFC and caudate nucleus is shown in D (Roberts

(i.e., extradimensional shift), the animals with lesions made fewer errors than control animals (see Fig. 13–1A and *D*). Thus, unlike patients with Parkinson's disease, marmosets with depleted dopamine levels were actually better at shifting an attentional set.

This unexpected enhancement in shifting an attentional set was later attributed to a deficit in acquiring an attentional set because a subsequent study revealed that 6-OHDA lesions of the PFC, made before any training, disrupted the acquisition of a series of discriminations requiring intradimensional shifts (Crofts et al., 2001) [see Fig 13–1 B and *E*]. Based on these findings, it was hypothesized that dopamine contributed to the process of attentional selection, and in the absence of prefrontal dopamine, animals were less able to attend to the relevant stimuli and more likely to attend to irrelevant stimuli. In other words, because the animals were not "tuned in" to the relevant features of the task in the first place, they subsequently found it easier to shift attention away from those features.

In support of this hypothesis, marmosets with 6-OHDA lesions were shown to be more susceptible to distraction than control animals (Crofts et al., 2001). Having learned to select an exemplar from the relevant dimension of a compound discrimination, the marmosets with 6-OHDA lesions were impaired at continuing to select this exemplar if the exemplars from the irrelevant dimension were replaced with novel exemplars (see Fig 13–1C and *F*).

---

et al., 1994) and *G* (Crofts et al., 2001), respectively. The expected increase in errors on the EDS, compared with the preceding IDS, seen in control animals and animals with 6-OHDA lesions of the caudate nucleus, is not seen in animals with 6-OHDA lesions of the PFC. The latter show a decrease in errors on the EDS. Examples of discriminations in which the same dimension remains relevant are shown in *B*, and the errors to criterion on the first and last discriminations, of a series of five, are shown for 6-OHDA lesions of the PFC and caudate nucleus in *E* and *H*, respectively (Crofts et al., 2001). The expected decrease in errors from the first to the last discrimination, reflecting acquisition of an attentional set, is not shown by animals with 6-OHDA lesions of the PFC, in contrast to control animals. To measure distractibility, novel exemplars from the irrelevant dimension are introduced into a discrimination that has been learned to a criterion level of performance, as depicted in *C*. The effects of 6-OHDA lesions of the PFC and caudate nucleus on this distractor test are shown in *F* and *I*, respectively (Crofts et al., 2001). Distractibility is reduced by 6-OHDA lesions of the caudate nucleus and enhanced by 6-OHDA lesions of the PFC. For comparison purposes, all data have been square root–transformed. However, where statistical significance between groups is indicated, this is based on the statistical analysis performed on the original data set described in full in the original publications. Control groups all received sham-operated control procedures. *Black lettering* indicates that shapes were the relevant dimension, and *white lettering* indicates that lines were the relevant dimension. bl, baseline performance at criterion; probe, performance on the day of the distractor probe; +, stimulus associated with reward; −, stimulus not associated with reward.

These findings provide empirical support for the computational models of prefrontal function proposed by Cohen and Durstewitz (Cohen and Servan-Schreiber, 1993; Braver and Cohen, 2000; Durstewitz et al., 2000). Their models suggest that dopamine plays a role in stabilizing representations within the PFC, as well as gating relevant and irrelevant information into the PFC—effects hypothesized to depend on tonic and phasic dopamine, respectively. Without dopamine in the PFC, the marmosets had difficulty gating the relevant and irrelevant features of the task and thus had difficulty ignoring changes to the irrelevant features.

Because 6-OHDA lesions of the PFC disrupted the ability to develop an attentional set, it was difficult to determine any involvement of dopamine in switching attentional sets in the same preparation. However, an improvement in attentional set-shifting, without any apparent effect on the acquisition of the attentional set, has been shown to occur after peripheral administration of tolcapone, an inhibitor to catechol-O-methyltransferase, an enzyme involved in catecholamine metabolism (Tunbridge et al., 2004). Inhibition of this enzyme resulted in marked elevations in stimulated dopamine release, but not in norepinephrine release, within the medial PFC of rats, thereby implicating prefrontal dopamine in set-shifting. More direct support for a role of dopamine in set-shifting has come from a series of studies investigating the behavioral effects of selective dopamine receptor agonists and antagonists infused directly into the rat medial PFC. Antagonists to both the D1 and D2 receptors have been shown to impair the ability of rats in a maze to shift from using a place to a visual cue strategy (or vice versa), whereas agonists to those same receptors were without effect (Ragozzino, 2002; Floresco et al., 2006). In contrast, an antagonist of the D4 receptor improved, whereas a D4 agonist impaired set-shifting ability. As discussed by Floresco and Magyar (2006), these effects may be understood in terms of the cooperative interaction between D1 and D2 receptor actions on the cellular activity of PFC neurons. Thus, the role of D2 receptors in increasing the excitability of PFC pyramidal neurons by decreasing inhibition, and thereby gating incoming information, may facilitate the ability of prefrontal networks to disengage from previously relevant cues and be activated by novel cues. These effects may be complemented by the role of D1 receptors in maintaining persistent levels of activity in prefrontal networks, acting to stabilize those representations that are currently task-relevant. For a review of the cellular actions of dopamine in the PFC, see Seamans and Yang (2004).

The factors that determine whether the effects seen after dopamine manipulations are primarily ones of distractibility, as seen in the attentional set-shifting studies in marmosets, or specifically in task set-shifting, as occurs after selective manipulations of D1 and D2 receptors in the medial PFC of rats, are unclear. Overall levels of dopaminergic tone may be a contributory factor because these will differ substantially between studies in which 6-OHDA has induced permanent reductions in prefrontal dopamine and those in which selective receptors have been temporarily inactivated. Certainly, the finding of

enhanced distractibility in marmosets with 6-OHDA PFC lesions is consistent with the proposal of Seamans and Yang (2004) that overall hypofunction of the prefrontal dopamine system would cause persistent activity states to be unstable to distractors. However, another contributory factor may be differences in the susceptibility to disruption of the acquisition and switching stages in different tasks. Thus, if competing stimuli are within the same sensory system (e.g., vision), as in the marmoset studies, then it is likely that there is considerably more interference, and thus more distraction at the acquisition stage, than if the stimuli are from distinct sensory systems (and thus more spatially separated), as in the rat studies. This may explain why the acquisition stages are more sensitive to disruption after dopamine manipulations in the marmoset studies than in the rat studies. In contrast, the opposite may be the case at the shift stage, when a switch in attention between sensory dimensions may be considerably more demanding than a switch within the same sensory dimension, and thus more vulnerable to dopamine manipulations. (This hypothesis is based on the assumption that the more spatially separate stimuli are, the less likely they are to interfere with one another, which is an advantage when one set of stimuli need to be ignored, as during an IDS, but is a disadvantage when the "ignored" stimuli subsequently require attention, as in an EDS). An additional factor that may contribute to the differences seen in set-shifting and set acquisition after prefrontal dopamine manipulations in rats and monkeys is the level of response conflict. This is greater in the rat studies because the same stimuli are present at the time of the switch. Thus, rats are not only required to switch at the level of attentional sets but also have to inhibit responding to a previously rewarded stimulus, similar to that in reversal learning, thereby confounding these two distinct processes.

Acquisition and Shifting of Attentional Sets
Are Insensitive to Serotonin Manipulations

In contrast to dopamine, there is little evidence to support a role for prefrontal serotonin in attentional set-shifting, although, as discussed later, serotonin does contribute to reversal learning. Reductions of central serotonergic function in humans, as a consequence of dietary tryptophan depletion, have no effect on the ability of subjects to acquire or shift attentional sets (Park et al., 1994; Talbot et al., 2006), even when the attentional demands are increased by asking subjects to learn discriminations composed of three, rather than two, dimensions (Rogers et al., 1999b). More specifically, when serotonin depletions restricted to the PFC have been induced in marmosets using 5,7, dihydroxytryptamine (5,7-DHT), they have had no effect on the ability of marmosets to shift an attentional set (see Fig. 13–2A and C), despite disrupting other aspects of prefrontal function (Clarke et al., 2004, 2005) [see Figs. 13–2B and D and 13–3C]. Subchronic administration of two selective 5-HT6 receptor antagonists in rats has been shown recently to improve attentional set-shifting performance (Hatcher et al., 2005). However, it is unlikely that these drug effects were very selective to set-shifting per se, because the drug-treated rats also showed an

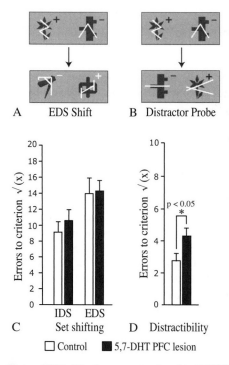

Figure 13–2 The effects of 5,7, dihydroxytryptamine (5,7-DHT) lesions of the pre-frontal cortex (PFC) on the shifting of attentional sets and on distraction (Clarke et al., 2005). An example of a discrimination requiring a shift of attentional set (i.e., intradimensional shift [IDS] and extradimensional shift [EDS]), from shapes to lines, is depicted in *A* and is equivalent to that depicted and described in Figure 13–1*A*. The mean number of errors to meet the criteria on each of these two types of discrimination (i.e., IDS and EDS), in animals with 5,7-DHT lesions of the PFC is shown in *C*. A comparable increase in errors on the EDS, compared with the preceding IDS, is seen in control animals and animals with 5,7-DHT lesions of the PFC. Introduction of novel exemplars from the irrelevant dimension into a discrimination that has been learned to a criterion level of performance is depicted in *B*. Distractibility is increased by 5,7-DHT lesions of the PFC (*D*) although this increase does not appear to be as great as that seen for 6-hydroxydopamine lesions of the PFC (see Fig. 13–1*F*). For comparison purposes, the data have been square root transformed. However, where statistical significance between groups is indicated, this is based on the statistical analysis performed on the original data set described in full in the original publications. Control groups all received sham-operated control procedures. *Black lettering* indicates that shapes were the relevant dimension, and *white lettering* indicates that lines were the relevant di-mension. +, stimulus was associated with reward; −, stimuli were not associated with reward.

overall improvement in performance across the task involving simple and compound discriminations, reversals, and intradimensional shifts. Indeed, these generalized improvements in task performance are consistent with a role for 5-HT6 antagonists in cognitive enhancement, an effect that may be due to alterations in the transmission of several transmitters, including acetylcholine (Mitchell and Neumaier, 2005). Such a lack of effect of serotonin manipulations on set-shifting may explain why atypical antipsychotics, such as clozapine, which have a strong affinity for 5-HT2a and 5-HT1a receptors (Ichikawa et al., 2001), have inconsistent effects on set-shifting deficits in patients with schizophrenia (Goldberg et al., 1993; Hagger et al., 1993; Lee et al., 1994).

Caudate Dopamine Loss Has No Effect on Attentional Set-Shifting Ability, But Induces a Form of Stimulus-Bound Behavior

In contrast to the effects of 6-OHDA lesions of the PFC on attentional selection and set-shifting ability, 6-OHDA lesions of the caudate nucleus are without effect on either the ability to shift an attentional set (Fig. 13–1*G*) or the ability to develop an attentional set (Crofts et al., 2001) [see Fig. 13–1*H*]. The same lesion, however, did disrupt spatial delayed response performance (Collins et al., 2000). This suggests that dopamine, at the level of the caudate nucleus, is not involved in higher-order rule-learning, at least that measured by this particular set-shifting task. It is consistent with the finding that set-shifting performance in patients with Parkinson's disease on the same task as that used in marmosets is also insensitive to whether the patients are on or off their dopamine medication (Cools et al., 2001; Lewis et al., 2005). The only behavior that distinguished the monkeys with 6-OHDA caudate lesions from both control animals and monkeys with 6-OHDA frontal lesions was their insensitivity to distraction when novel exemplars from the irrelevant dimension were introduced. Instead of being more distracted than control subjects, as was the case for marmosets with 6-OHDA frontal lesions, they were less distracted (see Fig 13–1*I*). However, because their attentional selection and set-shifting performance was equivalent to that of control subjects, any differences at the distractor stage were unlikely to have been due to changes at the level of dimensional selection. Instead, their responses, which appeared to be under greater control by the currently rewarded exemplar than that of the control group, could be described as "stimulus-bound." This implicates dopamine at the level of the striatum in certain aspects of cognitive flexibility, primarily at the level of concrete stimuli rather than at the level of higher-order abstract rules.

However, one study that has implicated striatal dopamine in attentional set-shifting is one in which unilateral activation of D2 receptors in the nucleus accumbens, in combination with inactivation of the contralateral medial PFC, disrupted the ability of rats to switch from using a visual cue to using an egocentric cue in a maze (Goto and Grace, 2005). It was hypothesized that this impairment was a direct result of an imbalance between limbic and cortical drive in favor of limbic input, because the activation of D2 receptors has been

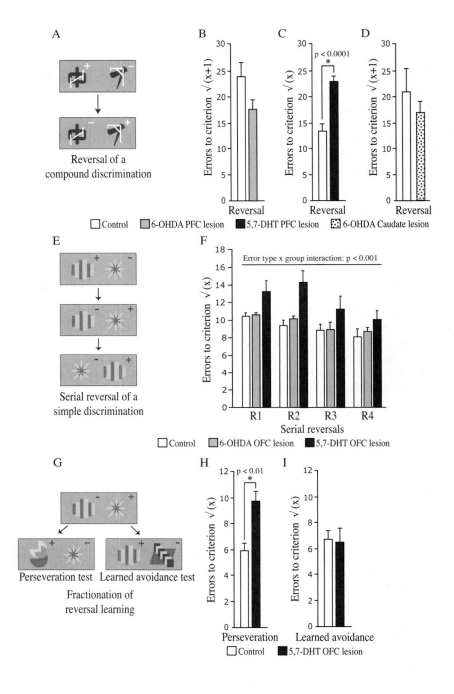

A

Reversal of a
compound discrimination

B

Errors to criterion √(x+1)

Reversal

C

p < 0.0001
*

Errors to criterion √(x)

Reversal

D

Errors to criterion √(x+1)

Reversal

☐ Control   ▨ 6-OHDA PFC lesion   ■ 5,7-DHT PFC lesion   ▨ 6-OHDA Caudate lesion

E

Serial reversal of a
simple discrimination

F

Error type x group interaction: p < 0.001

Errors to criterion √(x)

R1   R2   R3   R4

Serial reversals

☐ Control   ▨ 6-OHDA OFC lesion   ■ 5,7-DHT OFC lesion

G

Perseveration test   Learned avoidance test

Fractionation of
reversal learning

H

p < 0.01
*

Errors to criterion √(x)

Perseveration

I

Errors to criterion √(x)

Learned avoidance

☐ Control   ■ 5,7-DHT OFC lesion

298

shown to suppress medial PFC input, whereas activation of D1 receptors facilitates hippocampal input (Goto and Grace, 2005). Although these effects of dopamine on changing the balance between limbic and prefrontal inputs certainly support a role for striatal dopamine in switching, whether this is at the level of attentional sets is less certain. As described earlier, this particular switching task confounds attentional set-shifting with response inhibition at the level of concrete stimuli. See Chapter 14 for further discussion of these issues.

Neuromodulation of Discrimination Reversal

Prefrontal Serotonin, But Not Prefrontal
Dopamine, Facilitates Reversal Learning

There is considerable evidence that both dopamine and serotonin are implicated in discrimination reversal learning. Drugs that target the dopamine system have been shown to affect reversal performance in humans (Mehta et al., 2001), rats, and monkeys (Ridley et al., 1981; Mason et al., 1992; Smith et al., 1999; Jentsch et al., 2002). In addition, reversal learning is impaired in patients with PD who are on, but not off, dopaminergic medication, an effect that has been proposed to reflect supraoptimal dosing of the ventral PFC-striatal circuitry involved in reversal learning (Swainson et al., 2000; Cools et al., 2001). Similarly, manipulations of the serotonin system also affect reversal learning. Thus, dietary tryptophan depletion in humans, which reduces serotonin availability in the brain, impairs visual discrimination reversal learning (Park

◄────────────────────────────────────

Figure 13–3 The effects of 6-hydroxydopamine (6-OHDA) lesions of the prefrontal cortex (PFC) and the caudate nucleus and 5,7–dihydroxytryptamine (5,7-DHT) lesions of the PFC on visual discrimination reversal learning. The reversal of a compound discrimination is depicted in A, and the effects of 6-OHDA lesions and 5,7-DHT lesions of the PFC and 6-OHDA lesions of the caudate nucleus are shown in B (Roberts et al., 1994), C (Clarke et al., 2005), and D (Collins et al., 2000), respectively. Only 5,7-DHT lesions of the PFC increase the mean number of errors to meet the criterion. The neurochemical specificity of the deficit is shown in F (Clarke et al., 2006b), in which 5,7-DHT, but not 6-OHDA infusions into the orbitofrontal cortex (OFC) are seen to impair performance of a series of reversals of a simple pattern discrimination (R1–R4) depicted in E. The deficit in reversal learning after 5,7-DHT lesions of the PFC is dependent on the presence of the previously rewarded stimulus, as shown in H (Clarke et al., 2006b). In contrast, reversal performance is intact if the previously rewarded stimulus is replaced by a novel stimulus, as shown in I. The two types of reversal test depicted in G are named "perseverative" and "learned avoidance," respectively. As in Figure 13–1, the open bars in each graph represent performance of the sham-operated control groups. For comparison purposes, all data have been square root–transformed. However, where statistical significance between groups is indicated, this is based on the statistical analysis performed on the original data set described in full in the original publications. In the example given, the white lettering indicates that lines were the relevant dimension. +, stimulus was associated with reward; −, stimulus was not associated with reward.

et al., 1994; Rogers et al., 1999a). Peripheral administration of the 5-HT3 receptor antagonist ondansetron also improves visual discrimination reversal performance, although it also improves retention of the previously learned visual discrimination (Domeney et al., 1991). However, the neuroanatomical substrates of these dopaminergic and serotoninergic effects remain unknown. Previously, the same studies that investigated the effects of 6-OHDA lesions of the PFC in marmosets on attentional set-shifting also investigated their effects on visual discrimination reversal learning and found no effect (Roberts et al., 1994) [see Fig. 13–3B]. However, the level of dopamine depletion across the PFC was not uniform. Dopamine depletion was greater in the lateral PFC than in the OFC, but recall that the OFC was determined to be the PFC region crucial for mediating reversal learning. Thus, dopamine may not have been depleted sufficiently to disrupt reversal learning in those studies. Therefore, the effects of large depletions of dopamine within the OFC were investigated in a serial reversal task, and consistent with previous findings, the lesion did not affect reversal learning (Clarke et al., 2006b) [see Fig. 13–3F]. Thus, the disruption of reversal learning that has been reported to follow manipulations of the dopamine system is unlikely to be due to effects at the level of the PFC. Instead, as discussed later, these dopaminergic effects may be at other neural sites involved in reversal learning.

In contrast to the lack of effect of prefrontal dopamine depletions on reversal learning, there is a profound effect of prefrontal serotonin depletions. Large depletions of serotonin throughout the PFC (Fig. 13–3C), as well as more restricted lesions targeting the OFC (Fig. 13–3F), have resulted in marked perseverative behavior such that the marmosets with lesions display prolonged responding to the previously rewarded stimulus after a reversal of the reward contingencies (Clarke et al., 2004, 2005, 2006b). Moreover, this impairment has been present, regardless of whether animals have been performing a series of reversals of a simple visual discrimination (Clarke et al., 2004) or reversing a compound discrimination immediately after a shift of attentional set (Clarke et al., 2005). However, the deficit is abolished if the previously correct stimulus is no longer present at the time of the reversal and the subject has to choose instead between a novel stimulus and the previously unrewarded, but now rewarded, stimulus (Clarke et al., 2006b) [see Fig. 13–3I]. Intact performance on this version of reversal learning rules out any explanation of the reversal deficit in terms of a failure to respond to the previously unrewarded stimulus (learned avoidance). Instead, it supports the hypothesis that a failure to cease responding to the previously rewarded stimulus underlies the reversal deficit. Consistent with this, the reversal deficit is still present if the previously unrewarded stimulus is replaced with a novel stimulus and the subject must inhibit responding to the previously rewarded stimulus and choose instead the novel stimulus (see Fig. 13–3H).

Disruption of a number of mechanisms may be responsible for such apparently stimulus-bound behavior. A failure in error detection is one possibility, and the finding that the processing of negative feedback within the PFC

is modulated by serotonin depletion in humans (induced by a low tryptophan diet) is consistent with such an account (Evers et al., 2005). However, the
region most commonly activated by negative feedback is the dorsomedial
PFC, and although it was activation in this region that was modulated by
serotonin depletion in humans, this region was not depleted of serotonin in
marmosets. Alternatively, an altered responsiveness to punishment or aver-
siveness may have contributed to the failure to inhibit a prepotent response.
The lateral OFC is activated by aversive events, and serotonin has been implicated in the processing of aversive signals. For example, serotonin-
enhancing drugs attenuate the aversive effects of brain stimulation in animals
(Graeff et al., 1986; Smith and Kennedy, 2003), and serotonin has been extensively implicated in depression in humans (Deakin, 1991), depression being
associated with an oversensitivity to negative feedback (Elliott et al., 1997;
Murphy et al., 2003) and perceived failure (Beats et al., 1996). However, serotonin has also been implicated in the inhibitory control of behavior (Soubrie, 1986; Evenden, 1999), and a deficit in response inhibition could be an
alternative explanation for the reversal deficit. Thus, reductions in central serotonin are associated with impulsive pathology (Coccaro et al., 1989; Le-
Marquand et al., 1998, 1999; Cherek and Lane, 2000), and serotonergic drugs
decrease the hyperactivity of the lateral OFC associated with the perseverative
symptoms of obsessive-compulsive disorder (Saxena et al., 1998, 1999).

To summarize, in addition to their dependence on different prefrontal regions (discussed earlier), attentional set-shifting and discrimination reversal
are modulated by different neurochemical systems. Prefrontal dopaminergic
manipulations affect attentional set-shifting, but not discrimination reversal,
whereas the opposite pattern is observed for prefrontal serotonergic manipulations. However, there is one discrepant finding that still needs to be addressed.
Why do dopamine manipulations that do not specifically target the PFC affect
reversal learning?

Dopaminergic Modulation of Reversal Learning
at the Level of the Striatum and the Amygdala

Besides the OFC, other structures involved in reversal learning include the
ventral striatum, and under some circumstances, the amygdala. Because central dopamine manipulations affect reversal learning, but via mechanisms that
are not dependent on the actions of dopamine in the OFC, then a likely site of
action for these effects is the ventral striatum. Consistent with this proposal
are the results from a recent functional neuroimaging study in which dopaminergic medication modulated activity in the ventral striatum, but not in the
PFC, during reversal learning in patients with PD (Cools et al., 2007). However, whether this modulation is at the level of the caudate nucleus or the
nucleus accumbens is unclear (discussed earlier). Moreover, direct evidence
for a role of striatal dopamine in reversal learning is limited. Thus, deficits in
spatial reversal learning have been reported in rats with 6-OHDA lesions of the
nucleus accumbens, but as with excitotoxic lesions of this region, the deficit is

not specific to reversal learning (Taghzouti et al., 1985; Reading and Dunnett, 1991). Moreover, in marmosets, 6-OHDA lesions of the caudate nucleus that left dopamine in the nucleus accumbens relatively intact had no effect on reversal of a visual compound discrimination (Collins et al., 2000). Thus, although the effects of striatal dopamine on altering the balance between limbic and medial PFC inputs are certainly suggestive of a role in switching (and as described earlier, dopamine manipulations do affect response switching) [Goto and Grace, 2005], the specific behavioral contexts in which striatal dopamine plays such a role remain poorly specified. An important question to be addressed is how the balance of those striatal inputs from regions involved in discrimination reversal learning, including the OFC, amygdala, and sensory-related cortices, is modulated by dopamine.

Even more poorly specified are the effects, if any, of dopaminergic regulation of reversal learning at the level of the amygdala. Various aspects of reward processing have been shown to be affected by dopaminergic manipulation of the amygdala in rats (Phillips and Hitchcott, 1998; Di Ciano and Everitt, 2004). In humans, the level of amygdala activity in response to negative emotional stimuli is dependent on specific polymorphisms in the catechol-O-methyl-transferase gene (Smolka et al., 2005), which may affect both dopamine and noradrenaline levels. Moreover, as in the striatum, dopamine has been shown to play a role in altering the balance of inputs into the amygdala from the medial PFC and sensory-related regions. Thus, inputs from the medial PFC that inhibit amygdala output are suppressed by high levels of dopamine that, in turn, enhance sensory-related input (Grace and Rosenkranz, 2002). However, as in the striatum, the role of orbitofrontal inputs into the amygdala, and any modulation by dopamine, are unknown. Thus, any dopaminergic modulation of reversal learning at the level of the amygdala remains to be determined.

CONCLUSION AND FUTURE DIRECTIONS

In summary, it can be seen that the ability to shift attentional sets and reverse visual discriminations is dependent on distinct neural circuitry. Attentional set-shifting involves switching between higher-order rules, and this ability in humans and monkeys is critically dependent on the ventrolateral PFC. The ventrolateral PFC has also been implicated in the learning of higher-order rules, but the nature of the processing within this region that underlies these two functions is poorly understood. A slower rate of learning and a capacity to hold information online, not just within a trial, but between trials, are two aspects of prefrontal processing that, it has been suggested, support abstract rule-learning (see Chapter 18). The ability of the PFC to bias processing in posterior processing regions may also be a critical factor in both the learning of, and switching between, such rules. Whatever the specific processes, at least some of them are dependent on dopaminergic modulation. This chapter has reported the effects of prefrontal dopamine manipulations on the acquisition of an attentional set as well as on the shifting of an attentional set, effects

that may be explained in terms of a role for distinct dopaminergic receptors in the PFC in the stabilization of representations and the gating of incoming information. An imbalance in these two proposed functions can lead to either distractibility or rigidity. Distractibility can cause an impairment in the acquisition of an attentional set, but an apparent improvement when required to shift attentional sets. Rigidity can cause an impairment in shifting attentional sets. Other structures involved in attentional set-shifting remain to be determined. However, there appears to be convergent evidence that the striatum and its dopaminergic input are not involved in such higher-order rule-learning (discussed earlier; also see Chapters 2, 14, and 18). Only when set-shifting also involves response conflict does the striatum appear to be implicated.

Discrimination reversal learning, which does involve response conflict, depends on both the prefrontal cortex and the striatum, specifically, the OFC and the ventromedial sector of the striatum. Unlike attentional set-shifting, dopamine does not modulate reversal learning at the level of the prefrontal cortex. Instead, reversal learning is highly dependent on serotonin at the level of the OFC. Serotonin is critical, specifically, for cognitive processes that underlie the inhibition of a previously rewarded, but currently unrewarded, response. However, dopamine is implicated in reversal learning, and available evidence would suggest that at least some of its effects are at the level of the striatum. This is consistent with the findings that manipulations of dopamine via its different receptor subtypes can alter the effectiveness with which prefrontal inputs engage striatal processing and control response switching. Dopamine may also play a role in reversal learning at the level of the amygdala, because here, too, dopamine modulates the efficacy of prefrontal inputs, inputs that have been shown to suppress spontaneous and sensory-driven amygdala activity. However, any effects in the amygdala would be dependent on the reversal involving the suppression of amygdala-dependent affective responses, such as the conditioned behavioral and autonomic arousal that accompanies the presentation of a conditioned stimulus in an appetitive Pavlovian discrimination task. However, not all discrimination tasks depend on such associations for their successful performance, and so any involvement of the amygdala in reversal learning will depend on the type of discrimination task employed. Moreover, whether dopamine in the amygdala contributes to reversal learning remains to be determined, but if it does, then how such effects may interact with those of dopamine in the striatum becomes an important question to address. Indeed, future research needs to determine not only how the actions of neuromodulators, including dopamine and serotonin, complement or oppose one another within local circuits (e.g., the striatum), but also how their actions complement one another at different levels of a functional network, such as that underlying reversal learning, which may include the prefrontal cortex, striatum, and amygdala.

ACKNOWLEDGMENTS The research described here was funded by a Wellcome Trust Programme Grant awarded to T. W. Robbins, A. C. Roberts, B. J. Everitt, and B. J. Sahakian,

and a Medical Research Council (MRC) Programme Grant awarded to A. C. Roberts. The work was completed within the University of Cambridge Behavioural and Clinical Neuroscience Institute funded jointly by the MRC and the Wellcome Trust. I especially thank A. Newman for help preparing the figures and H. F. Clarke and T. W. Robbins for their helpful comments on the manuscript. I also thank all my colleagues for their efforts in these studies.

REFERENCES

Annett LE, McGregor A, Robbins TW (1989) The effects of ibotenic acid lesions of the nucleus accumbens on spatial learning and extinction in the rat. Behavioral Brain Research 31:231–242.

Aron AR, Robbins TW, Poldrack RA (2004) Inhibition and the right inferior frontal cortex. Trends in Cognitive Sciences 8:170–177.

Balleine BW, Dickinson A (1998) Goal-directed instrumental action: contingency and incentive learning and their cortical substrates. Neuropharmacology 37:407–419.

Baxter MG, Parker A, Lindner CC, Izquierdo AD, Murray EA (2000) Control of response selection by reinforcer value requires interaction of amygdala and orbital prefrontal cortex. Journal of Neuroscience 20:4311–4319.

Beats BC, Sahakian BJ, Levy R (1996) Cognitive performance in tests sensitive to frontal lobe dysfunction in the elderly depressed. Psychological Medicine 26:591–603.

Birrell JM, Brown VJ (2000) Medial frontal cortex mediates perceptual attentional set shifting in the rat. Journal of Neuroscience 20:4320–4324.

Botvinick MM, Braver TS, Barch DM, Carter CS, Cohen JD (2001) Conflict monitoring and cognitive control. Psychological Review 108:624–652.

Braesicke K, Parkinson JA, Reekie Y, Man MS, Hopewell L, Pears A, Crofts H, Schnell CR, Roberts AC (2005) Autonomic arousal in an appetitive context in primates: a behavioural and neural analysis. European Journal of Neuroscience 21:1733–1740.

Brass M, von Cramon DY (2004) Selection for cognitive control: a functional magnetic resonance imaging study on the selection of task-relevant information. Journal of Neuroscience 24:8847–8852.

Braver TS, Cohen JD (1999) Dopamine, cognitive control, and schizophrenia: the gating model. Progress in Brain Research 121:327–349.

Braver TS, Cohen JD (2000) On the control of control: the role of dopamine in regulating prefrontal function and working memory. In: Attention and performance (Monsell S, Driver J, eds.), pp 713–737. Cambridge: MIT Press.

Brown VJ, Bowman EM (2002) Rodent models of prefrontal cortical function. Trends in Neurosciences 25:340–343.

Brozoski TJ, Brown RM, Rosvold HE, Goldman PS (1979) Cognitive deficit caused by regional depletion of dopamine in prefrontal cortex of rhesus monkey. Science 205:929–932.

Burman KJ, Palmer SM, Gamberini M, Rosa MG (2006) Cytoarchitectonic subdivisions of the dorsolateral frontal cortex of the marmoset monkey (*Callithrix jacchus*), and their projections to dorsal visual areas. Journal of Comparative Neurology 495:149–172.

Butter CM (1969) Perseveration in extinction and in discrimination reversal tasks following selective frontal ablations in *Macaca mulatta*. Physiology and Behavior 4:163–171.

Canavan AG, Passingham RE, Marsden CD, Quinn N, Wyke M, Polkey CE (1989) The performance on learning tasks of patients in the early stages of Parkinson's disease. Neuropsychologia 27:141–156.

Cardinal RN, Parkinson JA, Lachenal G, Halkerston KM, Rudarakanchana N, Hall J, Morrison CH, Howes SR, Robbins TW, Everitt BJ (2002) Effects of lesions of the nucleus accumbens core, anterior cingulate cortex, and central nucleus of the amygdala on autoshaping performance in rats. Behavioral Neuroscience 116:553–567.

Cherek DR, Lane SD (2000) Fenfluramine effects on impulsivity in a sample of adults with and without history of conduct disorder. Psychopharmacology (Berlin) 152: 149–156.

Chudasama Y, Robbins TW (2003) Dissociable contributions of the orbitofrontal and infralimbic cortex to pavlovian autoshaping and discrimination reversal learning: further evidence for the functional heterogeneity of the rodent frontal cortex. Journal of Neuroscience 23:8771–8780.

Clarke HF, Dalley JW, Crofts HS, Robbins TW, Roberts AC (2004) Cognitive inflexibility after prefrontal serotonin depletion. Science 304:878–880.

Clarke HF, Robbins TW, Roberts AC (2006a) Reversal learning within orbitofrontal-subcortical networks: the roles of the ventromedial striatum and the amygdala. Society for Neuroscience Abstracts 571.2.

Clarke HF, Walker SC, Crofts HS, Dalley JW, Robbins TW, Roberts AC (2005) Prefrontal serotonin depletion affects reversal learning but not attentional set shifting. Journal of Neuroscience 25:532–538.

Clarke HF, Walker SC, Dalley JW, Robbins TW, Roberts AC (2007) Cognitive inflexibility after prefrontal serotonin depletion is behaviorally and neurochemically specific. Cerebral Cortex 17:18–27.

Coccaro EF, Siever LJ, Klar HM, Maurer G, Cochrane K, Cooper TB, Mohs RC, Davis KL (1989) Serotonergic studies in patients with affective and personality disorders: correlates with suicidal and impulsive aggressive behavior. Archives of General Psychiatry 46:587–599.

Cohen JD, Braver TS, Brown JW (2002) Computational perspectives on dopamine function in prefrontal cortex. Current Opinion in Neurobiology 12:223–229.

Cohen JD, Servan-Schreiber D (1993) A theory of dopamine function and its role in cognitive deficits in schizophrenia. Schizophrenia Bulletin 19:85–104.

Collins P, Wilkinson LS, Everitt BJ, Robbins TW, Roberts AC (2000) The effect of dopamine depletion from the caudate nucleus of the common marmoset (*Callithrix jacchus*) on tests of prefrontal cognitive function. Behavioral Neuroscience 114:3–17.

Cools R, Barker RA, Sahakian BJ, Robbins TW (2001) Enhanced or impaired cognitive function in Parkinson's disease as a function of dopaminergic medication and task demands. Cerebral Cortex 11:1136–1143.

Cools R, Clark L, Owen AM, Robbins TW (2002) Defining the neural mechanisms of probabilistic reversal learning using event-related functional magnetic resonance imaging. Journal of Neuroscience 22:4563–4567.

Cools R, Clark L, Robbins TW (2004) Differential responses in human striatum and prefrontal cortex to changes in object and rule relevance. Journal of Neuroscience 24:1129–1135.

Cools R, Ivry R, D'Esposito M (2006) The human striatum is necessary for responding to changes in stimulus relevance. Journal of Cognitive Neuroscience.18:1973–1983.

Cools R, Lewis S, Clark L, Barker R, Robbins T (20076) L-DOPA disrupts activity in the nucleus accumbens during reversal learning in Parkinson's disease. Neuropsychopharmacology 32:180–189.

Corbetta M, Miezin FM, Dobmeyer S, Shulman GL, Petersen SE (1991) Selective and divided attention during visual discriminations of shape, color, and speed: functional

anatomy by positron emission tomography. Journal of Neuroscience 11:2383–2402.

Crofts HS, Dalley JW, Collins P, Van Denderen JC, Everitt BJ, Robbins TW, Roberts AC (2001) Differential effects of 6-OHDA lesions of the frontal cortex and caudate nucleus on the ability to acquire an attentional set. Cerebral Cortex 11:1015–1026.

Deakin JF (1991) Depression and 5HT. International Clinical Psychopharmacology 6 (Supplement)3:23–28; discussion 29–31.

Delamater AR (2004) Experimental extinction in Pavlovian conditioning: behavioural and neuroscience perspectives. Quarterly Journal of Experimental Psychology Section B: Comparative and Physiological Psychology 57:97–132.

Dias R, Robbins TW, Roberts AC (1996a) Primate analogue of the Wisconsin Card Sorting Test: effects of excitotoxic lesions of the prefrontal cortex in the marmoset. Behavioral Neuroscience 110:872–886.

Dias R, Robbins TW, Roberts AC (1996b) Dissociation in prefrontal cortex of affective and attentional shifts. Nature 380:69–72.

Dias R, Robbins TW, Roberts AC (1997) Dissociable forms of inhibitory control within prefrontal cortex with an analog of the Wisconsin Card Sort Test: restriction to novel situations and independence from "on-line" processing. Journal of Neuroscience 17:9285–9297.

Di Ciano P, Everitt BJ (2004) Direct interactions between the basolateral amygdala and nucleus accumbens core underlie cocaine-seeking behavior by rats. Journal of Neuroscience 24:7167–7173.

Divac I, Rosvold HE, Szwarcbart MK (1967) Behavioral effects of selective ablation of the caudate nucleus. Journal of Comparative Physiological Psychology 63:184–190.

Domeney AM, Costall B, Gerrard PA, Jones DN, Naylor RJ, Tyers MB (1991) The effect of ondansetron on cognitive performance in the marmoset. Pharmacology Biochemistry and Behavior 38:169–175.

Downes JJ, Roberts AC, Sahakian BJ, Evenden JL, Morris RG, Robbins TW (1989) Impaired extra-dimensional shift performance in medicated and unmedicated Parkinson's disease: evidence for a specific attentional dysfunction. Neuropsychologia 27:1329–1343.

Durlach PJ, Mackintosh NJ (1986) Transfer of serial reversal-learning in the pigeon. Quarterly Journal of Experimental Psychology Section B: Comparative and Physiological Psychology 38:81–95.

Durstewitz D, Seamans JK, Sejnowski TJ (2000) Dopamine-mediated stabilization of delay-period activity in a network model of prefrontal cortex. Journal of Neurophysiology 83:1733–1750.

Eimas PD (1966) Effects of overtraining and age on intradimensional and extradimensional shifts in children. Journal of Experimental Child Psychology 3:348–355.

Elliott R, Sahakian BJ, Herrod JJ, Robbins TW, Paykel ES (1997) Abnormal response to negative feedback in unipolar depression: evidence for a diagnosis specific impairment. Journal of Neurology, Neurosurgery, and Psychiatry 63:74–82.

Evenden JL (1999) Varieties of impulsivity. Psychopharmacology 146:348–361.

Evers EA, Cools R, Clark L, van der Veen FM, Jolles J, Sahakian BJ, Robbins TW (2005) Serotonergic modulation of prefrontal cortex during negative feedback in probabilistic reversal learning. Neuropsychopharmacology 30:1138–1147.

Fellows LK, Farah MJ (2003) Ventromedial frontal cortex mediates affective shifting in humans: evidence from a reversal learning paradigm. Brain 126:1830–1837.

Ferry AT, Lu XC, Price JL (2000) Effects of excitotoxic lesions in the ventral striatopallidal-thalamocortical pathway on odor reversal learning: inability to extinguish an incorrect response. Experimental Brain Research 131:320–335.

Floresco SB, Magyar O (2006) Mesocortical dopamine modulation of executive functions: beyond working memory. Psychopharmacology (Berlin). 188:567–585.

Floresco SB, Magyar O, Ghods-Sharifi S, Vexelman C, Tse MT (2006) Multiple dopamine receptor subtypes in the medial prefrontal cortex of the rat regulate set-shifting. Neuropsychopharmacology 31:297–309.

Frank MJ (2005) Dynamic dopamine modulation in the basal ganglia: a neurocomputational account of cognitive deficits in medicated and nonmedicated Parkinsonism. Journal of Cognitive Neuroscience17:51–72.

Frank MJ, Claus ED (2006) Anatomy of a decision: striato-orbitofrontal interactions in reinforcement learning, decision making, and reversal. Psychological Review 113: 300–326.

Gaffan D, Harrison S (1987) Amygdalectomy and disconnection in visual learning for auditory secondary reinforcement by monkeys. Journal of Neuroscience 7:2285–2292.

Gallagher M, McMahan RW, Schoenbaum G (1999) Orbitofrontal cortex and representation of incentive value in associative learning. Journal of Neuroscience 19: 6610–6614.

Goldberg TE, Greenberg RD, Griffin SJ, Gold JM, Kleinman JE, Pickar D, Schulz SC, Weinberger DR (1993) The effect of clozapine on cognition and psychiatric symptoms in patients with schizophrenia. British Journal of Psychiatry 162:43–48.

Goto Y, Grace AA (2005) Dopaminergic modulation of limbic and cortical drive of nucleus accumbens in goal-directed behavior. Nature Neuroscience 8:805–812.

Grace AA, Rosenkranz JA (2002) Regulation of conditioned responses of basolateral amygdala neurons. Physiology & Behavior 77:489–493.

Graeff FG, Brandao ML, Audi EA, Schutz MT (1986) Modulation of the brain aversive system by GABAergic and serotonergic mechanisms. Behavioral Brain Research 21:65–72.

Hagger C, Buckley P, Kenny JT, Friedman L, Ubogy D, Meltzer HY (1993) Improvement in cognitive functions and psychiatric symptoms in treatment-refractory schizophrenic patients receiving clozapine. Biological Psychiatry 34:702–712.

Hampshire A, Owen AM (2006) Fractionating attentional control using event-related fMRI. Cerebral Cortex 16:1679–1689.

Hatcher PD, Brown VJ, Tait DS, Bate S, Overend P, Hagan JJ, Jones DN (2005) 5-HT6 receptor antagonists improve performance in an attentional set shifting task in rats. Psychopharmacology (Berlin) 181:253–259.

Hatfield T, Han JS, Conley M, Gallagher M, Holland P (1996) Neurotoxic lesions of basolateral, but not central, amygdala interfere with Pavlovian second-order conditioning and reinforcer devaluation effects. Journal of Neuroscience 16:5256–5265.

Hornak J, O'Doherty J, Bramham J, Rolls ET, Morris RG, Bullock PR, Polkey CE (2004) Reward-related reversal learning after surgical excisions in orbito-frontal or dorsolateral prefrontal cortex in humans. Journal of Cognitive Neuroscience 16:463–478.

Ichikawa J, Ishii H, Bonaccorso S, Fowler WL, O'Laughlin IA, Meltzer HY (2001) 5-HT(2A) and D(2) receptor blockade increases cortical DA release via 5-HT(1A) receptor activation: a possible mechanism of atypical antipsychotic-induced cortical dopamine release. Journal of Neurochemistry 76:1521–1531.

Iversen SD, Mishkin M (1970) Perseverative interference in monkeys following selective lesions of the inferior prefrontal convexity. Experimental Brain Research 11:376–386.

Izquierdo A, Murray EA. (2007) Selective bilateral amygdala lesions in rhesus monkeys fail to disrupt object reversal learning. Journal of Neuroscience 27:1054–1062.

Izquierdo A, Suda RK, Murray EA (2003) Effects of selective amygdala and orbital prefrontal lesions on object reversal learning in monkeys. Society for Neuroscience Abstracts 90.2.

Izquierdo A, Suda RK, Murray EA (2004) Bilateral orbital prefrontal cortex lesions in rhesus monkeys disrupt choices guided by both reward value and reward contingency. Journal of Neuroscience 24:7540–7548.

Jentsch JD, Olausson P, De La Garza R II, Taylor JR (2002) Impairments of reversal learning and response perseveration after repeated, intermittent cocaine administrations to monkeys. Neuropsychopharmacology 26:183–190.

Jones B, Mishkin M (1972) Limbic lesions and the problem of stimulus-reinforcement associations. Experimental Neurology 36:362–377.

Kazama A, Bachevalier J (2006) Selective aspiration or neurotoxic lesions of the orbital frontal areas 11 and 13 spared monkeys' performance on the object discrimination reversal task. Society for Neuroscience Abstracts 670.25.

Konishi S, Nakajima K, Uchida I, Kameyama M, Nakahara K, Sekihara K, Miyashita Y (1998b) Transient activation of inferior prefrontal cortex during cognitive set shifting. Nature Neuroscience 1:80–84.

Konishi S, Nakajima K, Uchida I, Kikyo H, Kameyama M, Miyashita Y (1999) Common inhibitory mechanism in human inferior prefrontal cortex revealed by event-related functional MRI. Brain 122 (Pt 5):981–991.

Konishi S, Nakajima K, Uchida I, Sekihara K, Miyashita Y (1998a) No-go dominant brain activity in human inferior prefrontal cortex revealed by functional magnetic resonance imaging. European Journal of Neuroscience 10:1209–1213.

Kowalska DM, Bachevalier J, Mishkin M (1991) The role of inferior prefrontal convexity in performance of delayed nonmatching-to-sample. Neuropsychologia 29:583–600.

Kringelbach ML, Rolls ET (2003) Neural correlates of rapid reversal learning in a simple model of human social interaction. Neuroimage 20:1371–1383.

Kringelbach ML, Rolls ET (2004) The functional neuroanatomy of the human orbitofrontal cortex: evidence from neuroimaging and neuropsychology. Progress in Neurobiology 72:341–372.

Lee MA, Thompson PA, Meltzer HY (1994) Effects of clozapine on cognitive function in schizophrenia. Journal of Clinical Psychiatry 55 (Supplement B):82–87.

LeMarquand DG, Benkelfat C, Pihl RO, Palmour RM, Young SN (1999) Behavioral disinhibition induced by tryptophan depletion in nonalcoholic young men with multigenerational family histories of paternal alcoholism. American Journal of Psychiatry 156:1771–1779.

LeMarquand DG, Pihl RO, Young SN, Tremblay RE, Seguin JR, Palmour RM, Benkelfat C (1998) Tryptophan depletion, executive functions, and disinhibition in aggressive, adolescent males. Neuropsychopharmacology 19:333–341.

Lewis SJ, Slabosz A, Robbins TW, Barker RA, Owen AM (2005) Dopaminergic basis for deficits in working memory but not attentional set-shifting in Parkinson's disease. Neuropsychologia 43:823–832.

Malkova L, Bachevalier J, Webster M, Mishkin M (2000) Effects of neonatal inferior prefrontal and medial temporal lesions on learning the rule for delayed nonmatching-to-sample. Developmental Neuropsychology 18:399–421.

Mason S, Domeney A, Costall B, Naylor R (1992) Effect of antagonists on amphetamine induced reversal learning impairments in the marmoset. Psychopharmacology 269:A68.

McAlonan K, Brown VJ (2003) Orbital prefrontal cortex mediates reversal learning and not attentional set shifting in the rat. Behavioral Brain Research 146:97–103.

Mehta MA, Swainson R, Ogilvie AD, Sahakian J, Robbins TW (2001) Improved short-term spatial memory but impaired reversal learning following the dopamine D(2) agonist bromocriptine in human volunteers. Psychopharmacology (Berlin) 159: 10–20.

Milner B (1963) Effects of different brain lesions on card sorting. Archives of Neurology 9:100–110.

Mitchell ES, Neumaier JF (2005) 5-HT6 receptors: a novel target for cognitive enhancement. Pharmacology and Therapeutics 108:320–333.

Murphy FC, Michael A, Robbins TW, Sahakian BJ (2003) Neuropsychological impairment in patients with major depressive disorder: the effects of feedback on task performance. Psychological Medicine 33:455–467.

Murray EA, Baxter MG, Gaffan D (1998) Monkeys with rhinal cortex damage or neurotoxic hippocampal lesions are impaired on spatial scene learning and object reversals. Behavioral Neuroscience 112:1291–1303.

Murray EA, Richmond BJ (2001) Role of perirhinal cortex in object perception, memory, and associations. Current Opinion in Neurobiology 11:188–193.

Nagahama Y, Okada T, Katsumi Y, Hayashi T, Yamauchi H, Oyanagi C, Konishi J, Fukuyama H, Shibasaki H (2001) Dissociable mechanisms of attentional control within the human prefrontal cortex. Cerebral Cortex 11:85–92.

Nelson HE (1976) A modified card sorting test sensitive to frontal lobe defects. Cortex 12:313–324.

O'Doherty J, Critchley H, Deichmann R, Dolan RJ (2003) Dissociating valence of outcome from behavioral control in human orbital and ventral prefrontal cortices. Journal of Neuroscience 23:7931–7939.

O'Doherty J, Kringelbach ML, Rolls ET, Hornak J, Andrews C (2001) Abstract reward and punishment representations in the human orbitofrontal cortex. Nature Neuroscience 4:95–102.

Ongur D, Price JL (2000) The organization of networks within the orbital and medial prefrontal cortex of rats, monkeys and humans. Cerebral Cortex 10:206–219.

Owen AM, Roberts AC, Polkey CE, Sahakian BJ, Robbins TW (1991) Extra-dimensional versus intra-dimensional set shifting performance following frontal lobe excisions, temporal lobe excisions or amygdalohippocampectomy in man. Neuropsychologia 29:993–1006.

Park SB, Coull JT, McShane RH, Young AH, Sahakian BJ, Robbins TW, Cowen PJ (1994) Tryptophan depletion in normal volunteers produces selective impairments in learning and memory. Neuropharmacology 33:575–588.

Phillips GD, Hitchcott PK (1998) Double dissociation of 7-OH-DPAT effects in central or basolateral amygdala nuclei on Pavlovian or instrumental conditioned appetitive behaviours. European Journal of Neuroscience 10:7903.

Pillon B, Dubois B, Lhermitte F, Agid Y (1986) Heterogeneity of cognitive impairment in progressive supranuclear palsy, Parkinson's disease, and Alzheimer's disease. Neurology 36:1179–1185.

Ragozzino ME (2002) The effects of dopamine D(1) receptor blockade in the prelimbic-infralimbic areas on behavioral flexibility. Learning and Memory 9:18–28.

Reading PJ, Dunnett SB (1991) The effects of excitotoxic lesions of the nucleus accumbens on a matching to position task. Behavioral Brain Research 46:17–29.

Reekie Y, Braesicke K, Man M, Cummings R, Roberts AC (2006) The role of the primate orbitofrontal cortex in emotional regulation: a behavioural and autonomic analysis of positive affect. Society for Neuroscience Abstracts 370.30.

Rescorla RA (2001) Experimental extinction. In: Handbook of contemporary learning theories (Mowrer RR, Klein SB, eds.), pp 119–154. Mahwah: Lawrence Erlbaum Associates.

Ridley RM, Haystead TA, Baker HF (1981) An analysis of visual object reversal learning in the marmoset after amphetamine and haloperidol. Pharmacology, Biochemistry, and Behavior 14:345–351.

Robbins TW, James M, Owen AM, Lange KW, Lees AJ, Leigh PN, Marsden CD, Quinn NP, Summers BA (1994) Cognitive deficits in progressive supranuclear palsy, Parkinson's disease, and multiple system atrophy in tests sensitive to frontal lobe dysfunction. Journal of Neurology, Neurosurgery, and Psychiatry 57:79–88.

Roberts AC (2006) Primate orbitofrontal cortex and adaptive behaviour. Trends in Cognitive Sciences 10:83–90.

Roberts AC, De Salvia MA, Wilkinson LS, Collins P, Muir JL, Everitt BJ, Robbins TW (1994) 6-Hydroxydopamine lesions of the prefrontal cortex in monkeys enhance performance on an analog of the Wisconsin Card Sort Test: possible interactions with subcortical dopamine. Journal of Neuroscience 14:2531–2544.

Roberts AC, Robbins TW, Everitt BJ (1988) The effects of intradimensional and extradimensional shifts on visual discrimination learning in humans and non-human primates. Quarterly Journal of Experimental Psychology B 40:321–341.

Rogers RD, Andrews TC, Grasby PM, Brooks DJ, Robbins TW (2000) Contrasting cortical and subcortical activations produced by attentional-set shifting and reversal learning in humans. Journal of Cognitive Neuroscience12:142–162.

Rogers RD, Blackshaw AJ, Middleton HC, Matthews K, Hawtin K, Crowley C, Hopwood A, Wallace C, Deakin JF, Sahakian BJ, Robbins TW (1999a) Tryptophan depletion impairs stimulus-reward learning while methylphenidate disrupts attentional control in healthy young adults: implications for the monoaminergic basis of impulsive behaviour. Psychopharmacology (Berlin) 146:482–491.

Rogers RD, Blackshaw AJ, Middleton HC, Matthews K, Hawtin K, Crowley C, Hopwood A, Wallace C, Deakin JFW, Sahakian BJ, Robbins TW (1999b) Tryptophan depletion impairs stimulus-reward learning while methylphenidate disrupts attentional control in healthy young adults: implications for the monoaminergic basis of impulsive behaviour. Psychopharmacology 146:482–491.

Rogers RD, Sahakian BJ, Hodges JR, Polkey CE, Kennard C, Robbins TW (1998) Dissociating executive mechanisms of task control following frontal lobe damage and Parkinson's disease. Brain 121 (Pt 5):815–842.

Rolls ET, Hornak J, Wade D, McGrath J (1994) Emotion-related learning in patients with social and emotional changes associated with frontal lobe damage. Journal of Neurology, Neurosurgery, and Psychiatry 57:1518–1524.

Rushworth MF, Buckley MJ, Gough PM, Alexander IH, Kyriazis D, McDonald KR, Passingham RE (2005) Attentional selection and action selection in the ventral and orbital prefrontal cortex. Journal of Neuroscience 25:11628–11636.

Saddoris MP, Gallagher M, Schoenbaum G (2005) Rapid associative encoding in basolateral amygdala depends on connections with orbitofrontal cortex. Neuron 46: 321–331.

Sakagami M, Niki H (1994) Encoding of behavioral significance of visual stimuli by primate prefrontal neurons: relation to relevant task conditions. Experimental Brain Research 97:423–436.

Sawaguchi T, Goldman-Rakic PS (1991) D1 dopamine receptors in prefrontal cortex: involvement in working memory. Science 251:947–950.

Sawaguchi T, Matsumura M, Kubota K (1990) Effects of dopamine antagonists on neuronal activity related to a delayed response task in monkey prefrontal cortex. Journal of Neurophysiology 63:1401–1412.

Saxena S, Brody AL, Maidment KM, Dunkin JJ, Colgan M, Alborzian S, Phelps ME, Baxter LR Jr (1999) Localized orbitofrontal and subcortical metabolic changes and predictors of response to paroxetine treatment in obsessive-compulsive disorder. Neuropsychopharmacology 21:683–693.

Saxena S, Brody AL, Schwartz JM, Baxter LR (1998) Neuroimaging and frontal-subcortical circuitry in obsessive-compulsive disorder. British Journal of Psychiatry 173:26–37.

Schoenbaum G, Chiba AA, Gallagher M (1998) Orbitofrontal cortex and basolateral amygdala encode expected outcomes during learning. Nature Neuroscience 1:155–159.

Schoenbaum G, Chiba AA, Gallagher M (1999) Neural encoding in orbitofrontal cortex and basolateral amygdala during olfactory discrimination learning. Journal of Neuroscience 19:1876–1884.

Schoenbaum G, Nugent SL, Saddoris MP, Setlow B (2002) Orbitofrontal lesions in rats impair reversal but not acquisition of go, no-go odor discriminations. Neuroreport 13:885–890.

Schoenbaum G, Setlow B (2003) Lesions of nucleus accumbens disrupt learning about aversive outcomes. Journal of Neuroscience 23:9833–9841.

Schoenbaum G, Setlow B, Nugent SL, Saddoris MP, Gallagher M (2003) Lesions of orbitofrontal cortex and basolateral amygdala complex disrupt acquisition of odor-guided discriminations and reversals. Learning and Memory 10:129–140.

Seamans JK, Yang CR (2004) The principal features and mechanisms of dopamine modulation in the prefrontal cortex. Progress in Neurobiology 74:1–58.

Servan-Schreiber D, Carter CS, Bruno RM, Cohen JD (1998a) Dopamine and the mechanisms of cognition, Part II: D-amphetamine effects in human subjects performing a selective attention task. Biological Psychiatry 43:723–729.

Servan-Schreiber D, Bruno RM, Carter CS, Cohen JD (1998b) Dopamine and the mechanisms of cognition, Part I: A neural network model predicting dopamine effects on selective attention. Biological Psychiatry 43:713–722.

Shepp BE, Schrier AM (1969) Consecutive intradimensional and extradimensional shifts in monkeys. Journal of Comparative and Physiological Psychology 67:199–203.

Slamecka NJ (1968) A methodological analysis of shift paradigms in human discrimination learning. Psychological Bulletin 69:423–438.

Smith RL, Kennedy CH (2003) Increases in avoidance responding produced by REM sleep deprivation or serotonin depletion are reversed by administration of 5-hydroxytryptophan. Behavioral Brain Research 140:81–86.

Smith AG, Neill JC, Costall B (1999) The dopamine D3/D2 receptor agonist 7-OH-DPAT induces cognitive impairment in the marmoset. Pharmacology, Biochemistry, and Behavior 63:201–211.

Smolka MN, Schumann G, Wrase J, Grusser SM, Flor H, Mann K, Braus DF, Goldman D, Buchel C, Heinz A (2005) Catechol-O-methyltransferase val158met genotype

affects processing of emotional stimuli in the amygdala and prefrontal cortex. Journal of Neuroscience 25:836–842.

Soubrie P (1986) Serotonergic neurons and behavior. Journal of Pharmacology 17:107–112.

Stern CE, Passingham RE (1995) The nucleus accumbens in monkeys (*Macaca fascicularis*). III: Reversal learning. Experimental Brain Research 106:239–247.

Stoet G, Snyder LH (2003) Executive control and task-switching in monkeys. Neuropsychologia 41:1357–1364.

Swainson R, Rogers RD, Sahakian BJ, Summers BA, Polkey CE, Robbins TW (2000) Probabilistic learning and reversal deficits in patients with Parkinson's disease or frontal or temporal lobe lesions: possible adverse effects of dopaminergic medication. Neuropsychologia 38:596–612.

Taghzouti K, Louilot A, Herman JP, Le Moal M, Simon H (1985) Alternation behavior, spatial discrimination, and reversal disturbances following 6-hydroxydopamine lesions in the nucleus accumbens of the rat. Behavioral and Neural Biology 44:354–363.

Talbot PS, Watson DR, Barrett SL, Cooper SJ (2006) Rapid tryptophan depletion improves decision-making cognition in healthy humans without affecting reversal learning or set shifting. Neuropsychopharmacology 31:1519–1525.

Taylor AE, Saint-Cyr JA, Lang AE (1986) Frontal lobe dysfunction in Parkinson's disease: the cortical focus of neostriatal outflow. Brain 109 (Pt 5):845–883.

Tunbridge EM, Bannerman DM, Sharp T, Harrison PJ (2004) Catechol-o-methyl transferase inhibition improves set-shifting performance and elevates stimulated dopamine release in the rat prefrontal cortex. Journal of Neuroscience 24:5331–5335.

Uylings HB, Groenewegen HJ, Kolb B (2003) Do rats have a prefrontal cortex? Behavioral Brain Research 146:3–17.

Wallis JD, Anderson KC, Miller EK (2001a) Single neurons in prefrontal cortex encode abstract rules. Nature 411:953–956.

Wallis JD, Dias R, Robbins TW, Roberts AC (2001b) Dissociable contributions of the orbitofrontal and lateral prefrontal cortex of the marmoset to performance on a detour reaching task. European Journal of Neuroscience 13:1797–1808.

14

Dopaminergic Modulation of Flexible Cognitive Control: The Role of the Striatum

Roshan Cools

The mesocorticolimbic dopamine system is known to play an important role in cognitive control processing. The effects of dopaminergic drugs on cognitive control are most commonly believed to be mediated by the prefrontal cortex (PFC), and a large body of evidence supports a role for prefrontal dopamine in the active maintenance of rule-relevant representations. In this chapter, I review studies that highlight a complementary role for the striatum in a different aspect of cognitive control. It is argued that the striatum mediates the dopaminergic modulation of flexible (as opposed to stable) control of relevant representations. Moreover, the role of the striatum is proposed to be restricted to the flexible control of concrete stimulus-response associations, and not to extend to the control of abstract rule representations.

INTRODUCTION

The ability to adapt to our constantly changing environment requires the maintenance of currently relevant representations in the face of irrelevant information. Such active maintenance is believed to facilitate goal-directed behavior by biasing processing in favor of task-relevant pathways, and is most commonly associated with the PFC (Miller and Cohen, 2001). The importance of the PFC for active maintenance was demonstrated by Jacobsen (1936), who revealed an impairment in monkeys with frontal lobe lesions on the now classic delayed response task. It was later shown that the deficit was alleviated by turning off the light in the testing room, suggesting that the frontal lobes are important for resisting visual distraction (Malmo, 1942). Online active maintenance has been associated with persistent neural activity in the PFC during cue-probe intervals in both humans and nonhuman primates (Fuster, 1989; Curtis and D'Esposito, 2003; Passingham and Sakai, 2004).

Active maintenance is critically dependent on dopamine (DA) in the PFC, as first demonstrated in 1979 by a landmark study by Brozoski and colleagues. These researchers found that DA and noradrenaline (NA) depletion in the

PFC of monkeys caused an impairment on the delayed response task that was almost as great as that seen after ablations of the PFC (Brozoski et al., 1979). Further research has revealed that injection of DA D1 receptor antagonists into the PFC dose-dependently impairs performance on the delayed response task (Sawaguchi and Goldman-Rakic, 1991). In addition, iontophoresis of DA and DA D1 antagonists alters the persistent firing of PFC neurons engaged specifically during the delay of the task (Sawaguchi et al., 1990). In monkeys, DA depletion in the PFC impairs the ability to maintain currently relevant information, not only in the context of a delayed response task, but also in the context of compound discrimination learning, suggesting a general role for prefrontal DA in the active protection of currently relevant information against distraction (Crofts et al., 2001; see also Chapter 13). This hypothesis concurs with theoretical models suggesting that enhanced DA (in particular, enhanced action at DA D1 receptors) increases the stability of PFC representations by increasing the resistance to susceptibility from distractors (Durstewitz et al., 2000). The necessity of DA for active maintenance in young human volunteers is substantiated by reports of beneficial and detrimental effects on delayed response tasks of DA-enhancing and DA-reducing drugs, respectively (e.g., Luciana et al., 1992).

High-level cognitive tasks require more than the ability to actively maintain relevant representations. Overly stable representations may lead behavior or thoughts to become overly focused, rigid, and perseverative. Mechanisms for the active maintenance of relevant representations (i.e., cognitive stability) must act in concert with mechanisms for the flexible updating of those representations in response to newly relevant information (i.e., cognitive flexibility) (Frank et al., 2001; Chapter 13). Cognitive flexibility may involve a system that releases stability, thereby allowing new learning from unexpected outcomes, and selective updating of currently relevant representations in the PFC in response to reward-predictive or otherwise salient cues. What might that system be?

Here, I will review four convergent lines of evidence from functional neuroimaging and neuropsychological studies that suggest that optimal levels of DA in the striatum are critical for at least certain forms of cognitive flexibility (compare with Floresco et al., 2006). (1) Neuropsychological studies have revealed that dopaminergic medication in patients with Parkinson's disease (PD), characterized primarily by DA depletion in the striatum, alters cognitive flexibility. (2) Functional neuroimaging studies with these patients have revealed that this modulation of cognitive flexibility is accompanied by changes at the level of the striatum and not in the PFC. (3) Pharmacological neuroimaging studies with healthy volunteers have revealed that dopaminergic drug administration to healthy people changes activity in the striatum, but not in the PFC, during tasks requiring cognitive flexibility. (4) Work with patients with focal brain lesions indicates that the striatum is not only involved, but also necessary for cognitive flexibility. Together, these data highlight the importance of DA in the striatum for at least some forms of cognitive flexibility. The conclusion that DA in the striatum is important for cognitive flexibility

will facilitate the reevaluation of current theories of basal ganglia function, and has implications for understanding the role of DA in the cognitive profile of PD.

COGNITIVE INFLEXIBILITY IN PARKINSON'S DISEASE IS DOPAMINE-DEPENDENT

One approach to addressing the role of DA in human cognition is by investigating disorders that implicate the DA system. One such disorder is PD, which is a progressive neurodegenerative disorder characterized by motor symptoms, such as tremor, rigidity, and bradykinesia. The core pathology underlying PD is the degeneration of the DA cells in the midbrain, leading to severe depletion of DA in the striatum. There is a spatiotemporal progression of DA depletion, such that in the early stages of the disease, DA levels are most severely depleted in the dorsal striatum (dorsolateral putamen and dorsal caudate nucleus), but relatively preserved in the ventral striatum (nucleus accumbens and ventral parts of the caudate nucleus and putamen) [Kish et al., 1988] (see Fig. 14–1). The degeneration of the ventral tegmental area, with consequent DA depletion in the PFC, is also less severe (Agid et al., 1993). The motor symptoms can be alleviated by replenishment of striatal DA through the oral administration of the DA precursor levodopa (l-3,4-dihydroxyphenylalanine) [l-dopa] or synthetic DA receptor agonists.

In addition to exhibiting motor symptoms, nondemented and nondepressed patients with PD also exhibit subtle cognitive problems, even in the earliest stages of the disease. These cognitive difficulties resemble, but are not identical to, those observed in patients with frontal lobe damage (e.g., Owen

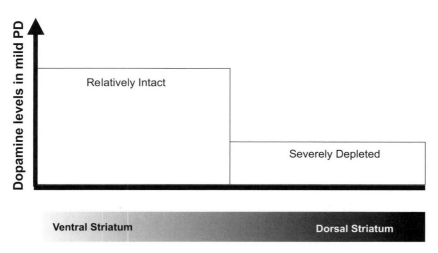

Figure 14–1 Schematic diagram of the imbalance of dopamine in the striatum in mild Parkinson's disease (PD).

et al., 1993). Particularly striking is the patients' inability to adapt flexibly to changes in task demands (e.g., Bowen et al., 1975; Cools et al., 1984; Owen et al., 1992). For example, patients have been observed to make an increased number of perseverative and nonperseverative errors on the Wisconsin Card Sorting Test (WCST), which requires the sorting of multidimensional stimuli according to different stimulus dimensions (i.e., color, shape, or number) [Grant and Berg, 1948; Bowen et al., 1975]. A cognitive switching deficit may also account, at least in part, for other cognitive deficits observed on learning and working memory tasks (e.g., Shohamy et al., 2004).

One major problem with a large number of studies reporting cognitive switching deficits in PD is that adequate performance on the switch paradigms that are typically used (e.g., WCST or the intradimensional-extradimensional set-shifting task) [ID/ED task] (Downes et al., 1989) requires not only cognitive switching but also other abilities. For example, the WCST critically requires working memory and concept formation in addition to cognitive switching. These working memory and learning demands were minimized in a series of studies using the task-switching paradigm (Hayes et al., 1998; Rogers et al., 2000; Cools et al., 2001a, b, 2003). In the task-switching paradigm, the acquisition of task sets is well learned beforehand, and switches are externally cued. The paradigm requires participants to switch continuously between two tasks, A and B (e.g., letter-naming and number-naming), and the sequence of trials (e.g., AABBAA, and so on) enables the measurement of switching against a baseline of nonswitching. The critical measure—the switch cost—is calculated by subtracting performance levels on nonswitch trials from that on switch trials.

Using such a paradigm, we and others have found that patients with mild PD exhibited significantly enhanced switch costs, compared with matched control participants (Hayes et al., 1998; Cools et al., 2001a). The deficit was specific to "crosstalk" conditions, in which stimuli primed both the relevant and the irrelevant task (e.g., "4 G'") and thus loaded highly on selection mechanisms. The deficit did not extend to no-crosstalk conditions, where stimuli primed only the relevant task (e.g., "4 #").

To test more directly the hypothesis that the cognitive switching deficit in PD is dependent on DA, a series of task-switching studies has been conducted with the controlled medication withdrawal procedure. In these studies, patients abstained from their dopaminergic medication for approximately 18 hours before assessment (Hayes et al., 1998; Cools et al., 2001b, 2003; Shook et al., 2005). This work has consistently revealed a significantly greater task-switching deficit in patients who were *off* their dopaminergic medication relative to both control subjects and patients who had taken their dopaminergic medication as usual. The consistently observed beneficial effect of dopaminergic medication on task-switching in PD suggests that the task-switching deficit is due to a lack of DA in severely depleted brain regions, such as the dorsal striatum and connected structures, which are replenished with DA by dopaminergic medication.

EFFECTS OF DOPAMINERGIC MEDICATION
ARE TASK-DEPENDENT

The relationship between cognitive flexibility and dopaminergic medication in PD is complex; contrasting effects of medication have been observed as a function of task demands, indicating that cognitive flexibility is a multicomponential construct. Although task-switching is remedied by dopaminergic medication, other forms of cognitive flexibility are unaffected by medication doses. In fact, certain forms of cognitive flexibility are *impaired* rather than remedied by medication. For example, unlike task-switching, WCST-like extradimensional set-shifting, as measured with the ID/ED set-shifting task, was shown to be insensitive to dopaminergic medication. Two medication withdrawal studies have revealed that extradimensional set-shifting does not depend on whether patients with PD are *on* or *off* their medication (Cools et al., 2001b; Lewis et al., 2005). By contrast, the same medication impaired feedback-based reversal learning (Cools et al., 2001b). Why would the same medication in the same patients improve one task of cognitive flexibility, while impairing another?[1]

To answer the question of why opposite effects of dopaminergic medication are seen on some tasks, we have turned to studies with experimental animals, which have revealed that a complex "inverted U-shaped" relationship exists between cognitive performance and DA, whereby excessive as well as insufficient DA levels impair cognitive performance (Arnsten, 1998). For example, using microdialysis in rats, Phillips et al. (2004) have shown that a DA D1 receptor agonist improved poor performance on a difficult task that was accompanied by low in vivo DA levels. Conversely, the same DA D1 receptor agonist impaired good performance on an easy task that was accompanied by high levels of DA.

The Medication Overdose Hypothesis

As noted earlier, PD is characterized by a spatiotemporal progression of DA depletion, so that, in the early stages of the disease, the depletion is most severe in the dorsal striatum, whereas DA levels in the ventral striatum are relatively intact (Kish et al., 1988). Based on this evidence and previous suggestions by Gotham et al. (1988), it was proposed that medication doses necessary to remedy functioning associated with the severely depleted dorsal striatum would detrimentally overdose functioning of the relatively intact ventral striatum (Swainson et al., 2000; Cools et al., 2001b). In other words, we hypothesized that the contrasting effects of medication reflected differential baseline DA levels in the neural circuitry underlying the distinct tasks of cognitive flexibility.

Evidence supporting this hypothesis came from a study by Swainson and colleagues (Mehta et al., 2001), who showed that, relative to never-medicated patients, medicated patients showed impaired probabilistic reversal learning, which has been associated with the relatively intact ventral striatum and

ventral PFC (Divac et al., 1967; Dias et al., 1996; Cools et al., 2002a; Fellows and Farah, 2003). In this task, participants are presented with two visual patterns. Choices of one stimulus are rewarded on 80% of trials, and choices of the other stimulus are rewarded on 20% of trials. After 40 trials of an initial acquisition stage, the probabilistic contingencies are reversed, and participants have to shift their responses according to these changes in reward values. The deficits in reversal learning correlated significantly with the medication (receptor agonist) dose, such that greater doses were associated with greater impairments in reversal learning. One potential caveat of this study was that the medicated patients were clinically more severely affected than the never-medicated patients. Therefore, the impairment could have been due to increased disease severity rather than to medication "overdose." However, additional support for the "overdose" hypothesis was obtained from studies employing controlled medication withdrawal procedures, in which patients were well matched in terms of disease severity.

In these studies, patients with mild PD were tested on different cognitive tasks, associated with distinct ventral and dorsal frontostriatal circuitry (Cools et al., 2001b, 2003). As predicted, medication withdrawal had contrasting effects on these tasks. On one hand, as described earlier, dopaminergic medication improved performance on the task-switching paradigm, which is known to involve the lateral PFC and posterior parietal cortex (Meyer et al., 1998; Dove et al., 2000; Sohn et al., 2000; Brass et al., 2003), both strongly connected to the severely depleted dorsal striatum. The beneficial effect of medication on task-switching was hypothesized to result from a remediation of DA levels in the severely depleted dorsal striatum. Conversely, the same medication impaired performance on the probabilistic reversal learning paradigm, which implicates the ventral striatum and connected cortical structures, such as the ventral and medial PFC. Thus, relative to patients *off* medication, patients *on* medication exhibited impaired reversal learning, although they performed better on the task-switching paradigm. This detrimental effect of dopaminergic medication was presumed to reflect "overdosing" of DA levels in relatively intact brain regions, such as the ventral striatum.

A second withdrawal study revealed that dopaminergic medication induced abnormally fast (impulsive) responses when participants placed bets in a gambling task; This task has also been shown to activate ventral frontostriatal circuitry (Rogers et al., 1999). Accordingly, the abnormal performance after medication may reflect a similar "over-dosing" of DA levels in the relatively intact ventral striatum. In addition, this second withdrawal study replicated our earlier observation that the same medication alleviated the task-switching deficit (Cools et al., 2003). These medication-induced deficits on the reversal learning and gambling tasks may well underlie the more severe decision-making abnormalities observed in a small sample of patients with PD. Indeed, in some patients, dopaminergic medication may contribute to the development of pathological gambling and compulsive drug intake (Seedat et al., 2000; Dodd et al., 2005; Evans et al., 2006). Together, the results suggest

that dopaminergic medication can improve or impair cognitive flexibility as a function of task demands. Differences in basal DA levels in dissociable (dorsal versus ventral) neural circuitries may account for the contrasting effects of DA.

Medication Effects in Parkinson's Disease Depend on Outcome Valence

Subsequent work has revealed that the effects of dopaminergic medication on reversal learning in PD depend on the motivational valence of the unexpected outcomes that signal the need to change behavior. Frank et al. (2004) have shown, using a probabilistic learning task, that patients *off* medication exhibit enhanced learning from negative feedback and display a persistent bias in favor of "no-go" learning. Conversely, patients *on* medication exhibit enhanced "go" learning from positive feedback.[2]

To test whether these contrasting effects on learning extend to the domain of cognitive flexibility, we investigated the role of DA in reversal learning as a function of motivational valence (reward versus punishment). We tested two groups of patients with mild PD: one *on* and one *off* dopaminergic medication (Cools et al., 2006a). Patients were presented with two stimuli on each trial of a novel adaptation of the reversal learning task. One of the stimuli was associated with reward (a smiley face, a pleasant tone, and an increase in points), whereas the other stimulus was associated with punishment or nonreward (a sad face, an unpleasant tone, and a decrease in points). On each trial, one of the two stimuli was highlighted and participants were required to predict, based on trial-and-error learning, whether the highlighted stimulus would lead to reward or punishment. After a number of consecutively correct trials, the outcome contingencies were reversed so that now the previously rewarded stimulus was associated with punishment and vice versa. The reversal was always signaled to participants by the presentation of an unexpected outcome. This outcome could be either an unexpected reward (paired with the previously punished stimulus) or an unexpected punishment (paired with the previously rewarded stimulus).

Analysis of accuracy on the trial after this unexpected reward or punishment indicated whether participants had learned to reverse the contingencies based on unexpected reward or punishment. The results extended the findings mentioned earlier by showing that the medication-induced deficit on reversal shifting was restricted to conditions in which reversals were signaled by unexpected punishment. Thus, patients *on* medication performed significantly more poorly than patients *off* medication and control subjects in the unexpected punishment condition. By contrast, there was no difference between the groups when the reversal was signaled by unexpected reward (Fig. 14–2). Hence, these data replicate findings from Frank et al. (2004), and further indicate that dopaminergic medication in PD impairs reversal-shifting, depending on the motivational valence of unexpected outcomes. Learning and reversal based on unexpected punishment (or reward omission) signals appear to be selectively vulnerable to excessive DA levels in the ventral striatum.

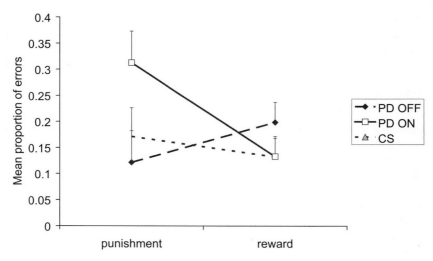

Figure 14–2 Contrasting effects of dopaminergic medication on punishment- and reward-based reversal learning in patients with mild Parkinson's disease (PD). Data represent the mean error rate on switch trials—trials after unexpected punishment (*left*) or unexpected reward (*right*). Patients who were taking medication (PD ON) were impaired on reversal learning based on unexpected punishment, but not when reversals were signaled by unexpected reward. Their performance was significantly different from that of control subjects (CS) and patients who were not taking medication (PD OFF) [for more details, see Cools et al., 2006b].

DOPAMINERGIC MODULATION OF BRAIN ACTIVITY DURING COGNITIVE FLEXIBILITY

Role of the Striatum in Patients with Parkinson's Disease

Do the medication-induced effects on cognitive flexibility reflect modulation at the level of the striatum or the PFC? PD is characterized by DA depletion not only in the striatum, but also, albeit to a lesser extent, in the PFC. Thus, the beneficial effects of dopaminergic medication on cognitive flexibility in PD may reflect effects on the striatum, the PFC, or both. Alternatively, they may reflect indirect effects on the PFC via direct effects on the striatum, which is strongly connected with the PFC in functionally specific circuitries (Alexander et al., 1986).

Functional neuroimaging studies have revealed that dopaminergic medication in patients with mild PD modulates brain activity in the dorsolateral PFC during the performance of complex working memory tasks, such as the n-back task or the Tower of London spatial planning task (Cools et al., 2002b; Mattay et al., 2002; Lewis et al., 2003). This observation concurs with overwhelming evidence for a role of PFC DA in working memory (discussed

earlier). However, the finding that medication modulates the PFC during working memory does not mean that the dopaminergic effects on cognitive flexibility are also mediated by the PFC. We propose here that the striatum plays a critical role in the dopaminergic modulation of cognitive flexibility (i.e., a function that is qualitatively different from—in some sense, computationally opposite to—the requirement of active maintenance in working memory tasks).

To test this hypothesis, we have recently conducted a pharmacological functional magnetic resonance imaging (fMRI) study in patients with mild PD. Specifically, we investigated whether the detrimental effect of dopaminergic medication in mild PD on reversal learning is mediated by the relatively intact ventral striatum and not by other areas, such as the severely depleted dorsal striatum or PFC. Eight patients with mild PD were scanned on two occasions, once *on* and once *off* their normal dopaminergic medication, while they performed a version of the above-described probabilistic reversal learning task, involving multiple reversals (Cools et al., 2007a). As predicted, we found that dopaminergic medication modulated the relatively intact ventral striatum, but not the severely depleted dorsal striatum or PFC during reversal learning. Specifically, patients *off* medication exhibited increased activity in the ventral striatum during the critical reversal errors (which led to behavioral adaptation), but not during the baseline correct responses. Similar reversal-related activity in the ventral parts of the striatum was observed in healthy volunteers in an earlier fMRI study using the same paradigm (Cools et al., 2002a). This concurs with evidence from animal work showing that the ventral striatum is necessary for reversal learning (Taghzouti et al., 1985; Annett et al., 1989, see Chapter 13). Conversely, reversal-related activity in the ventral striatum was abolished in patients *on* medication. Such drug-induced changes were not observed in the dorsal striatum or in any task-related area in the PFC (Fig. 14–3). These data support the hypothesis that the medication-induced impairment in

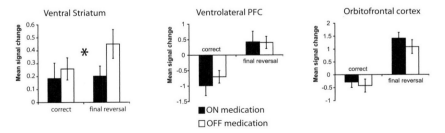

Figure 14–3 Effects of dopaminergic medication withdrawal on brain activity in patients with mild Parkinson's disease during probabilistic reversal learning. Medication abolished activity in the ventral striatum during the final reversal errors that led to behavioral adaptation, but not during baseline correct responses (for more details, see Cools et al., 2007a). PFC, prefrontal cortex.

reversal learning is accompanied by modulation of the relatively intact ventral striatum, possibly by detrimentally "overdosing" intact DA levels. Hence, our neuroimaging results converged with our neuropsychological findings, indicating that reversal learning in PD depends on medication status, task demands, and baseline DA levels in the underlying striatum. The neuroimaging study provided evidence that dopaminergic modulation at the level of the striatum, and not in the PFC, underlies at least some forms of cognitive flexibility. An outstanding question is whether the modulation of task-switching in PD is also modulated at the level of the striatum, but not in the PFC.

Role of the Striatum in Healthy Volunteers

The hypothesis that dopaminergic modulation of cognitive flexibility is mediated by the striatum is further substantiated by data from a recent pharmacological fMRI study performed in young, healthy volunteers (Cools et al., 2007b). The aim of this study was to assess the neural site of dopaminergic modulation of two distinct components of cognitive control: the flexible updating of task-relevant representations and the active maintenance of those representations in the face of distraction. To this end, we assessed the effects of DA receptor stimulation on a match-to-sample paradigm that enabled the separate assessment of cognitive flexibility and cognitive stability. Recent theorizing implicates a particularly important role of the D2 receptor in cognitive flexibility (Bilder et al., 2004; Seamans and Yang, 2004). Given this hypothesis and our primary interest in the role of the striatum, where D2 receptors are more abundant than in the PFC (Camps et al., 1990), we chose to investigate the effects of the D2 receptor agonist bromocriptine.

Based on previous theorizing and results (Crofts et al., 2001; Frank et al., 2001; see also Chapter 13), we hypothesized that the dopaminergic modulation of cognitive flexibility would be mediated by the striatum, whereas that of cognitive stability would be mediated by the PFC. Previous studies have revealed that large variation exists in terms of dopaminergic drug effects across different individuals (see Cools and Robbins, 2004; Cools, 2006), and such individual variation would have substantially reduced the power to detect significant changes.

In our pharmacological fMRI study, we aimed to control for this individual variation. We chose to do this by preselecting participants from a large pool of undergraduate students who had completed the Barratt Impulsiveness Scale (BIS) [Patton et al., 1995)], a self-report questionnaire of impulsive tendencies. The rationale for selection based on trait impulsivity was two-fold: (1) trait impulsivity is associated with reduced DA D2/D3 receptor binding as revealed by recent neurochemical imaging work (Dalley et al., 2007); (2) baseline performance levels in our paradigm were predicted to vary as a function of impulsivity. Therefore, one group of high-impulsive participants and another group of low-impulsive participants were selected from the tail ends of the distribution of total BIS scores (15th percentiles on each end). Both groups

(10 high-impulsive participants and 12 low-impulsive participants) were scanned twice, once after oral intake of a 1.25-mg dose of bromocriptine and once after placebo.

During scanning, participants were presented with four pictures—two faces and two scenes—arranged around a colored fixation cross (location randomized), which also served as an instruction cue. If the cross was green, they had to memorize the scenes; if the fixation cross was blue, they had to memorize the faces. The unpredictable sequence of blue (face) and green (scene) trials enabled the measurement of switching (face to scene or vice versa) against a background of nonswitching (face to face or scene to scene) (Fig. 14–4A).

The initial encoding period was followed by an 8-second delay period during which the stimuli were removed from the screen. After the delay period, a distractor was presented, which participants were instructed to ignore. This distractor was either a scrambled picture or a novel face or scene. The stimulus dimension of the novel picture was always congruent with the task-relevant stimulus dimension (i.e., both were faces or both were scenes). Relative to the scrambled picture, the congruent novel picture was expected to distract participants from their task of actively maintaining the task-relevant encoding stimuli (Yoon et al., 2006).The distractor was followed by a second delay period of 8 s, after which participants were presented with a final probe stimulus that required the pressing of a left or right button, depending on whether the stimulus matched one of the task-relevant encoding stimuli (Fig. 14–4A; see color insert).

Switch-related activity was assessed by comparing activity during the encoding period of switch trials with that of nonswitch trials. In addition, the task enabled assessment of distractor-related brain activity by comparing activity during the high distractors (novel pictures) with that during the low distractors (scrambled pictures). Analysis of performance data revealed higher behavioral switch costs (measured in terms of accuracy at probe) in the high-impulsive participants than in the low-impulsive participants, when they were scanned on placebo. The effects of the drug also depended on trait impulsivity, so that bromocriptine significantly reduced the switch cost in the high-impulsive participants, but if anything, enhanced the switch cost in the low-impulsive participants.

These drug effects on behavior were paralleled by selective effects on brain activity, specifically, the striatum. In the placebo session, switch-related activity (measured during encoding) in the striatum was lower in the high-impulsive participants relative to the low-impulsive participants. Again, the effects of the drug also depended on trait impulsivity, such that bromocriptine significantly potentiated switch-related activity in the striatum of high-impulsive participants, but if anything, attenuated switch-related activity in the low-impulsive participants. These drug effects were both regionally selective and process-specific. Bromocriptine potentiated switch-related activity in the striatum (putamen) [see Fig. 14–4B], but not in the PFC. Furthermore, these effects were seen only during cognitive switching: Distractor-related activity in the

A

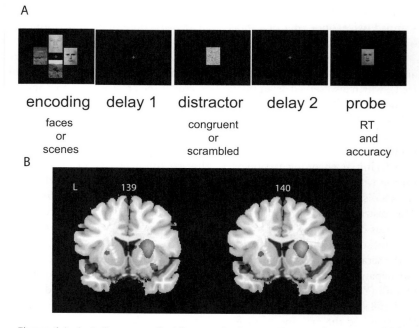

encoding   delay 1   distractor   delay 2   probe

faces   congruent   RT
or   or   and
scenes   scrambled   accuracy

B

Figure 14–4 *A.* Sequence of trial events in the paradigm used to assess which brain regions mediate the dopaminergic modulation of cognitive flexibility and cognitive stability. See text for a description of the task. *B.* Brain activity (contrast values) reflecting a significant interaction effect between impulsive personality (high versus low), drug (bromocriptine versus placebo), and trial-type (switch versus nonswitch). RT, response time.

striatum was unaltered. By contrast, bromocriptine modulated distractor-related activity in the PFC. Thus, in keeping with our prediction, bromocriptine modulated the striatum during the flexible updating of task-relevant representations, but modulated the PFC during distraction (Cools et al., 2007b).

These results support the hypothesis that flexible updating and active maintenance of task-relevant information (in the face of distraction) are mediated by dopaminergic modulation of the striatum and the PFC, respectively. Clearly, there are differences between the type of switching measured in classic task-switching paradigms and the type of switching measured in the current match-to-sample task. For example, this task requires only the switching of attention between stimulus features (and task rules), but not the direct resetting of response sets. The resetting of response sets is a central feature of classic task-switching paradigms. Nevertheless, these results strengthen the hypothesis that the effects on task-switching in patients with PD may also be mediated by modulation of the striatum. The observed effects of DA receptor activation were restricted to high-impulsive participants, who presumably have

DA-related abnormalities in the striatum, highlighting the importance of taking into account large individual variations in drug effects.

IS THE STRIATUM NECESSARY FOR COGNITIVE FLEXIBILITY?

The functional neuroimaging findings in patients with PD and healthy volunteers described earlier support the hypothesis that modulation of cognitive flexibility is mediated by the striatum. However, they cannot provide definitive evidence for the hypothesis that the striatum is necessary for cognitive flexibility. We recently compared the performance of six patients with focal, unilateral striatal lesions with that of six patients with unilateral frontal lobe lesions on a novel task-switching paradigm (Cools and Robbins, 2004; Cools et al., 2006b). The aim of this study was two-fold. First, the study allowed assessment of the *necessity* of the striatum for cognitive flexibility. Second, the study aimed to define more precisely the particular form of cognitive flexibility that is subserved by the striatum.

Earlier work with patients with PD had already indicated that some, but not all, forms of cognitive flexibility depend on DA in the striatum (discussed earlier). Task-switching appears to be particularly vulnerable to dopaminergic dysfunction in the striatum. However, task-switching is a multicomponential phenomenon and may depend on different mechanisms, depending on task demands. Thus, task-switching often requires switching between abstract task rules, which need not have direct instantiation in the motor or sensory domain. This form of flexibility based on abstract rules has been associated particularly strongly with the PFC (Wallis et al., 2001; Bunge et al., 2003). In addition, most task-switching paradigms also require the redirection of attention to different concrete stimuli or stimulus features. In a neuropsychological study, we employed a novel paradigm that enabled separate assessment of switching between abstract task rules and switching between concrete stimuli (Fig. 14–5).

Results revealed that both patients with striatal damage and those with frontal damage had considerable difficulty with the task. However, patients with striatal lesions exhibited a disproportionate switching deficit, whereas patients with lateral frontal lesions did not. Moreover, the switching deficit in patients with striatal damage was restricted to particular types of trials: They were impaired only when they had to redirect their attention to different response-relevant stimuli. The switching impairment did not extend to trials that required switching between abstract rules when there was no change in response-associated sensory input. Patients with much larger lesions in the lateral frontal lobe did not exhibit the same performance pattern, and in fact, relative to baseline nonswitch trials, did not exhibit a deficit in either stimulus-switching or rule-switching.

The dissociation between the striatal and frontal groups is particularly striking, given the fact that the frontal lesions were much larger than the striatal lesions. The lack of an abstract rule-switching deficit in the patients

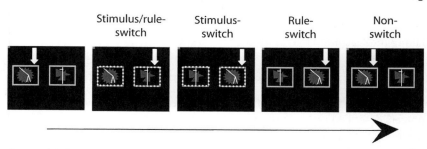

Figure 14–5 Sequence of trials in the paradigm used to assess the effects of striatal and frontal lesions on stimulus- and rule-based switching. On each trial, two abstract visual patterns were presented within blue (here: stippled) or yellow (here: solid) stimulus windows, with the color of the two windows identical for a given trial. Subjects were required to choose one of two stimuli, by making right or left button presses (corresponding to the location of the correct stimulus). The correct choice was determined by an abstract task-rule, which was signaled to subjects by the color of the stimulus. If the windows were yellow (here: solid), then the participant had to respond to the same stimulus as on the previous trial (i.e., matching rule). If the windows were blue (here: stippled), then the participant had to respond to the pattern that had not been selected on the previous trial (i.e., non-matching rule). Thus, some trials required that the participant switched responding between concrete stimuli (i.e., visual patterns), and some trials required that the participant switched responding between abstract rules (as indicated by the color of the boxes). More specifically, there were four trial-types: (1) non-switch trials: the rule and the target-stimulus were the same as on the previous trial, i.e., yellow trials following yellow trials; (2) stimulus-switch trials: the rule remained the same and the target-stimulus switched, that is, blue trials following blue trials; (3) rule-switch trials: the rule switched from the previous trial and the target-stimulus remained the same, that is, yellow trials following blue trials; (4) stimulus/rule-switch trials: the rule and the target-stimulus switched from the previous trial, that is blue trials following yellow trials.

with frontal lesions was not predicted, and this null effect does not provide definitive evidence against a role for the PFC in abstract rule-based cognitive flexibility. Although the latter issue awaits further investigation, we note that the group with frontal lesions did provide an interesting reference point for assessing the performance deficit of the patients with striatal lesions, which clearly was not simply due to nonspecific effects of brain damage.

Selective involvement of the striatum in switching between concrete stimuli, but not between abstract task rules, was also suggested by an earlier event-related fMRI study using the same paradigm in young, healthy volunteers (Cools et al., 2004). This study revealed significant activity in the striatum when participants switched between concrete stimuli compared with trials in which they switched between abstract rules. Finally, preliminary data from a group of patients with mild PD, tested *off* their dopaminergic medication, revealed that their performance pattern was similar to that seen in the patients with striatal lesions (Cools et al., 2007c). Therefore, this set of studies provides

converging evidence indicating an important role for the striatum in the behavioral adaptation to changes in stimulus, although not rule significance (see Chapters 2 and 18). Striatal lesions and PD diminish the efficacy of newly response-relevant stimuli for controlling behavior. These findings concur with observations that DA potentiates the salience of behaviorally relevant stimuli and the notion that DA and striatal neurons signal the behavioral relevance of environmental events (Hollerman and Schultz, 1998). Striatally mediated potentiation of stimulus salience may facilitate flexibility, but only when it requires redirecting of attention to response-associated sensory input.

CONCLUSION

The results reviewed in this chapter suggest that the striatum and its modulation by DA are critically involved in some forms of cognitive flexibility. At first sight, this conclusion may appear inconsistent with classic theory, according to which the striatum mediates the learning and memory of consistent relationships between stimuli and responses, leading to habitual or automatic "priming" of responses on stimulus presentation. For example, Mishkin and colleagues have suggested that the striatum subserves a slow, incremental "less cognitive, more rigid" form of memory, as opposed to the "more cognitive, flexible, and less rigid" form of memory subserved, for example, by the medial temporal lobes (Mishkin et al., 1984). By contrast, our findings suggest that the striatum also supports forms of flexible behavior. This point has been demonstrated repeatedly by the finding of DA-dependent deficits in patients with mild PD on task-switching paradigms that require rapid, flexible updating of task-relevant responses (Hayes et al., 1998; Cools et al., 2001a, b, 2003; Woodward et al., 2002; Shook et al., 2005). In addition, fMRI studies have shown that the dopaminergic modulation of cognitive flexibility in PD and in healthy volunteers is mediated by the striatum and not by the PFC (Cools et al., 2007a; Cools et al, 2007b).

The role of DA in the striatum may be restricted to particular forms of flexibility. Specifically, our data suggest that striatum-mediated flexibility is restricted to the selection of newly relevant response-associated stimuli. In other words, the role of the striatum in cognitive flexibility is limited to situations in which there is a change in response-relevant sensory input, and it does not extend to the updating of abstract rules. The type of switching (both task-switching and reversal learning) that is impaired by striatal lesions and PD involves consistent stimulus-response mappings, and does not require the resetting of links *between* stimuli and responses. What changes in these striatum-dependent tasks is the stimulus or stimulus feature (and, only indirectly, its associated response) that needs to be selected. Perhaps DA depletion in the striatum, as seen in PD, leads to reduced salience of stimuli and consequent stimulus-based inflexibility (i.e., impairment in the redirection to different stimuli that elicit behavioral responses), rather than reduced flexibility of the links between stimuli and responses. Indeed, our bromocriptine study

revealed that the striatum mediates the dopaminergic modulation of switching between behaviorally relevant stimuli, which affected consequent action only indirectly. In this sense, the role of the striatum in cognitive flexibility is not necessarily inconsistent, but rather may coexist, with a role for the striatum in the gradual formation of habits, or inflexible links *between* stimuli and responses.

OUTSTANDING ISSUES

There are a number of outstanding issues that must be addressed in future research. First, one might consider the alternative hypothesis that medication-induced impairments in PD patients relate, at least in part, to nondopaminergic mechanisms. Of particular interest is the serotonergic neurotransmitter system, which has been implicated in negative processing biases seen in anxiety and depression as well as punishment processing (Moresco et al., 2002; Abrams et al., 2004; Fallgatter et al., 2004; Harmer et al., 2004). Critically, l-dopa may inhibit the activity of tryptophan hydroxylase and interfere with serotonin synthesis (Maruyama et al., 1992; Naoi et al., 1994; Arai et al., 1995). Similarly, DA receptor agonists may decrease serotonergic turnover (Lynch, 1997). Accordingly, the medication-induced impairment, particularly in punishment-based reversal learning, may relate to medication-induced central serotonin depletion, biasing processing away from nonrewarded or punished events.

A second issue relates to the dependency of drug effects on trait impulsivity. It is unclear whether the low dose of bromocriptine acted primarily postsynaptically to enhance DA transmission, or whether it, in fact, reduced DA neurotransmission by acting presynaptically (see Frank and O'Reilly, 2006). Future studies may employ multiple doses to establish dose-response relationships.

The data from the pharmacological fMRI study in healthy volunteers suggest that high- and low-impulsive participants have differential baseline DA levels. This hypothesis is consistent with a recent positron emission tomography study by Dalley et al (2007), which revealed that impulsivity in rodents is associated with reduced uptake of the radioligand $[^{18}F]$ fallypride (which has high affinity for DA D2/D3 receptors) in the striatum. Reduced uptake may indicate reduced DA D2 receptor availability, or enhanced endogenous DA levels. Thus, it is unclear whether impulsivity is accompanied by increased or reduced baseline DA function, and whether bromocriptine reduced or increased DA transmission.

Finally, it will be interesting to reconcile observations that bromocriptine improves performance in high-impulsive healthy participants, while also improving performance in patients with PD, which has been associated with low novelty-seeking.

ACKNOWLEDGMENTS RC is supported by a Royal Society University Research Fellowship and a Junior Research Fellowship from St John's College, Cambridge. The

research was supported by a Welcome Trust Program Grant (no. 076274/4/Z/04) [to Trevor Robbins], an American Parkinson's Disease Association grant, NIH grants MH63901, NS40813 (to Mark D'Esposito), and the Veterans Administration Research Service. The work was completed within the Behavioral and Clinical Neurosciences Institute, supported by a consortium award from the Wellcome Trust and the MRC and the Helen Wills Neuroscience Institute, University of California, Berkeley. Scanning was completed at the Wolfson Brain Imaging Centre, Addenbrooke's Hospital, Cambridge, and the Brain Imaging Centre at Berkeley. I am grateful to Trevor Robbins, Mark D'Esposito, Richard Ivry, Roger Barker, Luke Clark, Lee Altamirano, Emily Jacobs, Margaret Sheridan, Elizabeth Kelley, Asako Miyakawa, Simon Lewis, and Barbara Sahakian for their support.

NOTES

1. There is indication that extradimensional set-shifting deficits in Parkinson's disease depend on nondopaminergic mechanisms and perhaps implicate noradrenergic dysfunction, which may be present in Parkinson's disease, but may not necessarily be normalized by dopaminergic medication (Middleton et al., 1999).

2. Frank likened these effects to the lay concept of "learning from carrots" versus "learning from sticks" (Frank, 2005). His later work has shown that there is considerable variation in "carrot" versus "stick "tendencies across healthy individuals (Frank MJ, O'Reilly RC (2006).

REFERENCES

Abrams JK, Johnson PL, Hollis JH, Lowry CA (2004) Anatomic and functional topography of the dorsal raphe nucleus. Annals of the New York Academy of Sciences 1018:46–57.

Agid Y, Ruberg M, Javoy-Agid, Hirsch E, Raisman-Vozari, R, Vyas S, Faucheux B, Michel P, Kastner A, Blanchard V, Damier P, Villares J, Zhang P (1993) Are dopaminergic neurons selectively vulnerable to Parkinson's disease? Advances in Neurology 60:148–164.

Alexander G, DeLong M, Stuck P (1986) Parallel organisation of functionally segregated circuits linking basal ganglia and cortex. Annual Review of Neuroscience 9:357–381.

Annett L, McGregor A, Robbins T (1989) The effects of ibutenic acid lesions of the nucleus accumbens on spatial learning and extinction in the rat. Behavioral Brain Research 31:231–242.

Arai R, Karasawa N, Geffard M, Nagatsu I (1995) L-DOPA is converted to dopamine in serotonergic fibers of the striatum of the rat: a double-labeling immunofluorescence study. Neuroscience Letters 195:195–198.

Arnsten AFT (1998) Catecholamine modulation of prefrontal cortical cognitive function. Trends in Cognitive Sciences 2:436–446.

Bilder R, Volavka K, Lachman H, Grace A (2004) The catechol-O-methyltransferase polymorphism: relations to the tonic-phasic dopamine hypothesis and neuropsychiatric phenotypes. Neuropsychopharmacology Advance (online publication):1–19.

Bowen FP, Kamienny RS, Burns MM, Yahr MD (1975) Parkinsonism: effects of levodopa treatment on concept formation. Neurology 25:701–704.

Brass M, Ruge H, Meiran N, Rubin O, Koch I, Zysset S, Prinz W, von Cramon DY(2003) When the same response has different meaning: recoding the response meaning in the lateral prefrontal cortex. Neuroimage 20:1036–1031.

Brozoski TJ, Brown R, Rosvold HE, Goldman PS (1979) Cognitive deficit caused by regional depletion of dopamine in the prefrontal cortex of rhesus monkeys. Science 205:929–931.

Bunge SA, Kahn I, Wallis JD, Miller EK, Wagner AD (2003) Neural circuits subserving the retrieval and maintenance of abstract rules. Journal of Neurophysiology 90: 3419–3428.

Camps M, Kelly P, Palacios J (1990) Autoradiographic localization of dopamine D1 and D2 receptors in the brain of several mammalian species. Journal of Neural Transmission: General Section 80:105–127.

Cools R (2006) Dopaminergic modulation of cognitive function: implications for L-DOPA treatment in Parkinson's disease. Neuroscience and Biobehavioral Reviews 30:1–23.

Cools R, Altamirano L, D'Esposito M (2006a) Reversal learning in Parkinson's disease depends on medication status and outcome valence. Neuropsychologia 44:1663–1673.

Cools R, Barker RA, Sahakian BJ, Robbins TW (2001a) Mechanisms of cognitive set flexibility in Parkinson's disease. Brain 124:2503–2512.

Cools R, Barker RA, Sahakian BJ, Robbins TW (2001b) Enhanced or impaired cognitive function in Parkinson's disease as a function of dopaminergic medication and task demands. Cerebral Cortex 11:1136–1143.

Cools R, Barker RA, Sahakian BJ, Robbins TW (2003) L-Dopa medication remediates cognitive inflexibility, but increases impulsivity in patients with Parkinson's disease. Neuropsychologia 41:1431–1441.

Cools R, Clark L, Owen AM, Robbins TW (2002a) Defining the neural mechanisms of probabilistic reversal learning using event-related functional magnetic resonance imaging. Journal of Neuroscience 22:4563–4567.

Cools R, Clark L, Robbins TW (2004) Differential responses in human striatum and prefrontal cortex to changes in object and rule relevance. Journal of Neuroscience 24:1129–1135.

Cools R, Ivry RB, D'Esposito M (2006b) The striatum is necessary for responding to changes in stimulus relevance. Journal of Cognitive Neurocience 18(12):1973–1983.

Cools R, Lewis SJ, Clark L, Barker RA, Robbins TW (2007a) L-DOPA disrupts activity in the nucleus accumbens during reversal learning in Parkinson's disease. Neuropsychopharmacology 32(1):180–189.

Cools R, Miyakawa A, Ivry RB, D'Esposito M (2007c). Cognitive inflexibility in Parkinson's disease reflects striatal or frontal dysfunction depending on medication status. Poster presentation at the 14th Annual Meeting of the Cognitive Neuroscience Society, New York City, May 5–8.

Cools R, Robbins TW (2004) Chemistry of the adaptive mind. Philosophical Transactions A 362:2871–2888.

Cools R, Sheridan M, Jacobs E, D'Esposito M (2007b) Impulsive personality predicts dopamine-dependent changes in fronto-striatal activity during component processes of working memory. J Neurosci, in press.

Cools R, Stefanova E, Barker RA, Robbins TW, Owen AM (2002b) Dopaminergic modulation of high-level cognition in Parkinson's disease: the role of the prefrontal cortex revealed by PET. Brain 125:584–594.

Cools AR, Van Den Bercken JHL, Horstink MWI, Van Spaendonck KPM, Berger HJC (1984) Cognitive and motor shifting aptitude disorder in Parkinson's disease. Journal of Neurology, Neurosurgery, and Psychiatry 47:443–453.

Crofts HS, Dalley JW, Van Denderen JCM, Everitt BJ, Robbins TW, Roberts AC (2001) Differential effects of 6-OHDA lesions of the frontal cortex and caudate nucleus on the ability to acquire an attentional set. Cerebral Cortex 11:1015–1026.

Curtis CE, D'Esposito M (2003) Persistent activity in the prefrontal cortex during working memory. Trends in Cognitive Sciences 7:415–423.

Dalley JW, Fryer TD, Brichard L, Robinson ES, Theobald DE, Laane K, Pena Y, Murphy ER, Shah Y, Probst K, Abakumova I, Aigbirhio FI, Richards HK, Hong Y, Baron JC, Everitt BJ, Robbins TW (2007) Nucleus accumbens D2/3 receptors predict trait impulsivity and cocaine reinforcement. Science 315(5816):1267–1270.

Dias R, Robbins TW, Roberts AC (1996) Dissociation in prefrontal cortex of affective and attentional shifts. Nature 380:69–72.

Divac I, Rosvold HE, Szwarcbart MK (1967) Behavioral effects of selective ablation of the caudate nucleus. Journal of Comparative and Physiological Psychology 63:184–190.

Dodd ML, Klos KJ, Bower JH, Geda YE, Josephs KA, Ahlskog JE (2005) Pathological gambling caused by drugs used to treat Parkinson disease. Archives of Neurology 62:1377–1381.

Dove A, Pollmann S, Schubert T, Wiggins CJ, Yves von Cramon D (2000) Prefrontal cortex activation in task-switching: an event-related fMRI study. Cognitive Brain Research 9:103–109.

Downes JJ, Roberts AC, Sahakian BJ, Evenden JL, Morris RG, Robbins TW (1989) Impaired extra-dimensional shift performance in medicated and unmedicated Parkinson's disease: evidence for a specific attentional dysfunction. Neuropsychologia 27:1329–1343.

Durstewitz D, Seamans J, Sejnowski T (2000) Dopamine-mediated stabilization of delay-period activity in a network model of prefrontal cortex. Journal of Neurophysiology 83:1733–1750.

Evans AH, Pavese N, Lawrence AD, Tai YF, Appel S, Doder M, Brooks DJ, Lees AJ, Piccini P (2006) Compulsive drug use linked to sensitized ventral striatal dopamine transmission. Annals of Neurology 59:852–858.

Fallgatter AJ, Herrmann MJ, Roemmler J, Ehlis AC, Wagener A, Heidrich A, Ortega G, Zeng Y, Lesch KP (2004) Allelic variation of serotonin transporter function modulates the brain electrical response for error processing. Neuropsychopharmacology 29:1506–1511.

Fellows L, Farah M (2003) Ventromedial frontal cortex mediates affective shifting in humans: evidence from a reversal learning paradigm. Brain 126:1830–1837.

Floresco SB, Magyar O, Ghods-Sharifi S, Vexelman C, Tse MT (2006) Multiple dopamine receptor subtypes in the medial prefrontal cortex of the rat regulate set-shifting. Neuropsychopharmacology 31:297–309.

Frank M (2005) Dynamic dopamine modulation in the basal ganglia: a neurocomputational account of cognitive deficits in medicated and non-medicated Parkinsonism. Journal of Cognitive Neuroscience 17(1):51–72.

Frank M, Loughry B, O'Reilly R (2001) Interactions between frontal cortex and basal ganglia in working memory: a computational model. Cognitive, Affective, and Behavioral Neuroscience 1:137–160.

Frank MJ, O'Reilly RC (2006) A mechanistic account of striatal dopamine function in human cognition: psychopharmacological studies with cabergoline and haloperidol. Behavioral Neuroscience 120:497–517.

Fuster J (1989) The prefrontal cortex. New York: Raven Press.

Gotham AM, Brown RG, Marsden CD (1988) 'Frontal' cognitive function in patients with Parkinson's disease 'on' and 'off' levodopa. Brain 111:299–321.

Grant DA, Berg EA (1948) A behavioural analysis of degree of reinforcement and ease of shifting to new responses in a Weigl-type card sorting problem. Journal of Experimental Psychology 38:404–411.

Harmer CJ, Shelley NC, Cowen PJ, Goodwin GM (2004) Increased positive versus negative affective perception and memory in healthy volunteers following selective serotonin and norepinephrine reuptake inhibition. American Journal of Psychiatry 161:1256–1263.

Hayes AE, Davidson MC, Keele SW (1998) Towards a functional analysis of the basal ganglia. Journal of Cognitive Neuroscience 10:178–198.

Hollerman JR, Schultz W (1998) Dopamine neurons report an error in the temporal prediction of reward during learning. Nature Neuroscience 1:304–309.

Jacobsen C (1936) Studies of cerebral functions in primates. Comparative Psychology Monographs 13:1–60.

Kish SJ, Shannak K, Hornykiewicz O (1988) Uneven patterns of dopamine loss in the striatum of patients with idiopathic Parkinson's disease. New England Journal of Medicine 318:876–880.

Lewis S, Dove A, Robbins T, Barker R, Owen A (2003) Cognitive impairments in early Parkinson's disease are accompanied by reductions in activity in frontostriatal neural circuitry. Journal of Neuroscience 23:6351–6356.

Lewis SJ, Slabosz A, Robbins TW, Barker RA, Owen AM (2005) Dopaminergic basis for deficits in working memory but not attentional set-shifting in Parkinson's disease. Neuropsychologia 43:823–832.

Luciana M, Depue RA, Arbisi P, Leon A (1992) Facilitation of working memory in humans by a D2 dopamine receptor agonist. Journal of Cognitive Neuroscience 4:58–68.

Lynch MR (1997) Selective effects on prefrontal cortex serotonin by dopamine D3 receptor agonism: interaction with low-dose haloperidol. Progress in Neuro-Psychopharmacology & Biological Psychiatry 21:1141–1153.

Malmo R (1942) Interference factors in delayed response in monkeys after removal of frontal lobes. Journal of Neurophysiology 5:295–308.

Maruyama W, Naoi M, Takahashi A, Watanabe H, Konagaya Y, Mokuno K, Hasegawa S, Nakahara D (1992) The mechanism of perturbation in monoamine metabolism by L-dopa therapy: in vivo and in vitro studies. Journal of Neural Transmission: General Section 90:183–197.

Mattay VS, Tessitore A, Callicott JH, Bertonlino A, Goldberg TE, Chase TN, Hyde TM, Weinberger DR (2002) Dopaminergic modulation of cortical function in patients with Parkinson's disease. Annals of Neurology 58:630–635.

Mehta MA, Swainson R, Ogilvie AD, Sahakian BJ, Robbins TW (2001) Improved short-term spatial memory but impaired reversal learning following the dopamine D2 agonist bromocriptine in human volunteers. Psychopharmacology 159:10–20.

Meyer DE, Evans JE, Lauber EJ, Gmeindl L, Rubinstein J, Junck L, Koeppe RA (1998) The role of dorsolateral prefrontal cortex for executive cognitive processes in task switching. In: Annual Meeting of the Cognitive Neuroscience Society. San Francisco, CA; 23–25 March.

Middleton HC, Sharma A, Agouzoul D, Sahakian BJ, Robbins TW (1999) Idoxan potentiates rather than antagonizes some of the cognitive effects of clonidine. Psychopharmacology 145:401–411.

Miller E, Cohen J (2001) An integrative theory of prefrontal cortex function. Annual Review of Neuroscience 24:167–202.

Mishkin M, Malamut B, Bachevalier J (1984) Memories and habits: two neural systems. In: Neurobiology of human learning and memory (Lynch G, McGaugh JL, Weinberger NM, eds.), pp 65–77. New York: Guilford Press.

Moresco FM, Dieci M, Vita A, Messa C, Gobbo C, Galli L, Rizzo G, Panzacchi A, De Peri L, Invernizzi G, Fazio F (2002) In vivo serotonin 5HT(2A) receptor binding and personality traits in healthy subjects: a positron emission tomography study. Neuroimage 17:1470–1478.

Naoi M, Maruyama W, Takahashi T, Ota M, Parvez H (1994) Inhibition of tryptophan hydroxylase by dopamine and the precursor amino acids. Biochemical Pharmacology 48:207–211.

Owen AM, James M, Leigh JM, Summers BA, Marsden CD, Quinn NP, Lange KW, Robbins TW (1992) Fronto-striatal cognitive deficits at different stages of Parkinson's disease. Brain 115:1727–1751.

Owen AM, Roberts AC, Hodges JR, Summers BA, Polkey CE, Robbins TW (1993) Contrasting mechanisms of impaired attentional set-shifting in patients with frontal lobe damage or Parkinson's disease. Brain 116:1159–1179.

Passingham D, Sakai K (2004) The prefrontal cortex and working memory: physiology and brain imaging. Current Opinion in Neurobiology 14:163–168.

Patton J, Stanford M, Barratt E (1995) Factor structure of the Barratt impulsiveness scale. Journal of Clinical Psychology 51:768–774.

Phillips A, Ahn S, Floresco S (2004) Magnitude of dopamine release in medial prefrontal cortex predicts accuracy of memory on a delayed response task. Journal of Neuroscience 14:547–553.

Rogers RD, Andrews TC, Grasby PM, Brooks DJ, Robbins TW (2000) Contrasting cortical and subcortical activations produced by attentional-set shifting and reversal learning in humans. Journal of Cognitive Neuroscience 12:142–162.

Rogers RD, Owen AM, Middleton HC, Williams EJ, Pickard JD, Sahakian BJ, Robbins TW (1999) Choosing between small, likely rewards and large, unlikely rewards activates inferior and orbitofrontal cortex. Journal of Neuroscience 20: 9029–9038.

Sawaguchi T, Goldman-Rakic PS (1991) D1 dopamine receptors in prefrontal cortex: involvement in working memory. Science 251:947–950.

Sawaguchi T, Matsumura M, Kubota K (1990) Effects of dopamine antagonists on neuronal activity related to a delayed response task in monkey prefrontal cortex. Journal of Neurophysiology 63:1401–1412.

Seamans JK, Yang CR (2004) The principal features and mechanisms of dopamine modulation in the prefrontal cortex. Progress in Neurobiology 74:1–58.

Seedat S, Kesler S, Niehaus DJ, Stein DJ (2000) Pathological gambling behaviour: emergence secondary to treatment of Parkinson's disease with dopaminergic agents. Depression and Anxiety 11:185–186.

Shohamy D, Myers C, Onlaor S, Gluck M (2004) Role of the basal ganglia in category learning: how do patients with Parkinson's disease learn? Behavioral Neuroscience 118:676–686.

Shook SK, Franz EA, Higginson CI, Wheelock VL, Sigvardt KA (2005) Dopamine dependency of cognitive switching and response repetition effects in Parkinson's patients. Neuropsychologia 43:1990–1999.

Sohn M, Ursu S, Anderson JR, Stenger VA, Carter CS (2000) The role of prefrontal cortex and posterior parietal cortex in task switching. Proceedings of the National Academy of Sciences U S A 97:13448–13453.

Swainson R, Rogers RD, Sahakian BJ, Summers BA, Polkey CE, Robbins TW (2000) Probabilistic learning and reversal deficits in patients with Parkinson's disease or frontal or temporal lobe lesions: possible adverse effects of dopaminergic medication. Neuropsychologia 38:596–612.

Taghzouti K, Louilot A, Herman J, Le Moal M, Simon H (1985) Alternation behaviour, spatial discrimination, and reversal disturbances following 6-hydroxydopamine lesions in the nucleus accumbens of the rat. Behavioral and Neural Biology 44:354–363.

Wallis J, Anderson K, Miller E (2001) Single neurons in prefrontal cortex encode abstract rules. Nature 411:953–956.

Woodward T, Bub D, Hunter M (2002) Task switching deficits associated with Parkinson's disease reflect depleted attentional resources. Neuropsychologia 40:1948–1955.

Yoon JH, Curtis CE, D'Esposito M (2006) Differential effects of distraction during working memory on delay-period activity in the prefrontal cortex and the visual association cortex. Neuroimage 29:1117–1126.

IV

BUILDING BLOCKS OF
RULE REPRESENTATION

15

Binding and Organization
in the Medial Temporal Lobe

Paul A. Lipton and Howard Eichenbaum

Just like the experience of a race car driver circling a racecourse, the routines of our everyday experience tend toward the repetitive. Consider the daily drive to and from work and our miraculous ability to distinguish each of these episodes in memory. The behavioral, sensory, cognitive, and emotional features that these episodes share, together with their unique, experience-specific elements, form the web of our own personal experience. Construction of and access to the contents of this web depend critically on unique contributions from and interactions between structures of the medial temporal lobe and prefrontal cortex. The ability to form associations between related events, remember their proper sequence, and distinguish one highly similar daily episode from another all are fundamentally decisive components of declarative memory, and they depend specifically on the hippocampus and related parahippocampal cortical structures.

Our goal in the current chapter is to present a conceptual framework within which the hippocampus and surrounding parahippocampal cortical structures support the binding and organization of information in memory. Contributions from structures beyond the medial temporal lobe, on the other hand, support our capacity to acquire, organize, manipulate, and call on at will—operations that are all critical to normal declarative memory—information that ranges from simplistic to remarkably complex that floods our everyday experience. Specifically, the convergence of multimodal sensory, affective, and cognitive input from the posterior cortical and subcortical areas, as well as crucial contributions about stimulus relationships from the medial temporal lobe memory system, allow the prefrontal cortex to generate abstract rules necessary for goal-directed behavior.

Over the last decade, data from studies on animals and humans have converged to yield considerable progress in our understanding of the mechanisms of declarative memory. Most prominent is an inherently relational and flexible expression of hippocampal-dependent memory. We present the current framework as a biologically plausible, mechanistic account of an information-processing syntax meant to apply to a broad range of phenomenon in declarative

memory, including episodic and semantic memory, and flexibility of memory expression. We refer to this combination as "relational memory."

It is important to keep in mind that, as we articulate our framework and review the literature, our reference to semantic or relational memory resembles what others throughout the book refer to as the "abstraction of rules" or "perceptual categorization." For example, Earl Miller and his colleagues have examined how neuronal activity reflects an animal's categorical representation of cats and dogs whose features have been morphed along some perceptual continuum (Freedman et al., 2003; see Chapter 17). Their findings demonstrate that, whereas the activity of posterior visual cortical neurons reflects a more veridical representation of sensory inputs, the activity of prefrontal cortical neurons tends toward a more binary, categorical representation of what, on the whole, appears to be a cat or a dog. Just as categorizing groups of stimulus percepts requires extracting regularities and differences among the defining features of those percepts, through the course of learning and experience, a semantic or relational memory structure likewise reflects a representational network of experience-dependent associations. A semantic structure, and its extensive network of related memories, may thus be used to abstract behaviorally relevant rules that are useful across a wide variety of novel and familiar situations. For example, four-legged house pets that bark are most likely dogs, whereas four-legged house pets that are indifferent to their owners are most likely cats. The same networking can be used to support logical generalizations across related instances. For example, if, in one experience, I find out that Sally knows Sue, and in another, I learn that Sue knows Fred, then I may be inclined to consider that Sally and Fred may have met.

BINDING AND ORGANIZATION

Our account explores the nature of memory representation mediated by the hippocampus and how these representations are used in the expression of memory. We begin with a brief sketch of this framework and its syntax, using the example introduced earlier (Fig. 15–1; see color insert). During the drive to work, the hippocampus receives a stream of highly preprocessed information about the events that compose that experience, and represents the flow of those events using a series of connected elements, represented as a series of snapshots or "frames" from a video camera (Fig. 15–1A, elements 1–4). Overlapping features across contiguous events provide the continuity of the representation and bind together sequential frames. This form of representation is seen as a basis for the encoding and retrieval of episodic memories.

Virtually all of our experiences share features with previous experiences. Although each new encounter is encoded as a separate sequence of events (Fig. 15–1B), overlapping elements from multiple experiences are encoded by the same frame (Fig. 15–1C). An extension of this representational overlap to multiple daily or weekly episodes that share common features is proposed to support a scaffold of memories bound to no one particular memory episode, that

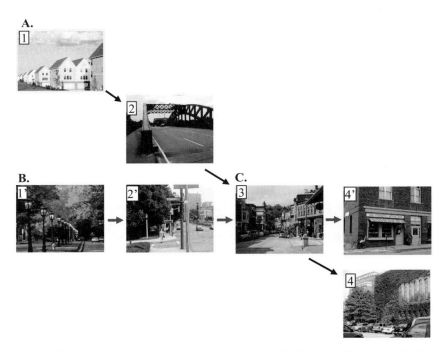

Figure 15–1 A sample relational network composed of two overlapping episodes (*A* and *B*), the first associated with a trip to work from home (*A*), and the second with a trip to the store from a friend's house (*B*). Each episode is construed as a sequence of elements that represent the conjunction of an event and the place where it occurred. *C* is an element that contains the same features in both episodes.

is, elements of semantic memory. Other elemental representations share not only commonalities, but also features that are distinct within each separate episode that serve to distinguish one episode from another. The combination of elements that represent overlap and distinctions between episodes mediate complementary processes in association and disambiguation, respectively, between related memories.

Related memories are linked by the representation of common features. Thus, activation of a particular memory, or component feature, will lead to the activation of multiple related memories through associated elements. Within the current framework, cortical areas use this information to compare, evaluate, and infer how multiple representations—that have never been explicitly experienced together—are related. This information-processing scheme is seen as underlying many of the memory phenomena observed at the behavioral level, including episodic memory, semantic memory, and inferences from memory discussed in greater detail later.

In the following sections, we will begin with a very brief outline of the brain system in which the hippocampus operates. This will be followed by a more

detailed outline of the relational memory framework introduced earlier, focusing on specific cognitive and neural mechanisms that define relational memory networks. In succeeding sections, we will summarize convergent evidence from neuropsychological studies in humans and animals, data from functional brain imaging in humans, and cellular recording studies in animals. Finally, we will conclude with a brief outline of how the hippocampus works within the larger cortical-hippocampal memory system to mediate its relational memory function.

THE HIPPOCAMPAL MEMORY SYSTEM

The hippocampus receives heavily processed cortical information relayed from and further processed by surrounding parahippocampal cortical structures (Suzuki and Amaral, 1994; Burwell and Amaral, 1998) [see Fig. 15–2A]. Cortical connectivity is both hierarchical and reciprocal, such that outputs of many neocortical unimodal and multimodal association areas converge first on the perirhinal and postrhinal cortices (called the "parahippocampal cortex" in primates), from which information is then sent to the entorhinal cortex before being relayed to the hippocampus. The output of hippocampal processing is projected back mainly to the parahippocampal cortical areas, and the outputs of those areas are directed back to the same neocortical areas that provided the initial inputs, although the specific output targets sometimes differ from the input origins within those areas (Lavenex et al., 2002).

Within this cortical-hippocampal pathway are two partially distinct, parallel channels through which different complements of neocortical input are transmitted through the perirhinal and postrhinal cortices (Suzuki and Amaral, 1994; Burwell and Amaral, 1998) [see Fig. 15–2B]. In the rat, the perirhinal cortex largely receives inputs from the polymodal ventral temporal association area, an area that disproportionately processes nonspatial information. In contrast, the postrhinal cortex is the recipient of principally spatial inputs from the posterior parietal cortex. This separation is partially maintained as information is sent on to the entorhinal cortex, such that the perirhinal cortex tends to project more to the lateral entorhinal cortex, and the postrhinal cortex tends to send its projections to the medial entorhinal cortex (Witter et al., 2000). In the last stage, entorhinal afferents are, for the most part, combined in the dentate gyrus and CA3 subregions of the hippocampus, although they are kept separate in CA1 and the subiculum (Witter et al., 2000), establishing an anatomical basis for a functional separation within specific hippocampal subregions.

It is generally considered that detailed representations of memories are stored at the level of the diverse neocortical areas, and the parahippocampal region and hippocampus represent successively more abstract representations of the convergence of cortical inputs. On a functional level, these areas form a highly interactive system in which the role of the hippocampus is perhaps best viewed as mediating the organization and persistence of the neocortical

A.

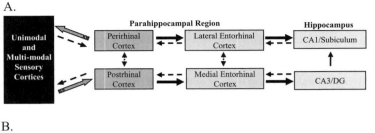

B.

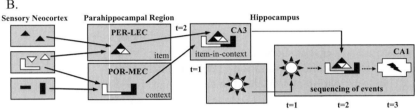

Figure 15–2 Functional and anatomical schematic diagram representing the flow of information through the medial temporal lobe. *A.* Preprocessed sensory information first converges on the perirhinal (PER) and postrhinal (POR) cortices, which have direct connections with specific areas of the entorhinal cortex (lateral [LEC] and medial [MEC], respectively). The CA3 and dentate gyrus (DG) subregions of the hippocampus receive the majority of their inputs from the medial entorhinal cortex, whereas the CA1 and subiculum subregions receive their major inputs from areas of the lateral entorhinal cortex. *B.* The largely parallel pathways through the parahippocampal cortex preserve a separation of item and context information that is refined and elaborated in the PER/LEC and POR/MEC, respectively. These areas are located within the CA3 subregion of the hippocampus to represent items in their context. CA1 may represent the order of events (t = 1, 2, . . .) based on individual representations of items in their respective temporal contexts.

representations. The purpose of this discussion is to consider the nature and mechanisms of this role.

Mechanisms of Relational Memory Representation

Declarative memory is characterized as unique both in its content and in its form of expression. A common view is that the content of declarative memory includes both episodic and semantic memory (Tulving, 1972). "Episodic memory" is our ability to recollect specific personal experiences, whereas "semantic memory" refers to our general knowledge about the world. The expression of declarative memory is typified by flexibility, that is, the use of previously acquired information in situations well outside repetition of the learning event. Cohen (1984) characterized declarative memories as "promiscuous" in that they influence and inform a broad range of relevant knowledge and other memories, and as accessible to many information-processing systems. Declarative memory also is defined as available to conscious recollection, in that we are

aware of the retrieved information as a memory of previous events or known facts.

Cognitive Mechanisms of Declarative Memory

In an early construal, Tulving (1983) contrasted the temporal dimension of episodic memory with the conceptual organization of semantic memory. Tulving (1983) argued that the central organizing feature of episodic memory is that "one event precedes, co-occurs, or follows another." This is reminiscent of Aristotle's (350 BC) characterization of vivid remembering: "Acts of recollection, as they occur in experience, are due to the fact that one thought has by nature another that succeeds it in regular order." The current account emphasizes the temporal organization of episodic memories.

This combination of considerations from cognitive science and philosophy suggests that the hippocampus encodes sequences of events that compose any attended experience (see Morris and Frey, 1997). In the scenario of driving to work introduced earlier, the representation of a single episode would consist of a series of connected "frames" that include a view of the local streets, street signs, landscape, and buildings. Each frame contains both the salient stimuli and events, such as choosing the correct street, and the background in which each event occurred, such as time of day. More generally, the hippocampal network represents the flow of all attended events in nearly any situation, and the contents of neuronal representations include the broadest possible combinations of spatial and nonspatial sensory information, such as an individual's actions, as well as what is common across repetitions of episodes.

A further consideration of the cognitive properties of episodic memory suggests that related episodic representations might be integrated with one another to support additional aspects of declarative memory, specifically, semantic memory and the flexibility of recollection. Referring to how different memories are integrated with one another, William James (1890) emphasized that "... in mental terms, the more other facts a fact is associated with in the mind, the better possession of it our memory retains. Each of its associates becomes a hook to which it hangs, a means by which to fish it up by when sunk beneath the surface. Together they form a network of attachments by which it is woven into the entire tissue of our thought." James saw semantic memory as a systematic organization of information wherein the usefulness of memories was determined by how well they are linked together. In our example, a drive to work may be linked to other experiences, such as driving to a shopping center or to a restaurant to have brunch with friends (Fig. 15–1B), by the common element of a particular street in each experience (Fig. 15–1C).

There are two main outcomes of linking representations of specific experiences. One is a network of associated elements independent of any episodic context. This network emerges when several experiences share considerable common information and the overlapping elements and common links among

them are reinforced, such that those items and associations become general regularities within a knowledge structure (one might even conceive of this as a "conceptual," as opposed to "perceptual," categorization). The representation of these general regularities constitutes semantic "knowledge" bound to no particular episode or learning context. Extending the example introduced earlier, every additional experience within the local environment on the way to work adds to the general knowledge about that local environment and can guide future excursions. The proposed networking of experiential memories by common elements provides a mechanism for the commonly held view that semantic knowledge is derived from information repeated within and abstracted from episodic memories. Importantly, for semantic memory to be derived this way, it is critical for experiences with the common information to be linked among many related representations to build the episode-independent, general (semantic) structure.

The second proposed outcome borne out of a network of linked memories is a capacity to use the common elements to retrieve multiple memories associated with that element. For example, one can use the linked network structure to access memories of specific experiences as well as the semantic information that is common among distinct experiences. Thus, cued by the mention of a local street, one can recall multiple trips to work. Reaching further, hippocampal representations could support a capacity to "surf" the network of linked memories and identify relationships and associations among items that were indirectly related through distinctly unrelated experiences. Thus, a single cue could generate the retrieval of multiple episodic and semantic memories, and cortical areas can access these multiple memories to analyze the consequential, logical, spatial, and other abstract relationships among items that appeared separately in distinct memories. These logical operations on indirectly related memories can support inferences from memory that mediate the flexible use of memory in situations outside repetition of one of the learning situations, for example, to find a new store for the first time. The organization of linked experience-specific and experience-general memories with the capacity for association and inference among memories is called a "relational memory network."

Biological Mechanisms

Are relational memory networks biologically plausible? The following well-known features of hippocampal circuitry can work in combination to support all of the properties of relational memory networks described earlier: (1) The hippocampus receives convergent afferents from virtually all cortical association areas, and these inputs are widely distributed onto the cell population in multiple subdivisions of the hippocampus (Amaral and Witter, 1995). Thus, the main afferents of hippocampal principle cells deliver high-level perceptual information about attended stimuli and spatial cues, as well as signals about emotions, actions, motivations, and virtually all forms of attended personal

information. (2) The hippocampus is noted for the prevalence of rapid synaptic plasticity, known as "long-term potentiation" (LTP) [Bliss and Collingridge, 1993], and is dependent on its wealth of excitatory glutamatergic synapses. In particular, a form of LTP that is dependent on N-methyl D-aspartate (NMDA) receptors has been strongly linked to memory (Martin et al., 2000) and to the memory-associated firing properties of hippocampal neurons (Shapiro and Eichenbaum, 1999).

These properties can work in combination to support key features of relational memory networks, specifically, the development of conjunctive representations of events, the sequential organization of event codings, and the linking of related memories. With regard to conjunctive representations, simultaneous activation of multiple high-level afferents to the pyramidal neurons of hippocampal CA fields could support rapid induction of associative LTP, such that the synapses of each of the inputs are all enhanced for an extended time. This associative LTP would support pattern completion, such that presentation of an elemental feature would activate associated elements of the network, and thus support retrieval of the whole pattern.

With regard to sequential organization, several recent computational models have emphasized temporal coding as a main organizing feature of the memory representations supported by the hippocampus and adjacent entorhinal cortex. The entorhinal cortex may encode and subsequently transmit information about the temporal context to the hippocampus (Lisman, 1999; Hasselmo and Eichenbaum, 2005), where unique anatomical properties may support sequence disambiguation (Levy, 1996). Thus, according to these models, when temporally patterned inputs reach the hippocampus, a rapid LTP mechanism enhances connections between cells that fire in sequence. When partial inputs are reproduced, the network is more likely to complete the sequence of the full initial input pattern.

With regard to linking memories, the same computational models that emphasize temporal organization in episodic memory representations provide a mechanism for joining memory representations and extracting the common information among them that is independent of their episodic context. Thus, the proposed networks include cells that receive no external inputs, but develop firing patterns that are regularly associated with a particular sequence or with overlapping sequences (Levy, 1996; Wallenstein et al., 1998; Sohal and Hasselmo, 1998). When episodes are repeated, these cells provide a local temporal context in which items within a particular sequence are linked. When these links incorporate events that are unique to a particular episode, they can assist the network in disambiguating successive patterns in overlapping, but distinct sequences. At the same time, when the links are activated similarly by separate episodes that share a series of overlapping features, they can allow the association of discontiguous episodes that share those features. Thus, the same network properties that support encoding episodes as sequences of events also contain means to link and disambiguate related episodes.

The Nature of "Relations"

The mechanisms proposed to mediate relational memory are simple associative and sequencing properties well known to hippocampal modelers. Nevertheless, when employed in concert with higher-order neocortical computations, relational networks can provide a critical contribution to the breadth of cognitive functions attributed to declarative memory. Consider the example of the transitive inference task where rats were tested for the capacity to learn and express flexibly nonspatial relationships (Dusek and Eichenbaum, 1997). In this task, normal rats and rats with hippocampal damage were trained on a series of four odor choices that involved overlapping items (A > B, B > C, C > D, D > E; where ">" means "is to be selected over"). Animals were tested for their ability to represent the items hierarchically, as implied by their relationships, by testing their judgment on the novel choice B > D. Although both groups acquired the appropriate responses on the elemental stimulus pairings, only the normal rats chose the correct item in novel probe trials. According to the relational memory model proposed here, each trial type (A > B, B > C, etc.) is encoded as a distinct type of episode. Stimuli that appear in multiple episodes (e.g., "C" in both B > C and C > D) are encoded by a single neural element common to each episodic representation. Thus, after accumulation of representations for all of the trial types, the hippocampus develops a network of episodic memories linked by the common stimulus representations. During the critical transitive inference test, presentation of a stimulus cue ("B and D") presumably engages the retrieval of all representations that contain those stimuli—in this case, all of the trial types ("B" would engage recovery of A > B and B > C; "D" would engage C > D and D > E).

According to this view, the hippocampus does not process this information further, except to transmit its retrieved memories to neocortical association areas with which the hippocampus is connected through the parahippocampal region. For example, the prefrontal cortex is a neocortical association area that receives hippocampal outputs and is likely critical to transitive inference (Waltz et al., 1999). It is also activated during transitive inference performance (Acuna et al., 2002; Hurliman et al., 2005). It is proposed that the hippocampus mediates the retrieval of details of all of the episodic representations contained in several cortical areas, and this information is conveyed to the prefrontal cortex, where judgments about the logical relations between the stimuli are identified (see Chapter 1 for a discussion of prefrontal mediation of conditional stimulus associations). Thus, according to the current proposal, the hippocampus does not compute or directly mediate transitive judgments. Rather, the hippocampus mediates only the retrieval of episodic and semantic information on which cortical areas might accomplish the critical judgment. The hippocampus does not directly compute transitive, spatial, familial, or any other type of abstract relationship. It merely supplies the information accumulated across distinct experiences on which such judgments may rely.

In the following sections, we consider, in a detailed review and analysis, the experimental evidence that validates key features of the theoretical framework described earlier. These features include how the hippocampus represents sequential events that compose unique experiences and that serve to disambiguate overlapping experiences, and how memories of particular experiences are linked to form relational networks that support flexibility of memory expression as a capacity for inferences from memory.

Episodic Memory, Semantic Memory, and the Hippocampus

Before we address how the hippocampus mediates aspects of the current conceptual framework, we will briefly review evidence that demonstrates that declarative memory relies on hippocampal function. Episodic and semantic memory, the two components of declarative memory (Tulving, 1972) differ so substantially that it is reasonable to ask whether they share sufficient features to have a common basis. Tulving and Markowitsch (1998) summarized their commonalities, pointing out that both are complex and multimodal, and both are characterized by fast encoding of vast amounts of new information. The contents of both are representational and propositional and can be accessed flexibly and used inferentially.

Evidence from Studies on Amnesia

Among the first studies to suggest the possibility of dissociating episodic and semantic memory by brain damage were Tulving's studies on the patient KC, who as a result of a closed head injury, suffered widespread damage to cortical, subcortical, and medial temporal lobe structures (Tulving and Moscovitch, 1998; Tulving, 2002). This patient has normal intelligence, language, and other cognitive capacities, including intact short-term memory. However, whereas his general knowledge acquired before the injury is largely intact, he has virtually no capacity for recollecting old experiences or forming new episodic memories. In tests of his capacity to learn new semantic information, KC struggled, but ultimately showed substantial success in learning to complete simple sentences and word definitions. However, because patient KC sustained diffuse damage, it was impossible to assign a special role in episodic memory to the hippocampus.

More specific to hippocampal function was the report of three patients, each of whom experienced transient anoxia early in life that led to selective hippocampal damage, sparing the surrounding cortical areas (Vargha-Khadem et al., 1997). These patients, tested in adulthood, were severely deficient in memory for everyday experiences. Nevertheless, they succeeded in acquiring language literacy and factual knowledge sufficient to allow them to attend mainstream schools. Their scores were within the normal range on standardized verbal IQ tests of semantic memory in vocabulary, information, and comprehension. They also performed normally on tests of recognition of words,

nonwords, and familiar and unfamiliar faces, as well as on several tests of associative recognition, including word pairs and face pairs. They were, however, impaired in learning word-voice and object-place associations.

Evidence from Studies of Functional Brain Imaging

Evidence from functional imaging studies in normal human subjects complements the studies on amnesic patients and likewise suggests an important role for the hippocampus in episodic memory. In one study, subjects first memorized a list of words. Then, during scanning, they were asked to recognize the old words and classify their remembering as either based on memory for the study experience or as a memory that lacks episodic detail (Eldridge et al., 2000). The hippocampus was activated relative to baseline only in association with correct episodic recollection, and not with errors or correct recollections that lacked episodic detail. Maguire et al. (2000) reported selective medial temporal lobe activation during retrieval of autobiographical events, but not retrieval of public events. The involvement of the hippocampus, however, in processing complex material is not limited to autobiographical details, but extends broadly, for example, to recollection of the context of learning in formal tests of memory (e.g., Davachi et al., 2003). Another recent study showed that the hippocampus is activated during encoding of multiple items, and more activated when subjects are required to link the items to one another by systematic comparisons, compared with rote rehearsal of the items (Davachi and Wagner, 2002). By contrast, greater activation of the surrounding cortical areas was associated with item-based processing rather than integration of the items. These observations are consistent with the findings from studies of amnesia that suggest differential roles for the hippocampus in linking multiple distinct items into an integrated whole (Cohen et al., 1999; Brasted et al., 2003) and for surrounding cortical areas in representing individual items (Stern et al., 1996; Kirchhoff et al., 2000).

Evidence from Animal Models

Although no doubt useful, due to variations in lesion size and location, as well as mnemonic demands, studies of amnesia or functional brain imaging do not provide unambiguous support for hippocampal mediation of episodic memory. Animal models, on the other hand, provide greater control as well as the chance for a detailed neurobiological investigation of the mechanisms of episodic memory. However, because awareness, a central feature of declarative memory in humans, is untestable in animals, we will focus on what is implicit in characterizations of episodic memory and prominent in complementary computational modeling efforts: the organization of an episode as a sequence of events that unfolds over time and space. Thus, rich episodic memories contain not only the particular item or items that one is attempting to recall, but also the experience of events that precede and follow. A consideration of memory for the orderliness of events in unique experiences, a capacity that can be

tested in animals, may provide a fruitful avenue for neurobiological explorations of episodic memory.

To investigate the specific role of the hippocampus in remembering the order of events in unique experiences, recent studies have employed a behavioral protocol that assesses memory for episodes composed of a unique sequence of olfactory stimuli (Fortin et al., 2002; Kesner et al., 2002). In one of these studies, memory for the sequential order of odor events was directly compared with recognition of the odors in the list, independent of memory for their order (Fig. 15–3). On each trial, rats were presented with a series of five odors, selected randomly from a large pool of common household scents. Memory for each series was subsequently probed using a choice test where the animal was reinforced for selecting the earlier of two of the odors that had appeared in the series, or in later testing, was reinforced for selecting a novel odor against one that had appeared in the series. Normal rats performed both tasks well. Rats with hippocampal lesions could recognize items that had appeared in the series, but were severely impaired in judging their order. Alternatively, although normal animals may have used relative strength of memory traces for the odors to judge sequential order, animals with hippocampal

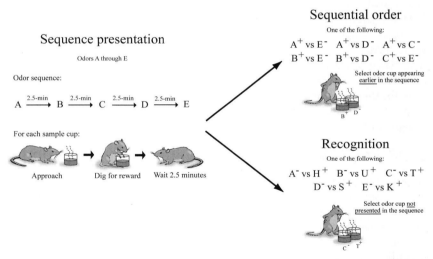

Figure 15–3 A schematic diagram of the odor-sequence task. For each unique sequence, animals are probed for their knowledge of the order of the elements through a choice between two nonadjacent items, or for knowledge about which of two odors appeared in the sequence. *Left.* Sequence of events in each trial. *Top right.* An example trial for the sequential order probes. *Bottom right.* An example trial for the recognition probes. A–E designates the order of presentation of odors in each series, with odor A presented first and odor E presented last. +, reinforced odor; −, nonreinforced odor. (Adapted with permission from Fortin et al., *Nature Neuroscience,* 5, 458–462. Copyright Macmillan Publishers, Ltd., 2002.)

lesions exhibited the same temporal gradient of recognition performance in the absence of above chance discrimination on sequential order probes. Contrary to the argument that animals lack episodic memory because they are "stuck in time" (Roberts, 2002; Tulving, 2002), these observations suggest that animals have the capacity to recollect the flow of events in unique experiences.

A robust model of episodic memory will depend on the capacity to develop representations that can distinguish two experiences that share common elements (Shapiro and Olton, 1994). Levy (1996) proposed that memory for the ordering of events mediated by the hippocampus may be especially important when the event sequences have overlapping elements through which memory of earlier elements must be remembered to complete each distinct sequence. To test whether sequence disambiguation is a fundamental feature of memory processing dependent on the hippocampus, Agster et al. (2002) trained rats with and without an intact hippocampus on a sequence disambiguation task designed after Levy's (1996) formal model that involved two series of events that overlap in the middle items (Fig. 15–4). The sequences were presented as a series of six pairwise odor choices in which, for each sequence, selection of the appropriate odor at each choice point was rewarded. Each trial began with

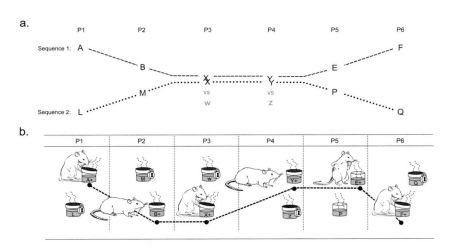

Figure 15–4 A schematic diagram of the sequence disambiguation task. A. The two sequences of odors are represented by A-B-X-Y-E-F and L-M-X-Y-P-Q. The rat begins each trial with a series of choices between odors at the same position in each sequence (e.g., A versus L, then B versus M, etc.), and must choose the odors for that sequence. B. On the first four pairs (*P1–P4*) and pair 6 (*P6*), the lid of the alternate, unrewarded choice is "locked." On pair 5 (*P5*), no lids are used, and the first choice is scored. After either no delay or a 30-min delay, the rat then makes a free choice between E and P. +, Reinforced odor. (Reprinted with permission from Agster et al., *Journal of Neuroscience*, 22, 5760–5768. Copyright Society for Neuroscience, 2002.)

two forced choices that initiated production of one of the two sequences. Then the animal was presented with two forced choices that were the same for both sequences. Subsequently, the subject was allowed a free choice, and was rewarded for selecting the odor assigned to the ongoing sequence. Finally, the animal completed that sequence with one more forced choice.

The critical feature of this task was the free choice. On that test, animals were required to remember their choices from the first two pairings of the current sequence during the ambiguous components of the trial, and then to use the earlier information to guide the correct odor selection. Pre- and postoperative performance of intact animals on the free choice (P5) [see Fig. 15–4] was equivalent and maintained at a high level. In contrast, compared with their preoperative performance, animals with selective hippocampal lesions performed significantly worse postoperatively. In an extension of this work to humans, the hippocampus is likewise implicated in mediating a declarative representation of sequence memory that can be established independent of conscious recollection (Keele et al., 2003; Schendan et al., 2003). The data support the view that the hippocampus is critical to the representation of the ordering of events in unique experiences, and to memory for early items in a sequence through the presentation of ambiguous events. Next we will consider how memories for specific experiences become linked to support the flexibility of declarative memory and the establishment of memory networks that mediate semantic memory.

LINKING AND FLEXIBILITY OF MEMORY EXPRESSION

Behavioral and Lesion Data

The notion that the hippocampus mediates a binding of disparate cortical representations of stimuli and contextual backgrounds (e.g., Squire et al., 1984) has been attributed to relational memory (Cohen et al., 1997, 1999; Davachi and Wagner, 2002). The hippocampal relational network mediates links between distinct episodes that may contain items experienced within different episodes or contexts that may support the abstraction of common features among related memories. By extension, the hippocampus contributes to semantic memory by constructing relational networks that coordinate memories stored in the cortex (Eichenbaum et al., 1999). As such, the hippocampus does not directly mediate semantic memory, but provides an architecture from which comparisons and generalizations can be made, albeit within a range of expression that differs across memories. Empirical support is provided by recent studies that note a relative sparing of semantic memory in amnesia associated with selective damage to the hippocampal region (Vargha-Khadem et al., 1997; Verfaellie et al., 2000; Holdstock et al., 2002; O'Kane et al., 2004). However, contrasting evidence suggests that normal acquisition and flexible expression of acquired semantic memories are very much dependent on the hippocampal region (Manns et al., 2003; Maguire and Frith, 2004).

A number of studies have examined how information processing by the hippocampus may enable the linking of memories and the use of resulting relational networks to make associational and logical inferences from memory. In one study, we trained normal rats and rats with hippocampal lesions on a series of olfactory "paired associates" (Bunsey and Eichenbaum, 1996), and asked whether an intact hippocampus was necessary to make an association between stimuli indirectly related through a common stimulus. Normal rats were able to form indirect relationships, whereas rats with selective hippocampal damage showed no capacity for this inferential judgment. Another study extended the range of networking mediated by the hippocampus to include a series of four hierarchically related odor choices, and to critical involvement of hippocampal connections via the fornix and parahippocampal region (Dusek and Eichenbaum, 1997). Combined, these studies demonstrate that rats with hippocampal damage can learn even complex associations, such as that embodied in odor-paired associates and conditional discriminations.

Studies on monkeys and humans have provided complementary evidence of information processing in the medial temporal lobe across species. For example, monkeys were trained on the same transitivity problems mentioned earlier, and those with damage to the adjacent entorhinal cortex were completely unable to express the transitivity judgments, in contrast to unimpaired performance by intact monkeys (Buckmaster et al., 2004). The results of two functional brain imaging experiments revealed selective hippocampal activation as subjects made transitive judgments about the relationship of items learned during an initial training session in comparison with nontransitive judgments (Heckers et al., 2004; Preston et al., 2004). The studies described earlier provide compelling evidence of hippocampal involvement across species in the flexible expression of memories using relational networks.

The capacity for flexible expression of memories acquired in a single experience also has been examined with a naturalistic form of learning that involves the social transmission of food preferences. In this experimental protocol, in a single experience of social interaction, rats learn an association between a food odor and the smell of rats' breath, and can express this memory flexibly by using the odor to guide subsequent food selection in the absence of social interaction (Strupp and Levitsky, 1984). Winocur (1990) initially characterized the expression of socially transmitted food preferences as dependent on the hippocampus, and in a further exploration, Bunsey and Eichenbaum (1995) showed that selective damage to the hippocampus is sufficient to produce the deficit. Other studies have replicated this finding (Alvarez et al., 2001; Clark et al., 2002), or have taken a step further to show that CA1 NMDA receptors are required (Rampon et al., 2000). These findings show that, even for a simple form of associative learning, the hippocampus is required for the organization of memories to support expression in a situation quite different from the original learning event.

Hippocampal Firing Patterns

In the remainder of this section, we will consider patterns of neuronal activation in humans, monkeys, and rats across a variety of behavioral protocols that demonstrate three general features of declarative memory discussed earlier: (1) encoding complex conjunctions of salient stimuli that compose the events that are represented by the hippocampus, (2) a representation of sequences of events, and (3) a representation of features common to overlapping events that could serve to link related experiences, and by extension, support a semantic network.

Conjunctive Coding

Although many consider hippocampal function primarily an agent of spatial mapping (Muller, 1996; Best et al., 2001), a number of studies have summarily reduced this stance to a byproduct of saliency (see Eichenbaum et al., 1999). Indeed, the activity of hippocampal neurons is often associated with ongoing behavior and the context of events, in conjunction with the animal's location (Eichenbaum et al., 1999). Two recent studies provide compelling evidence that hippocampal neurons encode associations of events and locations. In the first, rats were trained on an auditory fear conditioning task in which, before conditioning, few hippocampal cells responded to the auditory stimuli (Moita et al., 2003). After pairings of tone presentations and shocks, many cells fired briskly to the tone when the animal was in a particular place where the cell fired above baseline. In the second study, the activity of hippocampal neurons in monkeys was recorded while they rapidly learned to associate scenes and locations (Wirth et al., 2003). Just as the monkeys acquired a new response to a location in the scene, neurons in the hippocampus changed their firing patterns to become selective to particular scenes. These scene-location associations persist even long after learning is completed (Yanike et al., 2004).

Wood et al. (1999) directly compared spatial and nonspatial coding by hippocampal neurons by training animals to perform the same memory judgments at many locations in the environment. Rats performed a task in which they had to recognize any of nine olfactory cues placed in any of nine locations. Because the location of the discriminative stimuli was varied systematically, cellular activity related to the stimuli and behavior could be dissociated from that related to the animal's location. The activity of a large subset of hippocampal neurons was associated with a particular combination of odor, the place where it was sampled, and the match-nonmatch status of the odor. Similarly, Ekstrom et al. (2003) recorded the activity of hippocampal neurons in human subjects as they played a taxi driver game, searching for passengers picked up and dropped off at various locations in a virtual reality town. The activity of many of these cells was selectively associated with specific combinations of a place and the view of a particular scene or a particular goal. Hippocampal activity that represents specific salient objects in the context of a particular environment also has been observed in studies of rats engaged in

foraging (Gothard et al., 1996, Rivard, et al., 2004) and escape behavior (Hollup et al., 2001) in open fields. Thus, in rats, monkeys, and humans, a prevalent property of hippocampal firing patterns involves the representation of unique associations of stimuli, their significance, specific behaviors, and the places where these events occur.

Sequences of Events

It is also common to observe across species and behavioral protocols hippo-campal neuronal activity during virtually every aspect of task performance, including approach and stimulus-sampling behaviors, discriminative responses, and consummatory behaviors (Eichenbaum et al., 1999). This broad represen-tational coverage of task-related events extends to classical conditioning, dis-crimination learning, nonmatching- or matching-to-sample tasks, and a vari-ety of maze tasks (Berger et al., 1983; Eichenbaum et al., 1987; Deadwyler et al., 1996; McEchron and Disterhoft, 1997; Wiebe and Staubli, 1999). In these par-adigms, animals are repeatedly presented with specific stimuli and reinforcers, and they execute appropriate cognitive judgments and conditioned behaviors. Many hippocampal neurons are active during odor sampling, and some display striking specificity that corresponds to sequences of rewarded and nonrewarded cues or to particular spatial configurations of odors. Other cells display con-siderable generality, active throughout a sequence of trial events, or during all stimulus-sampling epochs, regardless of odor identity and reward contingency. This overall network activity can be characterized as a sequence of firings that represent step-by-step events in each repetitive behavioral episode. Many of the events were common across episodes (e.g., approach or odor sampling), but some events occurred only on a particular type of trial (e.g., a particular odor configuration).

One can envision that this pattern of sequential activity represents a series of events and locations that compose a meaningful episode, and the infor-mation contained therein both distinguishes and links related episodes. Re-cent studies on the spatial firing patterns of hippocampal neurons provide compelling data consistent with this characterization. In one study, rats were trained on the classic spatial alternation task on a modified T-maze (Wood et al., 2000). Performance on this task requires that the animal distinguish left-turn and right-turn episodes to guide each subsequent choice; thus, it effec-tively resembles a test of episodic memory. If hippocampal neurons encode each sequential behavioral event and its locus within one type of episode, then most cells should fire differentially across left-turn or right-turn episodes while occupying locations common to both trial types. Indeed, virtually all cells that were active as the rat traversed these overlapping locations fired differen-tially on left-turn versus right-turn trials. The majority of cells showed strong selectivity, some firing at more than ten times the rate on one trial type, sug-gesting that they were part of the representations of only one type of episode. Other cells fired substantially on both trial types, potentially providing a link

between left-turn and right-turn representations by the common places traversed on both trial types. Similar results have been observed in two other versions of this task (Frank et al., 2000; Ferbinteanu and Shapiro, 2003).

Relational Networks

As described elsewhere in this chapter, some hippocampal neurons encode features that are common among different experiences and could provide links between distinct memories; these representations are evident in virtually all of the studies described earlier. In the auditory fear conditioning study by Moita and colleagues (2003), a subset of cells responded to a tone only when it was presented as the animal occupied a particular location, whereas another group responded to the tone cue whenever or wherever it was presented. The odor-recognition memory study by Wood et al. (1999) reported that hippocampal neurons responded to the full range of task-related events. These include conjunctions of odors with their match-nonmatch status, with place, or with only one of those features across trials; differentially during odor sampling, regardless of location or match-nonmatch status; to location, independent of odor or match-nonmatch status; differentially to match-nonmatch status, regardless of odor or location. Similarly, in Ekstrom and colleagues' (2003) study of humans performing a virtual navigation task, whereas the activity of some hippocampal neurons was associated with combinations of views, goals, and places, other cells were active when subjects viewed particular scenes, occupied particular locations, or had particular goals in finding passengers or locations. Also, in Rivard and colleagues' (2004) study of rats exploring objects in open fields, whereas some cells were selectively active in response to an object in one environment, others responded to a particular object across environments.

The notion that these cells might reflect the linking of important features across experiences, and the abstraction of common (semantic) information, was highlighted in recent studies of monkeys and humans. Hampson et al. (2004) trained monkeys on matching-to-sample problems, then probed the nature of the representation of stimuli by recording from hippocampal cells when the animals were shown novel stimuli that shared features with the trained cues. They found many hippocampal neurons that encoded meaningful categories of stimulus features and appeared to employ these representations to recognize the same features across many situations. Kreiman et al. (2000a) characterized hippocampal firing patterns in humans during presentations of a variety of visual stimuli. They reported a substantial number of hippocampal neurons that were active when the subject viewed specific categories of material (e.g., faces, famous people, animals, scenes, houses) across many exemplars of each. A subsequent study showed that these neurons are activated when a subject simply imagines its optimal stimulus, supporting a role for hippocampal networks in the recollection of specific memories (Krieman et al., 2000b). This combination of findings across species provides compelling evidence for the notion that some

hippocampal cells represent common features among the various episodes that could serve to link memories obtained in separate experiences.

These observations are consistent with the notion that hippocampal neuronal representations are organized to represent behavioral sequences across a broad range of behavioral protocols and species. A subset of hippocampal neurons is selectively activated at every moment throughout task performance across a broad range of behavioral protocols. Furthermore, the full scope of information encoded by the hippocampal population is precisely as broad as the set of attended and regular events that compose the behavioral protocol. Hippocampal population activity can thus be viewed as a continuous and automatic recording of attended experiences (Morris and Frey, 1997) encoded as sequences of events that define both rare experiences and common stimuli, places, and events that are shared across episodes (Eichenbaum et al., 1999).

Additionally, within our current framework, hippocampally mediated conjunctive processing appears very similar to the rule abstraction of the prefrontal cortex described elsewhere in this book. Are these processes the result of a similar mechanism? It appears that hippocampal processing is important to establish a network of relationships based on similarities and differences among experiences, whereas the prefrontal cortex uses this network to abstract broad categorical similarities or differences to conditionally direct, in a task-relevant manner, subsequent behavior. Thus, the issue is who is doing what with the information. Both may evaluate similarities and differences; however, the prefrontal cortex may be the one to make behaviorally relevant decisions based on hippocampal and sensory cortical grunt work.

THE HIPPOCAMPAL MEMORY SYSTEM

This review has focused on the role of the hippocampus. However, a comprehensive understanding requires consideration of the neighboring parahippocampal cortical areas that provide the primary cortical inputs to the hippocampus and are the immediate cortical recipients of outputs of the hippocampus.

The parahippocampal region plays a critical role in the convergence of multisensory information (Bussey et al., 2002) and in mediating memory based on familiarity of stimuli (Eichenbaum, 2002). As alluded to earlier, two largely parallel processing streams converge on the hippocampus that together support an encoding of sequence information (Witter et al., 2000) [see Fig. 15–2]. The first transmits representations of single percepts and familiarity with those items through the perirhinal cortex and lateral entorhinal cortex, and is supported by anatomical (Burwell and Amaral, 1998), physiological (Young et al., 1997; Brown and Xiang, 1998; Henson et al., 2003), and neuropsychological data (Brown and Aggleton, 2001). Conversely, growing evidence for the second pathway through the postrhinal cortex and medial entorhinal cortex that represents contextual information comes from physiological (Quirk et al., 1992;

Wan et al., 1999; Davachi and Wagner, 2002; Burwell and Hafeman, 2003; Fyhn et al., 2004; Hargreaves et al., 2005) and neuropsychological (Charles et al., 2004; Alvarado and Bachevalier, 2005; Norman and Eacott, 2005) data. These representations are then combined in area CA3 (Witter et al., 2000), supporting the encoding of events as items in the context in which they were experienced. Event representations then may be temporally organized within CA1, potentially guided by information from the entorhinal cortex and CA3 (Hasselmo and Eichenbaum, 2005), to order the series of events that compose a complete episode.

The combination of observations from all of these studies suggests that multiple neocortical areas, the parahippocampal region, and the hippocampus work in concert to mediate relational memory (Eichenbaum, 2000). According to this view, neocortical areas mediate the representation of stimulus details, and outputs of these areas support parallel streams of information about objects ("what" information) and the context in which they were experienced ("where" information). The hippocampus combines these streams of information to compose representations of events as objects in their context, of episodes as sequences of events, and of relational networks as memories linked by their common features.

INTERACTIONS WITH THE PREFRONTAL CORTEX

Some of the functions we have attributed to hippocampal function have historically been associated with the prefrontal cortex, including source memory (Janowsky et al., 1989) and memory for temporal order (Shimamura et al., 1990; McAndrews and Milner, 1991). Our aim is not to strip the prefrontal cortex of these functions, but rather to reconcile their unique processing contributions in the context of prefrontal-medial temporal lobe interactions in memory. Surely, widespread neocortical areas play important roles in episodic and semantic memory (e.g., see reviews by Eichenbaum, 2000; Fuster, 1995; Buckner and Wheeler, 2001). The central question remains: What are the differential contributions of, and the nature of interactions between, diverse cortical and hippocampal areas?

Whereas the hippocampus and the surrounding parahippocampal cortex bind and organize high-level multimodal sensory information and distinguish overlapping episodic representations, one prominent view is that the prefrontal cortex regulates, or controls the gain of incoming sensory information to the medial temporal lobe (Miller and Cohen; 2001; Buckner, 2003). Consistent with this view, the encoding success of face-house paired associates varied as a function of regional activation within a network that included the posterior sensory cortices, prefrontal cortex, and medial temporal lobe (Summerfield et al., 2006). In addition, patients with prefrontal damage are impaired in the organization of their search strategies for the order or grouping of words in a list that they are attempting to recall (Milner et al., 1985; Gershberg and

Shimamura, 1995; Wheeler et al., 1995). Thus, top-down signals broadcast by the prefrontal cortex may control the flow of perceptual information supporting memory for source information and temporal order. In addition, areas of the human prefrontal cortex are strongly activated during retrieval of episodic memories in a variety of tasks. Thus, semantic analysis, recollective monitoring, and rehearsal—all attributed to the prefrontal cortex—may constitute key retrieval processes (Dobbins et al., 2002). Consistent with this view, activation of the prefrontal cortex reflects retrieval effort, rather than success in retrieval, consistent with the role of the prefrontal areas in working memory and rule-learning (Miller, 2000).

These considerations, combined with the role of the hippocampus and the neighboring parahippocampal region outlined earlier, suggest that the encoding and retrieval of declarative memories is a product of interactions between the prefrontal cortex and the hippocampal system. During encoding, the prefrontal cortex strongly influences the content and organization of information to be represented within the hippocampal system. During retrieval, the output of hippocampal representation is called up by strategic processing in the prefrontal cortex, which directs the contents and timing of recovery of the detailed cortical representations.

Finally, in deference to the connectionist perspective, consider the following analogy. Just as one issues Google a command to return all information pertaining to a specific query, the prefrontal cortex may "ask" the medial temporal lobe system what information it has about one's drive to work 2 days ago. The system regenerates the experience of driving to work that morning, including the route that was taken, items that were seen, and events that happened along the way. For example, it may recall that the road was out at a particular point and that you had to take a particular detour. Notably, the medial temporal system likely relies on reactivating the posterior cortical areas to recover details of what was seen and events that occurred, and these details may be sent directly from the posterior cortical areas to the prefrontal cortex. The medial temporal lobe system may also return other related memories, such as the fact that you read yesterday in the newspaper that the road would be out for the next several weeks. The prefrontal cortex searches and evaluates all of this information to generate rules that inform behavioral outcomes, such as, "That detour will still be there tomorrow, so I will need to take the alternate route." According to this conceptualization, the prefrontal cortex and medial temporal areas, together with the posterior cortical areas, contribute distinct information processing that is critical to generating decisions. The prefrontal cortex instigates the search for information in memory, and the representational provisions from the posterior, subcortical, and medial temporal lobe structures, together, can account for the phenomenology of declarative memory.

ACKNOWLEDGMENTS Preparation of this chapter was funded by the following grants: NIMH MH51570 and MH071702.

REFERENCES

Acuna BD, Eliassen JC, Donoghue JP, Sanes JN (2002) Frontal and parietal lobe activation during transitive inference in humans. Cerebral Cortex 12:1312–1321.

Agster KL, Fortin NJ, Eichenbaum H (2002) The hippocampus and disambiguation of overlapping sequences. Journal of Neuroscience 22:5760–5768.

Alvarado MC, Bachevalier J (2005) Comparison of the effects of damage to the perirhinal and parahippocampal cortex on transverse patterning and location memory in rhesus macaques. Journal of Neuroscience 25:1599–1609.

Alvarez P, Lipton PA, Melrose R, Eichenbaum H (2001) Differential effects of damage within the hippocampal region on memory for a natural non-spatial odor-odor association. Neurobiology of Learning and Memory 8:79–86.

Amaral DG, Witter MP (1995) Hippocampal formation. In: The rat nervous system (Pacinos G, ed.), pp 443–493, 2nd edition. San Diego: Academic Press.

Aristotle (350 BC) On memory and reminiscence (Beare JI, trans.). Retrieved February 3, 2003, from http://www.knuten.liu.se/~bjoch509/works/aristotle/memory.txt.

Berger TW, Rinaldi PC, Weisz DJ, Thompson RF (1983) Single-unit analysis of different hippocampal cell types during classical conditioning of rabbit nictitating membrane response. Journal of Neurophysiology 50:1197–1219.

Best PJ, White AW, Minai A (2001) Spatial processing in the brain: the activity of hippocampal place cells. Annual Review of Neuroscience 24:459–486.

Bliss TVP, Collinridge GL (1993) A synaptic model of memory: long-term potentiation in the hippocampus. Nature 361:31–39.

Brasted PJ, Bussey TJ, Murray EA, Wise SP (2003) Role of the hippocampal system in associative learning beyond the spatial domain. Brain 126(Pt 5):1202–1223.

Brown MW, Aggleton JP (2001) Recognition memory: what are the roles of the perirhinal cortex and hippocampus? Nature Reviews Neuroscience 2:51–61.

Brown MW, Xiang JZ (1998) Recognition memory: neuronal substrates of the judgment of prior occurrence. Progress in Neurobiology 55:149–189.

Buckmaster CA, Eichenbaum H, Amaral DG, Suzuki WA, Rapp P (2004) Entorhinal cortex lesions disrupt the relational organization of memory in monkeys. Journal of Neuroscience 24:9811–9825.

Buckner RL (2003) Functional-anatomic correlates of control processes in memory. Journal of Neuroscience 23:3999–4004.

Buckner RL, Wheeler ME (2001) The cognitive neuroscience of remembering. Nature Reviews Neuroscience 2:624–634.

Bunsey M, Eichenbaum H (1995) Selective damage to the hippocampal region blocks long term retention of a natural and nonspatial stimulus-stimulus association. Hippocampus 5:546–556.

Bunsey M, Eichenbaum H (1996) Conservation of hippocampal memory function in rats and humans. Nature 379:255–257.

Burwell RD, Amaral DG (1998) Cortical afferents of the perirhinal, postrhinal, and entorhinal cortices of the rat. Journal of Comparative Neurology 398:179–205.

Burwell RD, Hafeman DM (2003) Positional firing properties of postrhinal cortex neurons. Neuroscience 119: 577–588.

Bussey TJ, Saksida LM, Murray EA (2002) The role of perirhinal cortex in memory and perception: conjunctive representations for object identification. In: The parahippocampal region: organization and role in cognitive function (Witter MP, Wouterlood F, eds.), pp 239–254. Oxford, UK: Oxford University Press.

Charles DP, Browning PG, Gaffan D (2004) Entorhinal cortex contributes to object-in-place scene memory. European Journal of Neuroscience 20:3157–3164.

Clark RE, Broadbent NJ, Zola SM, Squire LR (2002) Anterograde amnesia and temporally graded retrograde amnesia for a nonspatial memory task after lesions of the hippocampus and subiculum. Journal of Neuroscience 22:4663–4669.

Cohen NJ (1984) Preserved learning capacity in amnesia: evidence for multiple memory systems. In: The neuropsychology of memory (Butters N, Squire LR, eds.), pp 83–103. New York: Guilford Press.

Cohen NJ, Poldrack RA, Eichenbaum H (1997) Memory for items and memory for relations in the procedural/declarative memory framework. Memory 5:131–178.

Cohen NJ, Ryan J, Hunt C, Romine L, Wszalek T, Nash C (1999) Hippocampal system and declarative (relational) memory: summarizing the data from functional neuroimaging studies. Hippocampus 9:83–98.

Davachi L, Wagner AG (2002) Hippocampal contributions to episodic encoding: insights from relational and item-based learning. Journal of Neurophysiology 88: 982–990.

Davachi L, Mitchell JP, Wagner AD (2003) Multiple routes to memory: distinct medial temporal lobe processes build item and source memories. Proceedings of the National Academy of Sciences U S A 100:2157–2162.

Deadwyler SA, Bunn T, Hampson RE (1996) Hippocampal ensemble activity during spatial delayed-nonmatch-to-sample performance in rats. Journal of Neuroscience 16:354–372.

Dobbins IG, Foley H, Schacter DL, Wagner AD (2002) Executive control during episodic retrieval: multiple prefrontal processes subserve source memory. Neuron 35: 989–996.

Dusek JA, Eichenbaum H (1997) The hippocampus and memory for orderly stimulus relations. Proceedings of the National Academy of Sciences U S A 94:7109–7114.

Eichenbaum H (2000) A cortical-hippocampal system for declarative memory. Nature Reviews Neuroscience 1:41–50.

Eichenbaum H (2002) Memory representations in the parahippocampal region. In: The parahippocampal region: organization and role in cognitive function (Witter M, Wouterlood F, eds.), pp 165–184. Oxford, UK: Oxford University Press.

Eichenbaum H, Dudchencko P, Wood E, Shapiro M, Tanila H (1999) The hippocampus, memory, and place cells: is it spatial memory or a memory space? Neuron 23: 209–226.

Eichenbaum H, Kuperstein M, Fagan A, Nagode J (1987) Cue-sampling and goal-approach correlates of hippocampal unit activity in rats performing an odor discrimination task. Journal of Neuroscience 7:716–732.

Ekstrom AD, Kahana MJ, Caplan JB, Fields TA, Isham EA, Newman EL, Fried I (2003) Cellular networks underlying human spatial navigation. Nature 425:184–188.

Eldridge LL, Knowlton BJ, Furmanski CS, Brookheimer SY, Engel SA (2000) Remembering episodes: a selective role for the hippocampus during retrieval. Nature Neuroscience 3:1149–1152.

Ferbinteanu J, Shapiro ML (2003) Prospective and retrospective memory coding in the hippocampus. Neuron 40:1227–1239.

Fortin NJ, Agster KL, Eichenbaum H (2002) Critical role of the hippocampus in memory for sequences of events. Nature Neuroscience 5:458–462.

Frank LM, Brown EN, Wilson M (2000) Trajectory encoding in the hippocampus and entorhinal cortex. Neuron 27:169–178.

Freedman DJ, Riesenhuber M, Poggio T, Miller EK (2003) A comparison of primate prefrontal and inferior temporal cortices during visual categorization. Journal of Neuroscience 23:5235–5246.

Fuster JM (1995) Memory in the cerebral cortex. Cambridge: MIT Press.

Fyhn M, Molden S, Witter MP, Moser EI, Moser M (2004) Spatial representation in the entorhinal cortex. Science 305:1258–1264.

Gershberg FB, Shimamura AP (1995) Impaired use of organizational strategies in free recall following frontal lobe damage. Neuropsychologia 33:1305–1333.

Gothard KM, Skaggs WE, Moore KM, McNaughton BL (1996) Binding of hippocampal CA1 neural activity to multiple reference frames in a landmark-based navigation task. Journal of Neuroscience 16:823–835.

Hampson RE, Pons TP, Stanford TR, Deadwyler SA (2004) Categorization in the monkey hippocampus: a possible mechanism for encoding information into memory. Proceedings of the National Academy of Sciences U S A 101:3184–3189.

Hargreaves EL, Rao G, Lee I, Knierim JJ (2005) Major dissociation between medial and lateral entorhinal input to dorsal hippocampus. Science 308:1792–1794.

Hasselmo ME, Eichenbaum H (2005) Hippocampal mechanisms for the context-dependent retrieval of episodes. Neural Networks 18:1172–1190.

Heckers S, Zalezak M, Weiss, AP, Ditman T, Titone D (2004) Hippocampal activation during transitive inference in humans. Hippocampus 14:153–162.

Henson RNA, Cansino S, Herron JE, Robb WGK, Rugg MD (2003) A familiarity signal in human anterior medial temporal cortex. Hippocampus 13:301–304.

Holdstock JS, Mayes AR, Isaac CL, Gong Q, Roberts N (2002) Differential involvement of the hippocampus and temporal lobe cortices in rapid and slow learning of new semantic information. Neuropsychologia 40:748–768.

Hollup SA, Molden S, Donnett JG, Moser MB, Moser EI (2001) Accumulation of hippocampal place fields at the goal location in an annular watermaze task. Journal of Neuroscience 21:1635–1644.

Hurliman E, Nagode JC, Pardo JV (2005) Double dissociation of exteroceptive and interoceptive feedback systems in the orbital and ventromedial prefrontal cortex of humans. Journal of Neuroscience 25:4641–4648.

James W (1918) The principles of psychology. New York: Holt (originally published in 1890).

Janowsky JS, Shimamura AP, Squire LR (1989) Source memory impairment in patients with frontal lobe lesions. Neuropsychologia 27:1043–1056.

Keele SW, Ivry R, Mayr U, Hazeline E, Heuer H (2003) The cognitive and neural architecture of sequence representation. Psychological Review 110:316–339.

Kesner RP, Gilbert PE, Barua LA (2002) The role of the hippocampus in memory for the temporal order of a sequence of odors. Behavioral Neuroscience 116:286–290.

Kirchhoff BA, Wagner AD, Maril A, Stern CE (2000) Prefrontal-temporal circuitry for novel stimulus encoding and subsequent memory. Journal of Neuroscience 20:6173–6180.

Kreiman K, Kock C, Fried I (2000a) Category specific visual responses of single neurons in the human medial temporal lobe. Nature Neuroscience 3:946–953.

Kreiman K, Kock C, Fried I (2000b) Imagery neurons in the human brain. Nature 408(6810):357–361.

Lavenex P, Suzuki WA, Amaral DG (2002) Perirhinal and parahippocampal cortices of the macaque monkey: projections to the neocortex. Comparative Neurology 447:394–420.

Levy WB (1996) A sequence predicting CA3 is a flexible associator that learns and uses context to solve hippocampal-like tasks. Hippocampus 6:579–590.

Lisman JE (1999) Relating hippocampal circuitry to function: recall of memory sequences by reciprocal dentate-CA3 interactions. Neuron 22:233–242.

Maguire EA, Frith CD (2004) The brain network associated with acquiring semantic knowledge. Neuroimage 22:171–178.

Maguire EA, Mummery CJ, Buchel C (2000) Patterns of hippocampal-cortical interaction dissociate temporal lobe memory subsystems. Hippocampus 10:475–482.

Manns JR, Hopkins RO, Squire LR (2003) Semantic memory and the human hippocampus. Neuron 38:127–133.

Martin SJ, Grimwood PD, Morris RGM (2000) Synaptic plasticity and memory: an evaluation of the hypothesis. Annual Review of Neuroscience 23:649–711.

McAndrews MP, Milner B (1991) The frontal cortex and memory for temporal order. Neuropsychologia 29:849–859.

McEchron MD, Disterhoft JF (1997) Sequence of single neuron changes in CA1 hippocampus of rabbits during acquisition of trace eyeblink conditioned responses. Journal of Neurophysiology 78:1030–1044.

Miller EK (2000) The prefrontal cortex and cognitive control. Nature Reviews Neuroscience 1:59–65.

Miller EK, Cohen JD (2001) An integrative theory of prefrontal cortex function. Annual Review of Neuroscience 24:167–202.

Milner B, Petrides M, Smith ML (1985) Frontal lobes and the temporal organization of memory. Human Neurobiology 4:137–142.

Moita MAP, Moisis S, Zhou Y, LeDoux JE, Blair HT (2003) Hippocampal place cells acquire location-specific responses to the conditioned stimulus during auditory fear conditioning. Neuron 37:485–497.

Morris RGM, Frey U (1997) Hippocampal synaptic plasticity: role in spatial learning or the automatic recording of attended experience? Philosophical Transactions of the Royal Society of London, Series B: Biological Sciences 352:1489–1503.

Muller RU (1996) A quarter of a century of place cells. Neuron 17:813–822.

Norman G, Eacott MJ (2005) Dissociable effects of lesions to the perirhinal cortex and the postrhinal cortex on memory for context and objects in rats. Behavioral Neuroscience 119:557–566.

O'Kane G, Kensinger EA, Corkin S (2004) Evidence for semantic learning in profound amnesia: an investigation with patient HM. Hippocampus 14:417–425.

Preston AR, Shrager Y, Dudukovic NM, Gabrieli JD (2004) Hippocampal contribution to the novel use of relational information in declarative memory. Hippocampus 14:148–152.

Quirk GJ, Muller RU, Kubie JL, Ranck JB Jr (1992) The positional firing properties of medial entorhinal neurons: description and comparison with hippocampal place cells. Journal of Neuroscience 12:1945–1963.

Rampon C, Tang YP, Goodhouse J, Shimizu E, Kyin M, Tsien J (2000) Enrichment induces structural changes and recovery from non-spatial memory deficits in CA1 NMDAR1-knockout mice. Nature Neuroscience 3:238–244.

Rivard B, Li Y, Lenck-Santini PP, Poucet B, Muller RU (2004) Representation of objects in space by two classes of hippocampal pyramidal cells. Journal of General Physiology 124:9–25.

Roberts WA (2002) Are animals stuck in time? Psychological Bulletin 128:473–489.

Schendan HE, Searl MM, Melrose RJ, Stern CE (2003) An fMRI study of the role of the medial temporal lobe in implicit and explicit sequence learning. Neuron 37:1013–1025.

Shapiro ML, Eichenbaum H (1999) Hippocampus as a memory map: synaptic plasticity and memory encoding by hippocampal neurons. Hippocampus 9:365–384.

Shapiro ML, Olton DS (1994) Hippocampal function and interference. In: Memory systems (Schacter DL, Tulving E, eds.), pp 87–117. Cambridge: MIT Press.

Shimamura AP, Janowsky JA, Squire LR (1990) Memory for the temporal order of events in patients with frontal lobe lesions and amnesic patients. Neuropsychologia 28:803–813.

Sohal VS, Hasselmo ME (1998) Changes in GABAb modulation during a theta cycle may be analogous to the fall of temperature during annealing. Neural Computation 10:889–902.

Squire LR, Cohen NJ, Nadel L (1984) The medial temporal region and memory consolidation: a new hypothesis. In: Memory consolidation (Weingartner H, Parker E, eds.), pp 185–210. Hillsdale, NJ: Lawrence Erlbaum Associates, Inc.

Stern CE, Corkin S, Gonzalez RG, Guimaraes AR, Baker JR, Jennings PJ, Carr CA, Sugiura RM, Vedantham V, Rosen BR (1996) The hippocampal formation participates in novel picture encoding: evidence from functional MRI. Proceedings of the National Academy of Sciences U S A 93:8660–8665.

Strupp BJ, Levitsky DA (1984) Social transmission of food preferences in adult hooded rats (*Rattus norvegicus*). Journal of Comparative Psychology 98:257–266.

Summerfield C, Greene M, Wager T, Enger T, Hirsch J, Mangels J (2006) Neocortical connectivity during episodic memory formation. PLoS Biology 4:e128.

Suzuki WA, Amaral DG (1994) Perirhinal and parahippocampal cortices of the macaque monkey: cortical afferents. Journal of Comparative Neurology 350:497–533.

Tulving E (1972) Episodic and semantic memory. In: Organization of memory (Tulving E, Donaldson W, eds.), pp 381–403. New York: Academic Press.

Tulving E (1983) Elements of episodic memory. New York: Oxford University Press.

Tulving E (2002) Episodic memory: From mind to brain. Annual Review of Psychology 53:1–25.

Tulving E, Markowitsch HJ (1998) Episodic and declarative memory: role of the hippocampus. Hippocampus 8:198–203.

Vargha-Khadem F, Gadin DG, Watkins KE, Connelly A, Van Paesschen W, Mishkin M (1997) Differential effects of early hippocampal pathology on episodic and semantic memory. Science 277:376–380.

Verfaellie M, Koseff P, Alexander MP (2000) Acquisition of novel semantic information in amnesia: effects of lesion location. Neuropsychologia 38:484–492.

Wallenstein GV, Eichenbaum H, Hasselmo ME (1998) The hippocampus as an associator of discontiguous events. Trends in Neurosciences 21:315–365.

Waltz JA, Knowlton BJ, Holyoak KJ, Boone KB, Mishkin FS, Sanbtos MM, Thomas CR, Miller BL (1999). A system for relational reasoning in human prefrontal cortex. Psychological Science 10:119–125.

Wan H, Aggleton JP, Brown MW (1999) Different contributions of the hippocampus and perirhinal cortex to recognition memory. Journal of Neuroscience 19:1142–1148.

Wheeler MA, Stuss DT, Tulving E (1995) Frontal lobe damage produces episodic memory impairment. Journal of the International Neuropsychological Society 1:525–536.

Wiebe SP, Staubli UV (1999) Dynamic filtering of recognition memory codes in the hippocampus. Journal of Neuroscience 19:10562–10574.

Winocur G (1990) Anterograde and retrograde amnesia in rats with dorsal hippocampal or dorsomedial thalamic lesions. Behavioral Brain Research 38:145–154.

Wirth S, Yanike M, Frank LM, Smith AC, Brown EN, Suzuki WA (2003) Single neurons in the monkey hippocampus and learning of new associations. Science 300: 1578–1581.

Witter MP, Naber A, van Haeften T, Machielsen WC, Rombouts SA, Barkhof F, Scheltens P, Lopes da Silva FH (2000) Cortico-hippocampal communication by way of parallel parahippocampal-subicular pathways. Hippocampus 10:398–410.

Wood E, Dudchenko PA, Eichenbaum H (1999) The global record of memory in hippocampal neuronal activity. Nature 397:613–616.

Wood E, Dudchenko P, Robitsek JR, Eichenbaum H (2000) Hippocampal neurons encode information about different types of memory episodes occurring in the same location. Neuron 27:623–633.

Yanike M, Wirth S, Suzuki WA (2004) Representation of well-learned information in the monkey hippocampus. Neuron 42:477–487.

Young BJ, Otto T, Fox GD, Eichenbaum H (1997) Memory representation within the parahippocampal region. Journal of Neuroscience 17:5183–5195.

16

Ventrolateral Prefrontal Cortex and Controlling Memory to Inform Action

David Badre

Humans rely on knowledge to guide action. On entering a room, for example, we immediately categorize the objects we perceive in action-relevant ways: objects to sit on, objects to eat, objects to talk to, and so on. Much of this action-relevant knowledge is declarative, in that it is consciously accessible and generally verbalizable. Declarative knowledge includes semantic memory—knowledge of facts—and episodic memory—knowledge of events (Tulving, 1972)—and it relies on the medial temporal lobe system for rapid associative learning and initial retrieval (Squire, 1992; Cohen et al., 1997). In this example, the knowledge comes to mind fairly automatically as we encounter various cues in the room (e.g., a chair, an olive, a friend). To be useful, however, our knowledge must be available to other systems, including the action system, when we need it. How, then, do we bring declarative knowledge to bear on our actions when it is most useful, rather than relying on a fortuitous encounter with a cue? It is the primary goal of this chapter to discuss those control processes, supported by left ventrolateral prefrontal cortex (VLPFC), that permit us to retrieve and select relevant declarative knowledge to guide action and meet our goals. Before discussing these prefrontal control processes, however, we must consider the relationship between declarative memory and action and to distinguish the types of knowledge that can constrain action.

RULES AND THE DECLARATIVE MEMORY SYSTEM

The relationship between our perceptions, our knowledge, and our actions may be expressed in terms of rules (Bunge, 2004). Importantly, however, not every type of declarative knowledge that is relevant to action should be called a "rule." Furthermore, because content does not determine the form of a representation (see Lovett and Anderson, 2005), not every type of action knowledge that can be expressed as a rule is necessarily declarative or is stored as an explicit rule (see Fig. 16–1). Hence, storage of action-relevant declarative memories in posterior neocortex and control mechanisms for accessing

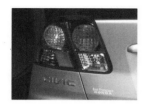 If light is on, then brake.

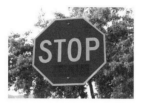 If you are driving and reach this sign and this is not an all-way stop, then stop and once stopped wait for cross traffic to clear before proceeding.

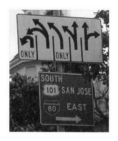 If you are driving in the far left lane then only make U-turn. If you are driving in the second lane, then make a U-turn or turn left. If you are in the third lane, then only turn left. If you are ...

Figure 16–1 The content of a representation does not determine the form of the representation. In the context of a well-proceduralized skill, such as driving, the response of braking when seeing an illuminated brake light is highly automatic. Even though one may be able to verbalize this behavior in terms of a rule (*right*), the representation governing the action, as in reflexively hitting the brake on seeing a brake light, may not be stored or implemented by the declarative system. The meanings of other action-relevant symbolic cues, such as a stop sign or a lane indicator, may indeed be stored declaratively. However, as demonstrated by the text on the *right,* even these declarative, symbolic representations may not be easily expressed as an explicit rule.

these memories in prefrontal cortex (PFC) may apply not only to knowledge easily amenable to expression as a rule, but also to declarative knowledge more generally.

Similar to the distinction between the content and form of rule representations, declarative knowledge relevant to action is not necessarily the same system as that which represents action knowledge itself. This difference is partially captured by the well-established distinction between declarative and nondeclarative memory. The nondeclarative memory system, also termed

procedural memory, refers to memory for skills, habits, stimulus-response relationships, and statistical properties of the environment that are not consciously accessible or readily verbalizable (Knowlton et al., 1994, 1996; Squire, 1994; Robbins, 1996; Poldrack et al., 1999a; Eichenbaum and Cohen, 2001). In other words, evidence of procedural memory is generally verifiable only through action, not through verbal report. Many forms of nondeclarative knowledge, such as stimulus-response associations, are rule-like in content (Fig. 16–1, top). However, in contrast to the rapid item-to-item associations formed by the declarative memory system, procedural memories are learned gradually, typically through feedback-based or reinforcement learning. Furthermore, they are encoded and retrieved independent of the medial temporal lobe memory system that is central to the encoding of declarative memories (Squire and Zola, 1996; Cohen et al., 1997). Rather, nondeclarative learning relies on corticostriatal circuitry (Knowlton et al., 1996; Poldrack et al., 1999a; Shohamy et al., 2004). Neuroimaging evidence from classification learning has further demonstrated that learning in the declarative and nondeclarative systems may even be competitive (Poldrack et al., 2001). Hence, in many cases, a stimulus-response production that might be described as a rule by an observer, such as learning over many trials to associate a complex visual display, a class of stimuli, or even a specific stimulus with a particular response, may be supported by a fundamentally different system than that used to acquire and store declarative knowledge of rules.

Beyond the declarative-nondeclarative distinction, it is also clear that intact declarative knowledge, even declarative knowledge of rules, is not necessarily a sufficient precondition for meaningful action. Apraxia, which typically results from damage to left inferior parietal cortex, is marked by the loss of the ability to produce complex or meaningful actions, often in the absence of deficits in comprehension (Leiguarda and Marsden, 2000). For example, apraxic patients will be unable to produce an appropriate action with an object on command or will demonstrate disturbances when pantomiming a particular action or gesture (Rothi et al., 1985). However, these patients are capable of naming objects and show otherwise intact lexical semantics and comprehension. Furthermore, this disorder is not due to muscle weakness or a loss of higher-level action productions, such as those stored by the nondeclarative system. Apraxic patients can produce actions that are triggered by a salient stimulus, as in covering their mouth when coughing, but they are unable to do so on command or intentionally (Grafton, 2003). Likewise, patients may perform a well-formed action, such as stirring their coffee, but may do so with an inappropriate implement, such as a bottle opener (De Renzi and Lucchelli, 1988). Based on these behaviors, some conceptualizations of apraxia characterize this disorder as a disconnection between declarative and action knowledge (Geschwind, 1965) or a disruption of an action portion of the conceptual system (Roy and Square, 1985).

Such perspectives do suggest that, although not sufficient for action, a route through the conceptual system is necessary for most object-oriented or

meaningful actions. However, reports of semantic dementia patients who have impaired knowledge of object functions, but intact object use (Buxbaum et al., 1997), suggest that semantic knowledge may not even be necessary for all complex actions. It is important to note that these cases are rare and somewhat controversial (e.g., Hodges et al., 2000), and impaired action semantics do impair much complex, goal-directed action. However, the existence of spared action in the presence of disrupted semantics argues against a unity between declarative action knowledge and actual stimulus-response productions, or even a mandatory path to action through the declarative memory system and its representations of rules and other action-relevant knowledge.

So, although actions are informed, constrained, and guided by long-term declarative knowledge, including rules, these are not necessarily the same systems or the same types of representations as productions that directly relate a cue to a response. Furthermore, declarative knowledge is not sufficient and may not even be necessary for storage and execution of all types of meaningful actions. Under what circumstances, then, is declarative knowledge important for action, and what types of knowledge are involved?

KNOWLEDGE-*FOR*-ACTION VERSUS KNOWLEDGE-*OF*-ACTION

Research into the relationship between declarative memory and action has focused primarily on what I will refer to as "knowledge-of-action," namely, which action or function is associated with a particular object, usually a tool, such as a hammer. This work has highlighted a distributed network of regions, including left lateral temporal regions commonly observed during semantic retrieval, but also left ventral PFC and premotor regions that might reflect the contribution of motor systems to the representation of action (Hauk et al., 2004; Johnson-Frey, 2004, 2005; Pulvermuller et al., 2005; Kan et al., 2006). However, it should be noted that activation of motor cortices during these tasks may also reflect an automatic attentional orientation to relevant motor systems in response to a salient stimulus, and so may not directly support the declarative knowledge of the function itself. Indeed, frontal cortex lesions do not impair knowledge-of-action to nearly the same extent as lateral temporal lobe damage (Goldenberg and Hagmann, 1998; Johnson-Frey, 2003).

An important question raised by these studies of knowledge-of-action is whether the regions of prefrontal and lateral temporal cortex activated in these experiments contribute specifically to the retrieval and representation of knowledge-of-action, or rather reflect more general declarative memory mechanisms, of which retrieving knowledge-of-action is one instance. A recent study by Kan et al. (2006) suggests that, whereas left ventral premotor cortex may indeed be sensitive to the retrieval of motor knowledge, the left VLPFC activation often observed in these studies reflects a more general process of selection from competition. Subjects were required to name pictures of action-relevant objects (i.e., tools) versus other objects (e.g., animals). The pictures

presented either had multiple candidate lexemes (low name agreement) or only a few candidate lexemes (high name agreement). Association with a larger number of candidate lexemes results in more competition at the lexical level on presentation of the stimulus (Levelt, 1999), making it more difficult to name the item. Critically, whereas ventral premotor cortex was differentially sensitive to tools relative to animals, it did not show a reliable effect of competition across these categories. By contrast, the opercular subdivision of left VLPFC was sensitive to competition across categories. Hence, although motor representations in premotor cortex may contribute to the representation of knowledge-of-action, activation in left VLPFC may reflect more general mnemonic control processes, such as selection from competition. Such a process would be employed during retrieval of knowledge-of-action, but also under most circumstances of lexical retrieval.

Following from this distinction, the remainder of this chapter will focus on the more general mnemonic control processes that support the retrieval and selection of knowledge-*for*-action rather than knowledge-*of*-action. Semantic knowledge relevant to action is not restricted to the common functions associated with tools. Rather, "knowledge-for-action" includes any property or association of a cue stored by the declarative memory system that might be relevant to one's goals or actions. This includes rules, such as the meanings of symbolic stimuli, such as road signs (Donohue et al., 2005), but also any other propositional knowledge stored by the declarative memory system. For instance, functional fixedness, in which a problem can be solved only by deriving an unusual use for an object, requires accessing general semantic knowledge of an object to assess its suitability for an alternative purpose. Using a shoe instead of a hammer to pound a nail is an example of applying task-relevant knowledge of a shoe (e.g., that it is hard and wieldy) for an atypical function. Furthermore, beyond a capacity to retrieve general declarative knowledge to inform higher planning and reasoning, an intact declarative memory system can select the relevant knowledge and action for the task at hand. For instance, patients with "frontal apraxia" are often bound by automatic retrieval, and consequently select the inappropriate features of objects to guide their action, such as spreading shaving cream on a toothbrush (Schwartz et al., 1995).

It follows from this discussion, then, that one does not necessarily need to propose a special system devoted only to the retrieval and representation of that subset of declarative knowledge directly relevant to action (e.g., rules or object functions). Rather, mnemonic processes generally involved in retrieving relevant semantic and perceptual features of objects, and one's particular temporal and spatial context, may also be called on to do so to guide action. The ability to strategically retrieve and select those features from semantic memory that are relevant to current actions and goals is the province of PFC. In the remainder of this chapter, I will consider the mnemonic control processes, supported by left VLPFC, that permit the retrieval and selection of task-relevant declarative knowledge. Note that, at the outset, these experiments consider the general case

of retrieval and can apply to declarative knowledge broadly, be it a rule, an action-relevant feature of an object, or any other task-relevant knowledge.

PREFRONTAL CORTEX AND THE CONTROL OF MEMORY

Humans store vast amounts of information (action-relevant and otherwise) about concepts, people, events, and object properties in a distributed network of posterior neocortical regions (Martin and Chao, 2001). Lateral temporal cortex, in particular, seems critical for the storage and retrieval of long-term semantic knowledge. Patients with damage to posterior temporal regions, typically inclusive of left posterior middle temporal gyrus (Gorno-Tempini et al., 2004), have the constellation of word-finding and semantic deficits in the presence of fluent language production that is the hallmark of Wernicke's aphasia. Similarly, degradation of the temporal pole results in semantic dementia, distinguished by word-finding deficits and loss of lexical, semantic, and object knowledge (Gorno-Tempini et al., 2004). Focal lesions in lateral temporal cortex can even result in impaired function within specific taxonomic categories (Damasio, 1990; Farah and McClelland, 1991; Martin and Chao, 2001; Thompson-Schill, 2003; Damasio et al., 2004).

Retrieval from this distributed store of information can occur automatically, in a bottom-up fashion and independent of PFC, on presentation of a cue. However, such bottom-up retrieval is obligatory and not strategic. To use declarative knowledge to full advantage in informing action, exclusive reliance on an encounter with a cue to retrieve relevant information can be problematic. Hence, PFC supports a control system that can guide retrieval and select information relevant to action goals, even when available cues are insufficient to do so automatically or lead to an inappropriate action.

Dissociable Mechanisms of Mnemonic Control in Left VLPFC

Considerable evidence has linked left ventrolateral prefrontal cortex with mnemonic control (Buckner, 1996; Gabrieli et al., 1998; Badre and Wagner, 2002; Petrides, 2002; Thompson-Schill, 2003; Poldrack and Wagner, 2004). VLPFC generally refers to the full extent of the inferior frontal gyrus anterior to premotor cortex and posterior to the frontal pole. Numerous neuroimaging studies involving word-reading, semantic decision tasks, long-term repetition priming, and other semantic retrieval manipulations have located activation in left VLPFC (Petersen et al., 1988; Kapur et al., 1994; Price et al., 1996; Poldrack et al., 1999b; Otten and Rugg, 2001; Roskies et al., 2001; Gold and Buckner, 2002; McDermott et al., 2003; Noesselt et al., 2003; Noppeney et al., 2004; Ruschemeyer et al., 2005; Wig et al., 2005). Furthermore, as reviewed earlier, left VLPFC may be involved in tasks requiring retrieval and selection of knowledge-*for*-action as well as knowledge-*of*-action, including, for example, comparisons of meaningful and meaningless gestures (Johnson-Frey et al., 2005). Damage to left VLPFC (Thompson-Schill et al., 1998) or intraoperative stimulation of left

VLPFC (Klein et al., 1997) results in disturbances on semantic tasks that require some form of control. Stimulation with transcranial magnetic stimulation in anterior VLPFC also results in disruption of decisions relying on semantic knowledge (Devlin et al., 2003), and stimulation in posterior VLPFC disrupts decisions relying on phonological knowledge (Gough et al., 2005). In addition, white matter tracts linking VLPFC with inferior and lateral temporal regions believed to store declarative knowledge have been identified in humans and nonhuman primates (Petrides and Pandya, 2002a, b; Croxson et al., 2005)—a connectivity pattern potentially consistent with this region's role in top-down control of these posterior neocortical regions.

Recent research efforts have focused on characterizing the mnemonic control processes supported by left VLPFC. With respect to rules and actions, such control processes may be important in guiding retrieval of knowledge-for-action. At least two functions have been attributed to left VLPFC computations (Wagner et al., 2001; Badre and Wagner, 2002; Thompson-Schill, 2003; Badre et al., 2005): (1) postretrieval selection and (2) controlled retrieval. Postretrieval selection is critical when multiple retrieved representations compete for processing (Thompson-Schill et al., 1999; Fletcher et al., 2000; Moss et al., 2005). Under such circumstances, selection processes bias relevant information over competitors. For example, selection is critical when naming pictures associated with multiple candidate lexemes (Levelt, 1999; Moss et al., 2005). Although names for a picture are retrieved relatively automatically, only one name is selected for production over the competitor lexemes. Hence, selection demands may be manipulated by increasing the number or strength of competitors during a memory task. Moreover, given its putative postretrieval nature, activation increases may be evident in left VLPFC under circumstances of competition, independent of activation differences in lateral temporal cortices associated with retrieval itself (Thompson-Schill et al., 1999).

The top-down or controlled retrieval of relevant semantic knowledge is necessary to the extent that relevant information does not become activated within long-term memory at retrieval (Wagner et al., 2001; Badre and Wagner, 2002). Under such circumstances, a control process that maintains relevant cues or retrieval plans could guide or bias retrieval to activate relevant knowledge. Controlled retrieval, then, should be more necessary to the extent that available cues are insufficient to elicit activation of target knowledge, such as under circumstances of low cue-target associative strength (Wagner et al., 2001). Notably, unlike selection that occurs postretrieval, controlled retrieval directly affects retrieval itself, and so should co-vary with activity in lateral temporal regions (Bokde et al., 2001).

Recently, my colleagues and I conducted a set of neuroimaging experiments that tested selection and controlled retrieval manipulations within subject (Badre et al., 2005). These experiments permitted dissociation of two subdivisions of left VLPFC and mid- and anterior VLPFC (Fig. 16–2) that were associated with selection and controlled retrieval, respectively.

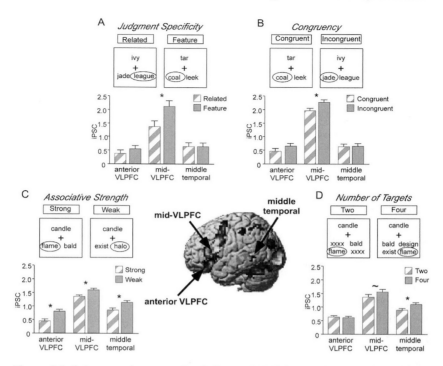

Figure 16–2 Integrated percent signal change (iPSC) in anterior ventrolateral pre-frontal cortex (VLPFC) [pars orbitalis, approximately BA 47], mid-VLPFC (pars tri-angularis, approximately BA 45), and posterior middle temporal cortex across four manipulations of semantic control. A. Judgment specificity manipulated whether par-ticipants made a global relatedness (related) or feature judgment (feature). B. Congru-ency manipulated whether the incorrect target during a feature judgment was a global associate of the cue (incongruent) or not (congruent). These manipulations resulted in activation in mid-VLPFC, but not in anterior VLPFC or middle temporal cortex. C. By contrast, manipulating associative strength, by making the correct target either a weak or a strong associate of the cue, resulted in greater activation in anterior and mid-VLPFC, as well as in middle temporal cortex. D. Finally, manipulating overall retrieval by varying the number of targets between two and four resulted in greater activation only in middle temporal and mid-VLPFC. (Adapted from Badre et al. *Neuron,* 47, 907–918. Copyright Elsevier, 2005.)

In all experiments, participants were presented with a cue word and either two or four target words, to which they made a judgment about semantic re-latedness. We employed two manipulations to vary selection demands directly. First, judgment specificity was manipulated such that participants were re-quired either to make a global relatedness judgment (i.e., which of the target words is most generally related to the cue word) or a similarity judgment along a particular feature dimension (i.e., which of the targets is most similar to the

cue with respect to color) [Fig. 16–2A]. The latter case, feature judgment, required participants to focus on a specific subset of retrieved knowledge, namely, the instructed feature (i.e., color), and so demanded increased selection (Thompson-Schill et al., 1997). Comparison of feature (high selection) and relatedness (low selection) judgments produced activation in posterior (approximately BA 44/6) [pars opercularis] and mid-VLPFC (approximately BA 45) [pars triangularis] (Fig. 16–2A).

We further manipulated selection demands within the feature judgment condition by varying the amount of automatically retrieved knowledge that is *irrelevant* to the current decision. Specifically, in half of the feature trials, the distractor, or incorrect target, was globally associated with the cue, but was not associated along the relevant dimension (e.g., banana-monkey, when the relevant dimension was color). During these incongruent trials (Fig. 16–2B), any information retrieved automatically because of the strong association between the cue and the distractor would be irrelevant to the current task and so would be expected to cause interference and increased selection demands. Consistent with the judgment specificity contrast, the contrast of incongruent to congruent trials produced activation in mid-VLPFC (Fig. 16–2B). Notably, neither of these contrasts was associated with increases in lateral temporal regions, potentially consistent with the postretrieval nature of these interference and selection effects.

Controlled retrieval was manipulated within the global relatedness judgment task by varying the associative strength of the correct target with the cue (Fig. 16–2C). Weak cue-target associative strength should elicit diminished bottom-up or cue-driven activation of relevant knowledge in memory, so choosing a response requires greater controlled retrieval (Wagner et al., 2001; Badre and Wagner, 2002; Bunge et al., 2005). It is important to note, however, that a manipulation of controlled retrieval may also increase selection demands because: (1) increases in retrieval will result in more relevant, but also more irrelevant, information from which to select, and (2) weak activation of relevant target knowledge makes this information less competitively viable, a case analogous to what has been recently termed an "underdetermined response" (Botvinick et al., 2004; Thompson-Schill et al., 2005). Hence, again, activation in posterior and mid-VLPFC was greater for weak–associative strength trials (high controlled retrieval and selection) than for strong–associative strength trials (low controlled retrieval and selection). Importantly, however, this effect was also evident in anterior VLPFC (approximately BA 47) [pars orbitalis], a region that showed no sensitivity to the selection manipulations (Fig. 16–2C).

Sensitivity to associative strength in posterior middle temporal cortex mirrored that observed in left VLPFC, consistent with the hypothesized interaction of controlled retrieval processes with long-term memory representations. However, middle temporal cortex was also active when comparing trials in which there were four (more overall retrieval) versus two targets (less overall retrieval). Anterior VLPFC, by contrast, showed no such sensitivity

(Fig. 16–2D). This is because the number of targets merely results in an increase in the amount of overall retrieval, not necessarily controlled retrieval. Indeed, pitting controlled retrieval against overall retrieval by contrasting weak, two-target trials (high controlled retrieval and low overall retrieval) with strong, four-target trials (low controlled retrieval and high overall retrieval) resulted in selective activation in anterior VLPFC (see Fig. 16–5B for a rendering of this contrast). This replicated a similar selective effect in anterior VLPFC of associative strength, independent of overall retrieval demands, reported by Wagner et al. (2001).

To summarize, anterior VLPFC was selectively responsive to increases in controlled retrieval demands, independent of retrieval-induced competition or the number of overall retrieval demands. Consistent with its role in storing long-term memory representations, posterior middle temporal cortex was sensitive to increases in controlled retrieval demands (associative strength) and overall retrieval (number of targets). Finally, mid-VLPFC was sensitive to all main effects, including those that did not elicit a retrieval response in posterior middle temporal cortex. Only when controlled retrieval was pitted against overall retrieval was mid-VLPFC not reliably active. This is theoretically consistent with a postretrieval selection process common to all of the manipulations.

Importantly, a common selection component, as predicted by this theoretical task analysis, should also be reflected by a common component in the behavioral variance across these manipulations. Reaction time (RT) and error rates across two independent sets of participants were assessed with principle-components analysis. A single component was extracted that accounted for more common variance across all of the manipulations than any of the individual measures in isolation. Such a common component might be reflective of a common selection process. A meta-variable that indexed this common "selection component" was computed for each participant and entered into our imaging analysis. Strikingly, the only region to co-vary with this index of a common "selection component" was, again, mid-VLPFC (see Fig. 16–5C). Hence, both qualitative and quantitative analyses implicated mid-VLPFC in a common postretrieval selection process.

Both selection and controlled retrieval should be critical in knowledge-for-action. As introduced earlier, the ability to interpret stimuli and extract relevant object properties, based on past experience with those objects or prior knowledge of those objects, is particularly important for action. Consider the example of functional fixedness described earlier. Here, controlled retrieval processes, supported by anterior VLPFC, might be important to bias retrieval of properties of shoes that were not retrieved automatically, such as the fact that they are easily and firmly held in one hand and light enough to be forcefully swung in a controlled manner. In addition, the automatic retrieval of irrelevant, but strongly associated, information about shoes, such as that they are worn on the feet, might compete for processing with the relevant information, and so require selection, supported by mid-VLPFC. Of course, this

example derives from the thesis that the same network characterized during general semantic retrieval tasks is important for knowledge-for-action, as well. Indeed, it is notable that rule retrieval, as indexed by identifying the meanings of unfamiliar road signs, implicates this same network of left anterior and mid-VLPFC and middle temporal cortex (Donohue et al., 2005). Hence, one might anticipate activation of these regions of anterior and mid-VLPFC when selection for action requires either the search of knowledge because available cues are insufficient, or when calls to memory are hindered by interference, and so require selection.

Proactive Interference and Left VLPFC

In the case of the congruency manipulation described earlier, we demonstrated that a pre-experimental association in semantic memory results in interference due to the automatic retrieval of irrelevant information. This irrelevant information interferes with target knowledge selection, and must be overcome by left mid-VLPFC control processes. However, it is also possible for associations among cues in a task to be built rapidly and to cause interference on subsequent encounters with those cues in a different context. As discussed later, this type of interference can be an obstacle to applying knowledge-for-action to current task goals.

Proactive interference (PI) occurs when prior learning negatively affects current processing (Brown, 1958; Peterson and Peterson, 1959; Keppel and Underwood, 1962). PI effects may be obtained even over a short time scale. One currently popular method of eliciting short-term PI uses a variant of a short-term item recognition test (Monsell, 1978; Jonides et al., 1998). In this experiment (Fig. 16–3A), participants are required to maintain a memory set of items over a brief delay and then indicate whether a probe item was (positive trials) or was not (negative trials) in the memory set. The critical PI manipulation is produced by varying whether the probe for the current trial overlaps with the memory set of the previous trial. A probe that is not a member of the current memory set (negative) but that was a member of the previous trial's memory set (recent) elicits PI. This interference is reflected in increased RT and sometimes errors when rejecting these negative recent probes.

Mid-VLPFC has been consistently observed to be more active in high-relative to low-overlap trials (Figure 16–3B) (Jonides et al., 1998; D'Esposito et al., 1999; Bunge et al., 2001; Mecklinger et al., 2003; Nelson et al., 2003; Postle et al., 2004; Badre and Wagner, 2005; Jonides and Nee, 2006), and a patient with damage to this region showed greatly enhanced PI effects (Thompson-Schill et al., 2002). Furthermore, interference in this task has been shown to arise from competing memory representations rather than opposing responses (Nelson et al., 2003). Hence, mid-VLPFC appears to play a role in resolving interference due to PI.

Recently, Anthony Wagner and I argued that PI in this task may arise from the automatic retrieval of irrelevant information required to assign a probe to

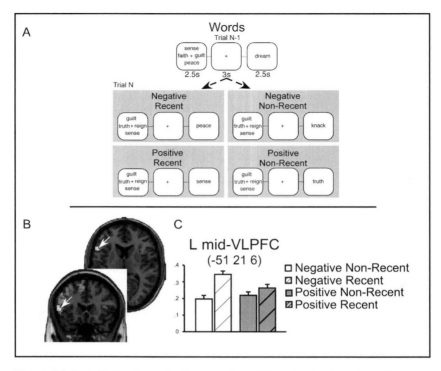

Figure 16–3 *A.* Task schematic diagram of conditions in the short-term item recognition experiment. Proactive interference is elicited by arranging an overlap of a target in trial N with a member of the memory set in trial N – 1. *B.* Overlap map of negative recent > negative nonrecent contrast and episodic context selection (Dobbins and Wagner, 2005). *Arrows* indicate the point of overlap in mid-ventrolateral prefrontal cortex (mid-VLPFC). *C.* Greater mid-VLPFC activation was evident for negative and positive recent trials relative to nonrecent trials. (Adapted from Badre and Wagner, *Cerebral Cortex,* 15, 2003–2012. Copyright Oxford University Press, 2005.)

a particular temporal context, thereby increasing selection demands and so requiring greater activation in left mid-VLPFC (Badre and Wagner, 2005). More specifically, we reasoned that the presentation of a probe, even in a short-term item memory test, requires assignment of the probe to a particular temporal context, such as the current trial, as opposed to the previous, trial. When encountering a probe that appeared in the previous trial, the participant retrieves irrelevant contextual information associated with that probe in the previous trial. To correctly assign the probe to the appropriate temporal context, the participant must select against this information, and so this selection demand elicits greater activation in left VLPFC.

One distinguishing implication of this hypothesis is the prediction that it makes for positive recent trials. Positive trials, although present in the cur-

rent trial's memory set, may also overlap with the previous trial's memory set. Whereas this arrangement ensures that familiarity with the probe is convergent with the correct response, any associations with the previous trial are still irrelevant and so should increase selection demands. Such an effect would produce increased activation in left VLPFC to positive recent trials.

To test our hypothesis, we designed a variant of the standard short-term item memory test and tested the effects of probe recency during positive as well as negative trials. As depicted in Figure 16–3C, both negative and positive recent trials resulted in increases in left mid-VLPFC activation. Importantly, this was not simply an effect of familiarity generally, because all positive trials are familiar, having been in the current set, and there was no difference between positive and negative low-overlap trials.

Following from the logic outlined earlier, one might further anticipate some convergence of mid-VLPFC and other regions observed in this task with those observed in tasks from other domains that require selection of details from memory to assign a probe to a given temporal context. In particular, episodic memory tasks often demand precisely this type of selection. Bearing in mind the limitations inherent in such analyses, there was, indeed, a high degree of convergence between mid-VLPFC activation in this task and an independent episodic memory task that directly manipulated the domain-general selection of contextual details (Figure 16–3B) (Dobbins and Wagner, 2005).

Hence, PI in this task may arise from the simultaneous activation of multiple contextually relevant details and may be overcome by a selection process in which relevant contextual representations are biased over irrelevant representations. Recently, Jonides and Nee (2006) have proposed a highly similar selection mechanism for left VLPFC function in this task, also conceptualizing it in terms of a biased competition framework, although in this case, emphasizing the selection of relevant attentional attributes, such as familiarity, rather than episodic details meant to assign a probe to a temporal context.

In general, however, left mid-VLPFC appears critical for the selection of relevant from irrelevant retrieved information. Moreover, the specific focus of activation in mid-VLPFC is highly convergent with that associated with the "selection component" from the study of semantic judgments (see Fig. 16–5C and D). To the extent that retrieval of knowledge-for-action depends on the same system that supports the storage and retrieval of declarative memories more generally, it follows that processes, such as selection, are also required to focus processing on relevant knowledge-for-action. In the next section, I will discuss how PI effects analogous to those investigated here can arise during task-switching, and how a selection process, supported by mid-VLPFC, may be critical in resolving this interference to select the relevant knowledge-for-action.

DECLARATIVE KNOWLEDGE AND CONTROL OF TASK SETS

As I have argued so far, the ability to strategically guide memory search and to select relevant retrieved representations for further processing are

general-purpose mnemonic control processes that should also play an important role in the retrieval and selection of knowledge-for-action. Our modern world of wireless Internet, cell phones, PDAs, and instant messaging can interrupt whatever task we were trying to complete (e.g., writing a book chapter) and force us to retrieve a whole new set of information, both episodic and semantic, about a more immediately pressing task. Hence, calls to memory are a fundamental part of shifting task sets, or task-switching, and so should be informed by research, such as that summarized earlier, on the controlled search, retrieval, and selection of task-relevant knowledge.

Our capacity to shift among different tasks may be studied in the laboratory by comparing trials during which a simple task is repeated with trials that entail a switch in task. Relative to repeat trials, switch trials are associated with an increase in RT and errors, known as the "behavioral switch cost" (Jersild, 1927; Allport et al., 1994; Rogers and Monsell, 1995; Logan and Bundesen, 2003; Monsell, 2003). Furthermore, preparation in advance of a switch can reduce, although not eliminate, the switch cost (Rogers and Monsell, 1995; Meiran et al., 2000).

The difficulty that we experience in switching tasks may be partially attributable to the demand to activate a new set of task-relevant representations from memory each time we engage in a new task. For this reason, some form of memory retrieval, or activation of a task set, is at the heart of most models of task-switching (Rogers and Monsell, 1995; Allport and Wylie, 2000; Mayr and Kliegl, 2000; Rubinstein et al., 2001), whether this retrieval is viewed as intentional and controlled or relatively automatic. Interestingly, a number of theorists have increasingly emphasized the resolution of interference from memory during task-switching paradigms as being a prime source of task switch costs (Allport et al., 1994; Allport and Wylie, 2000; Wylie and Allport, 2000; Dreher and Berman, 2002; Mayr, 2002).

One such interference theory, termed "task set priming," proposes that the automatic retrieval of irrelevant, competitive information may produce interference during a task switch (Allport and Wylie, 2000; Wylie and Allport, 2000; Waszak et al., 2003). From this perspective, task performance results in priming of the associations between available cues and any representations that enter processing. An additional encounter with these cues in the context of the same task will result in facilitated access to this information, an effect analogous to repetition priming. However, during a task switch, these primed associations result in facilitated retrieval of irrelevant information (e.g., Waszak et al., 2003), analogous to the instance of short-term PI described earlier. The activation of representations from the previous task competes with performance of the new task. Hence, as with the experiments focusing on short-term item recognition, one might anticipate involvement of mid-VLPFC to resolve this interference.

Consistent with this hypothesis, left VLPFC activation has been a common finding across studies of task-switching (Meyer et al., 1997, 1998; Dove et al., 2000; DiGirolamo et al., 2001; Brass and von Cramon, 2002, 2004a, b; Dreher

and Berman, 2002; Konishi et al., 2002; Luks et al., 2002; Shulman et al., 2002; Dreher and Grafman, 2003; Reynolds et al., 2004; Ruge et al., 2005). Moreover, patients with lesions broadly located in left lateral PFC show deficits in task-switching (Rogers et al., 1998; Mecklinger et al., 1999; Aron et al., 2003). Recently, Anthony Wagner and I conducted a functional magnetic resonance imaging (fMRI) study meant to draw a direct connection between mid-VLPFC activity during task-switching and the resolution of interference evoked from associative memory during a task switch (Badre and Wagner, 2006).

To study task-switching, we employed a standard explicit cueing variant (Meiran et al., 2000), in which participants were instructed as to which task (vowel-consonant letter or odd-even number decision) they would be required to perform before the presentation of an upcoming target (number-letter pair, such as "a1"). Categorizations were reported using a manual button press, and category-to-response mappings overlapped between tasks. For example, a left button press might mean "vowel" for the letter task and "odd" for the number task. Hence, this design allows us to manipulate task-switching (going from the letter to the number task, or vice versa), as well as the amount of preparation time (cue-to-stimulus interval).

To be theoretically explicit about our conception of memory-induced interference during task-switching and our predictions for the associated response in regions sensitive to interference, such as mid-VLPFC, we developed a simple computational model in which task switch costs arose from proactive interference among competing activated representations (Fig. 16–4A; see color insert). In our model, termed the "control of associative memory during task-switching," three layers represented the responses (left or right button press), semantic concepts ("odd," "even," "vowel," and "consonant"), and task goals (letter or number decision) in the explicit cueing task. Units within layers were mutually competitive, such that their simultaneous activation would result in greater conflict. Reciprocal connections between the layers meant that activation of a unit in the task layer (i.e., "letter task") would feed forward to activate relevant units in the concept layer (i.e., "vowel" and "consonant"), but also that activation of subordinate representations (e.g., left response) would feed back to activate associated superordinate representations (e.g., "vowel" and "odd" in the concept layer). Hence, these feedback connections ensured that there would be coactivation at multiple layers and so conflict during every trial, including repeat trials.

Greater conflict during switch trials occurred because of associative learning. Specifically, at each response, connections between coactive units were made stronger. During a task switch, then, connections between units of the previously relevant—but now irrelevant—task would be stronger and so would elicit stronger activation of these irrelevant units. The result is greater competition and interference in switch trials, and therefore a switch cost.

Control in the model took the form of a bias competition mechanism similar to that employed by others (Cohen et al., 1990; Botvinick et al., 2001).

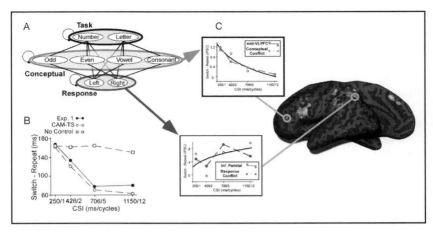

Figure 16–4 *A.* The model contains three reciprocally connected layers of units representing the task, conceptual, and response components of the explicit cueing task. *B.* Simulated switch costs and preparation costs track empirically derived behavioral responses very well. However, when control during the preparation period was turned off, there was no decline in switch costs with increased preparation. *C.* The switch versus repeat contrast revealed activation in left ventrolateral prefrontal cortex (VLPFC) [opercularis and triangularis], supplementary motor area (SMA), and parietal cortex. Responses across preparation intervals in mid-VLPFC matched the model's predicted conceptual conflict signal. This mid-VLPFC responses dissociated from the response in parietal cortex that appeared to match the predicted response conflict signal from the model. CSI, cue-to-stimulus interval; iPSC, integrated percent signal change. (Adapted from Badre and Wagner, *Proceedings of the National Academy of Sciences,* 103, 7186–7191. Copyright *PNAS,* 2006.)

An increase in the top-down bias of the task layer on the conceptual layer was applied during the preparation interval of each trial. At longer intervals of preparation, this increased top-down control permitted relevant representations to come to increasingly dominate the conceptual layer. The model produced switch costs and preparation curves consistent with behavioral data (Fig. 16–4*B*).

   To provide quantitative hypotheses about proactive interference among active representations across conditions of the task-switching fMRI experiment, we computed an index of conflict from different layers of the model using the Hopfield energy computation (Hopfield, 1982; Botvinick et al., 2001). Conflict in the conceptual layer was found to decrease with more preparation (Fig. 16–4*C*). By contrast, conflict in the response layer tended to increase with more preparation (Fig. 16–4*C*).

   These model indices of conflict fit the fMRI response during task-switching. Consistent with past reports, the switch versus repeat comparison produced

activation in mid-VLPFC. Critically, the model index of conflict from retrieved conceptual representations was characteristic of the decline in switching effects in left mid-VLPFC with increased preparation (Fig. 16–4C). This pattern of data dissociated this region from inferior parietal cortex, which appeared to track the ramping pattern of conflict from the response layer of the model. A transfer of processing from the conceptual to the response level may be consistent with event-related potential data, showing separable temporal components between early frontal and later parietal potentials (Lorist et al., 2000; Rushworth et al., 2002; Brass et al., 2005) and similar conflict-based dissociations during task-switching obtained with neuroimaging (Liston et al., 2006).

The mid-VLPFC focus identified in this experiment is highly convergent with that discussed in previous studies of semantic conflict and proactive interference resolution (Fig. 16–5C through E; see color insert). Hence, in addition to providing important support for interference theories of task-switching, these data also underscore the broader role for mid-VLPFC selection processes in the control of action.

CONCLUSIONS

The focus of this chapter has been on the relationship between declarative memory and action, and the contribution of left VLPFC in bringing declarative knowledge to bear on action. Rules, even when distinguished from nondeclarative productions as explicit constructs, are not the only type of declarative knowledge relevant to action. Mechanisms for retrieving rules may be the same as those required to retrieve task-relevant declarative knowledge more generally. Hence, understanding the general mechanisms by which PFC controls retrieval is fundamental to an understanding of rule-guided behavior, and indeed, more broadly, knowledge-guided behavior.

I have distinguished knowledge-for-action as the general case of retrieving declarative knowledge to constrain or guide action, and have summarized a line of research that specifies the mnemonic control processing in left VLPFC that is fundamental to this function. More specifically, left anterior VLPFC appears critical for the biased or controlled retrieval of long-term memory representations maintained in posterior neocortex, such as posterior middle temporal cortex (Fig. 16–5A and B). By contrast, left mid-VLPFC appears critical for resolving interference among retrieved representations (Fig. 16–5A, C, and D).

To the extent that one's knowledge of people, places, things, or the past is relevant to a task at hand, a call to memory is necessary. Hence, any such instance of action will be subject to the same obstacles as any act of memory retrieval. As with any act of retrieval, control will be important in guiding search and overcoming interference to focus processing on the most relevant information in memory. This was illustrated in the study on task-switching. Interference among automatically activated memory representations during

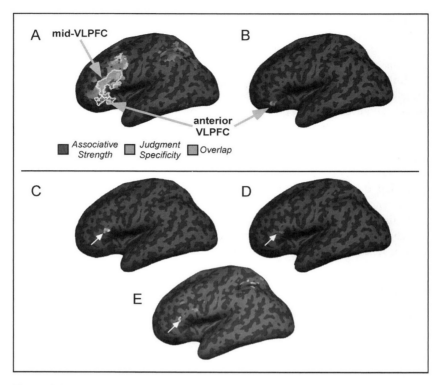

Figure 16–5 A. Overlap of judgment specificity (*red*) and associative strength (*blue*) manipulations on inflated canonical surface. Overlap in mid-ventrolateral prefrontal cortex (mid-VLPFC) to posterior VLPFC (*purple*). B. Contrast of weak–associative strength, two-target trials with strong–associative strength, four-target trials reveals activation in anterior VLPFC (Wagner et al., 2001; Badre et al., 2005). C–E. Inflated surface renderings demonstrate the high convergence in mid-VLPFC in response to selection demands across independent data sets, including "selection component" activation (Badre et al., 2005) [C], negative recent > negative nonrecent contrast (Badre and Wagner, 2005) [D], and switch minus repeat at the shortest cue-to-stimulus interval of 250 ms (Badre and Wagner, 2006) [E]. Note that the reference *arrow* is in the same position in each map.

a task switch was argued to be an important contributor to the switch cost. A left mid-VLPFC mechanism, in common with that required to select relevant retrieved representations, may thus be required to overcome this interference (Fig. 16–5C through E).

Left VLPFC control processes appear central to knowledge-guided action because they permit the retrieval and selection of task-relevant rules and general action-relevant knowledge. The characterization of these control processes is ongoing and controversial, and the progress of this research will likely

yield important insights into the manner by which knowledge is retrieved to inform action. Ultimately, however, the discussion of rule-guided behavior must lead to important and difficult questions about the interface between some of the systems mentioned in this chapter. How do retrieved declarative representations feed forward to influence the motor system? What is the relationship between the declarative and nondeclarative systems in influencing action? Are there important differences in action or rule representations between a human participant who is explicitly told the stimulus-response contingencies in a task a few minutes before beginning the task and a nonhuman primate that acquires the appropriate response contingencies over a long period of training? Future efforts may begin to address these fundamental questions about the relationship between memory and action.

ACKNOWLEDGMENTS Supported by NIH (F32 NS053337–03). I would like to acknowledge A. D. Wagner, my principal collaborator on the empirical work in this chapter. Thanks are also due to B. Buchsbaum and J. Rissman for their insightful comments on early drafts.

REFERENCES

Allport A, Styles EA, Hsieh S (1994) Shifting intentional set: exploring the dynamic control of tasks. In: Attention and performance XV: conscious and nonconscious information processing (Umilta C, Moscovitch M, eds.), pp 421–452. Cambridge, MA: MIT Press.

Allport A, Wylie G (2000) 'Task-switching,' stimulus-response bindings and negative priming. In: Control of cognitive processes: attention and performance XVIII (Monsell S, Driver J, eds.), pp 35–70. Cambridge, MA: MIT Press.

Aron AR, Watkins L, Sahakian BJ, Monsell S, Barker RA, Robbins TW (2003) Task-set switching deficits in early-stage Huntington's disease: implications for basal ganglia function. Journal of Cognitive Neuroscience 15:629–642.

Badre D, Poldrack RA, Pare-Blagoev EJ, Insler RZ, Wagner AD (2005) Dissociable controlled retrieval and generalized selection mechanisms in ventrolateral prefrontal cortex. Neuron 47:907–918.

Badre D, Wagner AD (2002) Semantic retrieval, mnemonic control, and the prefrontal cortex. Behavioral and Cognitive Neuroscience Reviews 1:206–218.

Badre D, Wagner AD (2005) Frontal lobe mechanisms that resolve proactive interference. Cerebral Cortex 15:2003–2012.

Badre D, Wagner AD (2006) Computational and neurobiological mechanisms underlying cognitive flexibility. Proceedings of the National Academy of Sciences U S A 103:7186–7191.

Bokde ALW, Tagamets M-A, Friedman RB, Horwitz B (2001) Functional interactions of the inferior frontal cortex during the processing of words and word-like stimuli. Neuron 30:609–617.

Botvinick MM, Braver TS, Barch DM, Carter CS, Cohen JD (2001) Conflict monitoring and cognitive control. Psychological Review 108:624–652.

Botvinick MM, Cohen JD, Carter CS (2004) Conflict monitoring and anterior cingulate cortex: an update. Trends in Cognitive Sciences 8:539–546.

Brass M, Ullsperger M, Knoesche TR, von Cramon DY, Phillips NA (2005) Who comes first? The role of the prefrontal and parietal cortex in cognitive control. Journal of Cognitive Neuroscience 17:1367–1375.

Brass M, von Cramon DY (2002) The role of the frontal cortex in task preparation. Cerebral Cortex 12:908–914.

Brass M, von Cramon DY (2004a) Selection for cognitive control: a functional magnetic resonance imaging study on the selection of task-relevant information. Journal of Neuroscience 24:8847–8852.

Brass M, von Cramon DY (2004b) Decomposing components of task preparation with functional magnetic resonance imaging. Journal of Cognitive Neuroscience 16: 609–620.

Brown J (1958) Some tests of the decay theory of immediate memory. Quarterly Journal of Experimental Psychology 10:12–21.

Buckner RL (1996) Beyond HERA: Contributions of specific prefrontal brain areas to long-term memory retrieval. Psychonomic Bulletin and Review 3:149–158.

Bunge SA (2004) How we use rules to select actions: a review of evidence from cognitive neuroscience. Cognitive, Affective, and Behavioral Neuroscience 4:564–579.

Bunge SA, Ochsner KN, Desmond JE, Glover GH, Gabrieli JD (2001) Prefrontal regions involved in keeping information in and out of mind. Brain 124:2074–2086.

Bunge SA, Wendelken C, Badre D, Wagner AD (2005) Analogical reasoning and the prefrontal cortex: evidence for separable retrieval and integration mechanisms. Cerebral Cortex 15:239–249.

Buxbaum LJ, Schwartz MF, Carew TG (1997) The role of semantic memory in object use. Cognitive Neuropsychology 14:219–254.

Cohen JD, Dunbar K, McClelland JL (1990) On the control of automatic processes: parallel distributed processing account of the Stroop effect. Psychological Review 97:332–361.

Cohen NJ, Eichenbaum H, Poldrack RA (1997) Memory for items and memory for relations in the procedural/declarative memory framework. Memory 5:131–178.

Croxson PL, Johansen-Berg H, Behrens TE, Robson MD, Pinsk MA, Gross CG, Richter W, Richter MC, Kastner S, Rushworth MF (2005) Quantitative investigation of connections of the prefrontal cortex in the human and macaque using probabilistic diffusion tractography. Journal of Neuroscience 25:8854–8866.

D'Esposito M, Postle BR, Jonides J, Smith EE (1999) The neural substrate and temporal dynamics of interference effects in working memory as revealed by event-related functional MRI. Proceedings of the National Academy of Sciences U S A 96:7514–7519.

Damasio AR (1990) Category-related recognition deficits as a clue to the neural substrates of knowledge. Trends in Neuroscience 13:95–98.

Damasio H, Tranel D, Grabowski T, Adolphs R, Damasio A (2004) Neural systems behind word and concept retrieval. Cognition 92:179–229.

De Renzi E, Lucchelli F (1988) Ideational apraxia. Brain 111 (Pt 5):1173–1185.

Devlin JT, Matthews PM, Rushworth MF (2003) Semantic processing in the left inferior prefrontal cortex: a combined functional magnetic resonance imaging and transcranial magnetic stimulation study. Journal of Cognitive Neuroscience 15:71–84.

DiGirolamo GJ, Kramer AF, Barad V, Cepeda NJ, Weissman DH, Milham MP, Wszalek TM, Cohen NJ, Banich MT, Webb A, Belopolsky AV, McAuley E (2001) General and task-specific frontal lobe recruitment in older adults during executive processes: a fMRI investigation of task-switching. Neuroreport 12:2065–2071.

Dobbins IG, Wagner AD (2005) Domain-general and domain-sensitive prefrontal mechanisms for recollecting events and detecting novelty. Cerebral Cortex 15: 1768–1778.

Donohue SE, Wendelken C, Crone EA, Bunge SA (2005) Retrieving rules for behavior from long-term memory. Neuroimage 26:1140–1149.

Dove A, Pollmann S, Schubert T, Wiggins CJ, von Cramon DY (2000) Prefrontal cortex activation in task switching: an event-related fMRI study. Brain Research: Cognitive Brain Research 9:103–109.

Dreher JC, Berman KF (2002) Fractionating the neural substrate of cognitive control processes. Proceedings of the National Academy of Sciences U S A 99:14595–14600.

Dreher J-C, Grafman J (2003) Dissociating the roles of the rostral anterior cingulate and the lateral prefrontal cortices in performing two tasks simultaneously or successively. Cerebral Cortex 13:329–339.

Eichenbaum H, Cohen NJ (2001) From conditioning to conscious recollection: memory systems of the brain. Oxford, UK: Oxford University Press.

Farah MJ, McClelland JL (1991) A computational model of semantic memory impairment: modality specificity and emergent category specificity. Journal of Experimental Psychology: General 120:339–357.

Fletcher PC, Shallice T, Dolan RJ (2000) 'Sculpting the response space'—an account of left prefrontal activation at encoding. Neuroimage 12:404–417.

Gabrieli JD, Poldrack RA, Desmond JE (1998) The role of left prefrontal cortex in language and memory. Proceedings of the National Academy of Sciences U S A 95: 906–913.

Geschwind N (1965) Disconnexion syndromes in animals and man, I. Brain 88:237–294.

Gold BT, Buckner RL (2002) Common prefrontal regions coactivate with dissociable posterior regions during controlled semantic and phonological tasks. Neuron 35: 803–812.

Goldenberg G, Hagmann S (1998) Tool use and mechanical problem solving in apraxia. Neuropsychologia 36:581–589.

Gorno-Tempini ML, Dronkers NF, Rankin KP, Ogar JM, Phengrasamy L, Rosen HJ, Johnson JK, Weiner MW, Miller BL (2004) Cognition and anatomy in three variants of primary progressive aphasia. Annals of Neurology 55:335–346.

Gough PM, Nobre AC, Devlin JT (2005) Dissociating linguistic processes in the left inferior frontal cortex with transcranial magnetic stimulation. Journal of Neuroscience 25:8010–8016.

Grafton ST (2003) Apraxia: a disorder of motor control. In: neurological foundations of cognitive neuroscience (D'Esposito M, ed.), pp 239–258. Cambridge: MIT Press.

Hauk O, Johnsrude I, Pulvermuller F (2004) Somatotopic representation of action words in human motor and premotor cortex. Neuron 41:301–307.

Hodges JR, Bozeat S, Lambon Ralph MA, Patterson K, Spatt J (2000) The role of conceptual knowledge in object use evidence from semantic dementia. Brain 123 (Pt 9):1913–1925.

Hopfield JJ (1982) Neural networks and physical systems with emergent collective computational abilities. Proceedings of the National Academy of Sciences U S A 79:2554–2558.

Jersild AT (1927) Mental set and shift. Archives of Psychology 89.

Johnson-Frey SH (2003) What's so special about human tool use? Neuron 39:201–204.

Johnson-Frey SH (2004) The neural bases of complex tool use in humans. Trends in Cognitive Sciences 8:71–78.

Johnson-Frey SH, Newman-Norlund R, Grafton ST (2005) A distributed left hemisphere network active during planning of everyday tool use skills. Cerebral Cortex 15: 681–695.

Jonides J, Nee DE (2006) Brain mechanisms of proactive interference in working memory. Neuroscience 139:181–193.

Jonides J, Smith EE, Marshuetz C, Koeppe RA, Reuter-Lorenz PA (1998) Inhibition in verbal working memory revealed by brain activation. Proceedings of the National Academy of Sciences U S A 95:8410–8413.

Kan IP, Kable JW, Van Scoyoc A, Chatterjee A, Thompson-Schill SL (2006) Fractionating the left frontal response to tools: dissociable effects of motor experience and lexical competition. Journal of Cognitive Neuroscience 18:267–277.

Kapur S, Rose R, Liddle PF, Zipursky RB, Brown GM, Stuss D, Houle S, Tulving E (1994) The role of the left prefrontal cortex in verbal processing: semantic processing or willed action? Neuroreport 5:2193–2196.

Keppel G, Underwood BJ (1962) Proactive inhibition in short-term retention of single items. Journal of Verbal Learning and Verbal Behavior 1:153–161.

Klein D, Olivier A, Milner B, Zatorre RJ, Johnsrude I, Meyer E, Evans AC (1997) Obligatory role of the LIFG in synonym generation: evidence from PET and cortical stimulation. Neuroreport 8:3275–3279.

Knowlton B, Mangels JA, Squire LR (1996) A neostriatal habit learning system in humans. Science 273:1399–1402.

Knowlton B, Squire LR, Gluck MA (1994) Probabilistic classification in amnesia. Learning and Memory 1:106–120.

Konishi S, Hayashi T, Uchida I, Kikyo H, Takahashi E, Miyashita Y (2002) Hemispheric asymmetry in human lateral prefrontal cortex during cognitive set shifting. Proceedings of the National Academy of Sciences U S A 99:7803–7808.

Leiguarda RC, Marsden CD (2000) Limb apraxias: higher-order disorders of sensorimotor integration. Brain 123 (Pt 5):860–879.

Levelt WJ (1999) Models of word production. Trends in Cognitive Sciences 3:223–232.

Liston C, Matalon S, Hare TA, Davidson MC, Casey BJ (2006) Anterior cingulate and posterior parietal cortices are sensitive to dissociable forms of conflict in a task-switching paradigm. Neuron 50:643–653.

Logan GD, Bundesen C (2003) Clever homunculus: is there an endogenous act of control in the explicit task-cuing procedure? Journal of Experimental Psychology: Human Perception and Performance 29:575–599.

Lorist MM, Klein M, Nieuwenhuis S, De Jong R, Mulder G, Meijman TF (2000) Mental fatigue and task control: planning and preparation. Psychophysiology 37: 614–625.

Lovett MC, Anderson JR (2005) Thinking as a production system. In: The Cambridge handbook of thinking and reasoning (Holyoak KJ, Morrison RG, eds.), pp 401–430. New York: Cambridge University Press.

Luks TL, Simpson GV, Feiwell RJ, Miller WL (2002) Evidence for anterior cingulate cortex involvement in monitoring preparatory attentional set. Neuroimage 17: 792–802.

Martin A, Chao LL (2001) Semantic memory and the brain: structure and processes. Current Opinion in Neurobiology 11:194–201.

Mayr U (2002) Inhibition of action rules. Psychonomic Bulletin and Review 9:93–99.

Mayr U, Kliegl R (2000) Task-set switching and long-term memory retrieval. Journal of Experimental Psychology: Learning, Memory, and Cognition 26:1124–1140.

McDermott KB, Petersen SE, Watson JM, Ojemann JG (2003) A procedure for identifying regions preferentially activated by attention to semantic and phonological relations using functional magnetic resonance imaging. Neuropsychologia 41:293–303.

Mecklinger AD, von Cramon DY, Springer A, Matthes-von Cramon G (1999) Executive control functions in task switching: evidence from brain injured patients. Journal of Clinical and Experimental Neuropsychology 21:606–619.

Mecklinger A, Weber K, Gunter TC, Engle RW (2003) Dissociable brain mechanisms for inhibitory control: effects of interference content and working memory capacity. Brain Research: Cognitive Brain Research 18:26–38.

Meiran N, Chorev Z, Sapir A (2000) Component processes in task switching. Cognitive Psychology 41:211–253.

Meyer DE, Evans JE, Lauber EJ, Gmeindl L, Rubinstein J, Junck L, Koeppe RA (1998, April 5–7). The role of dorsolateral prefrontal cortex for executive cognitive processes in task switching. Poster presented at the Cognitive Neuroscience Society. San Francisco, CA.

Meyer DE, Lauber EJ, Rubinstein J, Gmeindl L, Junck L, Koeppe RA (1997, March 23–25). Activation of brain mechanisms for executive mental processes in cognitive task switching. Poster presented at the Cognitive Neuroscience Society, Boston, MA.

Monsell S (1978) Recency, immediate recognition memory, and reaction time. Cognitive Psychology 10:465–501.

Monsell S (2003) Task switching. Trends in Cognitive Sciences 7:134–140.

Moss HE, Abdallah S, Fletcher P, Bright P, Pilgrim L, Acres K, Tyler LK (2005) Selecting among competing alternatives: selection and retrieval in the left inferior frontal gyrus. Cerebral Cortex 15:1723–1735.

Nelson JK, Reuter-Lorenz PA, Sylvester C-YC, Jonides J, Smith EE (2003) Dissociable neural mechanisms underlying response-based and familiarity-based conflict in working memory. Proceedings of the National Academy of Sciences U S A 100: 11171–11175.

Noesselt T, Shah NJ, Jancke L (2003) Top-down and bottom-up modulation of language related areas: an fMRI study. BioMed Central Neuroscience 4:13.

Noppeney U, Phillips J, Price C (2004) The neural areas that control the retrieval and selection of semantics. Neuropsychologia 42:1269–1280.

Otten LJ, Rugg MD (2001) Task-dependency of the neural correlates of episodic encoding as measured by fMRI. Cerebral Cortex 11:1150–1160.

Petersen SE, Fox PT, Posner MI, Mintun M, Raichle ME (1988) Positron emission tomographic studies of the cortical anatomy of single-word processing. Nature 331: 585–589.

Peterson LR, Peterson MJ (1959) Short-term retention of individual items. Journal of Experimental Psychology 58:193–198.

Petrides M (2002) The mid-ventrolateral prefrontal cortex and active mnemonic retrieval. Neurobiology of Learning and Memory 78:528–538.

Petrides M, Pandya DN (2002a) Comparative cytoarchitectonic analysis of the human and the macaque ventrolateral prefrontal cortex and corticocortical connection patterns in the monkey. European Journal of Neuroscience 16:291–310.

Petrides M, Pandya DN (2002b) Association pathways of the prefrontal cortex and functional observations. In: Principles of frontal lobe function (Stuss DT, Knight RT, eds.), pp 31–50. New York: Oxford University Press.

Poldrack RA, Clark J, Paré-Blagoev EJ, Shohamy D, Creso Moyano J, Myers C, Gluck MA (2001) Interactive memory systems in the human brain. Nature 414:546–550.

Poldrack RA, Prabhakaran V, Seger CA, Gabrieli JDE (1999a) Striatal activation during cognitive skill learning. Neuropsychology 13:564–574.

Poldrack RA, Wagner AD (2004) What can neuroimaging tell us about the mind? Insights from prefrontal cortex. Current Directions in Psychological Science 13: 177–181.

Poldrack RA, Wagner AD, Prull MW, Desmond JE, Glover GH, Gabrieli JD (1999b) Functional specialization for semantic and phonological processing in the left inferior prefrontal cortex. Neuroimage 10:15–35.

Postle BR, Brush LN, Nick AM (2004) Prefrontal cortex and the mediation of proactive interference in working memory. Cognitive, Affective, and Behavioral Neuroscience 4:600–608.

Price CJ, Wise RJ, Frackowiak RS (1996) Demonstrating the implicit processing of visually presented words and pseudowords. Cerebral Cortex 6:62–70.

Pulvermuller F, Shtyrov Y, Ilmoniemi R (2005) Brain signatures of meaning access in action word recognition. Journal of Cognitive Neuroscience 17:884–892.

Reynolds JR, Donaldson DI, Wagner AD, Braver TS (2004) Item- and task-level processes in the left inferior prefrontal cortex: positive and negative correlates of encoding. Neuroimage 21:1472–1483.

Robbins TW (1996) Refining the taxonomy of memory. Science 273:1353–1354.

Rogers RD, Monsell S (1995) Costs of a predictable switch between simple cognitive tasks. Journal of Experimental Psychology: General 124:207–231.

Rogers RD, Sahakian BJ, Hodges JR, Polkey CE, Kennard C, Robbins TW (1998) Dissociating executive mechanisms of task control following frontal lobe damage and Parkinson's disease. Brain 121 (Pt 5):815–842.

Roskies AL, Fiez JA, Balota DA, Raichle ME, Petersen SE (2001) Task-dependent modulation of regions of the left inferior frontal cortex during semantic processing. Journal of Cognitive Neuroscience 13:829–843.

Rothi LJ, Heilman KM, Watson RT (1985) Pantomime comprehension and ideomotor apraxia. Journal of Neurology, Neurosurgery, and Psychiatry 48:207–210.

Roy EA, Square PA (1985) Common considerations in the study of limb, verbal, and oral apraxia. In: Neuropsychological studies of apraxia and related disorders (Roy EA, ed.), pp 111–161. Amsterdam: North-Holland.

Rubinstein JS, Meyer DE, Evans JE (2001) Executive control of cognitive processes in task switching. Journal of Experimental Psychology: Human Perception and Performance 27:763–797.

Ruge H, Brass M, Koch I, Rubin O, Meiran N, von Cramon DY (2005) Advance preparation and stimulus-induced interference in cued task switching: further insights from BOLD fMRI. Neuropsychologia 43:340–355.

Ruschemeyer SA, Fiebach CJ, Kempe V, Friederici AD (2005) Processing lexical semantic and syntactic information in first and second language: fMRI evidence from German and Russian. Human Brain Mapping 25:266–286.

Rushworth MF, Passingham RE, Nobre AC (2002) Components of switching intentional set. Journal of Cognitive Neuroscience 14:1139–1150.

Schwartz MF, Montgomery MW, Fitzpatrick-DeSalme EJ, Ochipa C, Coslett HB, Mayer NH (1995) Analysis of a disorder of everyday action. Cognitive Neuropsychology 12:863–892.

Shohamy D, Myers CE, Grossman S, Sage J, Gluck MA, Poldrack RA (2004) Corticostriatal contributions to feedback-based learning: converging data from neuroimaging and neuropsychology. Brain 127:851–859.

Shulman GL, d'Avossa G, Tansy AP, Corbetta M (2002) Two attentional processes in the parietal lobe. Cerebral Cortex 12:1124–1131.

Squire LR (1992) Memory and the hippocampus: a synthesis from findings with rats, monkeys, and humans. Psychological Review 99:195–231.

Squire LR (1994) Declarative and nondeclarative memory: multiple brain systems supporting learning and memory. In: Memory systems (Schacter DL, Tulving E, eds.), pp 203–231. Cambridge: MIT Press.

Squire LR, Zola SM (1996) Structure and function of declarative and nondeclarative memory systems. Proceedings of the National Academy of Sciences U S A 93:13515–13522.

Thompson-Schill SL (2003) Neuroimaging studies of semantic memory: inferring 'how' from 'where.' Neuropsychologia 41:280–292.

Thompson-Schill SL, Bedny M, Goldberg RF (2005) The frontal lobes and the regulation of mental activity. Current Opinion in Neurobiology15:219–224.

Thompson-Schill SL, D'Esposito M, Aguirre GK, Farah MJ (1997) Role of left inferior prefrontal cortex in retrieval of semantic knowledge: a reevaluation. Proceedings of the National Academy of Sciences U S A 94:14792–14797.

Thompson-Schill SL, D'Esposito M, Kan IP (1999) Effects of repetition and competition on activity in left prefrontal cortex during word generation. Neuron 23: 513–522.

Thompson-Schill SL, Jonides J, Marshuetz C, Smith EE, D'Esposito M, Kan IP, Knight RT, Swick D (2002) Effects of frontal lobe damage on interference effects in working memory. Cognitive, Affective, and Behavioral Neuroscience 2:109–120.

Thompson-Schill SL, Swick D, Farah MJ, D'Esposito M, Kan IP, Knight RT (1998) Verb generation in patients with focal frontal lesions: a neuropsychological test of neuroimaging findings. Proceedings of the National Academy of Sciences U S A 95:15855–15860.

Tulving E (1972) Episodic and semantic memory. In: Organization of memory (Tulving E, Donaldson W, eds.), pp 382–403. New York: Academic Press.

Wagner AD, Paré-Blagoev EJ, Clark J, Poldrack RA (2001) Recovering meaning: left prefrontal cortex guides controlled semantic retrieval. Neuron 31:329–338.

Waszak F, Hommel B, Allport A (2003) Task-switching and long-term priming: role of episodic stimulus-task bindings in task-shift costs. Cognitive Psychology 46:361–413.

Wig GS, Grafton ST, Demos KE, Kelley WM (2005) Reductions in neural activity underlie behavioral components of repetition priming. Nature Neuroscience 8:1228–1233.

Wylie G, Allport A (2000) Task switching and the measurement of 'switch costs.' Psychological Research 63:212–233.

17

Exploring the Roles of the Frontal, Temporal, and Parietal Lobes in Visual Categorization

David J. Freedman

During a typical day, we are inundated with a continuous stream of sensory stimuli, ranging from ringing telephones and incoming e-mail messages to familiar faces in the hallway and numerous social interactions with colleagues and friends. Despite this barrage of sensory information, we easily and appropriately respond to the events of the day: answering the telephone, replying to messages, greeting friends, and making dinner plans. To behave appropriately in response to our surroundings, the brain must solve a series of enormously complex problems, including sensory processing of stimulus features, recognizing the behavioral significance or meaning of stimuli, and selecting motor responses that make sense, based on the current situation. Remarkably, the brain routinely solves each of these problems with ease. One of the central themes of this book is exploring how the brain learns and represents the rules and strategies that provide a context for incoming sensory stimuli, which in turn, provide the basis for efficient and successful goal-directed behavior. My research and this chapter focus on one aspect of this issue: the transformation of visual feature representations in sensory brain areas into more abstract encoding of the behavioral relevance, or meaning, of stimuli during visual categorization.

Our perception of the world around us is not a faithful representation of its physical features. Instead, we parse the world into meaningful groupings, or categories. This process of grouping stimuli into categories according to their functional relevance is fundamental to cognitive processing because it gives meaning to the sights and sounds around us. For example, recognizing that a particular device is a "telephone" instantly provides a great deal of information about its relevant parts and functions, sparing us from having to learn anew each time we encounter a new telephone. The ability to categorize stimuli is a cornerstone of complex behavior. Categories are evident in all sensory modalities, and category-based behaviors are evident in species throughout the animal kingdom, from insects, birds, and rats to monkeys and humans.

Although much is known about how the brain processes simple sensory features, such as color, orientation, and motion direction, much less is known

about how the brain learns and represents the meaning, or category, of stimuli. Categories often group items that have physically dissimilar features, but share a common function or meaning (e.g., "chairs," "mammals"). In addition, categories are often separated by sharp transitions or "category boundaries" (Barsalou, 1992; Ashby and Maddox, 2005), particularly in the case of lower-level perceptual categories (e.g. color perception). Because of this, neuronal category representations are unlikely to arise exclusively from neural "tuning" for basic visual features. Neurons in the early visual cortex exhibit gradual changes in neural activity that faithfully track changes in visual features, whereas physically similar stimuli may be treated very differently if they belong to different categories (e.g., "tables," "chairs"). Of course, we are not born with innate knowledge about higher-level and more abstract categories such as tables, chairs, and telephones. Instead, categories such as these are learned through experience. Thus, it is likely that the neural mechanisms underlying the acquisition and representation of categories are closely related to those involved in other types of visual learning.

The central goal of my research is to gain an understanding of how information about the behavioral relevance, or meaning, of visual stimuli is encoded by the brain. Through a series of experiments conducted in Earl Miller's laboratory at MIT and John Assad's laboratory at Harvard Medical School, our group recorded data from neurons in the prefrontal, posterior parietal, inferior temporal, and extrastriate visual cortices in monkeys trained to perform visual categorization tasks. These experiments revealed that neuronal activity in the prefrontal and posterior parietal cortices encoded the category membership, or meaning, of visual stimuli. In contrast, neurons in the inferior temporal and middle temporal areas seemed more involved in visual feature processing, and did not show explicit category encoding. Here, I will summarize the results of these experiments and those from several other laboratories that have given new insights into how the brain transforms sensory information into more meaningful representations that serve to guide complex goal-directed behaviors.

BEHAVIORAL EVIDENCE FOR CATEGORIZATION IN NONHUMAN ANIMALS

Perceptual categorization and category-based behaviors have been observed across a wide range of animals, from insects to primates. For example, it has been shown that crickets divide sound frequencies into two discrete categories. There are two sounds that are particularly relevant to crickets: mating calls (approximately 4 to 5 kHz) and echolocation signals (25 to 80 kHz) from predatory bats. Naturally, crickets try to maximize their chance of finding a mate and minimize their chance of being eaten. Wyttenbach and colleagues (1996) showed that crickets will approach tones with frequencies of less than 16 kHz and avoid those with frequencies of greater than 16 kHz, and that they sharply discriminate between frequencies near the 16 kHz boundary. This innate

categorization skill allows crickets to simply and efficiently maximize their chances of reproduction and survival.

Pigeons also exhibit an impressive ability to categorize sensory stimuli, particularly visual images. Decades of laboratory experiments have shown that pigeons can be trained to report (by pecking) whether a visual image contained objects of a particular category. For example, they can be taught to report, with surprising success, whether photographs contain items, such as trees (Herrnstein et al., 1976; Herrnstein, 1979), people (Herrnstein and Loveland, 1964), animals (Roberts and Mazmanian, 1988), or even manmade objects (Verhave, 1966). In some cases, their categorization abilities can even generalize to novel images that they have never seen before (Herrnstein and Loveland, 1964), indicating that they likely use a more flexible strategy than simple memorization of each visual image and its category label during learning. However, there are clear limitations to the flexibility and generality of category effects in pigeons. For example, it has proven difficult to train pigeons to apply more abstract categories or rules, such as "same" or "different," to novel, untrained stimuli (Edwards et al., 1983; Wright et al., 1983; for a more detailed review, see Cook, 2001).

Although insects and birds indeed have the capacity to categorize sensory stimuli, the complex range of behaviors in more advanced animals, such as monkeys and humans, must involve more sophisticated abilities to learn and represent categories and rules. The complexity of primate behavior likely depends on the ability to employ categories that are defined across multiple feature dimensions that may be difficult to define precisely, such as "tool." In addition, advanced animals have an impressive capacity to acquire new information and apply existing knowledge to new situations. Most of our categories, such as "chair," "house," and "mammal," are acquired by learning, and we can continually adapt, expand, and enhance these categories through further experience. Likewise, the complex range of behaviors of nonhuman primates suggests that they also can learn and recognize relatively complex categories and rules. For example, a number of studies have shown that monkeys have the ability to learn complex categories, such as animal versus non-animal (Roberts and Mazmanian, 1988), food versus non-food (Fabre-Thorpe et al., 1998), tree versus non-tree, fish versus non-fish (Vogels, 1999), ordinal numbers (Orlov et al., 2000), and more abstract categories, such as "same" and "different" (Premack, 1983; Wallis et al., 2001).

NEURONAL REPRESENTATIONS UNDERLYING VISUAL CATEGORIZATION

To fully understand how the brain processes visual categories, we must first determine which brain areas play a role in encoding the category membership of visual stimuli. One possibility is that areas involved in visual feature processing might also play a role in encoding more abstract and meaningful information about stimulus category. For example, the category membership of

visual shapes might be reflected in the activity of neurons along the ventral stream visual pathway (e.g., areas V4 and the inferior temporal cortex) that are known to be involved in the processing of visual shapes and shape recognition. Another possibility is that early sensory areas might show a veridical, or faithful, representation of stimulus features, whereas more abstract information about stimulus category emerges in downstream brain areas, such as the prefrontal cortex (PFC) and medial temporal lobe—areas that receive direct inputs from sensory areas, but are not believed to play a major role in sensory feature processing. In a series of experiments conducted in Earl Miller's laboratory at MIT, we tested these two hypotheses by recording the activity of PFC and inferior temporal cortex (ITC) neurons while monkeys performed a shape categorization task. These experiments revealed that PFC neurons showed robust category signals, whereas ITC activity did not show strong category encoding and seemed more suited to a role in visual feature processing.

Prefrontal Cortex

A substantial body of evidence suggests that the PFC plays a central role in guiding complex goal-directed behaviors. Neuropsychological studies of patients with PFC damage and neurophysiological investigations of PFC activity indicate that this area is centrally involved in the highest level of cognitive (executive) functions (Miller and Cohen, 2001). These include cognitive faculties that are neither purely sensory nor motor, such as short-term "working" memory, inhibition of prepotent responses, and the learning and representation of behavior-guiding rules. The PFC includes a collection of cortical areas that are directly interconnected with both cortical and subcortical brain areas that are involved in the processing of sensory, motor, emotional, and reward information. Thus, the PFC is ideally situated to integrate information across a wide range of brain systems and exert control over behavior. Correspondingly, PFC neurons are activated by stimuli from all sensory modalities (particularly when those stimuli are task-relevant), before and during a variety of actions, during memory for past events, and in anticipation of expected events and behavioral consequences. Additionally, PFC neurons are modulated by internal factors, such as motivational and attentional state (for a review, see Miller and Cohen, 2001). Therefore, the PFC is a likely candidate for playing a role in processing the behavioral relevance, or category, of stimuli.

Prefrontal Cortex and Visual Shape Categorization

To test for neural correlates of perceptual categories, we trained rhesus macaque monkeys to perform a novel visual shape categorization task and then recorded the activity of individual PFC neurons during task performance (Freedman et al., 2001, 2002). In this task, monkeys learned to group computer-generated stimuli into two categories, "cats" and "dogs" (Fig. 17–1). We employed a novel three-dimensional morphing system to create a large set of parametric blends of the six prototype images shown in Fig. 17–1A (three species

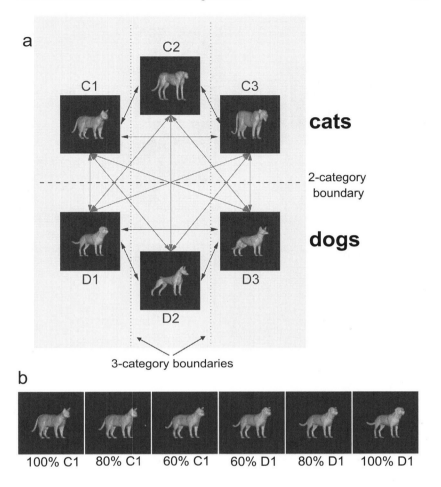

cats

2-category
boundary

dogs

3-category boundaries

100% C1   80% C1   60% C1   60% D1   80% D1   100% D1

Figure 17–1 The "cat" and "dog" stimulus set. *A*. The six prototype images and 15 morph lines. The sample stimulus set was composed of 54 unique images: six prototypes (as shown), four images evenly placed (20%, 40%, 60%, 80%) along the nine lines that cross the two-category boundary connecting each cat to each dog prototype, and two images (at 40% and 60%) along each of the six lines that do not cross the boundary between prototypes of the same category (with respect to the two-class boundary). The two *vertical dotted lines* indicate the two category boundaries used when the monkeys were retrained to group the stimuli into three categories. *B*. An example of the morphs generated between the C1 and D1 prototypes.

of cats and three breeds of dogs) [Beymer and Poggio, 1996; Shelton, 2000]. By varying the proportions of the six cat and dog prototype objects, we could smoothly vary stimulus shape and precisely define the category boundary (at the midpoint along cat-dog morph lines). Examples of the morphs generated along the morph-line between the C1 and D1 prototypes are shown in Fig. 17–1*B*. The

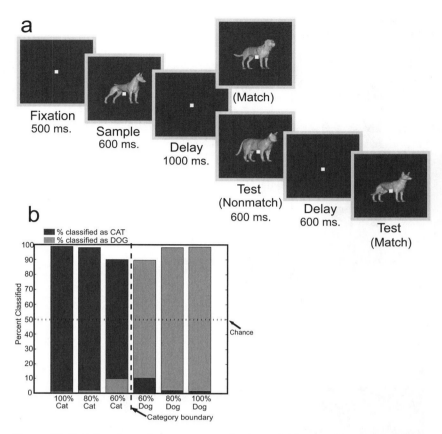

Figure 17–2 Delayed match-to-category task. *A.* A trial began with central fixation (500 ms), after which a sample stimulus appeared at the center of gaze for 600 ms. This was followed by a 1-s delay and then by a test stimulus (600 ms). If the category of the test matched that of the sample, monkeys had to release a lever to the test stimulus within 600 ms of its presentation to obtain a juice reward. If the test was a nonmatch, there was another delay interval (600 ms), followed by a presentation of a match, which required a lever release for a reward. There were an equal number of match and nonmatch trials, and they were randomly interleaved. *B.* Average performance of both monkeys during neurophysiological recordings for the two-category task. *Dark gray bars* indicate the percent of samples classified as cat, and *light gray bars,* the percent classified as dog.

category boundary divided the set of cat-dog images into two equal groups that the monkeys were trained to categorize. Through training, the monkeys learned that stimuli that were composed of more than 50% cat were in the "cat" category, and the remaining stimuli were "dogs." As a result, stimuli that were close to the boundary, but on opposite sides, could be visually similar, but belong to different categories, whereas stimuli that belonged to the same category could be

visually dissimilar (e.g., "cheetah" and "housecat"). This allowed us to dissociate the visual similarity and category membership of stimuli.

We trained monkeys to perform a delayed match-to-category task (DMC) [Fig. 17–2A], in which they were required to indicate whether successively presented sample and test stimuli belonged to the same category. For training, we chose stimuli from throughout the cat and dog morph space. After several months of training, the monkeys' categorization performance was excellent (approximately 90% correct), even for stimuli close to the category boundary. The monkeys classified dog-like cats (60% cat, 40% dog) correctly approximately 90% of the time, and misclassified them as dogs only 10% of the time, and vice versa (Fig. 17–2B). Thus, the monkeys' behavior indicated the sharp boundary that is diagnostic of a category representation.

After the monkeys were trained, we recorded data from 525 neurons in the lateral PFC, the PFC region directly interconnected with the ITC, and found many examples of neurons that seemed to encode category membership. An example is shown in Figure 17–3. Note that this neuron's activity discriminated sharply between dog-like (60%) cats and cat-like (60%) dogs, yet responded similarly to the three morph levels of stimuli within each category. In other words, PFC neurons showed the same sharp distinctions between categories that were evident in the monkey's behavior. Likewise, PFC neurons also

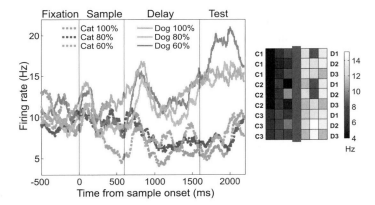

Figure 17–3 A spike-density histogram showing the mean firing rate across different conditions for a category-sensitive prefrontal cortex neuron. The grayscale plot to the *right* of the histogram shows the average activity of each neuron to each of the 42 stimuli along the nine between-class morph lines (see Fig. 17–1). The prototypes (C1, C2, C3, D1, D2, D3) are represented in the outermost columns; the category boundary is represented by the dark vertical line in the middle. Each prototype contributes to three morph lines. A gray scale indicates the activity level. For this plot, activity was averaged across the delay and test epochs.

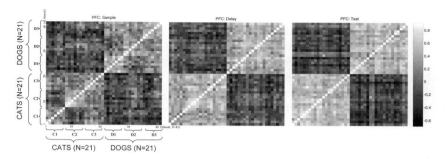

Figure 17–4 Average correlation matrix for the population of stimulus-selective prefrontal cortex (PFC) neurons. The *small patches* show pairwise correlation values between each stimulus and every other one. The stimuli are lined up in the same order on each axis so that the *diagonal white line* indicates the identity line. Across all stimulus-selective neurons during the sample ($N = 115$ neurons), delay ($N = 88$), and test ($N = 52$) epochs, the PFC shows four large "boxes" of high- versus low-correlation values, indicating similar activity within, but not between, categories, with significantly stronger category effects in the delay and test epochs.

mirrored the monkeys' behavior by responding similarly to stimuli that were in the same category.

Neuronal signals that reflected the stimulus category were evident in a substantial number of PFC neurons. Across the neural population, neuronal activity tended to reflect category membership rather than individual stimuli. This effect was further reflected by the correlation analysis shown in Figure 17–4. We applied the analysis to all of the stimulus-selective neurons (defined as neurons that showed significantly different activity among the sample stimuli according to a one-way analysis of variance [ANOVA]) in each time epoch. For each neuron, we calculated its average firing rate to each sample stimulus. Then, for the population, we determined the degree of correlation between the neuronal firing rates to every pair of sample stimuli. Category-selective neurons showed similar firing rates to pairs of stimuli in the same category (giving high correlation values for within-category stimulus pairs), whereas firing rates differed greatly for stimuli in different categories (giving low or negative correlation values for between-category stimulus pairs), and this effect is exactly what we saw across the neuronal population (Fig. 17–4). The small patches show pairwise correlation values between each stimulus and every other one during the sample (left), delay (middle), and test (right) epochs. The four large 21×21 square regions of high and low correlation values (light and dark gray regions, respectively) indicate similar neuronal activity within, but not between, categories. This shows that category (and not stimulus) information predominates in the PFC during all three time epochs, with especially strong category effects in the delay and test epochs.

When the test stimulus appeared, the monkeys needed to decide whether it was from the same category as the previously presented sample stimulus (and whether to release the lever). To determine whether PFC neurons carried information about the match-nonmatch status of the test stimulus, we computed a two-way ANOVA on each neuron's average activity during the test epoch. The factors were the match-nonmatch status and category of the test stimulus, and nearly 30% of PFC neurons ($n = 152$) showed a main effect of, or interaction between, these factors. Of these, one-third ($n = 48$) encoded the match-nonmatch status of the test stimulus. Approximately 20% ($n = 31$) of neurons encoded the category of the currently visible test stimulus. The remaining neurons showed an interaction between these two factors. This group included neurons that showed match-nonmatch effects that were stronger for one category than for the other, and also neurons that, during the test epoch, showed category selectivity for the previously presented sample stimulus (such as the neuron in Fig. 17–3). In sum, test epoch activity in the PFC encoded all of the behaviorally relevant factors that were necessary for solving the DMC task.

Because our monkeys had no experience with cats or dogs before training, it seemed likely that these effects resulted from training. To verify that these effects were due to learning, we retrained one monkey (one of the monkeys from the studies described above) to group the same cat-dog stimuli into three new categories that were defined by two new category boundaries that were orthogonal to the original boundary (Fig. 17–1). The two new category boundaries created three new categories, each containing morphs centered around one cat prototype and one dog prototype (e.g., "cheetah" and "Doberman"). After retraining, we recorded data from 103 PFC neurons and found that they were category-selective for the newly learned three categories, but no longer encoded the two old categories (that were no longer relevant for the task) [Freedman et al., 2001, 2002]. This demonstrated a dramatic plasticity of PFC stimulus selectivity as a result of several months of training, and indicated that PFC category effects were indeed a result of learning.

Recently, the results of several neurophysiological studies of PFC activity have reinforced the idea that PFC neurons can encode abstract information about the behavioral relevance of stimuli. For example, studies by Andreas Nieder and colleagues (2002) support a role for the PFC in encoding category-like information about the quantity of items visible on a computer screen. In this study, monkeys were trained to perform a number-matching task in which they had to report whether two sequentially presented arrays of stimuli (clusters of 1 to 5 visual shapes) contained the same number of stimuli. After training, the monkeys could perform the task well for small numbers of shapes (e.g., 1 to 3 items) [their performance dropped sharply for larger numbers], and lateral PFC recordings revealed neuronal activity that selectively grouped stimulus arrays according to their numerical quantity (even though, for example, arrays of three items could differ greatly in their visual appearance).

This suggests that PFC neurons can show a category-like encoding during a numerical matching task similar to that seen during visual shape categorization (e.g., the cats and dogs). Whether this reflects an innate numerical ability in monkeys or resulted entirely from training remains to be seen.

In another related study, Wallis et al. (2001) taught monkeys two rules: "match" and "nonmatch," and cued the monkeys to report (by releasing a lever) whether two sequentially presented stimuli were the same—if monkeys were cued to use the "match" rule on that trial—or different—if monkeys were cued to use the "nonmatch" rule. After the monkeys had learned these two rules, they could even apply them to novel stimuli that the monkeys had never seen before. Recordings from the PFC strikingly revealed a population of neurons that robustly encoded the rule ("match" or "nonmatch") that was currently in effect. This indicates an impressive ability for PFC neurons to encode abstract rules (that are not explicitly and rigidly tied to particular stimuli or features) as a result of learning, and it suggests that both high-level visual categories and abstract rules may share common underlying neurophysiological mechanisms in the PFC. To read more about this work, see Chapter 2.

Together, the results of these studies suggest that PFC activity encodes abstract information about the meaning, or category membership, of visual stimuli. PFC neurons responded similarly to stimuli of the same category, even if they differed greatly in visual appearance, and discriminated between visually similar stimuli in different categories. PFC category effects were also highly learning-dependent; retraining the monkeys to regroup the stimuli into new categories caused the PFC to reorganize their category representations and encode stimuli according to the new, now relevant, category boundaries.

However, important questions remain about how the brain learns and encodes categories. A primary goal of my research is to understand the progression from rigid encoding of stimulus features in primary sensory brain areas to more flexible cognitive representations, such as those observed in the PFC. One possibility is that category representations are encoded "upstream" from the PFC, perhaps in brain areas involved in high-level visual shape processing, such as the ITC, and then this information is merely copied to the PFC via direct interconnections between it and the ITC. Alternatively, the PFC may play a more active role in categorization, whereas the ITC primarily represents stimulus shape, not category. In the next section, I will describe experiments in which we directly compared PFC and ITC activity during the category task, and found that these two areas likely play different, although complimentary, roles in visual shape categorization.

Inferior Temporal Cortex

Decades of neuropsychological and neurophysiological studies suggest that the ITC plays a central role in visual form processing and object recognition. The ITC, located in the anterior ventral portion of the temporal lobe, receives inputs from "ventral stream" visual form processing areas, such as V4 and the

posterior inferior temporal cortex, and is interconnected with a large number of brain areas, including the medial temporal structures, the frontal lobe (including the PFC), and the parietal cortex (Ungerleider and Mishkin, 1982; Ungerleider et al., 1989; Webster et al., 1994; Murray et al., 2000). Damage to the ITC causes deficits in a variety of tasks that depend on discriminating and recognizing complex objects (Kluver and Bucy, 1938, 1939; Blum et al., 1950; Mishkin, 1954, 1966; Mishkin and Pribram, 1954), and in humans, it can cause category-specific agnosias (e.g., for faces) [Damasio et al., 1982].

In general, ITC neurons have properties that suggest involvement in high-level shape encoding; they exhibit broad neuronal selectivity for complex shapes (Gross, 1973; Bruce et al., 1981; Perrett et al., 1982; Desimone et al., 1984; Tanaka, 1996; Brincat and Connor, 2004). In addition, ITC shape selectivity can sometimes be highly specific for stimuli from a particular class, particularly for faces (Perrett et al., 1982; Desimone et al., 1984; Baylis et al., 1987; Tsao et al., 2006). A number of studies have shown that ITC shape selectivity can be modified by visual experience, typically resulting in sharpened tuning for familiar rather than novel stimuli (Logothetis et al., 1995; Booth and Rolls, 1998; Kobatake et al., 1998; Baker et al., 2002; Sigala and Logothetis, 2002; Freedman et al., 2005). ITC neurons develop similar responses to stimuli that are presented sequentially (Miyashita, 1993). Furthermore, prior exposure to a set of complex visual stimuli can cause a clustering of neurons with similar object preferences in the anterior ventral ITC (perirhinal cortex) [Erickson et al., 2000]. Thus, ITC shape selectivity and the observation that its shape representations can be modified through learning and experience suggest that the ITC could form the basis for the development of categorical neuronal representations.

Role of the Inferior Temporal Cortex in Visual Categorization

Until recently, the majority of previous neurophysiological studies of visual categorization focused on the temporal lobe. However, it remained uncertain whether ITC neurons would encode categories in the same way as in the PFC. There is evidence that categories are represented in the human medial temporal lobe (MTL), which is directly interconnected with the ITC. For example, several recent studies recorded data from MTL neurons in awake human patients with epilepsy who had MTL electrodes implanted to localize the focus of their seizures (Kreiman et al, 2000; Quiroga et al., 2005). They found single neurons that responded exclusively to stimuli from one category (e.g., famous people, tools), but showed little difference in their response to stimuli within the same category.

Several recent studies investigated the response of ITC neurons during visual categorization. In one study, Vogels (1999) trained monkeys to categorize trees versus non-trees and fish versus non-fish, and found a subset of ITC neurons that responded well to many of the stimuli from a given category (photographs of trees or fish), but weakly to a variety of stimuli from other categories (e.g., household items or scenes without trees). However, even the

best examples of category-selective neurons from this study did not exhibit the tight clustering of responses to stimuli within a category observed in the PFC, suggesting an intermixing of category and shape encoding. In a recent study by Sigala and Logothetis (2002), monkeys were trained to categorize line drawings of faces and fish. ITC recordings revealed enhanced tuning for the visual features that were relevant for the categorization task, but did not report finding more explicit and generalized encoding of categories. The categorization tasks and stimuli used in these studies differed substantially from the DMC task we had used in our PFC studies. For example, neither study used short-term memory delays or required the monkeys to match the category of two stimuli as in the DMC task. Thus, it remained unclear whether ITC neurons could encode more explicit information about stimulus category, as we observed in the PFC during the DMC task, or whether they are more involved in the high-level analysis of complex visual features.

Comparison of the Prefrontal and Inferior Temporal Cortices during Visual Shape Categorization

To investigate whether the activity of ITC neurons reflected the category membership of visual stimuli, we recorded 443 ITC neurons in area TE from two monkeys during performance of the cat versus dog categorization (DMC) task (Freedman et al., 2003). For a subset of these experiments, we recorded data simultaneously from both the PFC and ITC ($N = 130$ PFC and 117 ITC neurons). This allowed us to directly compare the patterns of PFC and ITC neuronal response properties and evaluate their respective roles in solving the DMC task. Specifically, we tested whether abstract category signals, such as those observed in the PFC, were evident in ITC activity and whether it seemed likely that PFC category selectivity was due to category-selective information relayed from the ITC. As I will describe later, these studies revealed that most ITC neurons did not show strong category selectivity, as in the PFC. Instead, the ITC seems more likely to play a role in shape or feature selectivity that does not generalize to include more abstract category encoding.

As in the PFC, a majority of ITC neurons were activated by the DMC task. However, the pattern of ITC activity differed from that in the PFC in several important ways. First, although there were several examples of neurons that showed strong category selectivity, most ITC neurons were selective among the sample stimuli, but did not show strong and explicit category-encoding. Instead, most ITC neurons were shape-selective, responding strongly to their preferred stimulus, with a gradual decrease in activity as the stimuli became more visually dissimilar (although we did find, on average, significantly sharper tuning across the category boundary than within each category). This trend toward shape and feature selectivity was even evident among the ITC neurons that showed the strongest category selectivity. For example, the ITC neuron in Figure 17–5 responded more strongly, on average, to stimuli in the "dog" category, although a closer look at the responses to the individual sample stimuli

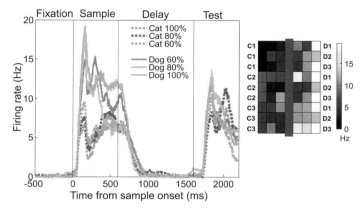

Figure 17–5 A spike-density histogram showing mean firing rate across different conditions for a category-sensitive inferior temporal cortex neuron. The grayscale plot to the right of the histogram shows the average activity of each neuron to each of the 42 stimuli along the nine between-class morph lines (see Fig. 17–1). The prototypes (C1, C2, C3, D1, D2, D3) are represented in the outermost columns; the category boundary is represented by the dark vertical line in the middle. Each prototype contributes to three morph lines. A gray scale indicates the activity level. For this plot, activity was averaged over the first half of the sample epoch.

(shown to the right of the average histogram) reveals a greater degree of variability among the sample stimuli (compared with the PFC neuron example in Figure 17–3), which might reflect the variability in the appearance of the stimuli within each category.

This trend toward weaker category effects and stronger selectivity for individual stimuli, compared with the PFC, was also evident across the ITC population. We applied the same correlation analysis as described earlier to the population of stimulus-selective ITC neurons during the sample, delay, and test epochs. As shown in Figure 17–6, the ITC showed a very different pattern of selectivity than was seen in the PFC. During the sample epoch (Fig. 17–6, *left*), the correlation analysis did not show strong correlations between all stimuli in the same category, as we had observed in the PFC (Fig. 17–4). Instead, ITC activity was highly correlated between visually similar stimuli. This is indicated by the six 7×7 regions of high correlation values along the diagonal in Figure 17–6 (*left*) [corresponding to the seven stimuli closest to, and visually similar to, each of the six prototype images]. In other words, ITC activity during stimulus presentation reflected the visual similarity between stimuli, and not their category membership. During the memory delay, there were relatively few neurons ($n = 38/443$) that were selective for the previously presented sample stimulus. Among those selective neurons, ITC selectivity was much weaker than in the PFC, showing only a hint of category selectivity (Fig. 17–6, *middle*). Interestingly,

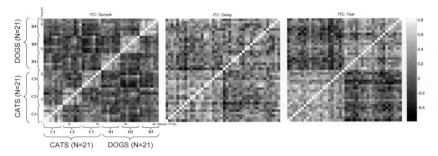

Figure 17–6 Average correlation matrix for the population of stimulus-selective inferior temporal cortex (ITC) neurons. During stimulus (sample) presentation, the population correlation values (across 186 stimulus-selective ITC neurons) form six small boxes lined up along the identity line. This corresponds to the six prototypes, and indicates that the ITC population responds similarly to stimuli that look similar. During the delay ($N = 38$), both stimulus and category selectivity were relatively weak (*middle*). Significant ITC category selectivity emerged during the test epoch ($N = 23$) of the trial, and even then, it was significantly weaker than that in the prefrontal cortex during the delay or test epoch.

significant category selectivity appeared in the ITC (among a small population of 23 stimulus-selective neurons) late in the trial, during the test epoch (Fig. 17–6, *right*), although it was still significantly weaker than that in the PFC during the delay and test epochs (Fig. 17–4, *right*). This suggests that category signals might first be encoded at the level of the PFC, and then feed back to the ITC during the decision (test) epoch of the task.

A third important difference between PFC and ITC activity was apparent during the test epoch of the task, when the monkeys viewed the test stimulus and had to decide whether it was a category match to the previously presented sample stimulus (and required a lever release). Although PFC activity during the test epoch reflected all factors relevant for solving the DMC task (sample category, test category, and match-nonmatch status of the test), a two-way ANOVA (as discussed earlier, with test-stimulus category and match-nonmatch status as factors) revealed that very few ITC neurons showed match-nonmatch effects (7%, or 10/151 neurons that showed any significant effects). Instead, the modal group of ITC neurons (59%, $n = 89/151$) encoded the category of the test stimulus. The remaining neurons showed an interaction between these two factors. This group primarily consisted of neurons that showed category selectivity for the previously presented sample stimulus (as suggested by the correlation analysis) [discussed earlier] (Fig. 17–6). Thus, ITC activity during the test epoch seemed most involved in the analysis of the currently visible test stimulus, and did not seem to encode factors directly related to match-nonmatch decisions or release-hold motor responses.

These results are compatible with those of previous neurophysiological studies of visual learning and categorization in the ITC (discussed earlier), and suggest that the PFC and ITC play distinct roles in category-based behaviors:

The ITC seems to be more involved in visual feature analysis of currently viewed shapes, whereas the PFC shows stronger category signals, memory effects, and a greater tendency to encode information in terms of its behavioral meaning. Although these studies indicate that the ITC is unlikely to provide explicit information about the category of visual stimuli to the PFC, it is possible, and even likely, that other brain areas play a direct role in visual categorization and the transformation from sensory to more cognitive stimulus representations. Other areas that are likely candidates for representing visual category information include medial temporal lobe areas, such as the perirhinal cortex and hippocampus, both of which receive input from the ITC.

Another candidate area is the posterior parietal cortex (PPC), which is directly interconnected with dorsal stream visual areas, such as the middle temporal (MT) and medial superior temporal areas (Lewis and Van Essen, 2000), and with a wide range of cortical and subcortical areas, including the PFC, ITC, basal ganglia, and areas involved in the control of eye movements (Felleman and Van Essen, 1991; Webster et al., 1994; Lewis and Van Essen, 2000). Traditionally, the PPC has been believed to play a central role in visuospatial processing, such as mediating spatial attention and eye movements. However, a number of recent studies suggest that the PPC may be involved in a more diverse set of cognitive functions, including shape processing, representations of task context or rules, and visual category representations.

Posterior Parietal Cortex

The PPC, particularly the lateral intraparietal (LIP) area, has been one of the most studied cortical areas among primate neurophysiologists in recent years. Decades of neurophysiological studies in monkeys have established that LIP neurons are selectively activated by a wide range of behaviors, particularly those involving visuospatial attention and visually guided actions (Colby and Goldberg, 1999; Andersen and Buneo, 2001).

Although the PPC has traditionally been studied in the context of visuospatial processing and spatial attention, a number of recent studies suggest that LIP neurons are also involved in visual or cognitive processing of nonspatial stimuli that cannot be explained by spatial attention or eye movement factors. For example, Sereno and Maunsell (1998) showed that LIP neurons can respond strongly and selectively to complex visual shapes, possibly due to direct interconnections with the ITC. Nieder and Miller (2004) trained monkeys to report the number of visible items during a number matching task (as in their studies of the PFC, discussed earlier), and found that many PPC neurons reflected the numerical quantity of stimuli.

In addition, several recent studies have found that PPC neurons are also sensitive to more abstract cognitive factors, such as the currently relevant task context or rule. For example, Toth and Assad (2002) trained monkeys to make an eye movement in one of two directions, based on either the location or color of a cue. At the beginning of each trial, monkeys were cued to attend to

either color or location on that trial. They found that LIP neurons can show color selectivity when the monkeys were cued to attend to color, but not when color was irrelevant for solving the task. In another study, Stoet and Snyder (2004) trained monkeys to perform a task in which they discriminated either the orientation or color of stimuli. Monkeys were cued at the start of each trial whether to attend to the color or orientation of the upcoming sample stimulus. PPC recordings revealed a population of neurons that selectively encoded the "rule" (attend to color or orientation) instructed by the cue (for more about this work, see Chapter 11). Together, these studies suggest that the PPC is likely involved in functions beyond spatial attention and the control of eye movements, and that PPC neurons can show surprising flexibility in their encoding of visual stimuli according to the demands of the task at hand.

Posterior Parietal Cortex and Visual Motion Categorization

The results from these prior studies raise the possibility that the PPC might also play a role in encoding more abstract information about the category membership, or meaning, of visual stimuli as a result of learning. To investigate whether PPC activity encodes the category membership of visual stimuli, we used a similar experimental design and behavioral paradigm (delayed match-to-category or DMC), as in the PFC and ITC. For two reasons, we chose visual motion patterns rather than complex shapes as stimuli. (1) LIP neurons are sensitive to the direction of visual motion, even for stimuli that are "passively viewed" outside the context of an active behavioral task (Fanini and Assad, submitted). This may be due to LIP's direct interconnection with MT and medial superior temporal areas (Lewis and Van Essen, 2000), which play a central role in visual motion processing (Born and Bradley, 2005). (2) The neuronal processing of simple visual motion patterns is better understood than that for complex shapes. Thus, it may be easier to identify how visual direction selectivity in the early visual areas is transformed into to more abstract and meaningful encoding of motion-based categories.

We trained monkeys to group 12 directions of motion into two categories that were separated by a learned "category boundary" (Fig. 17–7A). Monkeys performed a DMC task (Fig. 17–7B), in which they had to judge whether two successively presented (sample and test) stimuli were in the same category. To receive a reward, the monkeys had to release a lever if the direction of the test stimulus was in the same category as the sample. After training, the monkeys correctly categorized sample stimuli that were 75 degrees or 45 degrees from the category boundary with greater than 90% accuracy, on average, and performed at better than 70% correct for stimuli closest to (15 degrees) the category boundary (Fig. 17–7C). As with the cat versus dog DMC task, we could then determine whether neuronal activity reflected the visual features of the stimuli (e.g., direction of motion), their category membership, or both.

We recorded data from 156 LIP neurons from two monkeys during DMC task performance. A striking number of these neurons were category-selective:

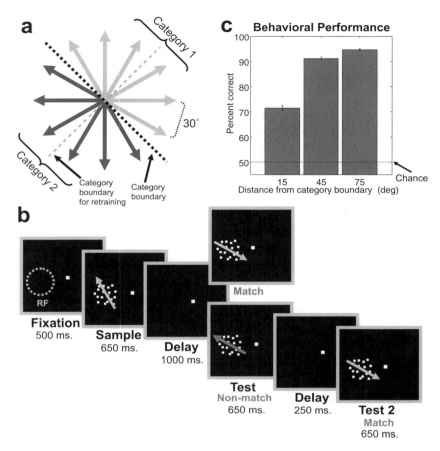

Figure 17–7 Visual motion stimuli and motion categorization task. *A.* Monkeys grouped 12 motion directions into two categories (*light* and *dark gray arrows*) separated by a "category boundary" (*black dotted line*). The *light gray dotted line* is the boundary used for retraining with the new categories. *B.* Delayed match-to-category (DMC) task. A sample stimulus was followed by a delay and test. If the sample and test were in the same category, monkeys were required to release a lever before the test disappeared. If the test was a nonmatch, there was a second delay, followed by a match (which required a lever release). *C.* Monkeys' average DMC task performance across all recording sessions was greater than chance (50%) for sample stimuli that were close to (15 degrees) and farther from (45 degrees or 75 degrees) the boundary.

They showed activity that differed sharply between categories and showed little variability in their responses to stimuli within a category (Freedman and Assad, 2006). Figure 17–8 (see color insert) shows the activity of two category-selective LIP neurons. The 12 traces correspond to the 12 motion directions used as samples, and are colored red (solid) and blue (dashed) according to their

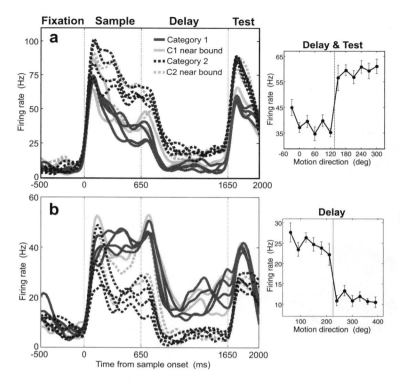

Figure 17–8 Examples of two category-selective lateral intraparietal (LIP) neurons. Average activity to the 12 sample directions for two LIP neurons is shown. The *red* and *blue traces* correspond to directions in the two categories (red [solid], category 1 or C1; blue [dashed], category 2 or C2), and *pale traces* indicate the directions closest to (15 degrees) the boundary. The three *vertical dotted lines* indicate (*left* to *right*) the timing of the sample onset, the sample offset, and the test stimulus onset. The neuron in *A* was recorded with the original category boundary. The neuron in *B* was recorded after the monkey had been retrained on the new categories. The plots at the *right* of each peristimulus time histogram show activity (mean ± standard error of the mean) for the 12 directions during the late delay and test epochs (*A*) and the delay epoch (*B*). C1, C2.

category membership. The pale red and blue traces indicate the four directions closest to (15 degrees) the category boundary. The neuron in Figure 17–8*A* showed a preference for category 2 during the sample, delay, and test epochs, whereas the neuron in Figure 17–8*B* responded preferentially to category 1 during the sample, delay, and test epochs.

To quantify the extent to which individual neurons responded more similarly to directions within each category than between categories, we computed a category tuning index using two parameters: (1) within-category difference

(WCD) [the average difference in firing rates between directions in the same category]; and (2) between-category difference (BCD) [the average difference in firing rates between directions in different categories] in the average firing rate to the 12 sample directions. We constructed a standard selectivity index from these values (WCD and BCD) that could range from -1.0 to 1.0, where positive values indicate larger activity differences between categories and more similar activity within categories. Across the population of direction-selective LIP neurons ($n = 122/156$ in sample, delay, or both), category indices were shifted toward positive values during both the sample and delay epochs, with the strongest category selectivity evident during the late delay and early test epochs. The time course of category selectivity (Fig. 17–9) shows a similar pattern to that in the PFC during visual shape categorization (Freedman et al., 2002)—selectivity that emerges during the sample epoch, persists throughout the memory delay epoch, and reaches peak values during the late delay and early test epochs.

To ensure that LIP category effects were due to learning the DMC task, we retrained both monkeys to group the same 12 directions into two new categories that were separated by a category boundary perpendicular to the original boundary. LIP population activity shifted dramatically after several weeks

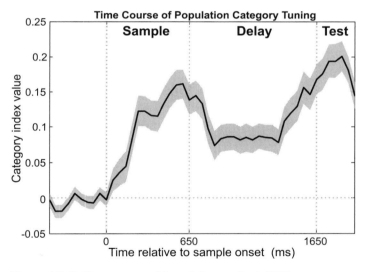

Figure 17–9 Time course of lateral intraparietal (LIP) category selectivity. A category index measured the strength of neuronal category selectivity. Positive index values indicate greater selectivity between categories or more similar activity within categories. The time course of average category index values across 122 direction-selective LIP neurons (during sample or delay) is shown. The *shaded area* around the *solid black line* indicates the standard error of the mean.

of retraining. After retraining, neurons reflected the new (now relevant) category boundary and not the old (now irrelevant) categories. We quantified this effect for each neuron by determining which of six possible category boundaries (that divided the 12 directions into two equal groups) gave the largest difference in average neuronal activity among the six directions on either side of the boundary. For neurons recorded using the original category boundary, sample and late delay activity for most neurons was best classified by the actual category boundary that the monkeys were using to solve the task, and not by the other five "irrelevant" boundaries. After retraining, neuronal activity during both the sample and late delay epochs no longer reflected the old category boundary, but rather was best divided by the new, now relevant, boundary (Freedman and Assad, 2006).

Our studies of the parietal cortex exhibit striking parallels with those of the PFC during shape (cat versus dog) categorization. Previously, it had been unclear whether neurons in brain areas considered to be closer to sensory processing areas (compared with the PFC), such as LIP, could encode information about the category of stimuli, or whether these abstract signals about stimulus category are exclusively encoded in executive areas, such as the PFC. These results also raised the possibility that motion categories might be encoded in motion processing areas, such as MT, that provide input to LIP. Alternatively, area MT may be primarily involved in basic visual motion processing, and more abstract signals about the behavioral relevance of motion direction might arise in downstream brain areas, such as LIP. To investigate the relative roles of areas MT and LIP in visual motion categorization, we compared the responses of LIP and MT neurons during visual motion categorization, as described in the next section.

Middle Temporal Area

Since its discovery more than 30 years ago (Allman and Kass, 1971; Dubner and Zeki, 1971), area MT of the macaque monkey has been one of the most extensively studied brain areas outside of the primary visual cortex. Area MT plays an important role in visual-motion processing. A primary feature of MT visual responses is that they respond strongly to moving spots, bars, and drifting gratings. Its neurons are typically highly sensitive, or tuned, to the direction and speed of visual motion. Area MT receives direct input from the primary visual cortex, in addition to inputs from areas V2 and V3, the lateral geniculate nucleus, and the pulvinar (Felleman and Van Essen, 1991). Its outputs include strong direct projections to the posterior parietal cortex, including area LIP (Lewis and Van Essen, 2000). For a recent review on MT, see Born and Bradley (2005).

Comparison of LIP and MT during Motion Categorization

To investigate the relative roles of areas LIP and MT during the visual motion DMC task, we recorded data from 67 MT neurons from the same two

monkeys used for the LIP studies, during DMC task performance. As in LIP, a majority of MT neurons were activated by the motion DMC task. During the sample epoch, most MT neurons were direction-selective: Nearly all MT neurons ($n = 66/67$) distinguished between the 12 directions of motion (one-way ANOVA, $p < 0.01$). However, the pattern of direction selectivity differed greatly from that in LIP: MT neurons did not group the motion directions according to their category membership. As the two single-neuron examples in Figure 17–10 (see color insert) illustrate, MT neurons showed classic direction-tuning: strong responses to motion in their preferred direction, and a gradual decrease in activity for directions that were progressively farther away from the

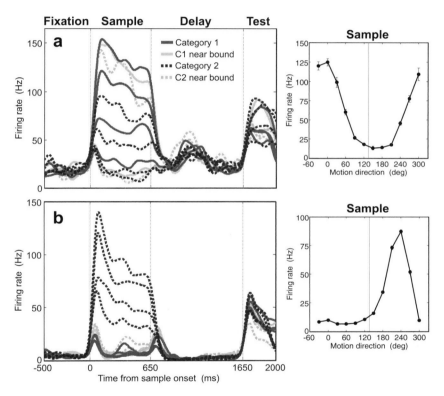

Figure 17–10 Examples of two direction-selective middle temporal (MT) neurons. *A* and *B*. Peristimulus time histograms show the average activity to the 12 sample stimulus directions for two single MT neurons. The red (solid) and blue (dashed) traces correspond to directions in the two categories. The *pale red* and *blue traces* indicate those directions that were close to (15 degrees) the category boundary. The three *vertical dotted lines* indicate (*left* to *right*) the timing of the sample onset, the sample offset, and the test stimulus onset. The plots at the *right* of each peri-stimulus time histogram (PSTH) show the average firing rate to the 12 directions during the sample epoch. *Error bars* indicate the standard error of the mean.

preferred direction. The neuron shown in Fig. 17–10A responded preferentially to directions near zero degrees, while the neurons in Fig. 17–10B preferred directions near 240 degrees.

To test whether MT neurons showed, on average, sharper selectivity across the category boundary and more similar activity within categories, we computed a category-tuning index in the same manner as for the LIP data. In contrast to LIP, category index values for area MT were not shifted toward positive values (Fig. 17–11). Instead, MT category indices were centered around zero, indicating that MT neurons did not, on average, show sharper direction-tuning around the category boundary. This indicates that MT responses during the DMC task did not explicitly represent the category of stimuli, but rather conveyed a more faithful veridical representation of visual motion direction.

Our combined results from these studies of motion categorization suggest that training monkeys to perform a motion categorization task causes LIP neurons to strongly and robustly reflect the category membership of visual motion direction. LIP neurons responded more similarly to motion directions of the same category, even when those directions were visually dissimilar, and they discriminated sharply between visually similar directions of different

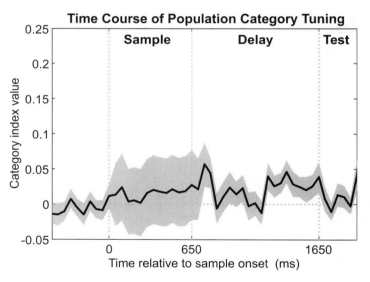

Figure 17–11 Time course of middle temporal (MT) category selectivity. A category index measured the strength of neuronal category selectivity. Positive index values indicate greater selectivity between categories or more similar activity within categories. The time course of average category index values across the entire population of 67 MT neurons is shown. In contrast with the lateral intraparietal area (Fig. 17–9), category selectivity was not observed in the MT during the sample, delay, or test epochs.

categories. In contrast, neurons in area MT, an important stage of visual motion processing that provides input to LIP, showed strong direction selectivity, but did not group directions according to their category membership. This suggests that, although LIP can show a great degree of visual plasticity as a result of learning, MT direction selectivity is comparatively rigid, and does not show dramatic changes in direction-tuning via experience.

DISCUSSION AND FUTURE DIRECTIONS

Together, the results of these studies indicate that visual categories are encoded in the activity of individual cortical neurons as a result of learning. We compared the responses of neurons in both the "ventral" and "dorsal" visual streams, which are believed to be specialized for shape and spatial motion processing, respectively, and found striking similarities in their patterns of neuronal activity during visual categorization. During the cat versus dog shape categorization task, PFC neurons encoded stimuli according to their category membership and were less sensitive to shape differences between stimuli in the same category. In contrast, ITC neurons (which provide input to the PFC) seemed to be more involved in visual shape feature analysis and did not show more generalized category encoding. In the motion-direction categorization task, LIP neurons reflected the category membership of visual motion, whereas MT neurons showed strong direction selectivity, but not more abstract category signals, consistent with a role in basic visual motion processing. This suggests that, for both visual shape and motion processing streams, there may be a distinct separation between the encoding of visual stimulus features and more abstract, learning-dependent representations about the behavioral relevance of stimuli.

Important questions remain about the role of the prefrontal, parietal, and temporal lobe areas in visual categorization. One question is whether PFC and LIP areas are "general-purpose" categorizers of many types of visual stimuli, or whether they are specialized for encoding the category of the specific types of stimuli used in our experiments. One possibility is that each of these areas is each specialized for visual shape (PFC) and motion (LIP) processing, and that category effects would not be observed in these areas for other types of stimuli. Alternatively, one or both of these areas might play a more general role in encoding the category membership of other types of stimuli. This seems especially likely in the PFC, because it receives projections from both the dorsal and ventral visual processing streams, in addition to both auditory and somatosensory processing areas (Pandya and Yeterian, 1998). Likewise, many studies have shown that PFC neurons can respond selectively to a wide range of visual, auditory, and tactile stimuli, particularly when those stimuli are task-relevant (Miller and Cohen, 2001). Thus, it seems likely that the PFC would reflect the category of motion direction, as in LIP. However, it is less clear whether LIP might encode the category membership of visual shapes. Although anatomical and neurophysiological studies suggest that LIP is more directly

linked with dorsal stream visual areas and oculomotor structures, such as the frontal eye fields and superior colliculus (Lewis and Van Essen, 2000), it is also interconnected with the PFC and temporal lobe shape processing areas, such as V4 and the ITC (Webster et al., 1994; Lewis and Van Essen, 2000). Several studies have found that posterior parietal neurons (including, in some cases, LIP neurons) can respond selectively to simple and complex shapes (Sereno and Maunsell, 1998; Nieder and Miller, 2004; Stoet and Snyder, 2004; Sereno and Amador, 2006), although further studies are needed to determine whether LIP neurons might encode shape categories, as we have observed in the PFC.

In some ways, it is surprising that ITC neurons did not show strong category signals. Before these studies, it had been assumed by many that the ITC was a likely—if not the most likely—candidate for the learning and storage of shape categories. This idea had developed because it was found that ITC damage in humans and monkeys resulted in behavioral impairments in high-level shape processing, and even category-specific, recognition deficits (e.g., facial agnosia). In addition, neurophysiological recordings from ITC neurons revealed selectivity for complex stimuli that was sometimes highly specific for stimuli from a specific category (especially faces). In contrast, damage to the PFC does not typically result in deficits in visual recognition or categorization, but instead, leads to impaired "executive" functions, such as deficits in short-term working memory, impaired rule learning, and inappropriate behaviors. This raises the possibility that the PFC is not the source of the category signals that we observed in our studies, but instead, may receive information about stimulus category via its inputs from other brain regions. One possibility is that more abstract category information is encoded elsewhere in the ITC, in regions that we did not record in our studies. Another possibility is that category signals emerge in more medial-temporal structures, such as the perirhinal cortex, that receive inputs from the ITC and are likely involved in both perceptual and memory-related functions (Murray et al., 2000). Additional experiments will be needed to fully understand how the brain transforms visual shape encoding (as in the ITC) into more abstract representations of their category membership.

Further studies are also needed to understand the neuronal processes that underlie category learning. In all of the studies described in this chapter, neuronal activity was recorded only after weeks or months of categorization training. Thus, the monkeys were expert categorizers at the time of neuronal recordings. Although PFC and LIP neurons conveyed reliable signals about the category of these highly familiar stimuli, they might show very different responses during the learning process. For example, some theories suggest that novel information is more actively processed by frontal lobe areas, and that neuronal processing shifts to more posterior brain areas for a more automatic and effortless encoding of familiar information (Miller and Cohen, 2001). This could explain the common experience that it is difficult to "multitask" when you are learning a new skill; for example, carrying on a conversation while learning to drive a car for the first time. In contrast, carrying out multiple tasks

that are highly familiar becomes a nearly effortless matter of routine. To better understand their respective roles in category learning, future studies are needed that monitor the activity of PFC and LIP neurons in real time, as monkeys learn new categories.

Visual categorization tasks have proven to be useful and productive tools for studying the relative roles of brain areas in visual learning and recognition. Of course, we are far from fully understanding how the brain learns and encodes the category membership of visual stimuli. Although further experiments may uncover more questions than answers, I am optimistic that this flavor of research will move us toward a better understanding of how the brain makes sense of the "blooming buzzing confusion" (James, 1890) that is the world around us.

ACKNOWLEDGMENTS I wish to thank John Assad, Jamie Fitzgerald, Constance Freedman, Todd Herrington, and Jonathan Wallis for their comments on an earlier version of this manuscript. I also thank Earl Miller and John Assad for numerous contributions, discussions, and support while I worked in their laboratories. In addition, Tomaso Poggio and Maximilian Riesenhuber made many contributions to the prefrontal cortex and inferior temporal cortex experiments during our collaborations at MIT. I was supported by a Kirschstein National Research Service Award postdoctoral fellowship.

REFERENCES

Allman JM, Kaas JH (1971) A representation of the visual field in the caudal third of the middle temporal gyrus of the owl monkey (*Aotus trivirgatus*). Brain Research 31:85–105.

Andersen RA, Buneo CA (2002) Intentional maps in posterior parietal cortex. Annual Review of Neuroscience 25:189–220.

Ashby FG, Maddox WT (2005) Human category learning. Annual Review of Psychology 56:149–178.

Baker CI, Behrmann M, Olson CR (2002) Impact of learning on representation of parts and wholes in monkey inferotemporal cortex. Nature Neuroscience 5:1210–1215.

Barsalou LW (1992) Cognitive psychology: an overview for cognitive scientists. Hillsdale, NJ: Lawrence Erlbaum Associates.

Baylis G, Rolls E, Leonard C (1987) Functional subdivisions of the temporal lobe neocortex. Journal of Neuroscience 7:330–342.

Beymer D, Poggio T (1996) Image representations for visual learning. Science 272: 1905–1909.

Blum JS, Chow KL, Pribram KH (1950) A behavioral analysis of the organization of the parieto-temporo-preoccipital cortex. Journal of Comparative Neurology 93:53–100.

Booth MC, Rolls ET (1998) View-invariant representations of familiar objects by neurons in the inferior temporal visual cortex. Cerebral Cortex 8:510–523.

Born RT, Bradley DC (2005) Structure and function of visual area MT. Annual Review of Neuroscience 28:157–189.

Brincat SL, Connor CE (2004) Underlying principles of visual shape selectivity in posterior inferotemporal cortex. Nature Neuroscience 7:880–886.

Bruce C, Desimone R, Gross CG (1981) Visual properties of neurons in a polysensory area in superior temporal sulcus in the macaque. Journal of Neurophysiology 46: 369–384.

Colby CL, Goldberg ME (1999) Space and attention in parietal cortex. Annual Review of Neuroscience 22:319–349.

Cook RG (2001). *Avian visual cognition.* Retrieved July, 2006 from http//www.pigeon .psy.tufts.edu/avc.

Damasio AR, Damasio H, Van Hoesen GW (1982) Prosopagnosia: anatomic basis and behavioral mechanisms. Neurology 32:331–341.

Desimone R, Albright TD, Gross CG, Bruce C (1984) Stimulus-selective properties of inferior temporal neurons in the macaque. Journal of Neuroscience 4:2051–2062.

Dubner R, Zeki SM (1971) Response properties and receptive fields of cells in an anatomically defined region of the superior temporal sulcus in the monkey. Brain Research 35:528–532.

Edwards CA, Jagielo JA, Zentall TR (1983) Same/different symbol use by pigeons. Animal Learning and Behavior 11:349–355.

Erickson CA, Jagadeesh, Desimone R (2000) Clustering of perirhinal neurons with similar properties following visual experience in adult monkeys. Nature Neuroscience 3:1066–1068.

Fabre-Thorpe M, Richard G, Thorpe SJ (1998) Rapid categorization of natural images by rhesus monkeys. Neuroreport 9:303–308.

Fanini and Assad (submitted).

Felleman DJ, Van Essen DC (1991) Distributed hierarchical processing in the primate cerebral cortex. Cerebral Cortex 1:1–47.

Freedman DJ, Assad JA (2006) Experience-dependent representation of visual categories in parietal cortex. Nature 443: 85-88.

Freedman DJ, Riesenhuber M, Poggio T, Miller EK (2001) Categorical representation of visual stimuli in the primate prefrontal cortex. Science 291:312–316.

Freedman DJ, Riesenhuber M, Poggio T, Miller EK (2002) Visual categorization and the primate prefrontal cortex: neurophysiology and behavior. Journal of Neurophysiology 88:914–928.

Freedman DJ, Riesenhuber M, Poggio T, Miller EK (2003) A comparison of primate prefrontal and inferior temporal cortices during visual categorization. Journal of Neuroscience 23:5235–5246.

Freedman DJ, Riesenhuber M, Poggio T, Miller EK (2005) Experience-dependent sharpening of visual shape selectivity in inferior temporal cortex. Cerebral Cortex 16: 1631–1644.

Gross CG (1973) Visual functions of inferotemporal cortex. In: Handbook of sensory physiology (Autrum H, Jung R, Lowenstein W, Mckay D, Teuber HL, eds.), pp 3–10, volume VII/3B. Berlin: Springer-Verlag.

Herrnstein RJ (1979) Acquisition, generalization, and discrimination reversal of a natural concept. Journal of Experimental Psychology: Animal Behavior Processes 5:116–129.

Herrnstein RJ, Loveland DH (1964) Complex visual concept in the pigeon. Science 146:549–551.

Herrnstein RJ, Loveland DH, Cable C (1976) Natural concepts in pigeons. Journal of Experimental Psychology: Animal Behavior Processes 2:285–302.

James W (1890) The principles of psychology. Cambridge, MA: Harvard University Press.

Kluver H, Bucy L (1938) An analysis of certain effects of bilateral temporal lobectomy in the rhesus monkey, with special reference to "psychic blindness." Journal of Psychology 5:33–54.

Kluver H, Bucy L (1939) Preliminary analysis of functions of the temporal lobes in monkeys. Archives of Neurology and Psychiatry 42:979–1000.

Kobatake E, Wang G, Tanaka K (1998) Effects of shape discrimination training on the selectivity of inferotemporal cells in adult monkeys. Journal of Neurophysiology 80:324–330.

Kreiman G, Koch C, Fried I (2000) Category-specific visual responses of single neurons in the human medial temporal lobe. Nature Neuroscience 3:946–953.

Lewis JW, Van Essen DC (2000) Corticocortical connections of visual, sensorimotor, and multimodal processing areas in the parietal lobe of the macaque monkey. Journal of Comparative Neurology 428:112–137.

Logothetis NK, Pauls J, Poggio T (1995) Shape representation in the inferior temporal cortex of monkeys. Current Biology 5:552–563.

Miller EK, Cohen JD (2001) An integrative theory of prefrontal cortex function. Annual Review of Neuroscience 24:167–202.

Mishkin M (1954) Visual discrimination performance following partial ablations of the temporal lobe, II: Ventral surface vs. hippocampus. Journal of Comparative and Physiological Psychology 47:187–193.

Mishkin M (1966) Visual mechanisms beyond the striate cortex. In: Frontiers in physiological psychology (Russell RW, ed.), pp 93–119. New York: Academic Press.

Mishkin M, Pribram K (1954) Visual discrimination performance following partial ablations of the temporal lobe, I: Ventral vs. lateral. Journal of Comparative and Physiological Psychology 47:14–20.

Miyashita Y (1993) Inferior temporal cortex: where visual perception meets memory. Annual Review of Neuroscience 16:245–263.

Murray EA, Bussey TJ, Hampton RR, Saksida LM (2000) The parahippocampal region and object identification. Annals of the New York Academy of Science 911:166–174.

Nieder A, Freedman DJ, Miller EK (2002) Representation of the quantity of visual items in the primate prefrontal cortex. Science 297:1708–1711.

Nieder A, Miller EK (2004) A parieto-frontal network for visual numerical information in the monkey. Proceedings of the National Academy of Sciences U S A 101:7457–7462.

Orlov T, Yakovlev V, Hochstein S, Zohary E (2000) Macaque monkeys categorize images by their ordinal number. Nature 404:77–80.

Pandya DN, Yeterian EH (1998) Comparison of prefrontal architecture and connections. In: The prefrontal cortex: executive and cognitive functions (Roberts AC, Robbins TW, Weiskrantz L, eds.), pp 51–66. Oxford, UK: Oxford University Press.

Perrett DI, Rolls ET, Caan W (1982) Visual neurones responsive to faces in the monkey temporal cortex. Experimental Brain Research 47:329–342.

Premack D (1983) Animal cognition. Annual Review of Psychology 34:351–362.

Quiroga RQ, Reddy L, Kreiman G, Koch C, Fried I (2005) Invariant visual representation by single neurons in the human brain. Nature 435:1102–1107.

Roberts WA, Mazmanian DS (1988) Concept learning at different levels of abstraction by pigeons, monkeys, and people. Journal of Experimental Psychology: Animal Behavior Processes 14:247–260.

Sereno AB, Maunsell JH (1998) Shape selectivity in primate lateral intraparietal cortex. Nature 395:500–503.

Sereno AB, Amador SC (2006) Attention and memory-related responses of neurons in the lateral intraparietal area during spatial and shape-delayed match-to-sample tasks. Journal of Neurophysiology 95: 1078-1098.

Shelton C (2000) Morphable surface models. International Journal of Computer Vision 38:75–91.

Sigala N, Logothetis NK (2002) Visual categorization shapes feature selectivity in the primate temporal cortex. Nature 415:318–320.

Stoet G, Snyder LH (2004) Single neurons in posterior parietal cortex (PPC) of monkeys encode cognitive set. Neuron 42:1003–1012.

Tanaka K (1996) Inferotemporal cortex and object vision. Annual Review of Neuroscience 19:109–139.

Toth LJ, Assad JA (2002) Dynamic coding of behaviorally relevant stimuli in parietal cortex. Nature 415:165–168.

Tsao DY, Freiwald WA, Tootell RB, Livingstone MS (2006) A cortical region consisting entirely of face cells. Science 311:670–674.

Ungerleider LG, Gaffan D, Pelak VS (1989) Projections from inferior temporal cortex to prefrontal cortex via the uncinate fascicle in rhesus monkeys. Experimental Brain Research 76:473–484.

Ungerleider LG, Mishkin M (1982) Two cortical visual systems. In: Analysis of visual behavior (Ingle DJ, Goodale MA, Mansfield RJW, eds.), pp 549–586. Cambridge: MIT Press.

Verhave T (1966) The pigeon as quality control inspector. American Psychologist 21: 109–115.

Vogels R (1999) Categorization of complex visual images by rhesus monkeys. European Journal of Neuroscience 11:1223–1238.

Wallis JD, Anderson KC, Miller EK (2001) Single neurons in prefrontal cortex encode abstract rules. Nature 411:953–956.

Webster MJ, Bachevalier J, Ungerleider LG (1994) Connections of inferior temporal areas TEO and TE with parietal and frontal cortex in macaque monkeys. Cerebral Cortex 4:470–483.

Wright AA, Santiago HC, Urcuioli PJ, Sands SF (1983) Monkey and pigeon acquisition of same/different concept using pictorial stimuli. In: Quantitative analyses of behavior (Commons ML, Herrnstein RJ, Wagner AR, eds.), pp 295–317, volume 4. Cambridge, MA: Ballinger.

Wyttenbach RA, May ML, Hoy RR (1996) Categorical perception of sound frequency by crickets. Science 273:1542–1544.

18

Rules through Recursion:
How Interactions between the
Frontal Cortex and Basal Ganglia
May Build Abstract, Complex Rules
from Concrete, Simple Ones

Earl K. Miller and Timothy J. Buschman

The brain has evolved to deal with two competing requirements—it must respond quickly to familiar situations while being able to adapt to novel ones and plan for the future. Quickly responding to the immediate environment in a reflexive, or habitual, fashion is relatively straightforward: Familiar stimuli activate well-established neural pathways that produce stereotyped behaviors. This is so-called "bottom-up," or "stimulus-driven," processing. These behaviors can be executed quickly and automatically because they are "concrete"; they rely on specific stimulus-response relationships, and the same cue always elicits the same response. It is an axiom of neuroscience that such reflexive reactions are formed by repeated activation of neural pathways, which strengthens their connections. Then, they can be simply triggered—fired off in an automatic fashion, with little variation and, hence, little need for internal oversight.

In contrast, truly sophisticated, goal-directed behavior requires a different mode of operation. Novel situations must be resolved, and goal direction requires the ability to act on, not just react to, a familiar environment. Navigating complex situations to achieve long-planned goals cannot rely on uncoordinated reactions. They must be orchestrated "top-down" from within oneself. By acquiring and building on knowledge of how the world works, we can predict what outcomes are desirable and determine what strategies will aid in attaining them. However, simply recording and replaying previous experiences does not suffice. Relevant relationships need to be sorted out from spurious coincidences, and smart animals get the "big picture" of the jigsaw puzzle of their experiences: They find the common structure across a wide range of experiences to form "abstract" rules—generalized principles that can be readily adapted to novel situations. These abstract rules are the overarching principles and general concepts that are the basis for high-level thought. They provide

the foresight needed for achieving distant goals; because abstract rules, by definition, are generalized across many past experiences, they provide the basis for generalizing to (predicting) future events.

The goal of this chapter is to review evidence that goal-directed behavior depends on interactions between two different "styles" of learning mechanisms in different frontal lobe systems. Specifically, we propose that ever more complex thoughts and actions can be bootstrapped from simpler ones through recursive interactions between fast, reward-based plasticity in the basal ganglia (BG) and slower, more Hebbian-based plasticity in the frontal cortex. By having these two systems interact in recursive processing loops, the brain can learn new concrete relationships quickly, but also can take the time to link in more experiences and more gradually build up abstract, big-picture thoughts and sophisticated actions.

ABSTRACT RULES AND THE PREFRONTAL CORTEX

Abstract rules lie at the center of the ability to coordinate thought and action and direct them toward a goal. Virtually all long-term, goal-directed behaviors are learned, and thus depend on a cognitive system that can acquire the rules of the game: what outcomes are possible, what actions might be successful at achieving them, what the costs of those actions might be, etc. Consider the set of rules invoked when we dine in a restaurant, such as "wait to be seated," "order," and "pay the bill." These rules are long divorced from the specific circumstances in which they were learned and thus give us an idea about what to expect (and what is expected of us) when we try a new restaurant. We have learned to generalize beyond specific experiences and construct a set of abstract rules that direct behavior. These rules orchestrate processing in diverse brain regions along a common, internal theme. It is widely accepted that the prefrontal cortex (PFC)—a neocortical region that finds its greatest elaboration in humans—is centrally involved in this process.

The PFC is situated at the anterior end of the brain and reaches its greatest elaboration and relative size in the primate, especially human, brain (Fuster, 1995). Thus, it is presumably involved in our advanced cognitive capabilities and goal-directed behaviors. Indeed, recent imaging work has suggested that the size of the PFC is directly correlated with intelligence in adult humans (Haier et al., 2004). The PFC seems anatomically well situated to play a role in the creation and implementation of abstract rules. As shown in Figure 18–1, the PFC receives and sends projections to most of the cerebral cortex (with the exception of primary sensory and motor cortices), as well as all of the major subcortical systems, such as the hippocampus, amygdala, cerebellum, and most importantly for this chapter, the BG (Porrino et al., 1981; Amaral and Price, 1984; Amaral, 1986; Selemon and Goldman-Rakic, 1988; Barbas and De Olmos, 1990; Eblen and Graybiel, 1995; Croxson et al., 2005). The PFC seems to be a hub of cortical processing, able to synthesize a wide range of external and internal information and also exert control over much of the cortex. Although

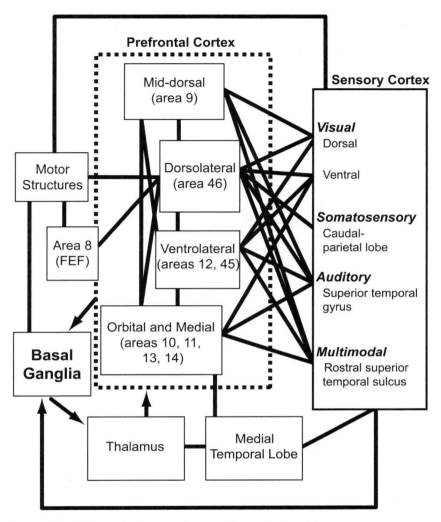

Figure 18–1 Schematic diagram of some of the extrinsic and intrinsic connections of the prefrontal cortex. The partial convergence of inputs from many brain systems and internal connections of the prefrontal cortex (PFC) may allow it to play a central role in the synthesis of diverse information needed for complex behavior. Most connections are reciprocal; the exceptions are indicated by *arrows*. The frontal eye field (FEF) has variously been considered either adjacent to, or part of, the PFC. Here, we compromise by depicting it as adjacent to, yet touching, the PFC. (Adapted from Miller and Cohen, *Annual Review of Neuroscience*, 24, 167–202.)

different PFC subdivisions have distinct patterns of interconnections with other brain systems (e.g., lateral—sensory and motor cortex; orbital—limbic), there are prodigious connections both within and between PFC subdivisions, ensuring a high degree of integration of information (Pandya and Barnes, 1987; Barbas and Pandya, 1989; Pandya and Yeterian, 1990; Barbas et al., 1991; Petrides and Pandya, 1999). Additionally, the heavy reciprocal interconnections between regions provide an infrastructure ideal for abstract learning— one that can act as a large associative network for detecting and storing associations between diverse events, experiences, and internal states. After learning, such a network can complete or "recall" an entire pattern given a subset of its inputs, an ability that may allow for a given situation to be recognized as a specific instance of an internal model of a more abstract one.

In addition to the anatomical evidence, there is a large amount of psychological, lesion, and neurophysiological evidence supporting the role of the frontal cortex in learning abstract rules (also see Chapter 2). Indeed, neurophysiological studies in animals and imaging studies in humans have shown that the PFC has many of the attributes necessary for representing abstract rules (Miller, 2000). First, the neurons sustain their activity across short, multisecond memory delays (Pribram et al., 1952; Fuster and Alexander, 1971; Fuster, 1973; Funahashi et al., 1989; Miller et al., 1996). This property is crucial for goal-directed behavior, which, unlike "ballistic" reflexes, typically extends over time. Second, neurons within the PFC are highly multimodal, representing a wide range of information, and the cells are plastic—with training, they learn to represent task-relevant information. For example, after training on a wide range of operant tasks, many PFC neurons (typically one-third to one-half of the population) reflect the learned task contingencies—the logic or rules of the task (White and Wise, 1999; Asaad et al., 2000; Wallis et al., 2001; Mansouri et al., 2006). For example, neurons have been found to represent visual categories (see Chapter 17) and small numbers (Nieder et al., 2002), whereas some neurons might activate in anticipation of a forthcoming expected reward or a relevant cue (Watanabe, 1996; Rainer et al., 1999; Wallis and Miller, 2003; Padoa-Schioppa and Assad, 2006). In short, the PFC does, indeed, act like a brain area that absorbs and reflects the abstract rules needed to guide goal-directed, volitional behavior.

Based on this evidence, Miller and Cohen (2001) argued that the cardinal PFC function is to acquire and actively maintain patterns of activity that represent goals and the means to achieve them ("rules") *and* the cortical pathways needed to perform the task ("maps"—together, "rulemaps") [Fig. 18–2]. Under this model, activation of a PFC rulemap sets up bias signals that propagate throughout much of the rest of the cortex, affecting sensory systems as well as systems responsible for response execution, memory retrieval, and emotional evaluation. The aggregate effect is to guide the flow of neural activity along pathways that establish the proper mappings between inputs, internal states, and outputs to best perform the task. Establishing the proper mapping is especially important whenever stimuli are ambiguous (i.e., they activate more

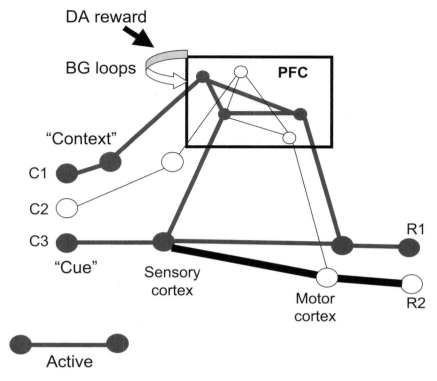

Figure 18–2 Schematic diagram illustrating the suggested role for the prefrontal cortex (PFC) in cognitive control adapted from Miller and Cohen (2001). Shown are processing units representing cues, such as sensory inputs, current motivational state, memories, and so on (C1, C2, and C3), and those representing two voluntary actions (e.g., "responses" R1 and R2). Also shown are internal, or "hidden," units that represent more central stages of processing. The PFC is not heavily connected with primary sensory or motor cortices, but instead is connected with higher-level "association" and premotor cortices. Via interactions with the basal ganglia (BG) [see text], dopaminergic (DA) reward signals foster the formation of a task model, a neural representation that reflects the learned associations between task-relevant information (as shown by the recursive arrow). A subset of the information (e.g., C1 and C2) can then evoke the entire model, including information about the appropriate response (e.g., R1). Thus, the PFC can coordinate processing throughout the brain and steer processing away from a prepotent (reflexive) response (C3 to R2) toward a weakly established, but more goal-relevant, response (C3 to R1). Excitatory signals from the PFC feed back to other brain systems to enable task-relevant neural pathways. *Thick lines* indicate well-established pathways mediating a prepotent behavior. *Solid circles* indicates active units or pathways.

than one input representation), or when multiple responses are possible and the task-appropriate response must compete with stronger, more habitual alternatives. In short, task information is acquired by the PFC, which provides support to related information in posterior brain systems, effectively acting as a global attentional controller.

However, as noted earlier, the PFC is heavily interconnected and does not work in isolation. Later in the chapter, we will review evidence that the PFC works in close collaboration with the BG in the learning of goal-directed behaviors. Specifically, we will argue that, through reciprocal connections between the PFC and BG, increasingly complex rules can be constructed.

CONCRETE RULES AND THE BASAL GANGLIA

The BG is a collection of subcortical nuclei that, similar to the PFC, have a high degree of cortical convergence. Cortical inputs arrive largely via the striatum (which includes both the caudate and the putamen); are processed through the globus pallidus, the subthalamic nucleus (STN), and the substantia nigra; and are then directed back into the cortex via the thalamus (Fig. 18–3). Although the PFC is believed to be involved in the creation and implementation of abstract rules, the BG is believed to be involved in the formation of concrete habits. We will review some anatomical and physiological evidence in support of this theory.

Early evidence about the function of the BG came from human patients with damage or dysfunction to this area. For example, both Parkinson's disease and Huntington's disease cause profound behavioral deficits, ranging from motor (e.g., difficulty initiating volitional movement) to cognitive (e.g., difficulty switching tasks) [Taylor et al., 1986; Cronin-Golomb et al., 1994; Lawrence et al., 1998]. Animal models of lesions of the striatum produce impairments in learning new operant behaviors (or concrete rules) and show that damage to different parts of the striatum generally causes deficits similar to those caused by lesions of the area of the cortex that loop with the affected region of the striatum (Divac et al., 1967; Goldman and Rosvold, 1972). For example, lesions of the regions of the caudate associated with the frontal cortex result in cognitive impairments, suggesting that the reciprocal connections between the BG and cortex play a significant role in the functioning of that cortical area.

Projections from the striatum are distributed along two parallel routes: the "direct" and "indirect" pathways (Fig. 18–3) [Mink, 1996; Graybiel, 2000]. The direct pathway leads from the striatum into the globus pallidus internal (GPi) and the substantia nigra pars reticulata (SNpr). These regions directly project onto the thalamus. All projections from the striatum release gamma-aminobutyric acid (GABA); therefore, they inhibit downstream neurons in the GPi/SNpr. Neurons in the GPi/SNpr inhibit the thalamus, making the direct pathway effectively excitatory—activity in the striatum releases inhibition on the thalamus. The indirect pathway involves striatal projections to the globus pallidus external (GPe), which in turn, projects to the STN, which

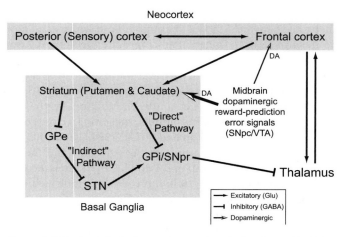

Figure 18–3 Simplified circuit diagram for the basal ganglia, illustrating the loops it makes with the frontal cortex. See text for explanation. The *heavy arrow* illustrates the much heavier projection of midbrain dopaminergic neurons to the striatum than to the cortex. DA, dopamine; GPe, globus pallidus external; STN, subthalamic nucleus; GPi, globus pallidus internal; SNpr, substantia nigra pars reticulata; SNpc, substantia nigra, pars compacta; VTA, ventral tegmental area; Glu, glutamate; GABA, gamma-aminobutyric acid.

projects onto the GPi/SNpr. Similar to the other connections in the BG, GPe inputs into the STN are inhibitory, but the STN provides glutamatergic, excitatory input into the GPi/SNpr. Due to the added inhibitory synapse, the indirect pathway increases inhibition on the thalamus. These two pathways are believed to exist in an equilibrium that allows for the release of desired patterns, while inhibiting unintended ones. Although cortical inputs into the striatum had a divergent nature, connections between the striatum and the GPi/SNpr and GPe are believed to be highly convergent (Flaherty and Graybiel, 1993, 1994; Parent and Hazrati, 1993). This convergence of inputs is effectively a reduction in the dimensionality of the patterns, and may allow for a certain degree of integration and generalization across specific cortical inputs.

Similar to the PFC, the structure of the BG is ideal for integrating information. Most of the cortex projects directly onto the striatum (Kemp and Powell, 1970; Kitai et al., 1976) in a divergent manner, so that cortical afferents make connections to multiple striatal neurons (Flaherty and Graybiel, 1991). The striatum is believed to be subdivided into striosomes and the matrix (Graybiel and Ragsdale, 1978), with striosomes preferentially receiving inputs from the entire cerebral cortex and the matrix primarily receiving inputs from the limbic and hippocampal systems and from the PFC (Donoghue and Herkenham, 1986; Gerfen, 1992; Eblen and Graybiel, 1995). Anatomical tracing techniques have suggested that functionally similar cortical areas project

into the same striosome (Yeterian and Van Hoesen, 1978; Van Hoesen et al., 1981; Flaherty and Graybiel, 1991). For example, both sensory and motor areas relating to the arm seem to preferentially innervate the same striosome. The segregated nature of BG inputs are maintained throughout the different nuclei such that the output from the BG (via the thalamus) is largely to the same cortical areas that gave rise to the initial inputs into the BG (Selemon and Goldman-Rakic, 1985; Parasarathy et al., 1992). Additionally, the frontal cortex receives the largest portion of BG outputs, suggesting a close collaboration between these structures (Middleton and Strick, 1994, 2000, 2002).

The majority of neurons found in both the striosome and the matrix are spiny cells (as high as 90%) [Kemp and Powell, 1971]. These neurons are so named for the high density of synaptic boutons along their dendritic arbor, due to the convergent nature of cortical inputs. Along with the cortical inputs, spiny cells receive a strong dopaminergic (DA) input from neurons in the midbrain. These DA neurons have been suggested to provide a reward-based "teaching signal" that gates plasticity in the striatum. All of this has suggested that the striatum has an ideal infrastructure for rapid, supervised learning (i.e., the quick formation of connections between cortical inputs that predict reward). This is exactly the type of learning that supports the imprinting of specific stimulus-response pairing that supports concrete rules. Finally, it is important to note that there are functional and anatomical differences between the dorsal and ventral striatum. The dorsal striatum is more associated with the PFC and the stimulus-response-reward learning that is the subject of this chapter. The ventral striatum is more connected with the sensory cortex and seems to be more involved in learning the reward value of stimuli (see O'Doherty et al., 2004).

DOPAMINERGIC TEACHING SIGNALS

The formation of rules requires guidance. Concrete rules are formed, through feedback, to actively bind neural representations that lead to reward and break associations that are ineffective. This direct form of plasticity can pair coactivated neurons to form specific rules and predictions. Abstract rules are also guided by feedback so that relevant events and predictive relationships can be distinguished from spurious coincidences. Although the form of plasticity is different for concrete and abstract rules, both need be guided by information about which associations are predictive of desirable outcomes. This guidance appears to come in the form of a "reinforcement signal" and is suggested to be provided by DA neurons in the midbrain.

Dopaminergic neurons are located in both the ventral tegmental area and the substantia nigra, pars compacta (Schultz et al., 1992, 1997; Schultz, 1998), and show activity that directly corresponds to the reward prediction error signals suggested by models of animal learning. These neurons increase activity whenever the animal receives an unexpected reward and will reduce activity if an expected reward is withheld. When active, these neurons release dopamine

onto downstream targets. Dopamine is a neuromodulator that has been suggested to regulate plasticity at the innervated site.

Midbrain DA neurons send heavy projections into both the frontal cortex and the striatum. The projections into the frontal cortex show a gradient connectivity with heavier inputs anteriorly that drop off posteriorly, suggesting a preferential input of reward information into the PFC (Thierry et al., 1973; Goldman-Rakic et al., 1989). However, the midbrain input of DA into the striatum is much heavier than that of the PFC, by as much as an order of magnitude (Lynd-Balta and Haber, 1994). Furthermore, recent evidence suggests that neither strengthening nor weakening of synapses in the striatum by long-term depression or potentiation can occur without DA input (Calabresi et al., 1992, 1997; Otani et al., 1998; Kerr and Wickens, 2001).

After training, DA neurons in the midbrain will learn to increase activity to an unexpected stimulus that directly predicts a reward: The event "stands in" for the reward (Schultz et al., 1993). DA neurons will now respond to the predictive event when it is unexpected, but will no longer respond to the actual, now expected, reward event. In short, the activity of these neurons seems to correspond to a teaching signal that says, "Something good happened and you did not predict it, so remember what just happened so you can predict it in the future." Alternatively, if a reward is expected, but not received, the signal provides feedback that whatever behavior was just taken is not effective in getting rewarded. If these reward signals affect connections within the PFC and BG that were recently active, and therefore likely involved in recent behavior, then the result may be to help to strengthen reward-predicting associations within the network, while reducing associations that do not increase benefits. In this way, the brain can learn what rules are effective in increasing desirable outcomes.

"FAST," SUPERVISED BASAL GANGLIA PLASTICITY VERSUS "SLOWER," LESS SUPERVISED CORTICAL PLASTICITY

One might expect that the greatest evolutionary benefit would be gained from learning as quickly as possible, and there are obvious advantages to learning quickly—adapting at a faster rate than competing organisms lends a definite edge, whereas missed opportunities can be costly (even deadly). However, there are also disadvantages to learning quickly because one loses the ability to integrate across multiple experiences to form a generalized, less error-prone prediction. Take the classic example of one-trial learning: conditioned taste aversion. Many of us have had the experience of eating a particular food and then becoming ill for an unrelated reason. However, in many cases, the person develops an aversion to that food, even though the attribution is erroneous. Extending learning across multiple episodes allows organisms to detect the regularities of predictive relationships and leave behind spurious associations and coincidences. In addition to avoiding errors, slower, more deliberate learning also provides the opportunity to integrate associations across many different experiences to detect common structures.

It is these regularities and commonalities across specific instances that form abstractions, general principles, concepts, and symbolisms that are the medium of the sophisticated, "big-picture" thought needed for truly long-term goals. Indeed, this is fundamental to proactive thought and action. Generalizing among many past experiences gives us the ability to generalize to the future, to imagine possibilities that we have not yet experienced—but would like to—and given the generalized rules, we can predict the actions and behaviors needed to achieve our goal. In addition, abstraction may aid in cognitive flexibility, because generalized representations are, by definition, concise because they lack the details of the more specific representations. Based on the compressed representations, it is probably easier to switch between, and maintain, multiple generalized representations within a given network than to switch between representations when they are elaborate and detailed.

Networks that learn at a slower rate also tend to be more stable. It is believed that fast versus slow learning correlates with large versus small changes in synaptic weights, respectively. Artificial neural networks with small changes in synaptic weights at each learning episode converge very slowly, whereas large synaptic weight changes can quickly capture some patterns, the resulting networks tend to be more volatile and exhibit erratic behavior. This is due to the fact that a high learning rate can overshoot minima in the error function, even oscillating between values on either side of the minima, but never reaching the minima (for more information on artificial neural networks, see Hertz et al., 1991; Dayan and Abbott, 2001).

Given the advantages and disadvantages associated with both forms of learning, the brain must balance the obvious pressure to learn as quickly as possible with the advantages of slower learning. One possible solution to this conundrum comes from O'Reilly and colleagues, who suggested that fast learning and slow learning systems interact with one another (McClelland et al., 1995; O'Reilly and Munakata, 2000). Studying the consolidation of long-term memories, McClelland et al. (1995) specifically suggested that fast plasticity mechanisms within the hippocampus are able to quickly capture new memories while "training" the slower-learning cortical networks. In this way, the brain is able to balance the need to initially grasp new memories with the advantages of a generalized, distributed representation of long-term memories. The idea is that the hippocampus is specialized for the rapid acquisition of new information; each learning trial produces large weight changes. The output of the hippocampus will then repeatedly activate cortical networks that have smaller weight changes per episode. Continued hippocampal-mediated reactivation of cortical representations allows the cortex to gradually connect these representations with other experiences. That way, the shared structure across experiences can be detected and stored, and the memory can be interleaved with others so that it can be readily accessed.

We propose that a similar relationship exists between the PFC and BG. A recent experiment by our laboratory provides suggestive evidence (Pasupathy and Miller, 2005) [see Fig. 18–4]. Monkeys were trained to associate a visual

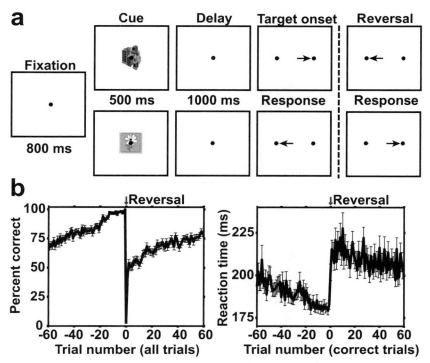

Figure 18–4 *A.* One of two initially novel cues was briefly presented at the center of gaze, followed by a memory delay and then presentation of two target spots on the right and left. Saccade to the target associated with the cue at that time was rewarded (as indicated by arrow). After this was learned, the cue-saccade associations were reversed and relearned. *B.* Average percentage of correct performance on all trials (*left*) and average reaction time on correct trials (*right*) across sessions and blocks as a function of trial number during learning for two monkeys. Zero (*downward arrow*) represents the first trial after reversal. *Error bars* show standard error of the mean.

cue with a directional eye movement over a period of trials (Fig. 18–4*A*). Once performance reached criterion and plateaued, the stimulus-response associations were reversed and the animals were required to relearn the pairings (Fig 18–4*B*). During the task, single neurons were recorded in both the PFC and the BG to determine the selectivity for the cue-direction association in each area. Over the period of a few tens of trials, the animals quickly learned the new cue-direction pairing (Fig 18–4*B*), and selectivity in both the striatum and PFC increased. As can be seen in Figure 18–5*A*, neural activity in the striatum showed rapid, almost bistable, changes in the timing of selectivity. This is in contrast to the PFC, where changes were much slower, with selective responses slowly advancing across trials (Fig 18–5*B*). Interestingly, however, the slower PFC seemed to be the final arbiter of behavior; the monkeys'

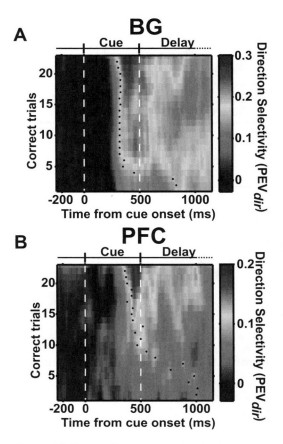

Figure 18–5 *A and B.* Selectivity for the direction of
eye movement associated with the presented cue. Selectivity was measured as the percent of explained variance by direction (PEV$_{dir}$), and is shown in the color
gradient across time for both the basal ganglia (BG)
[*A*], and prefrontal cortex (PFC) [*B*]. *Black dots* show
the time of rise, as measured by the time to half-peak.

improvement in selecting the correct response more closely matched the timing of PFC changes than striatum changes.

These results may reflect a relationship between the BG and PFC that is
similar to the relationship between the hippocampus and cortex, as suggested
by O'Reilly. As the animals learned specific stimulus-response associations,
these changes are quickly represented in the BG, which in turn, slowly trains
the PFC. In this case, the fast plasticity in the striatum (strong weight changes)
is better suited to the rapid formation of concrete rules, such as the associations between a specific cue and response. However, as noted earlier, fast

learning tends to be error-prone, and indeed, striatal neurons began predicting the forthcoming behavioral response early in learning, when that response was often wrong. By contrast, the smaller weight changes in the PFC may have allowed it to accumulate more evidence and arrive at the correct answer more slowly and judiciously. Interestingly, during this task, behavior more closely reflected the changes in the PFC, possibly due to the fact that the animals were not under enough pressure to change its behavior faster, choosing instead the more judicious path of following the PFC.

The faster learning-related changes in the striatum reported by Pasupathy and Miller (2005) are consistent with our hypothesis that there is stronger modulation of activity in the striatum than in the PFC during performance of these specific, concrete rules. But what about abstracted, generalized rules? Our model of fast BG plasticity versus slower PFC plasticity predicts the opposite, namely, that abstract rules should have a stronger effect on PFC activity than on BG activity because the slower PFC plasticity is more suited to this type of learning. A recent experiment by Muhammad et al. (2006) showed just that. Building on the work of Wallis et al. (2001), in this experiment, monkeys were trained to apply the abstract rules "same" and "different" to pairs of pictures. If the "same" rule was in effect, monkeys responded if the pictures were identical, whereas if the "different" rule was in effect, monkeys responded if the pictures were different. The rules were abstract because the monkeys were able to apply the rules to novel stimuli—stimuli for which there could be no pre-existing stimulus-response association. This is the definition of an abstract rule. Muhammad et al. (2006) recorded neural activity from the same PFC and striatal regions as Pasupathy and Miller (2005), and found that, in contrast to the specific-cue response associations, the abstract rules were reflected more strongly in PFC activity (more neurons with effects and larger effects) than in BG activity, the opposite of what Pasupathy and Miller (2005) reported for the specific cue-response associations.

In fact, this architecture (fast learning in more primitive, noncortical structures training the slower, more advanced, cortex) may be a general brain strategy; in addition to being suggested for the relationship between the hippocampus and cortex, it has also been proposed for the cerebellum and cortex (Houk and Wise, 1995). This makes sense: The first evolutionary pressure on our cortex-less ancestors was presumably toward faster learning, whereas only later did we add on a slower, more judicious and flexible cortex. These different styles of plasticity in the striatum versus PFC might also be suited to acquiring different types of information beyond the distinction between concrete and abstract discussed so far. This is illustrated in a recent proposal by Daw et al. (2005).

THE PREFRONTAL CORTEX AND STRIATUM: MODEL-BUILDING VERSUS "SNAPSHOTS"

Daw et al. (2005) proposed functional specializations for the PFC and BG (specifically, the striatum) that may be in line with our suggestions. They

suggested that the PFC builds models of an entire behavior—it retains information about the overall structure of the task, following the whole course of action from initial state to ultimate outcome. They liken this to a "tree" structure for a typical operant task: Behaviors begin in an initial state, with two or more possible response alternatives. Choosing one response leads to another state, with new response alternatives, and this process continues throughout the task, ultimately leading to a reward. The PFC is able to capture this entire "tree" structure, essentially providing the animal with an internal model of the task. By contrast, the striatum is believed to learn the task piecemeal, with each state's response alternatives individually captured and separate from the others. This "caching reinforcement learning" system retains information about which alternative is "better" in each state, but nothing about the overall structure of the task (i.e., the whole "tree").

This is believed to explain observations of tasks that use reinforcer devaluation. In such tasks, you change the value of the reward by saturating the animal on a given reward (e.g., overfeeding on chocolate if chocolate is a reward in that task). This has revealed two classes of behavior. Behaviors that are affected by reinforcer devaluation are considered goal-directed because changing the goal changes the behavior. As mentioned earlier, goal-directed behaviors depend on the PFC. By contrast, overlearned behaviors whose outcomes remain relatively constant can become habits, impervious to reinforcer devaluation. Because these behaviors are not affected by changing the goal, they seem to reflect control by a caching system in which the propensity for a given alternative in each situation is stored independently of information about past or future events (states). Habits have long been considered a specialization of the BG. Daw et al. (2005) proposed that there is arbitration between each system based on uncertainty; whichever system is most accurate is the one deployed to control behavior.

We believe that this maps well onto our notion of the fast, supervised, BG plasticity versus slow, more-Hebbian, PFC plasticity. Fast plasticity, such as the nearly bistable changes that Pasupathy and Miller (2005) observed in the striatum, would seem ideal for learning the reinforcement-related snapshots that capture the immediate circumstances and identify which alternative is preferable for a particular state. The slow plasticity in the PFC seems more suited for the linking in of additional information about past states that is needed to learn and retain an entire model of the task and thus predict future states.

The interactions of these systems might explain several aspects of goal-directed learning and habit formation. The initial learning of a complex operant task invariably begins with the establishment of a simple response immediately proximal to reward (i.e., a single state). Then, as the task becomes increasingly complex as more and more antecedents and qualifications (states and alternatives) are linked in, the PFC shows greater involvement. It facilitates this learning via its slower plasticity, allowing it to stitch together the relationships between the different states. This is useful because uncertainty about the

correct action in a given state adds up across many states in a complex task. Thus, in complex tasks, the ability of the reinforcement to control behavior would be lessened with the addition of more and more states. However, model-building in the PFC may provide the overarching infrastructure—the thread weaving between states—that facilitates learning of the entire course of action. This may also explain why, when complex behaviors are first learned, they are affected by reinforcer devaluation and susceptible to disruption by PFC damage. Many tasks will remain dependent on the PFC and the models it builds, especially those requiring flexibility (e.g., when the goal often changes or there are multiple goals to choose among), or when a strongly established behavior in one of the states (e.g., a habit) is incompatible with the course of action needed to obtain a specific goal. However, if a behavior, even a complex one, is unchanging, then all of the values of each alternative at each juncture are constant, and once these values are learned, control can revert to a piecemeal caching system in the BG. That is, the behavior becomes a "habit," and it frees up the more cognitive PFC model-building system for behaviors requiring the flexibility it provides.

Note that this suggests that slower plasticity in the PFC might sometimes support relatively fast learning on the behavioral level (i.e., faster than relying on the BG alone) because it is well suited to learning a complex task. This distinction is important, because thus far, we have been guilty of confusing learning on the neuronal level and learning on the behavioral level. Although it is true that small changes in synaptic weights might often lead to slow changes in behavior and vice versa, this is too simplistic. Certain tasks might be learned better and faster through the generalized, model-based learning seen in the PFC than through the strict, supervised learning observed in the striatum.

RECURSIVE PROCESSING AND BOOTSTRAPPING IN CORTICO-GANGLIA LOOPS

"Bootstrapping" is the process of building increasingly complex representations from simpler ones. The recursive nature of the anatomical loops between the BG and PFC may lend itself to this process. As described earlier, anatomical connections between the PFC and BG seem to suggest a closed loop—channels within the BG return outputs, via the thalamus, into the same cortical areas that gave rise to their initial cortical input. This recursive structure in the anatomy may allow for learned associations from one instance to be fed back through the loop for further processing and learning. In this manner, new experiences can be added onto previous ones, linking in more and more information to build a generalized representation. This may allow the bootstrapping of neural representations to increasing complexity, and with the slower learning in the PFC, greater abstractions.

A hallmark of human intelligence is the propensity for us to ground new concepts in familiar ones because it seems to ease our understanding of novel ideas. For example, we learn to multiply through serial addition and we begin

to understand quantum mechanisms through analogies to waves and particles. The recursive interactions between the BG and PFC may support this type of cognitive bootstrapping—initial, simple associations (or concrete rules) are made in the BG and fed back into the PFC. This feedback changes the representation of the original association in the PFC, helping to encode the concrete rule in both the BG and PFC. Additional concrete associations through different experiences can also be made and modified in a similar manner. The associative nature of the PFC will begin to bind across experiences, finding similarities in both the cortical inputs into the PFC as well as the looped inputs from the BG. This additional generalization is the basis for the formation of abstract rules based on the concrete rules that are first learned in the BG. As this process continues, new experiences begin to look "familiar" to the PFC, and a more generalized representation of a specific instance can be constructed. This generalized representation can now be looped through the BG to make reliable predictions of associations based on previously learned concrete rules.

Reward processing is a specific instance where recursive processing might provide the framework necessary for the observed neuronal behavior. As previously described, midbrain DA neurons respond to earlier and earlier events in a predictive chain leading to a reward. Both the frontal cortex and the striatum send projections into the midbrain DA neurons, possibly underlying their ability to bootstrap to early predictors of reward. However, although this is suggestive, it is still unknown whether these descending projections are critical for this behavior.

Additionally, the PFC-BG loops suggest an autoassociative type of network, similar to that seen in the CA3 of the hippocampus. The outputs looping back on the inputs allow the network to learn to complete (i.e., recall) previously learned patterns, given a degraded version or a subset of the original inputs (Hopfield, 1982). In the hippocampus, this network has been suggested to play a role in the formation of memories; however, BG-PFC loops are heavily influenced by DA inputs, and therefore may be more goal-oriented.

An intriguing feature of autoassociative networks is their ability to learn temporal sequences of patterns and thus make predictions. This feature relies on feedback of the activity pattern into the network with a temporal delay, allowing the next pattern in the sequence to arrive as the previous pattern is fed back, building an association between the two (Kleinfeld, 1986; Sompolinsky and Kanter, 1986).

The PFC-BG loops have two mechanisms by which to add this lag in feedback. One possibility is through the use of inhibitory synapses, which are known to have a slower time constant than excitatory ones. The "direct" pathway has two inhibitory synapses, the result being a net excitatory effect on the cortex via disinhibition of the thalamus, whereas the "indirect" one has three inhibitory synapses, making it net inhibitory. These two pathways are believed to exist in balance—activity in the indirect pathway countermands current processing in the direct loop. But why evolve a loop out of inhibitory synapses? First, it can prevent runaway excitation and thus allow greater control

over processing (Wong et al., 1986; Connors et al., 1988; Wells et al., 2000), but it is also possible that inhibitory synapses are used to slow the circulation of activity through the loops and allow for the binding of temporal sequences. Many inhibitory synapses are mediated by potassium channels with slow time courses (Couve et al., 2000). A second way to add lag to the recursion is through a memory buffer. The PFC is well known for this type of property; its neurons can sustain their activity to bridge short-term memory delays. This can act as a bridge for learning contingencies across several seconds, or even minutes. The introduction of lag into the recursive loop through either mechanism (or both) may be enough to tune the network for sequencing and prediction.

After training, a lagged autoassociative network that is given an input will produce, or predict, the next pattern in the sequence. This is a fundamentally important feature for producing goal-directed behaviors, especially as they typically extend over time. Experimental evidence for the role of the BG in sequencing and prediction comes from neurophysiological observations that striatal neural activity reflects forthcoming events in a behavioral task (Jog et al., 1999) and that lesions of the striatum can cause a deficit in producing learned sequences (Miyachi et al., 1997; Bailey and Mair, 2006).

SUMMARY: FRONTAL CORTICAL–BASAL GANGLIA LOOPS CONSTRUCT ABSTRACT RULES FOR COGNITIVE CONTROL

In this chapter, we have proposed that the learning of abstract rules occur through recursive loops between the PFC and BG. The learning of concrete rules, such as simple stimulus-response associations, is more a function of the BG, which—based on anatomical and physiological evidence—is specialized for the detection and storage of specific experiences that lead to reward. In contrast, abstract rules are better learned slowly, across many experiences, in the PFC. The recursive anatomical loops between these two areas suggest that the fast, error-prone learning in the BG can help train the slower, more reliable, frontal cortex. Bootstrapping from specific instances and concrete rules represented and stored in the BG, the PFC can construct abstract rules that are more concise, more predictive, and more broadly applicable; it can also build overarching models that capture an entire course of action. Note that we are not suggesting that there is serial learning between the BG and PFC; we are not suggesting that the BG first learns a task and then passes it to the PFC. Goal-directed learning instead depends on a highly interactive and iterative processing between these structures, working together and in parallel to acquire the goal-relevant information.

The result of this learning can be thought of as creating a "rulemap" in the PFC that is able to capture the relationships between the thoughts and actions necessary to successfully achieve one's goals in terms of which cortical pathways are needed (Miller and Cohen, 2001) [see Fig. 18–2]. The appropriate rulemap can be activated when cognitive control is needed: in situations in

which the mapping between sensory inputs, thoughts, and actions either is weakly established relative to other existing ones or is rapidly changing. Activation of the PFC rulemaps establishes top-down signals that feed back to most of the rest of the cortex, dynamically modulating information flow through the brain to best regulate important information and generate appropriate goal-directed thoughts and actions.

ACKNOWLEDGMENTS This work was supported by the National Institute of Mental Health, the National Institute of Neurological Disorders and Stroke, and the RIKEN-MIT Neuroscience Research Center. The authors thank M. Wicherski for helpful comments.

REFERENCES

Amaral DG (1986) Amygdalohippocampal and amygdalocortical projections in the primate brain. Advances in Experimental Medicine and Biology 203:3–17.

Amaral DG, Price JL (1984) Amygdalo-cortical projections in the monkey (*Macaca fascicularis*). Journal of Comparative Neurology 230:465–496.

Asaad WF, Rainer G, Miller EK (2000) Task-specific activity in the primate prefrontal cortex. Journal of Neurophysiology 84:451–459.

Bailey KR, Mair RG (2006) The role of striatum in initiation and execution of learned action sequences in rats. Journal of Neuroscience 26:1016–1025.

Barbas H, De Olmos J (1990) Projections from the amygdala to basoventral and mediodorsal prefrontal regions in the rhesus monkey. Journal of Comparative Neurology 300:549–571.

Barbas H, Henion TH, Dermon CR (1991) Diverse thalamic projections to the prefrontal cortex in the rhesus monkey. Journal of Comparative Neurology 313:65–94.

Barbas H, Pandya DN (1989) Architecture and intrinsic connections of the prefrontal cortex in the rhesus monkey. Journal of Comparative Neurology 286:353–375.

Calabresi P, Maj R, Pisani A, Mercuri NB, Bernardi G (1992) Long-term synaptic depression in the striatum: physiological and pharmacological characterization. Journal of Neuroscience 12:4224–4233.

Calabresi P, Saiardi A, Pisani A, Baik JH, Centonze D, Mercuri NB, Bernardi G, Borrelli E, Maj R (1997) Abnormal synaptic plasticity in the striatum of mice lacking dopamine D2 receptors. Journal of Neuroscience 17:4536–4544.

Connors B, Malenka R, Silva L (1988) Two inhibitory postsynaptic potentials, and GABAA and GABAB receptor-mediated responses in neocortex of the rat and cat. Journal of Physiology (London) 406:443–468.

Couve A, Moss SJ, Pangalos MN (2000) GABAB receptors: a new paradigm in G protein signaling. Molecular and Cellular Neuroscience 16:296–312.

Cronin-Golomb A, Corkin S, Growdon JH (1994) Impaired problem solving in Parkinson's disease: impact of a set-shifting deficit. Neuropsychologia 32:579–593.

Croxson PL, Johansen-Berg H, Behrens TEJ, Robson MD, Pinsk MA, Gross CG, Richter W, Richter MC, Kastner S, Rushworth MFS (2005) Quantitative investigation of connections of the prefrontal cortex in the human and macaque using probabilistic diffusion tractography. Journal of Neuroscience 25:8854–8866.

Dayan P, Abbott L (2001) Theoretical neuroscience: computational and mathematical modeling of neural systems. Cambridge: MIT Press.

Daw ND, Niv Y, Dayan P (2005) Uncertainty-based competition between the pre-frontal and dorsolateral striatal systems for behavioral control. Nature Neuroscience 8:1704–1711.

Divac I, Rosvold HE, Szwarcbart MK (1967) Behavioral effects of selective ablation of the caudate nucleus. Journal of Comparative and Physiological Psychology 63:184–190.

Donoghue JP, Herkenham M (1986) Neostriatal projections from individual cortical fields conform to histochemically distinct striatal compartments in the rat. Brain Research 365:397–403.

Eblen F, Graybiel A (1995) Highly restricted origin of prefrontal cortical inputs to striosomes in the macaque monkey. Journal of Neuroscience 15:5999–6013.

Flaherty AW, Graybiel AM (1991) Corticostriatal transformations in the primate soma-tosensory system: projections from physiologically mapped body-part representations. Journal of Neurophysiology 66:1249–1263.

Flaherty A, Graybiel A (1993) Output architecture of the primate putamen. Journal of Neuroscience 13:3222–3237.

Flaherty A, Graybiel A (1994) Input-output organization of the sensorimotor striatum in the squirrel monkey. Journal of Neuroscience 14:599–610.

Funahashi S, Bruce CJ, Goldman-Rakic PS (1989) Mnemonic coding of visual space in the monkey's dorsolateral prefrontal cortex. Journal of Neurophysiology 61:331–349.

Fuster JM (1973) Unit activity in prefrontal cortex during delayed-response perfor-mance: neuronal correlates of transient memory. Journal of Neurophysiology 36:61–78.

Fuster JM (1995) Memory in the cerebral cortex. Cambridge: MIT Press.

Fuster JM, Alexander GE (1971) Neuron activity related to short-term memory. Science 173:652–654.

Gerfen CR (1992) The neostriatal mosaic: multiple levels of compartmental organi-zation. Trends in Neurosciences 15:133–139.

Goldman PS, Rosvold HE (1972) The effects of selective caudate lesions in infant and juvenile rhesus monkeys. Brain Research 43:53–66.

Goldman-Rakic PS, Leranth C, Williams SM, Mons N, Geffard M (1989) Dopamine synaptic complex with pyramidal neurons in primate cerebral cortex. Proceedings of the National Academy of Sciences U S A 86:9015–9019.

Graybiel AM (2000) The basal ganglia. Current Biology 10:R509–R511.

Graybiel AM, Ragsdale CW Jr (1978) Histochemically distinct compartments in the striatum of humans, monkeys, and cats demonstrated by acetylthiocholinesterase staining. Proceedings of the National Academy of Sciences U S A 75:5723–5726.

Haier RJ, Jung RE, Yeo RA, Head K, Alkire MT (2004) Structural brain variation and general intelligence. Neuroimage 23:425–433.

Hertz J, Palmer R, Krogh A (1991) Introduction to the theory of neural computation. Redwood City, Calif.: Addison-Wesley Pub. Co.

Hopfield JJ (1982) Neural networks and physical systems with emergent collective com-putational abilities. Proceedings of the National Academy of Sciences U S A 79:2554–2558.

Houk JC, Wise SP (1995) Distributed modular architectures linking the basal ganglia, cerebellum, and cerebral cortex: their role in planning and controlling action. Ce-rebral Cortex 5:95–110.

Jog MS, Kubota Y, Connolly CI, Hillegaart V, Graybiel AM (1999) Building neural representations of habits. Science 286:1745–1749.

Kemp JM, Powell TP (1970) The cortico-striate projection in the monkey. Brain 93: 525–546.

Kemp JM, Powell TP (1971) The structure of the caudate nucleus of the cat: light and electron microscopy. Philosophical Transactions of the Royal Society of London B 262:383–401.

Kerr JND, Wickens JR (2001) Dopamine D-1/D-5 receptor activation is required for long-term potentiation in the rat neostriatum in vitro. Journal of Neurophysiology 85:117–124.

Kitai ST, Kocsis JD, Preston RJ, Sugimori M (1976) Monosynaptic inputs to caudate neurons identified by intracellular injection of horseradish peroxidase. Brain Research 109:601–606.

Kleinfeld D (1986) Sequential state generation by model neural networks. Proceedings of the National Academy of Science USA 83:9469–9473.

Lawrence AD, Hodges JR, Rosser AE, Kershaw A, French-Constant C, Rubinsztein DC, Robbins TW, Sahakian BJ (1998) Evidence for specific cognitive deficits in pre-clinical Huntington's disease. Brain 121:1329–1341.

Lynd-Balta E, Haber SN (1994) The organization of midbrain projections to the ventral striatum in the primate. Neuroscience 59:609–623.

Mansouri FA, Matsumoto K, Tanaka K (2006) Prefrontal cell activities related to monkeys' success and failure in adapting to rule changes in a Wisconsin Card Sorting Test analog. Journal of Neuroscience 26:2745–2756.

McClelland J, McNaughton B, O'Reilly R (1995) Why there are complementary learning systems in the hippocampus and neocortex: insights from the successes and failures of connectionist models of learning and memory. Psychological Review 102:419–457.

Middleton FA, Strick PL (1994) Anatomical evidence for cerebellar and basal ganglia involvement in higher cognitive function. Science 266:458–461.

Middleton FA, Strick PL (2000) Basal ganglia and cerebellar loops: motor and cognitive circuits. Brain Research Reviews 31:236–250.

Middleton FA, Strick PL (2002) Basal-ganglia 'projections' to the prefrontal cortex of the primate. Cerebral Cortex 12:926–935.

Miller EK (2000) The prefrontal cortex and cognitive control. Nature Reviews Neuroscience 1:59–65.

Miller EK, Cohen JD (2001) An integrative theory of prefrontal function. Annual Review of Neuroscience 24:167–202.

Miller EK, Erickson CA, Desimone R (1996) Neural mechanisms of visual working memory in prefrontal cortex of the macaque. Journal of Neuroscience 16:5154–5167.

Mink J (1996) The basal ganglia: focused selection and inhibition of competing motor programs. Progress in Neurobiology 50:381–425.

Miyachi S, Hikosaka O, Miyashita K, Karadi Z, Rand MK (1997) Differential roles of monkey striatum in learning of sequential hand movement. Experimental Brain Research 115:1–5.

Muhammad R, Wallis JD, Miller EK (2006) A comparison of abstract rules in the prefrontal cortex, premotor cortex, inferior temporal cortex, and striatum. Journal of Cognitive Neuroscience 18:974–989.

Nieder A, Freedman DJ, Miller EK (2002) Representation of the quantity of visual items in the primate prefrontal cortex. Science 297:1708–1711.

O'Doherty J, Dayan P, Schultz J, Deichmann R, Friston K, Dolan RJ (2004) Dissociable roles of ventral and dorsal striatum in instrumental conditioning. Science 16: 452–454.

O'Reilly RC, Munakata Y (2000) Computational explorations in cognitive neuroscience: understanding the mind. Cambridge: MIT Press.

Otani S, Blond O, Desce JM, Crepel F (1998) Dopamine facilitates long-term depression of glutamatergic transmission in rat prefrontal cortex. Neuroscience 85:669–676.

Padoa-Schioppa C, Assad JA (2006) Neurons in the orbitofrontal cortex encode economic value. Nature 41(7090):223–226.

Pandya DN, Barnes CL (1987) Architecture and connections of the frontal lobe. In: The frontal lobes revisited (Perecman E, ed.), pp 41–72. New York: IRBN Press.

Pandya DN, Yeterian EH (1990) The prefrontal cortex in relation to other cortical areas in rhesus monkey: architecture and connections. Progress in Brain Research 85:63–94.

Parasarathy H, Schall J, Graybiel A (1992) Distributed but convergent ordering of corticostriatal projections: analysis of the frontal eye field and the supplementary eye field in the macaque monkey. Journal of Neuroscience 12:4468–4488.

Parent A, Hazrati LN (1993) Anatomical aspects of information processing in primate basal ganglia. Trends in Neurosciences 16:111–116.

Pasupathy A, Miller EK (2005) Different time courses of learning-related activity in the prefrontal cortex and striatum. Nature 433:873–876.

Petrides M, Pandya DN (1999) Dorsolateral prefrontal cortex: comparative cytoarchitectonic analysis in the human and the macaque brain and corticocortical connection patterns. European Journal of Neuroscience 11:1011–1036.

Porrino LJ, Crane AM, Goldman-Rakic PS (1981) Direct and indirect pathways from the amygdala to the frontal lobe in rhesus monkeys. Journal of Comparative Neurology 198:121–136.

Pribram KH, Mishkin M, Rosvold HE, Kaplan SJ (1952) Effects on delayed-response performance of lesions of dorsolateral and ventromedial frontal cortex of baboons. Journal of Comparitive and Physiological Psychology. 45:565–575.

Rainer G, Rao SC, Miller EK (1999) Prospective coding for objects in the primate prefrontal cortex. Journal of Neuroscience 19:5493–5505.

Schultz W (1998) Predictive reward signal of dopamine neurons. Journal of Neurophysiology 80:1–27.

Schultz W, Apicella P, Ljungberg T (1993) Responses of monkey dopamine neurons to reward and conditioned stimuli during successive steps of learning a delayed response task. Journal of Neuroscience 13:900–913.

Schultz W, Apicella P, Scarnati E, Ljungberg T (1992) Neuronal activity in monkey ventral striatum related to the expectation of reward. Journal of Neuroscience 12: 4595–4610.

Schultz W, Dayan P, Montague PR (1997) A neural substrate of prediction and reward. Science 275:1593–1599.

Selemon L, Goldman-Rakic P (1988) Common cortical and subcortical targets of the dorsolateral prefrontal and posterior parietal cortices in the rhesus monkey: evidence for a distributed neural network subserving spatially guided behavior. Journal of Neuroscience 8:4049–4068.

Selemon LD, Goldman-Rakic (1985) Longitudinal topography and interdigitation of corticostriatal projections in the rhesus monkey. Journal of Neuroscience 5:776–794.

Sompolinsky H, Kanter II (1986) Temporal association in asymmetric neural networks. Physical Review Letters 57:2861–2864.

Taylor AE, Saint-Cyr JA, Lang AE (1986) Frontal lobe dysfunction in Parkinson's disease: the cortical focus of neostriatal outflow. Brain 109:845–883.

Thierry AM, Blanc G, Sobel A, Stinus L, Glowinski J (1973) Dopaminergic terminals in the rat cortex. Science 182:499–501.

Van Hoesen GW, Yeterian EH, Lavizzo-Mourey R (1981) Widespread corticostriate projections from temporal cortex of the rhesus monkey. Journal of Comparative Neurology 199:205–219.

Wallis JD, Miller EK (2003) Neuronal activity in the primate dorsolateral and orbital prefrontal cortex during performance of a reward preference task. European Journal of Neuroscience 18:2069–2081.

Wallis JD, Anderson KC, Miller EK (2001) Single neurons in the prefrontal cortex encode abstract rules. Nature 411:953–956.

Watanabe M (1996) Reward expectancy in primate prefrontal neurons. Nature 382: 629–632.

Wells JE, Porter JT, Agmon A (2000) GABAergic inhibition suppresses paroxysmal network activity in the neonatal rodent hippocampus and neocortex. Journal of Neuroscience 20:8822–8830.

White IM, Wise SP (1999) Rule-dependent neuronal activity in the prefrontal cortex. Experimental Brain Research 126:315–335.

Wong RK, Traub RD, Miles R (1986) Cellular basis of neuronal synchrony in epilepsy. Advances in Neurology 44:583–592.

Yeterian EH, Van Hoesen GW (1978) Cortico-striate projections in the rhesus monkey: the organization of certain cortico-caudate connections. Brain Research 139:43–63.

19

The Development of Rule Use in Childhood

Philip David Zelazo

Rule use unfolds in time; that much is obvious. It takes time to turn an intention into an action. It takes time to switch between task sets. What may be less obvious is that the capacity for rule use is itself continually in flux: It improves gradually, albeit in a saltatory fashion, during childhood and adolescence, and it deteriorates in the same way—gradually, and then suddenly—during senescence. These changes mirror the development of prefrontal cortex (PFC), and developmental investigations of rule use therefore provide an opportunity not only to understand rule use in an additional temporal dimension, but also to examine the way in which rule use depends on underlying neural mechanisms.

In developmental cognitive neuroscience, rule use is typically studied under the rubric of executive function—the processes underlying the conscious control of thought, action, and emotion. Indeed, according to one theory, the Cognitive Complexity and Control-revised (CCC-r) theory (Zelazo et al., 2003), conscious control is *always* mediated by rules—symbolic representations of means, ends, relations between means and ends, and the contexts in which these relations obtain. This theory, which has its origins in the work of Vygotsky (e.g., 1934/1986) and Luria (e.g., 1961), holds that the development of conscious control in childhood consists mainly of age-related increases in the complexity of the rule systems that children are able to formulate and maintain in working memory. Together with a number of related proposals (e.g., Zelazo and Müller, 2002; Zelazo, 2004; Bunge and Zelazo, 2006; Zelazo and Cunningham, 2007), CCC-r theory provides a comprehensive framework that addresses not only rule use and its development, but also (1) the role of self-reflection in bringing about age-related increases in rule complexity (discussed in terms of the "levels of consciousness" model), and (2) the way in which the development of rule use depends on the development of neural systems involving specific regions of PFC. Empirical support for this theory is reviewed in detail elsewhere (e.g., Zelazo et al., 2003). This chapter summarizes the theory, provides examples to illustrate key claims, and highlights several predictions for future research.

COGNITIVE COMPLEXITY AND CONTROL-REVISED THEORY

The CCC-r theory was initially designed to account for behavioral data showing that, with age, children are able to use increasingly complex representations to guide their actions. In infancy, the use of representations to guide behavior has been examined using search tasks, such as "delayed response" (Hunter, 1917) and "A-not-B" (Piaget, 1952). In a typical "A-not-B" task, for example, infants watch as an object is conspicuously placed at one of two or more hiding locations (i.e., at location A versus location B). After a delay, the infants are allowed to search for the object. This is repeated a number of times, with the object being hidden at location A in each trial. Then, in the crucial switch trial, infants watch as the object is hidden conspicuously at location B. Nine-month-old infants often search incorrectly (and perseveratively) at location A in this trial—evidently failing to keep a representation of the object at its current location (i.e., the goal) in mind and use it to guide search. Instead, their behavior seems to be determined by their prior experience of reaching to the A location—it seems to be determined by the stimulus-reward association established during performance of the A trials. Older infants are more likely to search correctly (see Marcovitch and Zelazo, 1999, for a meta-analysis).

Beyond infancy, conscious control may also be studied by providing children with various types of verbal instruction and examining the circumstances in which they can follow these instructions—the so-called "rule use paradigm" pioneered by Luria. For example, Luria (e.g., 1959) reported that 2-year-olds often failed to obey a single, conditional rule (e.g., "When the light flashes, you will press the ball" Luria, 1959). Younger 2-year-olds simply ignored the conditional prerequisite of the rule and acted immediately. Older 2-year-olds, in contrast, successfully refrained from responding until the first presentation of the light, although many of them then proceeded to respond indiscriminately. Following a single rule involves keeping in mind a representation of a conditionally specified response (i.e., a relation between a stimulus and a response), and considering this relation relative to a goal (e.g., the goal of pleasing the experimenter). Whereas 1-year-old infants are able to keep a simple goal in mind, 2-year-olds are also able to represent a conditionally specified means for obtaining that goal.

Following Luria's seminal work on the subject (see Zelazo and Jacques, 1996, for a review), Zelazo and Reznick (1991) investigated the development of rule use in 2.5- to 3-year-olds using a card sorting task in which children were presented with not just one, but two ad hoc rules (e.g., "If it's something found inside the house, then put it here. If it's something found outside the house, then put it there."), and then were asked to use these rules to separate a series of 10 test cards. Target cards were affixed to each of two sorting trays—for example, a sofa on one tray and a swing set on the other. Children were told the rules, and then the experimenter provided a demonstration, sorting one test card according to each rule. Then, in each test trial, children were shown a test card (e.g., a refrigerator), told, "Here's a refrigerator," and then asked,

"Where does this go?" The younger children often erred, despite possessing knowledge about the cards, whereas 3-year-olds performed well. Knowledge about the cards was demonstrated by correct responses to direct questions: "Here's a refrigerator. Does it go inside the house or outside the house?" Analyses of children's errors revealed a tendency to repeat responses: Children rarely put all of the cards into the same box, but when they made an error, it usually involved putting a card into the box in which they had put a card in the previous trial (Zelazo et al., 1995). These results suggest that 2.5-year-olds understood the task and the rules, and actually started to use the rules, but had difficulty keeping two rules in mind and using them contrastively.

By approximately 3 years of age, most children switched flexibly between the two rules; they seemed to appreciate the need to consider carefully which of the two antecedent conditions was satisfied. Because successful responding was underdetermined by the nonlinguistic aspects of the task (e.g., the perceptual similarity of the exemplars), rule use in this task implies that children were representing the rules, keeping them in mind, and using them to govern their behavior. (In fact, when children were given the same target and test cards and simply told to put the test cards with the ones they go with, 3-year-olds failed to create the categories spontaneously). Three-year-olds still have difficulty using more complex rules, however.

Limitations on 3-year-olds' rule use have been investigated using the Dimensional Change Card Sort (DCCS) [see Fig. 19–1; see color insert], in which children are shown two target cards (e.g., a blue rabbit and a red boat) and asked to sort a series of bivalent test cards (e.g., red rabbits and blue boats), first according to one dimension (e.g., color), and then according to the other dimension (e.g., shape). Regardless of which dimension is presented first, the majority of typically developing 3-year-olds perseverate during the post-switch phase, continuing to sort test cards by the first dimension (e.g., Zelazo et al., 2003). Moreover, they do this despite being told the new rules in every trial, despite having sorted cards by the new dimension on other occasions, and despite correctly answering questions about the post-switch rules (e.g., "Where do the rabbits go in the shape game?"). They also do this despite being able, at this age, to keep four ad hoc rules in mind. In contrast, by 5 years of age, most children switch immediately on the DCCS when instructed to do so. Like adults, they seem to recognize immediately that they know two ways of sorting the cards: "If I'm playing the color game, and if it's a red rabbit, then it goes here..."). Despite this accomplishment, however, the ability to switch rapidly between bivalent pairs of rules continues to improve beyond 5 years of age (Frye et al. [experiment 3], 1995; Cepeda et al., 2001; Zelazo et al., 2004; Crone et al., 2006).

According to the CCC-r theory, the age-related improvements in rule use illustrated by these examples are brought about by developmental changes in the complexity of the representations that children are able to formulate and use, as well as increases in the proficiency of using rules at a particular level of complexity. Toward the end of the first year of life, infants acquire the ability

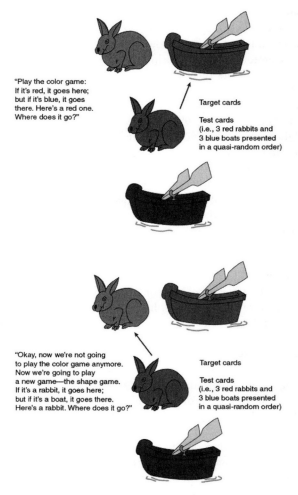

"Play the color game:
If it's red, it goes here;
but if it's blue, it goes
there. Here's a red one.
Where does it go?"

Target cards

Test cards
(i.e., 3 red rabbits and
3 blue boats presented
in a quasi-random order)

"Okay, now we're not going
to play the color game anymore.
Now we're going to play
a new game—the shape game.
If it's a rabbit, it goes here;
but if it's a boat, it goes there.
Here's a rabbit. Where does it go?"

Target cards

Test cards
(i.e., 3 red rabbits and
3 blue boats presented
in a quasi-random order)

Figure 19–1 Sample target and test cards in the standard version of the Dimensional Change Card Sort (DCCS). (Reprinted with permission from Zelazo, *Nature Protocols*, 1, 297–301. Nature Publishing Group, 2006).

to keep a goal in working memory and use it to guide their response, even when there is interference from prepotent stimulus-response associations, as in the "A-not-B" task. During the second year, children become able to represent a conditionally specified response (i.e., a single rule, considered against the background of a goal kept in mind). By approximately 3 years of age, children are able to represent a pair of rules and consider them contrastively.

It is not until approximately age 4 years that most children are able to formulate a hierarchical system of rules that allows them to select among bivalent rules. Subsequent development involves increases in the proficiency of using complex systems of rules—increases in the speed and efficiency with which children can navigate through complex hierarchies of rules and foreground appropriate information.

The tree diagrams in Figure 19–2 illustrate rules at different levels of complexity, and show how more complex hierarchal systems of rules can be established by the formulation of higher-order rules for selecting among rules. Two-year-old children are able to formulate a rule, such as rule A in Figure 19–2A, which indicates that response 1 (r_1) should follow stimulus 1 (s_1). However, to switch flexibly between two univalent stimulus-response associations—rules in which each stimulus is uniquely associated with a different response, such as rules A and B in Figure 19–2B—a higher-order rule, such as rule E, is required. Rule E is used to select rule A or B, depending on which antecedent conditions are satisfied. Figure 19–2C shows two incompatible pairs of bivalent rules, in

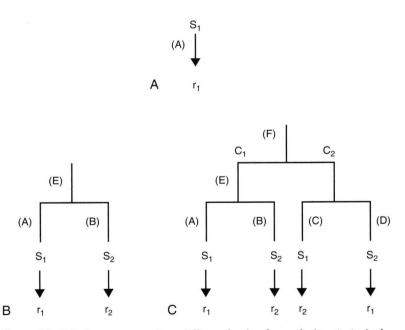

Figure 19–2 Rule systems at three different levels of complexity. A. A single, univalent rule (rule A) linking a stimulus to a response. B. A pair of univalent rules (rules A and B), and a higher-order rule (rule E) for selecting between them. C. A hierarchical system of rules involving two pairs of bivalent rules (rules A and B versus rules C and D) and a higher-order rule (rule F) for selecting between them. s_1 and s_2, stimuli; r_1 and r_2, responses; c_1 and c_2, contexts or task sets.

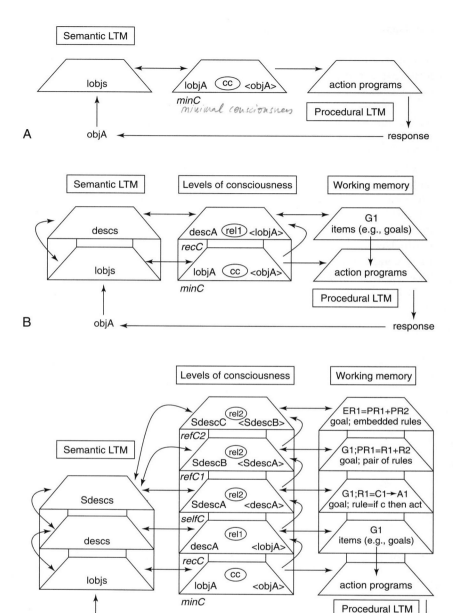

Figure 19–3 The implications of reflection (levels of consciousness) for rule use. *A.* Automatic action on the basis of unreflective consciousness (minC). An object in the environment (objA) triggers an intentional representation of that object (IobjA) in semantic long-term memory (LTM); this IobjA, which is causally connected (cc) to a bracketed objA, becomes the content of consciousness (referred to at this level as "minimal consciousness") [minC]. *B.* Action on the basis of one degree of reflection.

which the same stimuli are linked to different responses in different rules (e.g., s_1 in rule A versus C). These incompatible rule pairs may be referred to as "task sets," or ways of construing a set of stimuli (e.g., in terms of different dimensions). When using one task set (involving rules C and D), one has to ignore interference from any tendency to use the competing task set (involving rules A and B) instead. To do so, one has to formulate a still higher-order rule (rule F) that can be used to select the discrimination between rules A and B, as opposed to the discrimination between rules C and D. This higher-order rule makes reference to setting conditions or contexts (c_1 and c_2) that condition the selection of lower-order rules, and that would be taken for granted in the absence of a higher-order rule.

According to the theory, these increases in the complexity of children's rule systems are made possible by age-related increases in the highest degree of conscious reflection (or "level of consciousness") [Zelazo, 2004] that children can muster in response to situational demands. Reflection on rules formulated at one level of complexity is required to formulate higher-order rules that control the selection and application of these rules. Rather than taking rules for granted and simply assessing whether their antecedent conditions are satisfied, reflection involves making those rules themselves an object of consideration and considering them in contradistinction to other rules at the same level of complexity. The top-down selection of certain rules within a complex system of rules then results in the goal-directed amplification and diminution of attention to potential influences on thought (inferences) and action when multiple possible influences are present. This, in turn, allows for greater cognitive flexibility in situations where behavior might otherwise be determined by the bottom-up activation of rules that have been primed through previous experience.

Figure 19–3 contrasts three cases in which action is based on different levels of consciousness. In Figure 19–3*A*, action occurs in the absence of any reflection at all—it occurs on the basis of what is referred to as "minimal consciousness"

After minC processing of objA, the contents of minC are then fed back into minC via a re-entrant feedback process, producing a new, more reflective level of consciousness referred to as "recursive consciousness" (recC). The contents of recC can be related (rel1) in consciousness to a corresponding description (descA), or label, which can then be decoupled from the experience, labeled, and deposited into working memory, where it can serve as a goal (G1) to trigger an action program in a top-down fashion from procedural LTM. *C.* Subsequent (higher) levels of consciousness, including self-consciousness (selfC), reflective consciousness 1 (refC1), and reflective consciousness 2 (refC2). Each level of consciousness allows for the formulation and maintenance in working memory of more complex systems of rules. descs, descriptions; Iobjs, intentional objects; Sdescs, self-descriptions; ER1, system of embedded rules; PR, pair of rules; R, rule; C, condition; A, action. (Reprinted with permission from Zelazo, *Trends in Cognitive Sciences*, 8, 12–17. Copyright Elsevier, 2004).

(minC). An object in the environment (objA) triggers a salient, low-resolution "description" from semantic long-term memory. This description ("intentional object") [IobjA] then becomes an intentional object of minC, and it automatically triggers the most strongly associated action program in procedural long-term memory or elicits a stored stimulus-reward association. A telephone, for example, might be experienced by a minC infant as "suckable thing," and this description might trigger the stereotypical motor schema of sucking. In another example, a particular hiding location may have been associated with an interesting activity (e.g., a hiding event) or a reward (e.g., retrieving an object), and so, when seen, may elicit reaching toward that location.

In Figure 19–3*B*, action is based on one degree of reflection, resulting in a higher level of consciousness called "recursive consciousness" (recC). Now when objA triggers IobjA and becomes the content of minC, instead of triggering an associated action program directly, IobjA is fed back into minC (at a subsequent moment), where it can be related to a label (descA) from semantic long-term memory. This descA can then be decoupled from the minC experience, labeled, and deposited in long-term memory (where it provides a potentially enduring trace of the experience) and into working memory, where it can serve as a goal (G1) that triggers an action program, even in the absence of objA, and even if IobjA would otherwise trigger a different action program. For example, when presented with a telephone, a toddler operating at this level of consciousness may activate a specific semantic association and put the telephone to his or her ear (functional play) instead of putting the telephone in his or her mouth (a generic, stereotypical response). In the "A-not-B" task, the toddler may respond on the basis of a representation (in working memory) of the object at its current B location and avoid responding on the basis of an acquired tendency to reach toward location A. The toddler responds *mediately* to the decoupled label in working memory rather than *immediately* to a superficial gloss of the situation. This reflective mediation of responding has consequences not only for action but also for recollection. In the absence of reflection, the contents of minC are continually replaced by new intero- and exteroceptor stimulation, and no symbolic trace of the experience is available for subsequent recollection; the experience is exclusively present-oriented, moment-by-moment.

Figure 19–3*C* shows that more deliberate action occurs in response to a more carefully considered construal of the same situation, brought about by several degrees of reprocessing the situation. The higher level of consciousness depicted in Figure 19–3*C* allows for the formulation (and maintenance in working memory) of a more complex and more flexible system of rules or inferences. With each increase in level of consciousness, the same basic processes are recapitulated, but with distinct consequences for the quality of the subjective experience (richer because of the incorporation of new elements), the potential for episodic recollection (greater because information is processed a deeper level) [Craik and Lockhart, 1972], the complexity of children's explicit knowledge structures, and the possibility of the conscious control of thought,

action, and emotion. In general, however, as level of consciousness increases, reflective processing is interposed between a stimulus and a response, creating *psychological distance* from what Dewey (1931/1985) called the "exigencies of a situation."

Because levels of consciousness are hierarchically arranged, one normally operates on multiple levels of consciousness simultaneously—with processing at all levels focused on aspects of this same situation. In some cases, however, processing at different levels may be dissociated. For example, when we drive a car without full awareness because we are conducting a conversation, our driving is based on a relatively low level of consciousness (and our experience of driving is likely to be forgotten), but our conversation is likely to be based on a higher, more reflective level.

According to the CCC-r theory, language plays a key role in rule use. First, the formulation of rules is hypothesized to occur primarily, if not exclusively, in potentially silent, self-directed speech. People need to talk their way through rule use tasks—and more generally, through problems requiring conscious control. We often do not notice (or remember) that we are using private speech, but research on the effects of articulatory suppression is consistent with this claim (e.g., Emerson and Miyake, 2003). Second, the use of language, and in particular, labeling one's subjective experiences, helps to make those experiences an object of consideration at a higher level of consciousness (within developmental constraints on the highest level of consciousness that children are able to obtain). The effect of labeling on levels of consciousness and flexibility can be illustrated by work by Jacques et al. (2007), using the Flexible Item Selection Task. In each trial of the task, children are shown sets of three items designed so that one pair matches on one dimension, and a different pair matches on a different dimension (e.g., a small yellow teapot, a large yellow teapot, and a large yellow shoe). Children are first told to select one pair (i.e., selection 1), and then asked to select a different pair (i.e., selection 2). To respond correctly, children must represent the pivot item (i.e., the large yellow teapot) according to both dimensions. Four-year-olds generally perform well on selection 1, but poorly on selection 2, indicating inflexibility. Asking 4-year-old children to label their perspective on selection 1 (e.g., "Why do those two pictures go together?") makes it easier for them to adopt a different perspective on selection 2. This finding is consistent with the hypothesis that labeling their initial subjective perspective places children at a higher level of consciousness, from which it is possible to reflect on their initial perspective, and from which it is easier to access an alternative perspective on the same situation.

On this account, the reprocessing of information through levels of consciousness, the formulation of more complex rule systems, and the maintenance of these rule systems in working memory are believed to be mediated by thalamocortical circuits involving PFC, although different regions of PFC play different roles at different levels of complexity (and consciousness). Bunge (2004) and Bunge and Zelazo (2006) summarized evidence that PFC plays a

key role in rule use, and that different regions of PFC are involved in representing rules at different levels of complexity—from simple stimulus-reward associations (orbitofrontal cortex [OFC]), to sets of conditional rules (ventrolateral prefrontal cortex [VLPFC] and dorsolateral prefrontal cortex [DLPFC]), to explicit consideration of task sets (rostrolateral prefrontal cortex [RLPFC]) [see Fig. 19–4].

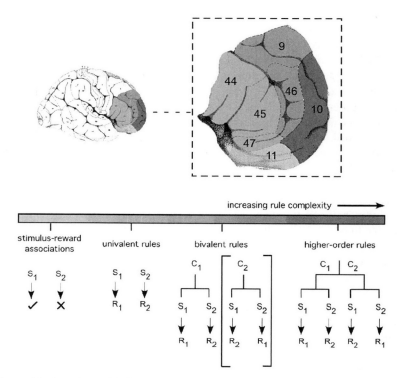

Figure 19–4 A hierarchical model of rule representation in lateral prefrontal cortex. *Top.* Lateral view of the human brain, with regions of prefrontal cortex identified by the Brodmann areas (BA) that comprise them: orbitofrontal cortex (BA 11), ventrolateral prefrontal cortex (BA 44, 45, 47), dorsolateral prefrontal cortex (BA 9, 46), and rostrolateral prefrontal cortex (BA 10). The prefrontal cortex regions are shown in various *shades of gray,* indicating which types of rules they represent. *Bottom.* Rule structures, with *darker shades of gray* indicating increasing levels of rule complexity. The formulation and maintenance in working memory of more complex rules depends on the reprocessing of information through a series of levels of consciousness, which in turn, depends on the recruitment of additional regions of prefrontal cortex into an increasingly complex hierarchy of prefrontal cortex activation. S, stimulus; check, reward; X, nonreward; R, response; C, context, or task set. Brackets indicate a bivalent rule that is currently being ignored. (Reprinted with permission from Bunge and Zelazo, *Current Directions in Psychological Science,* 15, 118–121. Copyright Blackwell Publishing, 2006.)

The function of PFC is proposed to be hierarchical in a way that corresponds roughly to the hierarchical complexity of rule use, as shown in Figure 19–4. As individuals engage in reflective processing, ascend through levels of consciousness, and formulate more complex rule systems, regions of lateral PFC are integrated into an increasingly elaborate hierarchy of PFC function via thalamocortical circuits. As the hierarchy unfolds, information is first processed via circuits connecting the thalamus and OFC. OFC generates learned approach-avoidance (stimulus-reward) rules. If these relatively unreflective processes do not provide an adequate response to the situation, then anterior cingulate cortex (ACC), serving as a performance monitor (e.g., Ridderinkhof et al., 2004), signals the need for further reflection, and the information is then reprocessed via circuits connecting the thalamus and VLPFC. Further processing—as required, for example, when prepotent response tendencies elicited by bivalent rules need to be ignored—occurs via circuits connecting the thalamus to DLPFC. Thalamocortical circuits involving RLPFC play a role in the explicit consideration of task sets at each level in the hierarchy. Iterations of this mechanism of reprocessing information underlie the ascent through levels of consciousness, with VLPFC, DLPFC, and RLPFC playing distinct roles in the representation and maintenance of rules in working memory.

As Bunge and Zelazo (2006) noted, developmental research suggests that the order of acquisition of rule types shown in Figure 19–4 corresponds to the order in which corresponding regions of PFC mature. The volume of gray matter reaches adult levels earliest in OFC, followed by VLPFC, and then by DLPFC (Giedd et al., 1999; Gogtay et al., 2004). Measures of cortical thickness suggest that DLPFC and RLPFC exhibit similar, slow rates of structural change (O'Donnell et al., 2005). With development, children are able to engage neural systems involving the hierarchical coordination of more regions of PFC—a hierarchical coordination that develops in a bottom-up fashion, with higher levels in the hierarchy operating on the products of lower levels through thalamocortical circuits.

IMPLICATIONS AND PREDICTIONS

Key aspects of this model have been captured in mathematical and computational models, leading to testable predictions that have since received empirical support; this material has been reviewed elsewhere (e.g., see Zelazo et al., 2003). This final section highlights implications that may be particularly relevant to the developmental cognitive neuroscience of rule use.

1. As children develop, they will be more likely to engage in reflective processing during challenging measures of rule use. This should result in increasing reliance on more anterior regions of PFC (i.e., frontalization) [see Rubia et al., 2000]. Consistent with this prediction, Lamm et al. (2006) used a high-density (128-channel) electroencephalogram to measure event-related potentials as children and

adolescents performed a "go/no-go" task, which involves a simple pair of univalent rules, and collected a number of independent measures of executive function. The source of the N2 component, an index of cognitive control measured on correct "go" trials, was more anterior in those children who performed well on the executive function tasks than it was in those children who performed poorly.

2. Reflective processing and the use of higher-order rules take time to occur, so the theory makes predictions about the time course of rule use and the consequences of requiring rapid responses. Response deadlines will interrupt the cycles of reprocessing involved in reflection and the formulation of higher-order rules, resulting in action based on lower levels of consciousness and less complex hierarchies of rules, as well as decreases in activation in anterior regions of lateral PFC. Older children and adults should look like younger children when required to respond quickly, resulting not only in poorer performance but also in characteristic errors (e.g., perseverative errors versus random errors) and relatively immature patterns of neural activation. Given that PFC-mediated reprocessing is effortful, manipulations such as divided attention would also be predicted to result in decreases in rule complexity as well as decreases in activation in anterior regions of lateral PFC.

3. Reflective processing and the use of higher-order rules are hypothesized to be mediated by language. In children, performance on measures of rule use is consistently found to be related to measures of language acquisition or skill (e.g., Jacques et al., 2006), and similar results would be expected for adults. In addition, articulatory suppression should have predictable effects on rule complexity and patterns of neural activation.

4. Different regions of PFC will be involved in working memory at different levels of rule complexity. Working memory has traditionally been linked to DLPFC function using a number of different neuropsychological methods, including functional magnetic resonance imaging and lesion studies (e.g., Braver et al., 1997; Smith and Jonides, 1999). Given the way in which working memory is typically assessed in human adults—as the ability to maintain and manipulate information to control responses across a series of trials in a single context—this evidence is consistent with the hypothesis that DLPFC plays a key role in following bivalent rules: using one rule while ignoring a competing alternative. That is, measures of working memory require participants to work on some information (e.g., trial-unique information) while ignoring other information (e.g., information from previous trials). The theory suggests, however, that other regions of PFC will play a key role in the maintenance in working memory of other types of rules. For example, VLPFC will play a fundamental role in the maintenance in working memory of univalent conditional rules (e.g., Bunge et al., 2003; Crone et al., 2006).

5. Finally, the model speaks to the distinction between relatively "hot," motivationally significant aspects of executive function more associated with OFC, and the more clearly cognitive, "cool" aspects more associated with lateral PFC (Miller and Cohen, 2001; Zelazo and Müller, 2002). In terms of the hierarchical model of lateral PFC function (Fig. 19–4), it is not that ventral regions, such as OFC, are exclusively involved in hot executive function, but rather that they remain more activated, even as a hierarchy of lateral PFC regions is elaborated. Simple rules for approaching versus avoiding concrete stimuli (the provenance of OFC) are more difficult to ignore in motivationally significant situations, so in effect, hot executive function involves increased bottom-up influences on PFC processing, with the result that hot executive function (versus cool executive function) requires relatively more attention to (and activation of) lower levels in rule hierarchies—discriminations at that level become more salient. Thus, this model views hot-cool as a continuum that is correlated with the degree of reflection and rule complexity made possible by the reprocessing of information in lateral PFC.

CONCLUSION

The development of rule use in childhood follows a protracted course that mirrors the slow development of PFC. In the account summarized here, age-related improvements in rule use are brought about via increases in the complexity of the rule systems that children are able to formulate and maintain in working memory. These increases in rule complexity, in turn, are made possible by increases in the highest level of consciousness that children are able to muster. The need for reprocessing rules is signaled by ACC activation, indicating that OFC-mediated stimulus-reward rules are inadequate in the current situation. ACC recruits more lateral areas of PFC associated with higher levels of consciousness and the formulation (and maintenance in working memory) of increasingly complex rule hierarchies. More complex rule systems allow for more flexible selection among competing task sets, and improvements in the ability to ignore irrelevant information. As outlined here, research on rule use has the potential to shed light on fundamental topics, such as the role of consciousness in the development of cognitive control.

ACKNOWLEDGMENTS The preparation of this chapter was supported in part by a grant from NSERC of Canada. The author thanks Silvia Bunge for providing very helpful comments on an earlier draft of this manuscript.

REFERENCES

Braver TS, Cohen JD, Nystron LE, Jonides J, Smith EE, Noll DC (1997) A parametric study of prefrontal cortex involvement in human working memory. Neuroimage 5:49–62.

Bunge SA (2004) How we use rules to select actions: a review of evidence from cognitive neuroscience. Cognitive, Affective, and Behavioral Neuroscience 4:564–579.

Bunge SA, Kahn I, Wallis JD, Miller EK, Wagner AD (2003) Neural circuits subserving the retrieval and maintenance of abstract rules. Journal of Neurophysiology 90: 3419–3428.

Bunge SA, Zelazo PD (2006) A brain-based account of the development of rule use in childhood. Current Directions in Psychological Science 15:118–121.

Cepeda NJ, Kramer AF, Gonzalez de Sather JCM (2001) Changes in executive control across the life-span: examination of task switching performance. Developmental Psychology 37:715–730.

Craik F, Lockhart R (1972) Levels of processing: a framework for memory research. Journal of Verbal Learning and Verbal Behavior 11:671–684.

Crone EA, Bunge SA, Van der Molen MW, Ridderinkhof KR (2006) Switching between tasks and responses: a developmental study. Developmental Science 9:278–287.

Crone EA, Wendelken C, Donohue SE, Bunge SA (2006) Neural evidence for dissociable components of task switching. Cerebral Cortex 16:475–486.

Dewey J (1985) Context and thought. In: John Dewey: the later works 1925–1953, 1931–1932 (Boydston JA, Sharpe A, eds.), pp 3–21, volume 6. Carbondale, IL: Southern Illinois University Press (original work published in 1931).

Emerson MJ, Miyake A (2003) The role of inner speech in task switching: a dual-task investigation. Journal of Memory and Language 48:148–168.

Frye D Zelazo PD, Palfai T (1995) Theory of mind and rule-based reasoning. Cognitive Development 10:483–527.

Giedd JN, Blumenthal J, Jeffries NO, Castellanos FX, Liu H, Zijdenbos A, Paus T, Evans AC, Rapoport JL (1999) Brain development during childhood and adolescence: a longitudinal MRI study. Nature Neuroscience 2:861–863.

Gogtay N, Giedd JN, Lusk L, Hayashi KM, Greenstein D, Vaituzis AC, Nugent TF III, Hunter WS (1917) Delayed reaction in a child. Psychological Review 24:74–87.

Jacques S, Zelazo PD, Lourenco SF, Sutherland AE (2007) The roles of labeling and abstraction in the development of cognitive flexibility. (Manuscript under review)

Lamm C, Zelazo PD, Lewis MD (2006) Neural correlates of cognitive control in childhood and adolescence: disentangling the contributions of age and executive function. Neuropsychologia 44:2139–2148.

Luria AR (1959) The directive function of speech in development and dissolution, Part I: Development of the directive function of speech in early childhood. Word 15: 341–352.

Luria AR (1961) Speech and the regulation of behaviour. London: Pergamon Press.

Marcovitch S, Zelazo PD (1999) The A-not-B error: results from a logistic meta-analysis. Child Development 70:1297–1313.

Miller EK, Cohen JD (2001) An integrative theory of prefrontal cortex function. Annual Review of Neuroscience 24:167–202.

O'Donnell S, Noseworthy MD, Levine B, Dennis M (2005) Cortical thickness of the frontopolar area in typically developing children and adolescents. Neuroimage 24: 948–954.

Piaget J (1952) The construction of reality in the child (Cook M, trans.) New York: Basic Books.

Ridderinkhof KR, Ullsperger M, Crone EA, Nieuwenhuis S (2004) The role of the medial frontal cortex in cognitive control. Science 306:443–447.

Rubia K, Overmeyer S, Taylor E, Brammer M, Williams SCR, Simmons A, Andrew C, Bullmore ET (2000) Functional frontalisation with age: mapping neurodevelopmental trajectories with fMRI. Neuroscience and Biobehavioral Reviews 24:13–19.

Smith EE, Jonides J (March 1999) Storage and executive processes in the frontal lobe. Science 283:1657–1661.

Vygotsky LS (1986) Thought and language (Kozulin A, ed.). Cambridge: MIT Press (original work published in 1934).

Zelazo PD (2004) The development of conscious control in childhood. Trends in Cognitive Sciences 8:12–17.

Zelazo PD, Craik FIM, Booth L (2004) Executive function across the life span. Acta Psychologica 115:167–184.

Zelazo PD, Cunningham W (2007) Executive function: mechanisms underlying emotion regulation. In: Handbook of emotion regulation (Gross J, ed.), pp 135–158. New York: Guilford.

Zelazo PD, Jacques S (1997) Children's rule use: representation reflection and cognitive control. Annals of Child Development 12:119–176.

Zelazo PD, Müller U (2002) Executive functions in typical and atypical development. In: Handbook of childhood cognitive development (Goswami U, ed.), pp 445–469. Oxford: Blackwell.

Zelazo PD, Müller U, Frye D, Marcovitch S (2003) The development of executive function in early childhood. Monographs of the Society for Research on Child Development 68:vii-137.

Zelazo PD, Reznick JS (1991) Age related asynchrony of knowledge and action. Child Development 62:719–735.

Zelazo PD, Reznick JS, Piñon DE (1995) Response control and the execution of verbal rules. Developmental Psychology 31:508–517.

Index

Abstract information encoding, 38–40, 40t
Abstraction. *See also* Categorization; Visual
    categorization
  prefrontal topography and, 107, 108f,
    119–123, 121f
  theories of, 107–111
  varying levels of, and rule use, 113–119
Abstraction of rules
  encoding in prefrontal-associated regions,
    31–37, 33–36f
  future research needs, 37, 40–41
  hippocampal processing and, 337, 355
  prefrontal cortex and, 24–25, 30, 31t,
    286–287, 302
  prefrontal cortex neuronal representation
    of, 27–31, 30f, 31t
  relational memory and, 338
  species comparisons of, 25–27
  stimulus-response associations compared
    to, 23, 37–38
  utility of, 23–24, 39–40
Abstract mental representation, 107–123
  lateral prefrontal cortex in, 107, 111–118,
    116f, 120f
  prefrontal topography and, 107, 108f,
    119–123, 121f
  process-based vs. representation-based
    organization in, 121–123
  theories of, 107–111
Abstract response strategies, 81–102
  adaptive advantage of, 100–102
  comparison of studies of, 96–99
  description of, 82
  repeat-stay/change-shift strategy studies
    conditional motor learning and,
      83–86, 84f
    physiology of, 86–95, 87f, 89–91f,
      93–94f
  vs. rule encoding, 95–96, 96f
Abstract rules. *See also* Abstraction of rules
  goal-directed behavior and, 419–420, 428
  prefrontal cortex–basal ganglia
    interactions and, 428–431, 435
  prefrontal cortex and, 420–424, 421f, 423f

ACC. *See* Cingulate cortex, anterior (ACC)
Action effects vs. action outcomes, 272
Action goals, 256, 266, 267–268, 277, 278f.
    See also Goal-response associations
Action knowledge, 368–369, 382–383. *See
    also* Knowledge-for-action
Action outcome associations, anterior
    cingulate and, 145–148, 146f,
    147f, 151
Action-relevant declarative memory,
    365–366, 368–370, 381–383
Action representation
  vs. function knowledge, 49–50, 50f
  long-term storage
    imagery vs. semantic retrieval and,
      49–51, 50f
    parietal cortex in, 49, 52
    posterior middle temporal gyrus and,
      45–50, 46f, 48f, 50f
    premotor cortex and, 49–50, 51–52, 51f
    ventrolateral prefrontal cortex in,
      45–46, 46f
  retrieval, selection, and maintenance
    of rules
    mid-dorsolateral prefrontal cortex in,
      53, 57–61, 59f, 60f
    ventrolateral prefrontal cortex in,
      52–57, 55f, 56f, 58–61, 60f
Action selection, 129–151. *See also* Decision-
    making
  action outcome associations and,
    145–148, 146f, 147f
  action values and, 148–150, 149f, 151f
  attention and stimulus selection and,
    135–139, 137f, 139f
  changing between rules and, 129,
    140–145, 141f, 142f, 143f, 151
  dorsomedial frontal cortex and
    anterior cingulate cortex, 129, 130f,
      144–150, 147f, 149f, 151, 151f
    pre-supplementary motor area,
      129, 130f, 140–144, 141f, 142f,
      143f, 151
  intentional control of, 256, 266–268, 277

457

Action selection (*continued*)
    interface with motor planning, 268–271,
        269f, 271f
    internally/externally-guided, 267–268
    strategies and, 139–140
    ventrolateral prefrontal cortex and, 129,
        130f, 131–135, 134f
Action sequencing, pre-supplementary
    motor area and, 143–144, 143f
Action values, anterior cingulate and,
    148–150, 149f
Active maintenance, dopamine and,
    313–315
Adaptation to changing task demands,
    211–216
Advance-target preparation study
    congruent vs. incongruent, 268–269, 269f
    participant strategies, 270–271, 271f
aIFG. *See* Frontal gyrus, anterior inferior
    (aIFG)
Allocentric cues, 287
Amnesia, hippocampal function and,
    346–347
Amygdala
    anterior cingulate connections of,
        150, 151f
    dopaminergic modulation in, 302, 303
    prefrontal connections of, 134f, 135
    in reversal learning, 289–290, 291
Anagrams, 116–117, 118f
Anatomical connectivity, 207, 209, 210, 211
Animal models. *See also* Monkeys; Primates,
    non-human
    in abstract rule use studies, 25–27
    in hippocampal function studies,
        347–350, 348f, 349f
    in switch-cost investigations, 246, 250
Animals
    abstract rule use in, 25–27
    categorization by, 392–393
Anterior cingulate cortex. *See* Cingulate
    cortex, anterior (ACC)
Antipsychotics, atypical, 297
APF. *See* Prefrontal cortex, anterior (APF)
Apraxia, 52, 367, 369
Arcuate sulcus, 12
Arm movement. *See* Reaching movement
Artificial neural networks, 428
Associations. *See also* Mappings
    action outcome, 145–148, 146f, 147f, 151
    goal-response, 266, 268, 277. *See also*
        Action goals; Intentional control
    object-outcome, 288

stimulus-response, 23, 37–38, 426.
    See also Concrete rules
stimulus-reward, 38. *See also* Reversal
    learning
Associative learning, conditional. *See*
    Conditional associative responses
Attention
    in conditional rule learning, 135–139,
        137f, 139f
    in extracting abstract ideas, 109, 110
    selective
        in abstraction, 109, 110, 122–123
        event-related optical signal studies,
            205–206
        executive function and, 204
        reciprocal inhibition and, 211
Attentional control of action selection, 256,
    266–268, 277
Attentional selection, 102, 286
Attentional-set shifting
    behavioral considerations, 284–285
    lateral prefrontal cortex and, 283,
        285–287, 302
    neuromodulation of, 302–303
        caudate dopamine and, 297–299, 298f,
            301–303
        prefrontal dopamine and, 291–295,
            292f, 302–303
        serotonin and, 295–297, 296f
    neuronal networks in, 285–287
    Parkinson's disease and, 318
Attention sets
    acquisition of, dopamine and, 293
    definition of, 67
    maintenance of, 286
    tonic top-down vs. phasic bottom-up
        signals and, 77–78
Auditory sensory memory, 204–205
Autoassociative networks, 434–435
Aversive signal processing, 301
Axons, optical properties of, 199

Basal ganglia. *See also specific structures,*
    e.g., Striatum
    anatomical connectivity of, 424–426,
        425f, 434–435
    concrete rules and, 424–426
    dopaminergic teaching signals in,
        426–427, 434
    plasticity in, 427–431, 429f, 430f,
        432–433
    prefrontal cortex relationships of,
        428–431

in bootstrapping, 433–436
in model-building, 431–433
Behavior
    goal-directed
        abstraction and, 419–420, 428
        of lagged autoassociative networks in
            production, 435
        in model-building, 431–433
        prefrontal cortex properties and,
            422–424
        of top-down orchestration, 419–420
    motor. *See* Motor behavior
    stimulus-bound, 297, 300
Behavioral flexibility. *See* Attentional-set
    shifting; Reversal learning
Behavioral preparation effect, 71–73, 72f
Behavioral switch costs. *See* Switch costs
Behaviorism, influence of, 81
Bias signals, 422
Bicuculline, 16
Bidimensional task cues, 186–187
Birds, abstract rule use in, 25, 26
Birefringence, 199
Blood-oxygen level–dependent (BOLD)
    fMRI
        event-related optical signal validation by,
            202, 203
        preparation interval analysis by, 259, 260f
        switch cost analysis by, 258
Bootstrapping in cortico-ganglia loops, 420,
    433–436
Bottom-up processing, 419
Brain imaging. *See* Imaging methods
Broca's speech area, 4, 268
Brodmann areas (BA)
    topography of, 108f
    BA 4, 161
    BA 6, 17, 49–50, 50f, 51f, 52, 60f, 72, 73f,
        129, 161, 179
    BA 6 + 8, 114
    BA 6/8/9, 88
    BA 6/8A, 12, 13f, 14, 15f, 19
    BA 6/44, 51
    BA 7, 60f
    BA 8, 57, 69, 70f
    BA 9, 58, 59f, 60, 179, 210, 450f
    BA 9/46, 12, 13f, 15f, 16, 17, 30, 57, 108
    BA 10, 15f, 61, 69, 70f, 73f, 108, 112,
        114, 450f
    BA 10/46, 118
    BA 11, 450f
    BA 11 + 13, 30
    BA 11/47, 114

    BA 12, 86
    BA 12/47, 285
    BA 21, 45, 46f, 48f, 50f, 60f
    BA 24c and 24c', 129
    BA 40, 49, 50f, 52, 60f
    BA 44, 69, 179, 268, 450f
    BA 44/6, 373
    BA 44/45, 58
    BA 44/45/47, 45, 46f, 60f
    BA 45, 15f, 54–56, 55f, 56f, 59f, 69, 108,
        114, 132, 187, 372f, 373, 450f
    BA 45 + 47/12, 15f, 18
    BA 46, 88, 108, 118, 450f
    BA 47, 55–56, 72, 73f, 114, 372f,
        373, 450f
    BA 47/11, 108, 118
    BA 47/12, 15f, 30, 129, 132
Bromocriptine, 322, 323–324, 327, 328

Catechol-O-methyltransferase inhibition,
    294
Categorization. *See also* Abstraction
    in cognitive processing, 391–392
    evidence for, in nonhuman animals,
        392–393
    future research needs, 413–415
    visual. *See* Visual categorization
Category boundaries, 392
Caudate nucleus
    dopaminergic modulation in, 297–299,
        298f, 301–302
    in reversal learning, 289, 290
CC (corpus callosum), 208–209, 210
CCC-r theory. *See* Cognitive Complexity
    and Control-revised (CCC-r) theory
Childhood, development of rule use in.
    See Cognitive Complexity and
    Control-revised (CCC-r) theory
Cingulate cortex, anterior (ACC)
    action outcome associations and,
        145–148, 146f, 147f, 151
    action selection based on reward history
        and, 129–130, 130f
    action values and, 148–150, 149f
    changing between rules and, 144–145
    in complex rule use, 451, 453
    connections of, 150, 151f
    intentional task set selection and,
        188, 189f
    in learning of stimulus-response
        associations, 38
Cingulate zone, rostral, 188, 189f
Clozapine, 297

Cognitive Complexity and Control-revised
    (CCC-r) theory, 441–453
  implications and predictions of, 451–453
  language and, 449, 452
  levels of consciousness model, 441, 446f,
    447–449, 451
  overview, 441
  prefrontal cortex in rule representation,
    449–451, 450f
  representation complexity development
    in childhood, 442–445
  tree diagrams of rule complexity,
    445–447, 445f
Cognitive control. *See also* Attentional-set
    shifting; Executive function; Reversal
    learning
  frontal and parietal cortices in, 188–190,
    190f, 394
  high-level, prefrontal cortex and,
    38–40, 40t
Cognitive deficits, in Parkinson's disease,
    314, 315–316
Cognitive flexibility/inflexibility
  in children, 449
  dopaminergic modulation of, 320–325,
    321f, 324f, 328
  in Parkinson's disease
    deficits in, 314, 315–316
    dopaminergic medication and, 314,
      317–319
    motivational valence and, 319, 320f
  prefrontal cortex in, 283, 313–315,
    325–326, 326f
  striatum and, 314–315, 325–328, 326f
Cognitive mechanisms of declarative
    memory, 342–343
Cognitive neurophysiology, 81
Cognitive neuroscience, developmental. *See*
    Cognitive Complexity and Control-
    revised (CCC-r) theory
Cognitive processes
  categorization in, 391–392
  in repeat-stay/change-shift strategies,
    86
Cognitive stability, 314, 322, 324, 324f
Cognitive theories of abstraction,
    110–111
Comparative psychology of abstract rule use,
    25–27
Competition-resolution explanation of
    switch costs, 257–258
Conceptual clustering, in extracting abstract
    ideas, 111

Concrete rules
  vs. abstract rules, 419
  basal ganglia and, 424–426
Conditional associative responses, 3–19
  frontal cortex and
    motor responses, 3–4, 6–10, 8f, 10f
    spatial responses, 10–12, 11f, 12f
  hippocampal system and, 7–8, 8f, 10, 10f,
    11, 12f, 18, 19
  mid-ventrolateral prefrontal cortex and,
    15f, 16–18, 19
  posterior lateral frontal cortex and, 12–16,
    13f, 15f, 19
  ventrolateral prefrontal cortex/temporal
    lobe interactions and, 130, 132–135,
    134f
Conditional motor learning. *See also* Motor
    behavior, rules-based
  repeat-stay/change-shift strategies and,
    83–86, 84f
Conditional rules
  use of, by children, 442–445
  ventral prefrontal cortex and, 131–132,
    151
Conflicting cues, 186–187
Congruency. *See also* Incongruency costs
  advance-target preparation study,
    268–269, 269f, 271f
  encoding of, 239–244, 241f, 242f, 244f,
    247–248
Congruency-sensitivity/insensitivity,
    270–271, 271f
Connectivity, 207, 208–211, 217. *See also*
    Inter-regional interactions
Conscious accessibility of preparatory
    processes, 273–274, 275f, 276–277,
    278n
Consciousness, levels of. *See* Levels of
    consciousness model
Corpus callosum (CC), 208–209, 210
Cortical stimulation, and alteration of
    decision-making strategy by, 96
Corvids, abstract rule use in, 25, 26
Cost-benefit tradeoff
  in decision-making, 39
  medial frontal cortex in, 276
  in motor planning, 268–270, 269f, 278
  volition and, 266, 272
Crickets, categorization by, 392–393
Cue alternation, 181–182
Cue-based processes, 256
  conscious accessibility of preparation in,
    274, 275f

and inferior frontal junction activation, 262–263, 263f
and task priority, 258–259, 260f
voluntary control during, 274, 276–277, 278
Cued task-switching paradigm, 228. *See also* Task-switching
Cue-related activation, 182f
Cues. *See also* Stimuli
bidimensional, 186–187
egocentric vs. allocentric, 287
Cue-target-response mappings, compound, 265
Cumulative prioritization model of executive function, 263–265, 264f

DA. *See* Dopamine (DA)
DCCS (Dimensional Change Card Sort), 443, 444f–445f
Decision-making. *See also* Action selection
abstract information and, 38–40, 40t
basic parameters of, 39
cortical stimulation alteration of, 96
prefrontal cortex in, 96–99
Declarative memory. *See also* Relational memory
action-relevant, 365–366, 368–370, 381–383
cognitive mechanisms of, 342–343
features of, 341–342, 352
hippocampal function and, 337–338, 346–350
prefrontal cortex/hippocampal interactions and, 357
relational memory networks and, 345–346
and task set control, 377–382
Declarative memory system, rules and, 365–368, 381–383
Delayed match-to-category task (DMC)
motion stimuli, 406, 407f
shape stimuli, 396f, 397
Depression, 301
Development. *See* Neurodevelopment
5,7-DHT (5,7-dihydroxytryptamine), 295–297, 296f
Difference task, 27–28, 29f
"Different" rule, 27–31
Diffusion tensor imaging, 217
Diffusion weighted magnetic resonance imaging. *See* Magnetic resonance imaging, diffusion weighted (DWI)

5,7-Dihydroxytryptamine (5,7-DHT), 295–297, 296f
Dimensional Change Card Sort (DCCS), 443, 444f
Discrimination reversal learning. *See* Reversal learning
Distractibility, dopamine and, 293–294, 297, 314, 324
DLPFC. *See* Prefrontal cortex, dorsolateral (DLPFC, PFdl)
DMC. *See* Delayed match-to-category task (DMC)
Dolphins, abstract rule use in, 25
Domain-general/domain-specific processes, 198, 211–216, 213f, 217
Dopamine (DA)
in active maintenance, 313–315
in attentional-set acquisition, 292f, 293, 295
in attentional-set shifting, 291–295, 292f, 297
and cognitive inflexibility, 320–325, 321f, 324f
future research needs, 328
in Parkinson's disease, 314–315, 315f
depletion of, in striatum, 314–315, 315f
and impulsivity, 322, 324f, 328
in reinforcement signaling, 426–427, 434
in reversal learning, 298f, 299–302, 303
Dopamine receptor agonists
cognitive flexibility/stability studies, 314, 322–325
for Parkinson's disease, 315, 317
Dopamine receptors, 291, 294, 297–299
Dopaminergic medication
cognitive flexibility and, 314, 317–319
and serotonin depletion, 328
Dopaminergic teaching signals, 426–427, 434
DWI. *See* Magnetic resonance imaging, diffusion weighted (DWI)
Dysexecutive syndrome, 24

EEG (electroencephalography), 189–190, 258
Effective connectivity, 209
Egocentric cues, 287
Electroencephalography (EEG), 189–190, 258
Empirical knowledge, exemplars and, 100

Encoding. *See also* Rule encoding
    abstract information encoding, 38–40, 40t
    of congruency, 239–244, 241f, 242f, 244f,
        247–248
    neural encoding of task rules, 234–238,
        236–238f, 246–247
    shape encoding, 400–402
    strategy encoding, 95–96, 96f
Entorhinal cortex, 340, 355
Episodic memory
    definition of, 341
    hippocampal function and, 346–350
    organization of, 338–339
    temporal dimension of, 342, 344,
        348–350, 348f, 349f, 353–354
EROS. *See* Event-related optical
        signal (EROS)
ERPs. *See* Event-related brain potentials
        (ERPs)
Error-guided action-reversal task,
        148–150
Essay Concerning Human Understanding
        (Locke), 109
Event-related brain potentials (ERPs), 198,
        204–205, 206, 216
Event-related optical signal (EROS)
    compared to other imaging methods,
        198–199, 203, 216
    connectivity of brain regions and, 207,
        208–211, 217
    coordination of brain region activity
        studies, 209–211
    experimental background, 201–203
    general vs. specific processes, 211–216,
        212f, 213f, 217
    in individual subject studies, 216
    limitations of, 216, 217
    mechanisms of, 199–200, 201f
    selective attention studies, 204, 205–206
    sensory memory studies, 204, 205
    working memory studies, 204, 206–209
Excitotoxic lesions, 290, 301
Executive function. *See also* Cognitive
        control; Voluntary control
    adaptive organization of, 211–216
    connectivity of brain regions and, 207,
        208–211, 217
    coordination of brain region activity and,
        209–211
    definition of, 197
    development of, in children. *See*
        Cognitive Complexity and Control-
        revised (CCC-r) theory

    domain-specific vs. domain-general
        processes, 198, 211–216, 213f, 217
    evaluative vs. action-oriented aspect
        of, 197
    event-related optical signal studies and,
        203–204
    frontal and parietal cortices in, 188–190,
        190f, 394
    hot vs. cool aspects of, 453
    in humans vs. monkeys, 228, 245–246
    models of
        compound cue-target-response
            mappings, 265
        cumulative prioritization, 263–265,
            264f
        hierarchial, 261–263, 263f, 277
        nonhierarchical, 263–265, 264f,
            277, 278n
    selective attention and, 204
    working memory and, 197, 204–208
Exemplars, empirical knowledge and, 100
Extradimensional shifts, 284, 291, 292f, 293,
        296f, 317
Extreme capsule, prefrontal connections of,
        133, 134f, 135
Eye field
    frontal, 17, 37, 78, 138, 421f
    supplementary, 141–142, 141f

FG (fusiform gyrus), 74f, 75, 76f
Flexibility, cognitive. *See* Cognitive
        flexibility/inflexibility
Flexible Item Selection Task, 449
fMRI. *See* Magnetic resonance imaging,
        functional (fMRI)
Food preferences, socially transmitted, 351
FPN. *See* Frontoparietal network (FPN)
Frontal cortex. *See also* Prefrontal cortex
        (PFC)
    in cognitive control, 188–190, 190f
    frontomedial vs. frontolateral, in
        cognitive control, 184, 187–188, 191
    functional parcellation of, 3, 190–191
    medial
        dopamine depletion in, 293–294
        in intentional control of action
            selection, 267, 269f, 270–271,
            276, 278
    posterior frontolateral. *See also* Frontal
        junction, inferior (IFJ)
        functional parcellation of, 190–191
        structural neuroanatomy of, 178–180,
            178f

studies showing activation of, 182–183, 184f
posterior lateral, in conditional associative responses, 12–16, 13f, 15f, 19
Frontal cortical excisions
conditional associative responses and animal study localization of, 12–16, 13–15f
motor responses, 3–4, 6–10, 8f, 10f
spatial responses, 10–12, 11f, 12f
deficits from, 3–5
examples of, 4, 4f
Frontal eye field, 17, 37, 78, 138, 421f
Frontal gyrus
anterior inferior (aIFG)
activity correlation with task set activity, 74f, 75, 76f
inter-regional interactions, 72
inferior, cue alternation activity, 182
middle, in task-general processing, 213–214, 213f
posterior inferior (pIFG), inter-regional interactions, 69, 70f
Frontal junction, inferior (IFJ)
in cognitive control paradigms, 182–183, 184f, 190f, 191
in conditional associative responses, 19
connectivity of, 180
dissociation from more anterior regions, 186–187, 191
in executive control, 262–263, 262f, 263f
and exogenous vs. endogenous components of task set updating, 187–188
functional relationships of, 184–186
location of, 177
structural neuroanatomy of, 178–180, 178f
in updating of task representations, 180–182, 182f
Frontal sulcus
inferior (IFS), 177, 178, 178f
dissociation from inferior frontal junction, 186–187, 191
superior (SFS), inter-regional interactions, 69, 70f
Frontoparietal network (FPN)
organization of, 214–215
specialization within, 208–209
in task-general processing, 213–214, 213f
in working memory and executive function, 207

Functional connectivity, 209–211, 217. See also Inter-regional interactions
Functional magnetic resonance imaging. See Magnetic resonance imaging, functional (fMRI)
Fusiform gyrus (FG), 74f, 75, 76f

Gating signal, voluntary, in cue-based tasks, 276
Generalization. See Abstraction
Geniculate nucleus, lateral (LGN), 206, 410
Globus pallidus (GP), 424. See also Basal ganglia
Glutamatergic synapses, 344, 425
Goal-directed behavior
abstraction and, 419–420, 428
lagged autoassociative networks in production of, 435
model-building in, 431–433
prefrontal cortex properties and, 422–424
top-down orchestration of, 419–420
Goal-directed movement, planning of, 52
Goal-response associations, 266, 268, 277. See also Action goals; Intentional control
Go/no-go task, 58
GP. See Globus pallidus (GP)

Habit formation, 432–433
Hand postures, 6f
Hebbian plasticity, 420, 432
Higher-order task rules, anterior prefrontal cortex and, 75–77
Hippocampal system, 340–350
cognitive mechanisms of declarative memory and, 342–343
in conditional associative responses, 7–8, 8f, 10, 10f, 11, 12f, 18, 19
experimental studies of, 346–350
information flow in, 337, 340–341, 341f, 355–356
relational memory networks and, 343–344
relational memory representation and, 341–342
temporal lobe excisions and, 5, 5f
Hippocampus
in declarative memory, 337–338, 346–350
input/output pathways to neocortex, 340–341, 341f, 355–356
neuronal activation patterns in, 350–355
prefrontal cortex interactions, 337, 356–357, 428

Hippocampus (*continued*)
  in relational memory, 350–351, 354–355
  in retrieval of episodic representations,
      345–346
  and spatial mapping, 343, 345, 352–355
Honeybees, abstract rule use in, 26–27
5-HT. *See* Serotonin (5-HT)
Human studies
  action outcome association, 145–148,
      146f, 147f
  conditional associative responses
    motor responses, 3–4, 6–10, 8f, 10f
    spatial responses, 10–12, 11f, 12f
  congruent vs. incongruent target studies,
      268–271, 269f, 271f
  dopaminergic modulation of cognitive
      flexibility, 321, 321f, 322–325, 324f
  event-related optical signal usefulness in,
      202–203
  frontal and parietal cortices in cognitive
      control, 188–190, 190f
  functional study of inferior frontal
      junction, 180–182, 182f
  intentional task set selection study,
      188, 189f
  prefrontal cortex organization, by level of
      abstraction, 112–119, 116f, 120f
  selective attention, 206
  supplementary eye field lesions, 141–142,
      141f
  task-switching compared to monkeys,
      231–234, 232f, 244–246
  task-switching studies in, limitations
      of, 227
  ventrolateral prefrontal cortex in
      attentional-set shifting, 285–287
  on volition, 272–274, 275f
Huntington's disease, 424
6-Hydroxydopamine (6-OHDA) lesions
  of caudate nucleus, 297, 298f
  of nucleus accumbens, 301–302
  of prefrontal cortex, 291–295, 292f
5-Hydroxytryptamine. *See* Serotonin
      (5-HT)

Ideomotor apraxia, 52
IFJ. *See* Frontal junction, inferior (IFJ)
IFS. *See* Frontal sulcus, inferior (IFS)
Imagery vs. semantic retrieval, 49–51, 50f
Imaging methods. *See also names of specific*
      techniques, e.g., Magnetic resonance
      imaging
  comparison of, 198–199, 203, 216

spatial and temporal resolution of,
      198–199, 217
  switch cost analysis disparity between,
      258
Impulsivity. *See* Trait impulsivity
Incongruency costs, 229, 233–234, 245–246.
      See also Congruency
Inflexibility. *See* Cognitive flexibility/
      inflexibility
Inhibition
  in discrimination reversal, 287
  reciprocal, 207, 210–211
Inhibitory rules, 58–61, 60f
Inhibitory synapses, in prefrontal
      cortex–basal ganglia loops,
      434–435
Insects, abstract rule use in, 26–27
Instruction delay
  activity during, 69, 70f, 78–79
  length of, and reaction time, 71–73, 72f
Intention, definition of, 266, 272
Intentional control, 256, 266–268, 277.
      See also Goal-directed behavior
Intentional task set selection, 188, 189f
Intention-based conflict resolution, 266
Interference, in task-switching, 378–382.
      See also Proactive interference
Inter-regional interactions. *See also*
      Connectivity
  imaging studies of, 69–70, 70f
  rule-specific activity and, 67–69, 68f
Intradimensional shifts, 284, 291, 292f, 293,
      296f, 297
Intraparietal (LIP) area, lateral
  research on, 405–406
  visual categorization and, 406–413, 408f,
      409f, 413–415
Intraparietal sulcus (IPS)
  action representation and, 52
  task rule encoding in, 235, 236–238,
      238f, 246
IPL. *See* Parietal lobule, inferior (IPL)
IPS. *See* Intraparietal sulcus (IPS)
ITC. *See* Temporal cortex, inferior (ITC)

Knowledge-for-action, 369–370. *See also*
      Action knowledge
  controlled (top-down) retrieval, 371, 373,
      374, 381
  postretrieval selection, 371, 373, 374,
      377, 381
  retrieval of, 371–375, 381–383
Knowledge-of-action, 368–369

Labeling, and levels of consciousness, 449
Language, 85, 248–250, 449, 452. *See also*
    entries beginning with Verbal
Latency
    congruent vs. incongruent stimuli and,
        239–244, 241f, 242f, 244f, 247–248
    of picture selectivity, 35, 36f
    of rule selectivity, 34, 34f
L-dopa. *See* Levodopa (l-dopa)
Learning. *See also* Reversal learning
    abstract rule, 422, 435–436
    of categorization, 391–392, 393, 399–400,
        409–410, 414–415
    new, prefrontal cortex in, 37
    rapid vs. slow, 428
    visual discrimination test emphasis on, 285
Learning sets, 25–26
Learning systems, low-level, 38
Levels of consciousness model, 441, 446f,
    447–449, 451
Levodopa (l-dopa)
    for Parkinson's disease, 315
    serotonin synthesis and, 328
LGN (lateral geniculate nucleus), 206, 410
Linguistics, developmental, 85
LIP. *See* Intraparietal (LIP) area, lateral
Location–event associations, hippocampus
    and, 352–353
Long-term potentiation, 344

Macaque monkeys
    anterior cingulate lesions in, 144–145,
        148–150, 149f
    attention and stimulus selection in,
        135–139, 137f, 139f
    conditional associative learning in, 3,
        12–16, 13–15f
    dorsolateral prefrontal cortex lesions
        in, 131
    frontotemporal interactions in, 133–135
    as model system for motor behavior
        studies, 160
    visual categorization in, 394–400
Magnetic resonance imaging, diffusion
    weighted (DWI), 148
    anterior cingulate cortex, 150, 151f
    extreme capsule, uncinate fascicle, and
        amygdala, 134f, 135
Magnetic resonance imaging, functional
    (fMRI). *See also* Blood-oxygen
        level–dependent (BOLD) fMRI
    action representation studies, 47–50, 48f,
        50f, 58–61, 59f

    dopaminergic modulation of cognitive
        flexibility, 322–325, 324f
    in executive function studies, 216
    frontal and parietal cortices in cognitive
        control, 188–190, 190f
    functional study of inferior frontal
        junction, 180–182, 182f
    hippocampus in episodic recollection, 347
    intentional task set selection study, 188,
        189f
    of inter-regional interactions, 69–70, 70f
    of mid-dorsolateral prefrontal cortex,
        17–18
    neuronal networks underlying
        attentional-set shifting, 285
    Parkinson's disease and reversal learning
        study, 321, 321f
    prefrontal cortex organization, by level
        of abstraction, 113–115, 116f,
        118, 120f
    selective attention studies, 206
    spatial resolution of, 198
    switch cost analysis by, 258
Magnetoencephalography (MEG), 199
Mappings. *See also* Associations
    cue-target-response, 265
    spatial, 343, 345, 352–353
    visuomotor, 184–185, 191
Marmosets, prefrontal dopamine depletion
    in, 291–295
Matching-to-sample task, 25, 26f, 27
Mechanical knowledge, 47. *See also* Action
    representation
Medication overdose hypothesis, 317–319
MEG (magnetoencephalography), 199
Memory
    control mechanisms of, anterior frontal
        cortex in, 76–77
    declarative. *See* Declarative memory
    episodic. *See* Episodic memory
    long-term, 428
    non-declarative, procedural, 366–367
    relational. *See* Relational memory
    retrieval of, ventrolateral prefrontal cortex
        activation and, 53
    semantic. *See* Semantic memory
    sensory. *See* Sensory memory
    ventrolateral prefrontal cortex in
        formation of, 57
    verbal, ventrolateral prefrontal cortex in,
        58, 60–61, 60f
    visual sensory, 205
    working. *See* Working memory

Memory representation, hippocampus and,
    338–340, 341–342. *See also*
    Hippocampal system
Mental representations, abstract. *See*
    Abstract mental representation
Metaphorical concepts, abstract ideas and,
    110
N-Methyl D-aspartate (NMDA) receptors,
    344, 351
Middle temporal area (MT), in visual
    feature processing, 410–413, 411f,
    412f
mid-DLPFC. *See* Prefrontal cortex,
    mid-dorsolateral (mid-DLPFC)
mid-VLPFC. *See* Prefrontal cortex,
    mid-ventrolateral (mid-VLPFC)
Mirror neurons, 268
Mismatch negativity, 204–205
Model-building, goal-directed behavior and,
    431–433
Monkeys. *See also* Macaque monkeys
    abstract rule use in, 25–26
        prefrontal-associated regions and,
            31–37, 33–36f
        prefrontal cortex and, 27–31, 30f, 31t
    conditional associative learning in, 3,
        12–16, 13–15f
    conditional motor learning in, 83–86, 84f
    executive control in, 227, 228
    higher-order vs. lower-order rules in,
        99–100
    hippocampal function studies, 351
    as model of human cognitive function,
        246, 250
    prefrontal cortex in decision making,
        97–99, 97f
    prefrontal dopamine depletion in, 291–295
    rule representation and application in,
        246
    task-switching compared to humans,
        231–234, 232f, 244–246
    task-switching paradigm for, 228–231,
        230f
    visual categorization in, 394–400
Motion categorization
    middle temporal area and, 410–413, 411f,
        412f
    posterior parietal cortex and, 405–410,
        408f, 409f
Motivational valence, and learning, in
    Parkinson's disease, 319, 320f
Motor behavior, rules-based, 159–173
    brain regions involved in, 162

    execution of, 170, 171f, 172–173
    hierarchial organization of, 160–161,
        160f, 172f
    planning of, 166–168, 168f, 169f, 172
    target selection for, 163–166, 163f, 165f,
        166f, 172
Motor cortices. *See also* Premotor cortex;
    Primary motor cortex
    anatomical organization of, 161, 161f
    prefrontal cortex projections to,
        24, 162
Motor knowledge. *See* Action knowledge
Motor planning stage, interface with action
    selection, 268–271, 269f, 271f
Motor responses, conditional associative
    learning and, 3–4, 6–10, 8f, 10f
MT. *See* Middle temporal area (MT)

N1/N100 component of event-related
    potential, 204–205
N-back task, 183, 208–209
Near-infrared light, penetration of, 200
Negative feedback, and reversal learning,
    319, 320f
Neural encoding, of task rules, 234–238,
    236–238f, 246–247
Neural networks
    artificial, 428
    autoassociative, 434–435
    underlying attentional-set shifting,
        285–287
Neurodevelopment
    in children. *See* Cognitive Complexity and
        Control-revised (CCC-r) theory
    prefrontal organization and, 122–123
Neuroimaging. *See* Imaging methods
Neuromodulation. *See also* Dopamine (DA);
    Serotonin (5-HT)
    of attentional-set shifting
        dopamine and, 291–295, 292f, 297–
            299, 302–303
        serotonin and, 295–297, 296f
    dopaminergic. *See* Dopamine (DA)
    of reversal learning, 298f, 299–302, 303
Neuronal latency, 239–244, 241f, 242f, 244f,
    247–248
Neuronal representation
    of abstract rule encoding
        in prefrontal-associated regions, 31–37,
            33–36f
        in prefrontal cortex, 27–31, 30f, 31t,
            38–39
        inter-regional interactions, 67–70, 68f, 70f

in repeat-stay/change-shift strategies
average population activity, 92–95,
96f, 97f
individual cells, 88–92, 89f, 90f, 91f
stimulus-response associations and,
37–38
in visual categorization
posterior parietal cortex and, 405–410,
408f, 409f
prefrontal cortex and, 394–400, 397f,
398f, 402–405, 413–415
in visual feature processing
inferior temporal cortex and, 400–405,
403f, 404f, 413, 414
middle temporal area and, 410–413,
411f, 412f
Neurons
dopaminergic, 426–427, 434. See also
Dopamine (DA)
of prefrontal cortex, 422
of striatum, 424–425, 426–427
Neuropharmacology. See Neuromodulation
Neurophysiology
of abstract response strategies. See
Abstract response strategies
cognitive, 81
NMDA (N-Methyl D-aspartate) receptors,
344, 351
Nondeclarative memory. See Procedural
memory
Non-human primates. See Primates,
non-human
Nonspatial information, hippocampal
pathways for, 340
Nonverbal vs. verbal rules, 249–250
Noradrenaline, depletion of, in prefrontal
cortex, 313–314
Nucleus accumbens, 289, 290, 301–302

Object manipulation, 47, 51. See also Action
representation
Object-outcome associations, 288
Object recognition, 400–402
Obsessive-compulsive disorder, 301
Occipital-temporal junction, in task-general
processing, 213, 213f
OFC. See Orbitofrontal cortex (OFC)
6-OHDA lesions. See 6-Hydroxydopamine
(6-OHDA) lesions
Ondansetron, 300
Optical imaging, 199–200. See also
Event-related optical signal (EROS)
Optical properties of axons, 199

Optical signal measurement, continuous-
wave vs. frequency-domain
methods, 200
Orbitofrontal cortex (OFC)
in abstraction of rules, 30, 31t
differentiation of rule types and, 61
object-outcome associations and, 288
in reversal learning, 283, 287–289, 291
neuromodulation of, 300–301, 303
rule complexity and, 450, 450f
thalamocortical circuits, 451

Parahippocampal cortex, 337, 340, 355–356
Parietal cortex/lobe. See also Frontoparietal
network (FPN); Intraparietal (LIP)
area, lateral; Intraparietal sulcus
(IPS)
in executive control, 188–190, 190f,
191, 227
in neural representations of action, 49, 52
posterior (PPC)
and integration of cortical processes,
227
task rule encoding in, 235, 236–238,
238f, 246–247
in visual categorization, 408f, 409f,
410–413
Parietal lobule, inferior (IPL), 49, 52,
213f, 214
Parkinson's disease (PD)
attentional-set shifting and, 291, 318
dopamine-dependent cognitive
inflexibility in, 314–316, 315f
dopaminergic medication effects, 314,
317–319
reversal learning and, 299, 317, 318,
319, 320f
Pars orbitalis, 372f, 373
Pars triangularis, 372f, 373
Patient studies. See Human studies
Payoff (reward), in decision-making, 39
PD. See Parkinson's disease (PD)
Perceptual categorization, relational
memory and, 338
Periarcuate lesions, in conditional
associative responses, 12–16, 13f,
15f, 19
Perirhinal cortex, 340, 355
PFC. See Prefrontal cortex (PFC)
PFdl. See Prefrontal cortex, dorsolateral
(DLPFC, PFdl)
PFv. See Prefrontal cortex, ventrolateral
(VLPFC, PFv)

PFv+o. *See* Prefrontal cortex, ventrolateral
 with orbital areas (PFv+o)
Philosophical theories of abstraction,
 108–109
Phonological tasks, 71–73, 72f, 73f
Picture selectivity, 35, 35f, 36f
pIFG. *See* Frontal gyrus, posterior inferior
 (pIFG)
Pigeons, categorization by, 393
Planning. *See* Goal-directed behavior;
 Intentional control
Plasticity, of frontal cortex vs. basal ganglia,
 427–431, 429f, 430f, 432–433
Plato, 108–109
PMd. *See* Premotor cortex, dorsal (PMd)
PMv. *See* Premotor cortex, ventral (PMv)
Positive feedback. *See also* Reward
 processing
 in decision-making, 39
 and reversal learning, 319, 320f
Positron emission tomography, of striatum,
 285–286
postMTG. *See* Temporal gyrus, posterior
 middle (postMTG)
Postretrieval selection, 371, 373, 374,
 377, 381
Postrhinal cortex, 340, 355
PPC. *See* Parietal cortex, posterior (PPC)
Precentral sulcus, inferior, 177,
 178–179, 178f
Prefrontal cortex (PFC). *See also* Frontal
 cortex
 abstract information encoding by, 38–40,
  40t
 abstract rule encoding in
  anatomical connectivity and, 420–422,
   421f
  neuronal representation of, 27–31, 31t,
   36–37
  prefrontal-associated regions and,
   31–37, 31t, 33–35f
  research evidence for, 422–424, 423f
 anatomical connectivity of, 420–422, 421f
 anatomy of, 24
 anterior (APF)
  higher-order task rules and, 75–77
  inter-regional interactions, 69–73, 70f,
   75, 76f
 basal ganglia relationships of, 428–431
  in bootstrapping, 433–436
  in model-building, 431–433
 in cognitive flexibility, 283, 313–315,
  325–326, 326f

 in conditional associative responses, 10,
  12–18, 13f, 15f, 19
 in decision-making, 96–99. *See also*
  Action selection
 dopaminergic modulation in, 291–295,
  298f, 302–303, 313–315, 324
 dorsolateral (DLPFC, PFdl)
  in abstraction of rules, 30, 31t
  abstract mental representations and,
   112, 118, 120
  in conditional associative responses, 10,
   12–16, 13f, 15f
  deficits due to lesions of, 131
  dopamine modulation in, and working
   memory, 320–321
  mid-dorsolateral (mid-DLPFC). *See*
   Prefrontal cortex, mid-dorsolateral
   (mid-DLPFC)
  rule complexity and, 450, 450f, 451
 dorsomedial
  anterior cingulate cortex in action
   selection, 129, 130f, 144–150, 147f,
   149f, 151, 151f
  pre-supplementary motor area in
   action selection, 129, 130f, 140–144,
   141f, 142f, 143f, 151
 hierarchial model of rule representation
  in, 449–451, 450f, 452
 higher-order task rules and, 75–77
 hippocampal interactions with, 337,
  356–357
 integration of low-level learning systems
  by, 38
 lateral
  abstract mental representation and,
   107, 111–118, 116f, 120f
  anatomical organization of, 161–162,
   161f
  in arm movement, 162
  in execution of motor behavior, 170,
   171f
  in executive control, 261–263, 262f,
   263f
  functional organization of, 162–170
  in target selection for motor behavior,
   163–166, 163f, 165f, 166f, 172
  topographical organization of, 107,
   108f, 111–112, 115, 118, 120f
 left/right differences in task-switching,
  210–211, 215
 mid-dorsolateral (mid-DLPFC)
  in action representation, 57–61,
   59f, 60f

in conditional associative responses, 12–13, 13f, 15f, 16–18
inferior frontal junction and, 186–187
in intentional control of action selection, 266–268, 269f
in rule retrieval, 53
mid-ventrolateral (mid-VLPFC)
  in conditional associative responses, 15f, 16–18, 19
  in mnemonic control, 372f, 373, 375–377, 381
  in task-switching, 378, 380f, 381, 382
in mnemonic control, 370–377, 381–383
in neural representations of action, 45–46, 46f, 52–57, 55f, 56f, 58–61, 60f
in new learning, 37
orbitofrontal region. See Orbitofrontal cortex (OFC)
organization of
  hierarchial model of rule representation in, 449–451, 450f, 452
  process-based vs. representation-based, 121–123, 121f
  topographical, by level of abstraction, 107, 108f, 113–119, 114–120f
plasticity in, 427–431, 429f, 430f, 432–433
posterior lateral, in conditional associative responses, 12–16, 13f, 15f, 19
primary motor cortex connections of, 162
regional interactivity of, and task sets, 71–73, 72f, 73f
roles of, 101, 394, 420–424
rostrolateral (RLPFC)
  abstract mental representations and, 112, 114, 117f, 118, 119
  rule complexity and, 450, 450f, 451
serotonergic regulation in, 296f, 298f, 303
in stimulus-response associations, 37–38
unconscious processing in, 276–277, 278n
ventrolateral (VLPFC, PFv)
  in abstraction of rules, 24–25, 30, 31t, 286–287, 302
  abstract mental representations and, 114, 117f, 118, 120
  in action selection, 129, 130f, 131–135, 134f, 151
  anterior ventrolateral, in mnemonic control, 372f, 373, 381
  in attentional-set shifting, 283, 285–287, 290, 302

and declarative knowledge in guiding action, 365–368
inferior frontal junction and, 186–187
lesions of, deficits from, 53
mid-ventrolateral. See Prefrontal cortex, mid-ventrolateral (mid-VLPFC)
in mnemonic control, 370–375, 381–382
motor knowledge and, 368–369
in neural representations of action, 45–46, 46f
with orbital areas (PFv+o), in action selection, 129, 130f, 133, 139–140
proactive interference and, 375–377, 376f
rule complexity and, 450, 450f, 451
in rule retrieval, selection, and maintenance, 52–57, 55f, 58–61, 60f
in semantic knowledge retrieval, 56–57, 56f
temporal lobe connections of, 130, 132–135, 134f
ventrolateral with orbital areas (PFv+o), in action selection, 129, 130f, 133, 139–140
in visual shape categorization, 394–400, 397f, 398f, 402–405, 413–415
Premotor cortex
  activity correlation with task set activity, 74f, 75, 76f
  anatomy of, 161f
  dorsal (PMd)
    action representations and, 49, 52
    action selection and, 130f
    inferior frontal junction and, 184–186, 191
    in neural representations of action, 49–50, 51–52, 51f
    in planning motor behavior, 166–168, 168f, 169f, 172
  ventral (PMv), action representations and, 50, 51, 51f
Preparation interval
  neural activity analysis during, 257–258
  self-paced, response time and, 273–274, 275f
Preparatory processes
  conscious accessibility of, 273–274, 275f, 276–277, 278n
  optional engagement of, 272
  target-specific, 256–271, 269f, 271f, 278

Pre-supplementary motor area (pre-SMA)
   action sequencing and, 143–144, 143f
   activation in cognitive control, 190
   changing between rules and, 129, 130f,
     140–144, 141f, 142f, 151
   cue-related activation of, 181
   and exogenous vs. endogenous
     components of task set updating,
     187–188
Primary motor cortex
   anatomy of, 161f
   in execution of motor behavior, 170,
     172–173
   somatotopic organization of, 161
Primates, non-human. See also Monkeys
   abstract rule use in, 25–26
   categorization by, 393
   prefrontal cortex organization, by
     level of abstraction, 112–113,
     119–120, 121f
   rule representation in, dorsolateral
     prefrontal cortex and, 57
   ventrolateral prefrontal cortex in
     attentional-set shifting, 285–287
Proactive interference
   in task-switching, 378–381
   ventrolateral prefrontal cortex and,
     375–377, 376f
Probabilistic tractography
   anterior cingulate cortex, 150, 151f
   extreme capsule, uncinate fascicle, and
     amygdala, 134f, 135
Procedural memory, mechanisms of,
   366–367
Process-based organization of prefrontal
   cortex, 121–123, 121f
Progressive nuclear palsy, 291
Psychological distance, 449
Punishment. See Negative feedback
Putamen, 323, 424, 425f. See also Striatum
   (STR)

Rabies virus, 162
Rational knowledge, abstraction and, 100
Rats
   hippocampal function studies, 348–350,
     348f, 349f, 351
   impaired attentional-set shifting in, 285
   prefrontal dopamine depletion in,
     294–295
Reaching movement
   brain regions involved in, 162
   execution of, 170, 171f, 172–173

   hierarchial organization of, 160–161,
     160f, 172f
   planning of, 166–168, 168f, 169f, 172
   target selection for, 163–166, 163f, 165f,
     166f, 172
Reaction time (RT), 71–73, 72f
Receiver operating characteristic (ROC)
   analysis
   quantification of task rule encoding,
     237–238, 238f
   strategy vs. rule encoding, 32–33, 95–96,
     96f
Reciprocal inhibition, 207, 210–211
Reconfiguration explanation of switch costs,
   257–258
Recursive consciousness, 446f, 448
Recursive processing in cortico-ganglia
   loops, 420, 433–436
Region-of-interest (ROI) analysis, 50f,
   56, 60
Reinforcement signals, dopaminergic,
   426–427, 434
Reinforcer devaluation, 432
Relational memory, 338. See also Declarative
   memory
Relational memory networks
   binding and organization of, 338–340
   biological mechanisms of, 343–344
   cognitive mechanisms of, 342–343
   components of, 356
   hippocampus in, 350–351, 354–355
   nature of, 337–338, 345–346
Relational memory representation,
   mechanisms of, 341–342
Repeat-stay/change-shift strategies
   cognitive processes in, 86
   conditional motor learning and,
     83–86, 84f
   neurophysiology of
     average population activity, 92–95,
       96f, 97f
     individual cells, 88–92, 89f, 90f, 91f
Representation. See also Abstract mental
   representation; Action
   representation; Neuronal
   representation
   memory representation, 338–340,
     341–342. See also Hippocampal
     system
   rule representation, 249–250
   semantic representation, 46, 49, 60f,
     61, 339
   symbolic representation, 366f, 441

working memory representation, 112, 113, 120–121
Representation-based organization of prefrontal cortex, 122–123
Response ambiguity, 239
Responses, competing, conditional rules and. *See* Conditional associative responses
Response switching task, pre-supplementary motor area and, 141–142, 141f
Reversal learning
 neuromodulation of, 298f, 299–302, 303, 320–321, 321f
 orbitofrontal cortex and, 283, 287–289, 291, 300–301
 Parkinson's disease and, 317, 318, 319, 320f
 subcortical mechanisms in, 289–290, 301–302, 320–321, 321f
 visual discrimination, 289–290, 298f, 299–300
Reward processing
 anterior cingulate and, 130
 dopaminergic neurons and, 426–427, 434
Rhesus monkeys. *See* Macaque monkeys
Rigidity. *See also* Cognitive flexibility/ inflexibility
Risk, in decision-making, 39
RLPFC. *See* Prefrontal cortex, rostrolateral (RLPFC)
Road sign study, 47–49, 48f, 51, 51f, 53–56
ROC analysis. *See* Receiver operating characteristic (ROC) analysis
ROI analysis. *See* Region-of-interest (ROI) analysis
RT (reaction time), 71–73, 72f
Rule abstraction. *See* Abstraction of rules
Rule encoding
 abstract, 31–37, 31t, 33f, 35f, 36f
 vs. strategy encoding, 95–96, 96f
Rule knowledge
 long-term storage of
  imagery vs. semantic retrieval and, 49–51, 50f
  parietal cortex in, 49, 52
  posterior middle temporal gyrus and, 45–50, 46f, 48f, 50f
  premotor cortex and, 49–50, 51–52, 51f
  ventrolateral prefrontal cortex in, 45–46, 46f
 retrieval, selection, and maintenance of mid-dorsolateral prefrontal cortex in, 53, 57–61, 59f, 60f

ventrolateral prefrontal cortex in, 52–57, 55f, 56f, 58–61, 60f
Rule learning, strategies and, 139–140
Rulemaps, 422–424, 423f, 435–436
Rule representation, verbal vs. nonverbal, 249–250
Rule retrieval, effortful, 53–56
Rule-reversal task. *See also* Reversal learning levels of abstraction and, 113–116, 114f, 115f, 116f, 119
Rules
 abstract. *See* Abstract rules
 changing between. *See* Task-switching
 complexity of
  childhood development and, 442–445
  tree diagrams of, 445–447, 445f
 concrete
  vs. abstract, 419
  basal ganglia and, 424–426
 conditional, competing response selection and. *See* Conditional associative responses
 declarative memory system and, 365–368, 381–383
 development of rule use in children. *See* Cognitive Complexity and Control-revised (CCC-r) theory
 differentiation of types of, 57–61, 59f, 60f
 higher-order vs. lower-order, 99–100, 445–446, 445f, 452
 inhibitory vs. noninhibitory, 58–61, 60f
 vs. strategies, 99–100
 verbal vs. nonverbal, 249–250
 well-known vs. recently learned, 47–49, 48f
Rule selection, 54–56

Sameness rule, 25–27
Scattering, of light, 199
Sea lions, abstract rule use in, 25
SEF (supplementary eye field), 141–142, 141f
Selective attention
 in abstraction, 109, 110, 122–123
 event-related optical signal studies, 205–206
 executive function and, 204
 reciprocal inhibition and, 211
Self-paced preparation time, response time and, 273–274, 275f
Self-reflection, in rule use development in children, 441, 447–449. *See also* Levels of consciousness

Semantic dementia, 368, 370
Semantic knowledge
  controlled retrieval of, 371–374
  hippocampus and, 343, 354–355
  retrieval of, 56–57, 56f, 60f, 61
    vs. imagery, in long-term rule storage,
      49–51, 50f
Semantic memory
  abstraction of rules and, 338
  definition of, 341
  episodic memory vs., 342
  hippocampal function and, 346–350
  as systemic organization of information,
    342
Semantic representation
  organization of, 339
  posterior middle temporal gyrus and, 46,
    49, 60f, 61
Semantic tasks
  instructional delay, neural correlation of,
    72–73, 73f
  instruction delay vs. reaction time in,
    71–72, 72f
Sensory memory
  event-related optical signal studies of, 205
  event-related potential studies, 204–205
Sequence of events. See also Temporal
    dimension of episodic memory
Serotonin (5-HT)
  in attentional-set shifting, 295–297, 296f
  functions of, 301
  medication-induced depletion of, 328
  in reversal learning, 298f, 299–301, 303
Serotonin receptor antagonists, 300
SFS. See Frontal sulcus, superior (SFS)
Shape categorization. See under Visual
    categorization
Shape encoding, 400–402
Shifts. See also Attentional-set shifting;
    Repeat-stay/change-shift strategies;
    Task-switching
  extradimensional, 284, 291, 292f, 293,
    296f, 317
  intradimensional, 284, 291, 292f, 293,
    296f, 297
Short-term item recognition test, 375,
    376f, 377
Simulators, in extracting abstract ideas, 111
Single neuron activity. See Neuronal
    representation
SN. See Substantia nigra (SN)
Spatial information, hippocampal pathways
    for, 340

Spatially tuned response, congruency and,
    239–244, 241f, 242f, 244f
Spatial mapping, hippocampus and, 343,
    345, 352–353
Spatial matching-to-sample task, strategies
    for, 82
Spatial resolution of imaging techniques,
    198–199, 209, 217
Spatial responses, conditional associative
    learning and, 10–12, 11f, 12f
Spatial tasks, superior frontal sulcus and,
    69, 70f
Spatial working memory, dopamine and,
    291
Spatiotemporal functional studies, 198–199,
    209–211
Spiny cells, 426
Stimuli. See also Cues
  congruent vs. incongruent, 239–244, 241f,
    242f, 244f, 247–248
Stimulus-bound behavior, 297, 300
Stimulus-driven processing, 419
Stimulus-response associations. See also
    Concrete rules
  vs. abstract rules, 23, 37–38
  striatum and, 426
Stimulus-response rules, vs. task rules,
    185, 186
Stimulus-reward associations
  anterior cingulate and, 38
  reversal of. See Reversal learning
Stimulus selection, in conditional rule
    learning, 135–139, 137f, 139f
STN. See Subthalamic nucleus (STN)
STR. See Striatum (STR)
Strategies. See also Repeat-stay/change-shift
    strategies
  abstract response. See Abstract response
    strategies
  conditional rule learning and, 135–149
  deficits in implementation of, 98–99
  description of, 82–83
  of participants, in advance-target
    preparation study, 270–271, 271f
  and rule learning, 139–140
  vs. rules, 99–100
Strategy encoding vs. rule encoding, 95–96,
    96f
Strategy task, 86–88, 87f
Striatum (STR). See also Basal ganglia
  abstract rule encoding and, 31–37, 31t,
    33–35f
  in attentional-set shifting, 285–286, 290

concrete rules and, 424–426
direct and indirect pathways of, 424–425,
    434–435
dopamine depletion in Parkinson's
    disease, 314–315, 315f
dopaminergic modulation in, 297–299,
    298f, 301–302, 303
    cognitive flexibility and, 314–315,
        325–328, 326f
    medication overdose hypothesis and,
        317–319
    reversal learning and, 320–321, 321f
    switch-related activity and, 323–324,
        324f
    and teaching signals, 426–427, 434
plasticity in, 427–431, 429f, 430f, 432
in reversal learning, 289, 291, 320–321,
    321f
in stimulus-response associations,
    37–38
Striosomes, 425–426
Stroop task, 58, 59f, 183
Substantia nigra (SN), 424. See also Basal
    ganglia
Subthalamic nucleus (STN), 424. See also
    Basal ganglia
Sulcus principalis, 12
Supplementary eye field (SEF), 141–142,
    141f
Switch costs
    in humans vs. monkeys, 232–233,
        245–246
    interference and, 378, 379–380
    mechanisms of, 181, 233
    Parkinson's disease alterations of, 316
    task-switching paradigms as measure
        of, 229
    theoretical explanations of, 257–258
Switch trials. See Task-switching
Symbolic representations, 366f, 441

Target-based processes, 256
    conscious accessibility of preparation in,
        274, 275f
    and inferior frontal junction activation,
        262–263, 263f
    levels of processing in, 266
    and task priority, 259, 260f
    voluntary control during, 274, 275–276,
        278
Targets
    congruent vs. incongruent, 268–271, 269f,
        271f

selection of, for motor behavior, 163–166,
    163f, 165f, 166f, 172
Target-specific preparatory processes,
    265–271, 269f, 271f, 278
Task difficulty vs. abstraction level, 115–119,
    119f
Task-general vs. task-specific processes,
    211–216, 212f, 213f
Task preparation, 228, 231, 233, 234–235
Task prioritization, 259–260, 261f
Task rules
    higher-order, anterior prefrontal cortex
        and, 75–77
    neural encoding of, 234–238, 236–238f,
        246–247
    vs. stimulus-response rules, 185, 186
Task set priming, 378
Task sets, 67–79
    definition of, 67
    and development of rule use in children,
        445, 447
    functional significance of prefrontal
        activity and, 71–73, 72f, 73f
    intentional selection of, 188, 189f
    inter-regional interactions and, 67–70,
        68f, 70f
    task performance prediction and, 73–75,
        74f, 79
    tonic top-down vs. phasic bottom-up
        signals and, 77–78
    updating of, exogenous vs. endogenous
        components in, 187–188
Task-switching. See also Attentional-set
        shifting; Repeat-stay/change-shift
        strategies; Reversal learning
    anterior cingulate and, 144–145
    attentional vs. intentional control of, 256,
        266–268, 277
    in children, 442–445
    cingulate cortex, anterior and, 144–145
    cue-based vs. target-based. See Cue-based
        processes; Target-based processes
    declarative knowledge and, 377–382
    dopamine modulation in striatum and,
        314, 315–316, 318, 324, 325–327,
        326f
    encoding of congruency and, 239–244,
        241f, 242f, 244f, 247–248
    event-related optical signal studies of,
        210, 211–216, 212f, 213f
    functional study of inferior frontal
        junction, 180–182, 180f, 183
    literature review, 256–258

Task-switching (*continued*)
  in monkeys vs. humans, 231–234, 232f,
    244–246
  preparatory control mechanisms. *See*
    Preparatory processes
  pre-supplementary motor area and, 129,
    130f, 140–144, 141f, 142f, 151
  task-general vs. task-specific processes,
    211–216, 212f, 213f
  task rule encoding, 234–238, 236–238f
Task-switching paradigms, 228–231, 230f
  cued vs. uncued, 228
  experimental use of, 255
  in Parkinson's disease studies, 316
  Wisconsin Card Sorting Task,
    228–229
Teaching signals, 426–427, 434
Temporal area, middle (TM), in visual
    feature processing, 410–413, 411f,
    412f
Temporal cortex/lobe
  anterior
    conditional associative responses and,
      7–8, 8f, 10, 10f, 11, 12f
    excisions of, examples of, 4–5, 5f
    in semantic knowledge control, 372f
  inferior (ITC)
    in abstract rule encoding, 31–37, 31t,
      33f, 35f, 36f
    in visual feature processing, 400–405,
      403f, 404f, 413, 414
  lateral, in semantic knowledge storage and
    retrieval, 368, 370, 371
  medial. *See also* Hippocampus;
    Parahippocampal cortex; *other*
    specific structures, e. g., Perirhinal
    cortex
    in associative learning and retrieval,
      365
    in categorization, 401, 405
    middle, and memory retrieval, 372f, 373,
      374–375, 381
  ventrolateral prefrontal cortex
    interactions of, conditional
    associative responses and, 130,
      132–135, 134f
Temporal dimension of episodic memory,
    342, 344, 348–350, 348f, 349f,
    353–354
Temporal gyrus, posterior middle
    (postMTG)
  action vs. function knowledge in, 49–50,
    50f

  in neural representations of action, 45–59,
    46f, 48f, 60f, 61
  Wernicke's aphasia and, 370
Temporal integration of information, 186
Temporal lobe. *See* Temporal cortex/lobe
Temporal resolution, of imaging techniques,
    198–199, 207, 209, 217
Thalamocortical circuits, in complex rule
    use, 449–451
Thalamus, 206, 424, 451
Theory of forms, 109
TMS (transcranial magnetic stimulation),
    96, 141–142, 141f
Tolcapone, 294
Tool use, 47, 51. *See also* Action
    representation
Top-down task control. *See* Executive
    function
Tractography, probabilistic
  anterior cingulate cortex, 150, 151f
  extreme capsule, uncinate fascicle, and
    amygdala, 134f, 135
Trait impulsivity, 322–325, 324f, 328
Transcranial magnetic stimulation (TMS),
    96, 141–142, 141f
Transitive inference, 345–346, 351
Transneuronal transport, retrograde, 162
Treatise Concerning the Principles of Human
    Knowledge (Berkeley), 109
Tree diagrams of rule complexity, 445–447,
    445f
Trial-and-error procedure, 6–9, 7f, 8f
Tryptophan depletion, dietary, 295, 299, 301

Uncinate fascicle
  prefrontal connections of, 134f, 135
  transection of, and conditional rule
    use, 133
Unconscious processing, in prefrontal
    cortex, 276–277, 278n
Uncued task-switching paradigm,
    description of, 228

Verbal memory, ventrolateral prefrontal
    cortex in, 58, 60–61, 60f
Verbal n-back task, 183
Verbal-problem solving task, 116–118, 118f
Verbal tasks, posterior inferior frontal gyrus
    and, 69, 70f
Verbal vs. nonverbal rules, 249–250
Visual attention tasks, set activity and, 77–78
Visual categorization, 391–415
  in cognitive processing, 391–392

evidence for, in nonhuman animals,
  392–393
future research needs, 413–415
motion categorization
  middle temporal area and, 410–413,
    411f, 412f
  posterior parietal cortex and, 405–410,
    408f, 409f
shape categorization
  inferior temporal cortex and, 400–405,
    403f, 404f, 413, 414
  prefrontal cortex and, 394–400, 397f,
    398f, 402–405, 413–415
Visual discrimination reversal learning,
  289–290, 298f, 299–300
Visual discrimination test, 284–285
Visual feature processing
  inferior temporal cortex and, 400–405,
    403f, 404f
  middle temporal area and, 410–413, 411f,
    412f
Visual judgment condition, 71–73, 72f, 73f
Visual-motor conditional task, 3–4, 6–10
  demonstration procedure, 9–10, 10f
  in monkey studies, 13, 14f
  trial-and-error procedure, 6–9, 7f, 8f
Visual-motor tasks, ventrolateral prefrontal
  cortex and, 52–53, 57
Visual sensory memory, 205
Visual-spatial conditional task, 10–12,
  11f, 12f
Visual spatial selective attention, 206
Visuomotor mappings, 184–185, 191
Vividness of Visual Imagery Questionnaire,
  50f, 51

VLPFC. See Prefrontal cortex, ventrolateral
  (VLPFC, PFv)
Volition, definition of, 266, 272
Voluntary control, 272–276. See also
  Cognitive control; Executive
  function
  of action selection–motor planning
    interface, 269f, 270–271, 271f
  during cue-based preparation, 274,
    276–277, 278
  experimental approaches to, 272–273
  semiautomatic vs. fully controlled modes
    of, 274–277
  during target-based preparation, 274,
    275–276, 278

Wernicke's aphasia, 370
Wisconsin Card Sorting Task (WCST),
  24–25, 228–229, 284, 316
Working memory
  connectivity and, 208–209
  dopaminergic modulation and, 291, 316,
    320–321
  executive function and, 197, 204–208,
    210
  and levels of rule complexity, 441, 446f,
    448
    prefrontal cortex regions and, 449–450,
      450f, 451, 452
  as principal prefrontal cortex function,
    101, 102
  spatial, 291
Working memory representation, prefrontal
  cortex organization and, 112, 113,
  120–121